Physical Activity and Health

AN INTERACTIVE APPROACH

Physical Activity and Health

AN INTERACTIVE APPROACH

Kelli McCormack Brown
Department of Community and Family Health
University of South Florida

David Q. Thomas
School of Kinesiology and Recreation
Illinois State University

Jerome E. Kotecki
Department of Physiology and Health Science
Ball State University

JONES AND BARTLETT PUBLISHERS
Sudbury, Massachusetts
BOSTON TORONTO LONDON SINGAPORE

World Headquarters
Jones and Bartlett Publishers
40 Tall Pine Drive
Sudbury, MA 01776
978-443-5000
info@jbpub.com
www.jbpub.com

Jones and Bartlett Publishers Canada
2406 Nikanna Road
Mississauga, ON L5C 2W6
CANADA

Jones and Bartlett Publishers International
Barb House, Barb Mews
London W6 7PA
UK

Production Credits
Chief Executive Officer: Clayton E. Jones
Chief Operating Officer: Donald W. Jones, Jr
V.P., Senior Managing Editor: Judith H. Hauck
V.P., Design and Production: Anne Spencer
V.P., Manufacturing and Inventory Control: Therese Bräuer
Editor in Chief, College: Michael Stranz
Sponsoring Editor: Suzanne Jeans
Senior Production Editor: Lianne Ames
Developmental Editor: Ohlinger Publishing Services
Editorial/Production Assistant: Amanda Green
Design and Composition: Seventeenth Street Studios
Editorial Production Service: Seventeenth Street Studios
Cover Design: Anne Spencer
Cover Illustration: ©Peter Hurley
Printing and Binding: Courier Companies
Cover Printing: Lehigh Press

Library of Congress Cataloging-in-Publication Data
Brown Kelli McCormack.
Physical activity and health: an interactive approach / Kelli McCormack Brown, David Q. Thomas, Jerome E. Kotecki.
p. cm.
Includes bibliographical references and index.
ISBN 0-86720-936-4
1. Exercise. 2. Physical fitness. 3. Health. I. Thomas, David Q. II. Kotecki, Jerome Edward. III. Title.

RA 781 .K763 2001
613.7'1—dc21

2001046194

Printed in the United States of America
05 04 03 02 01 10 9 8 7 6 5 4 3 2 1

Brief Contents

Contents

UNIT 2: ENHANCING QUALITY OF LIFE

UNIT 3: ENERGIZING YOUR BODY

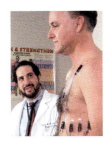

CHAPTER 9

Achieving and Maintaining a Healthy Body Fatness 193

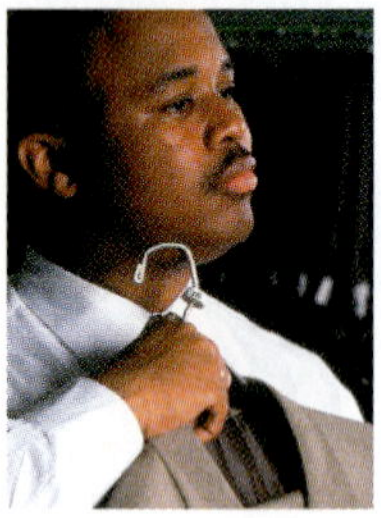

UNIT 4: BUILDING A STRONG BODY

CHAPTER 10

Achieving Optimal Bone Health 221

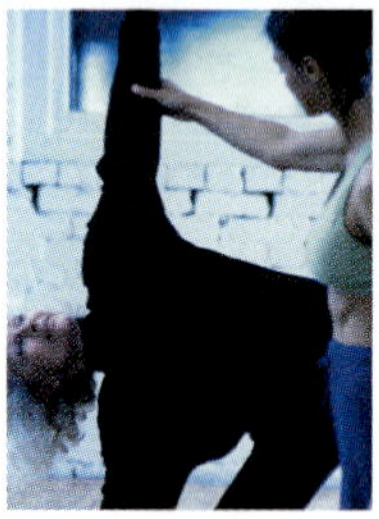

CHAPTER 11

Muscular Strength and Endurance 235

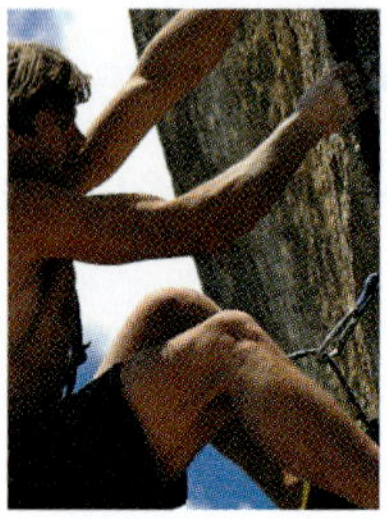

CHAPTER 12

Stretching and Flexibility 263

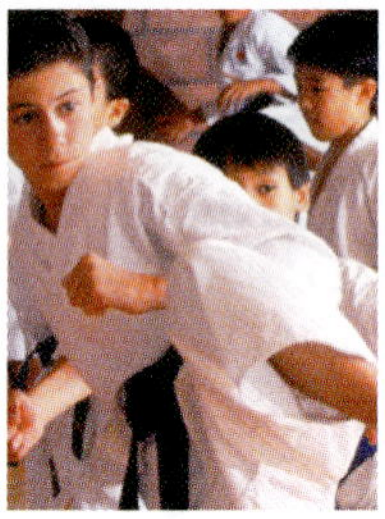

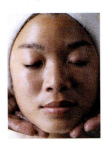

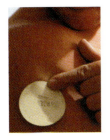

Instructor's Introduction

"No less than two hours a day should be devoted to exercise."

Thomas Jefferson (1743–1826)

"If the man who wrote the Declaration of Independence, was Secretary of State, and twice President could give it two hours, our children can give it ten or fifteen minutes."

John F. Kennedy (1917–1963)

The concept that people need physical activity is not new. What is new is the idea that activity need not be overly strenuous to provide benefit. Traditionally, people have been given advice on how much **exercise** they should perform, usually including recommendations to work out at vigorous intensities for prolonged periods of time. It was thought that this kind of exercise was necessary to improve health and physical fitness.

Physical activity, however, can include any bodily movement that results in the expenditure of energy. In addition to exercise, physical activity may include behavior such as housework, gardening, strolling, hiking and a wide variety of other activities. Recent research has indicated that the accumulation of thirty minutes of moderate intensity physical activity on most if not all days of the week will provide significant health benefits and a great deal of protection against most of the degenerative diseases our population faces.

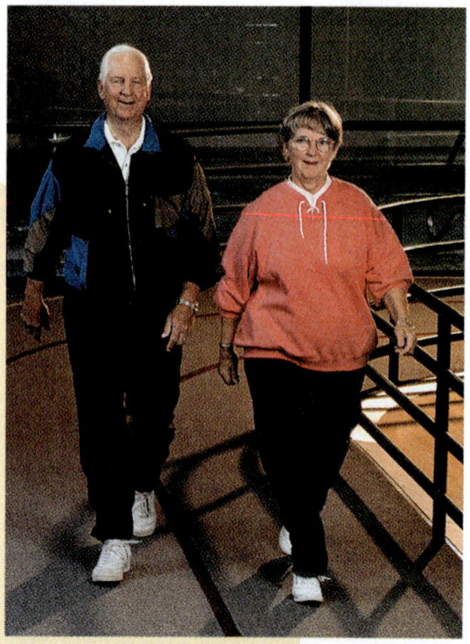

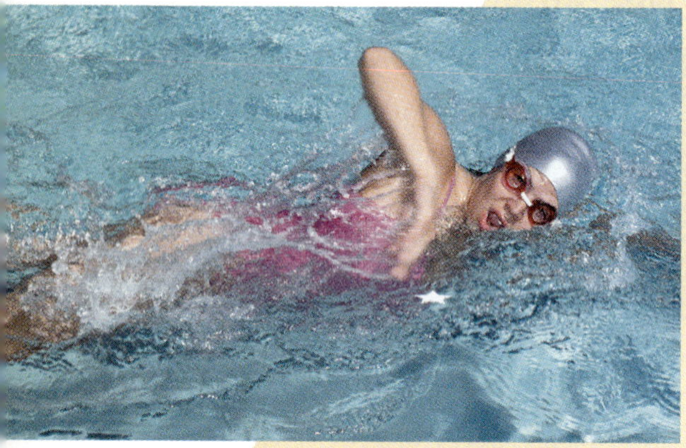

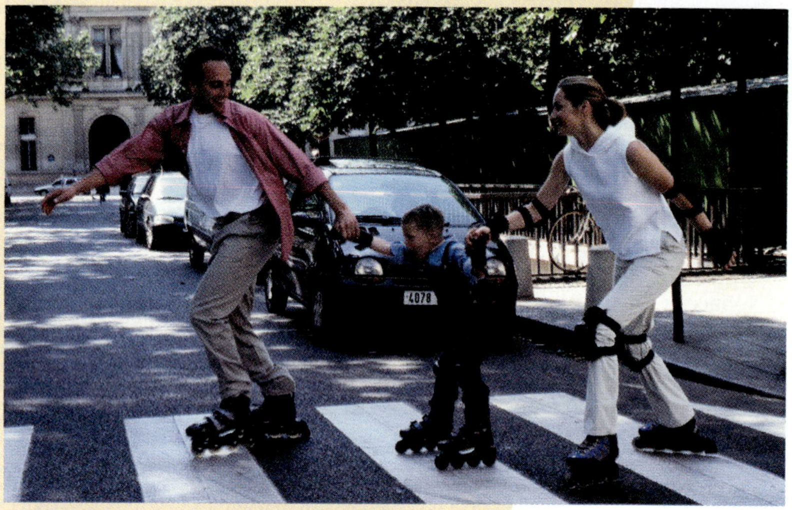

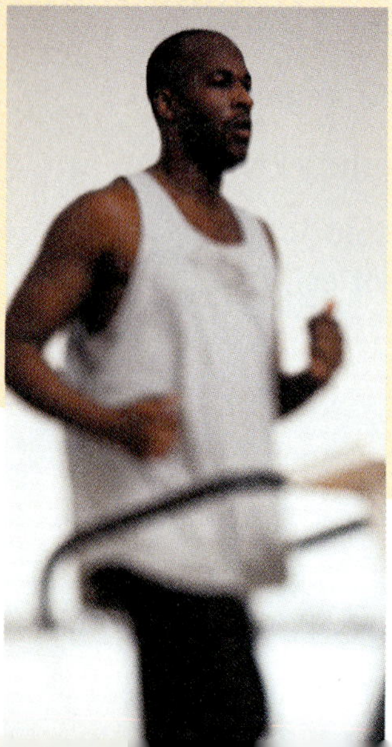

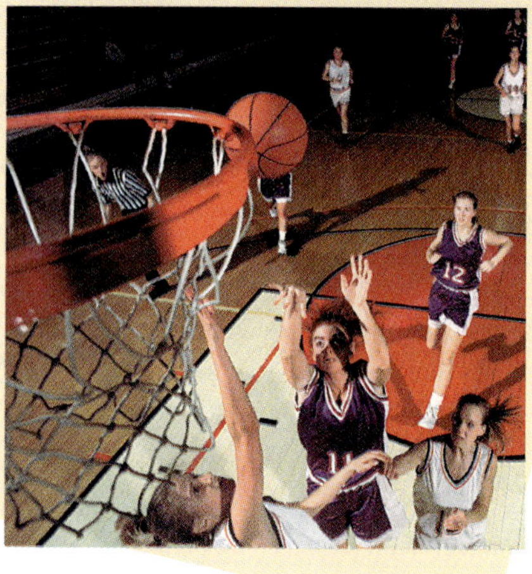

OUR APPROACH

The Physical Activity and Health Connection Our goal in this book is to demonstrate how physical activity and good health are inseparable. This is not a fitness book in the traditional sense. **Physical fitness** is a product of being physically active. Our emphasis is on the process of being active: if the process is engaged in, the product will result. By focusing on the process, we hope to show that it is more important to be active than it is to achieve any preconceived level of fitness. Not all people are capable of achieving the same level of fitness. However, most people are capable of being physically active, and are, therefore, capable of improving their health. How much improvement they see will depend on how much and what kind of physical activity they perform.

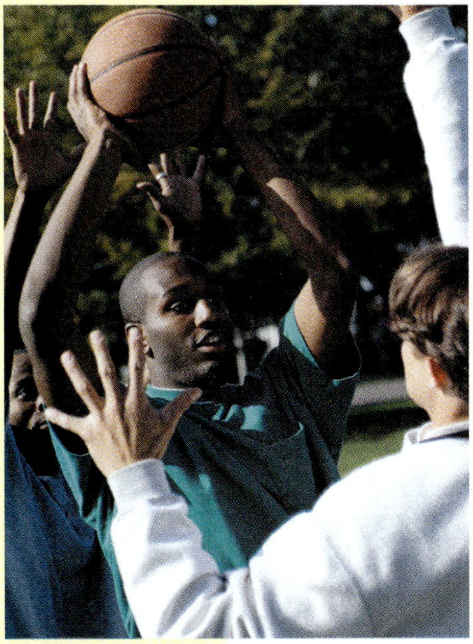

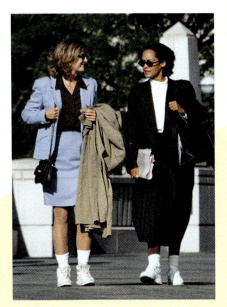

Traditional fitness books provide you with multiple chapters on fitness and one or two chapters about health. Traditional health books provide you with multiple chapters on health and only a brief mention of fitness. This book is designed to be a hybrid of the two. We focus on the interconnectedness of health and being physically active. It is our opinion that the two cannot be separated. Every chapter and section is designed to reinforce this connection.

An Interactive Approach We also use a distinctive interactive approach to convey our message. This interactive approach supports our beliefs about the connection between physical activity and health and our strong belief that each individual must take an active role in achieving a healthy lifestyle. Self-responsibility is a central focus of this book, as we arm each individual with the knowledge and skills necessary to become independent, active, and healthy. Following this theme, the book provides sound behavior-change theories to assist readers in developing a personalized physical activity and health plan.

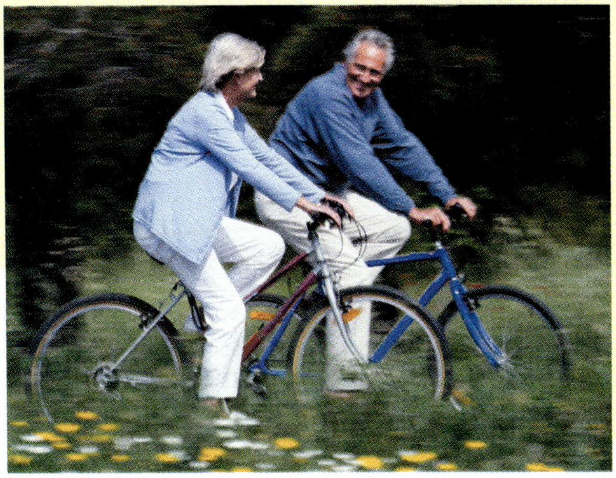

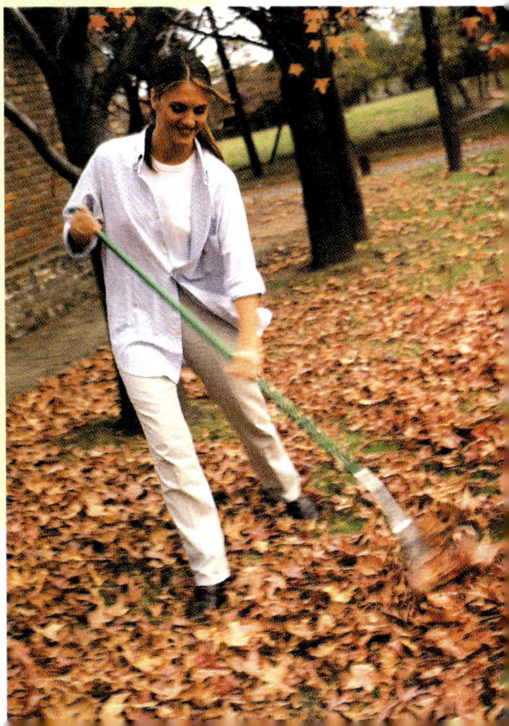

FEATURES

Each chapter begins with the **Concept Connection**, which is a numbered list of the chapter's key points. Numbered icons identify each concept as it appears in the chapter. The concepts reappear at the end of the chapter in a numbered summary.

What's the Connection?, at the start of each chapter, presents a short scenario about someone who wants to change a specific behavior. At the end of the chapter, **Making the Connection** shows what the characters have learned about the behaviors they want to change.

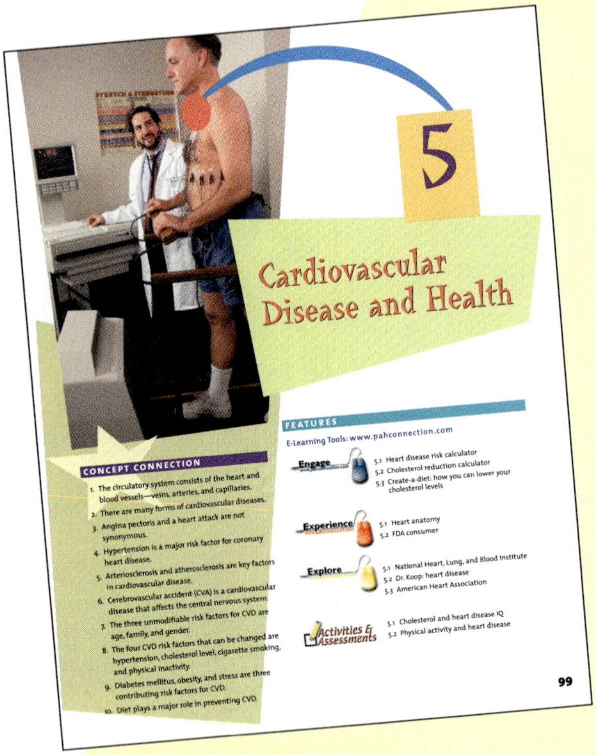

5

Cardiovascular Disease and Health

CONCEPT CONNECTION

1. The circulatory system consists of the heart and blood vessels—veins, arteries, and capillaries.
2. There are many forms of cardiovascular diseases.
3. Angina pectoris and a heart attack are not synonymous.
4. Hypertension is a major risk factor for coronary heart disease.
5. Arteriosclerosis and atherosclerosis are key factors in cardiovascular disease.
6. Cerebrovascular accident (CVA) is a cardiovascular disease that affects the central nervous system.
7. The three unmodifiable risk factors for CVD are age, family, and gender.
8. The four CVD risk factors that can be changed are hypertension, cholesterol level, cigarette smoking, and physical inactivity.
9. Diabetes mellitus, obesity, and stress are three contributing risk factors for CVD.
10. Diet plays a major role in preventing CVD.

FEATURES

E-Learning Tools: www.pahconnection.com

Engage
5.1 Heart disease risk calculator
5.2 Cholesterol reduction calculator
5.3 Create-a-diet: how you can lower your cholesterol levels

Experience
5.1 Heart anatomy
5.2 FDA consumer

Explore
5.1 National Heart, Lung, and Blood Institute
5.2 Dr. Koop: heart disease
5.3 American Heart Association

Activities & Assessments
5.1 Cholesterol and heart disease IQ
5.2 Physical activity and heart disease

99

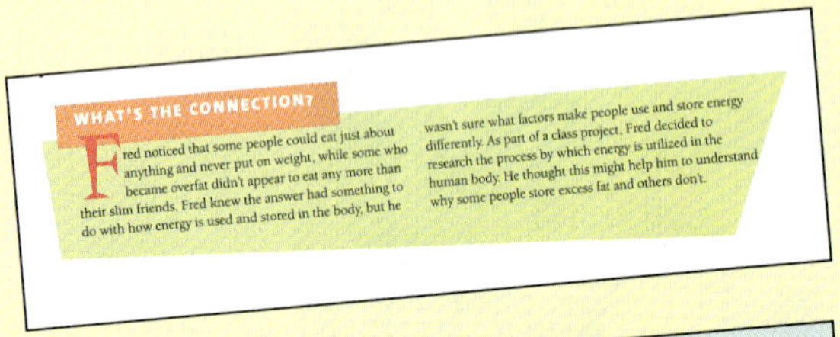

WHAT'S THE CONNECTION?

Fred noticed that some people could eat just about anything and never put on weight, while some who became overfat didn't appear to eat any more than their slim friends. Fred knew the answer had something to do with how energy is used and stored in the body, but he wasn't sure what factors make people use and store energy differently. As part of a class project, Fred decided to research the process by which energy is utilized in the human body. He thought this might help him to understand why some people store excess fat and others don't.

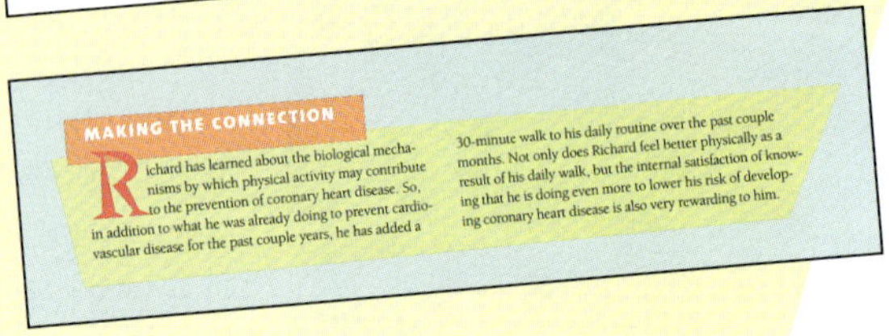

MAKING THE CONNECTION

Richard has learned about the biological mechanisms by which physical activity may contribute to the prevention of coronary heart disease. So, in addition to what he was already doing to prevent cardiovascular disease for the past couple years, he has added a 30-minute walk to his daily routine over the past couple months. Not only does Richard feel better physically as a result of his daily walk, but the internal satisfaction of knowing that he is doing even more to lower his risk of developing coronary heart disease is also very rewarding to him.

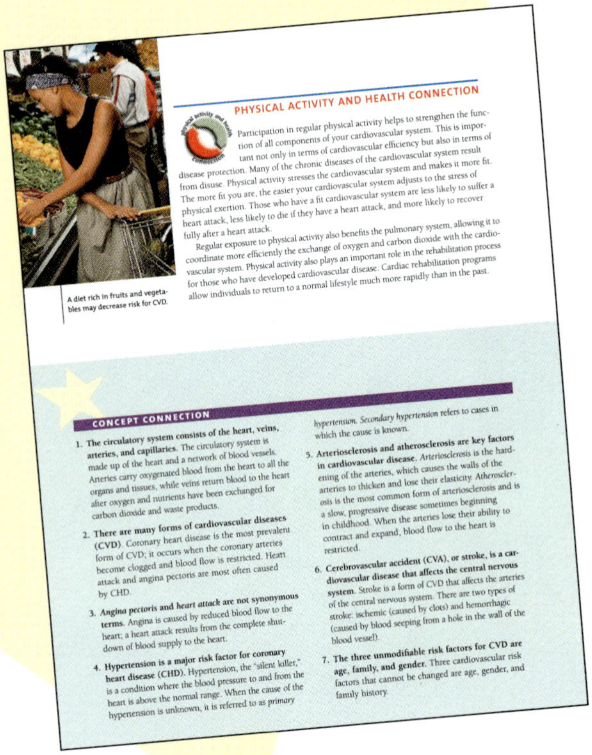

PHYSICAL ACTIVITY AND HEALTH CONNECTION

Participation in regular physical activity helps to strengthen the function of all components of your cardiovascular system. This is important not only in terms of cardiovascular efficiency but also in terms of disease protection. Many of the chronic diseases of the cardiovascular system result from disuse. Physical activity stresses the cardiovascular system and makes it more fit. The more fit you are, the easier your cardiovascular system adjusts to the stress of physical exertion. Those who have a fit cardiovascular system are less likely to suffer a heart attack, less likely to die if they have a heart attack, and more likely to recover fully after a heart attack.

Regular exposure to physical activity also benefits the pulmonary system, allowing it to coordinate more efficiently the exchange of oxygen and carbon dioxide with the cardiovascular system. Physical activity also plays an important role in the rehabilitation process for those who have developed cardiovascular disease. Cardiac rehabilitation programs allow individuals to return to a normal lifestyle much more rapidly than in the past.

A diet rich in fruits and vegetables may decrease risk for CVD.

CONCEPT CONNECTION

1. **The circulatory system consists of the heart, veins, arteries, and capillaries.** The circulatory system is made up of the heart and a network of blood vessels. Arteries carry oxygenated blood from the heart to all the organs and tissues, while veins return blood to the heart after oxygen and nutrients have been exchanged for carbon dioxide and waste products.
2. **There are many forms of cardiovascular diseases (CVD).** Coronary heart disease is the most prevalent form of CVD; it occurs when the coronary arteries become clogged and blood flow is restricted. Heart attack and angina pectoris are most often caused by CHD.
3. ***Angina pectoris* and *heart attack* are not synonymous terms.** Angina is caused by reduced blood flow to the heart; a heart attack results from the complete shutdown of blood supply to the heart.
4. **Hypertension is a major risk factor for coronary heart disease (CHD).** Hypertension, the "silent killer," is a condition where the blood pressure to and from the heart is above the normal range. When the cause of the hypertension is unknown, it is referred to as *primary hypertension*. *Secondary hypertension* refers to cases in which the cause is known.
5. **Arteriosclerosis and atherosclerosis are key factors in cardiovascular disease.** *Arteriosclerosis* is the hardening of the arteries, which causes the walls of the arteries to thicken and lose their elasticity. *Atherosclerosis* is the most common form of arteriosclerosis and is a slow, progressive disease sometimes beginning in childhood. When the arteries lose their ability to contract and expand, blood flow to the heart is restricted.
6. **Cerebrovascular accident (CVA), or stroke, is a cardiovascular disease that affects the central nervous system.** Stroke is a form of CVD that affects the arteries of the central nervous system. There are two types of stroke: ischemic (caused by clots) and hemorrhagic (caused by blood seeping from a hole in the wall of the blood vessel).
7. **The three unmodifiable risk factors for CVD are age, family, and gender.** Three cardiovascular risk factors that cannot be changed are age, gender, and family history.

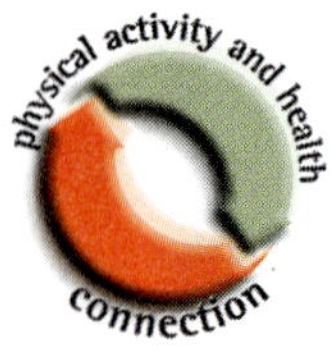

A **Physical Activity and Health Connection** icon appears in the margin of the text whenever the material highlights the link between physical activity and health. These points are summarized in the last section of every chapter.

Activities and Assessments accompany each chapter, and students are prompted to complete the activity or assessment by a margin icon next to the material that relates to it. These activities and assessments appear at the end of the chapter.

PAHConnection.com offers a variety of resources to students, including a behavioral change contract and an anatomy review. Icons in the text also direct students to the site for text-specific exercises, assessments, and activities.

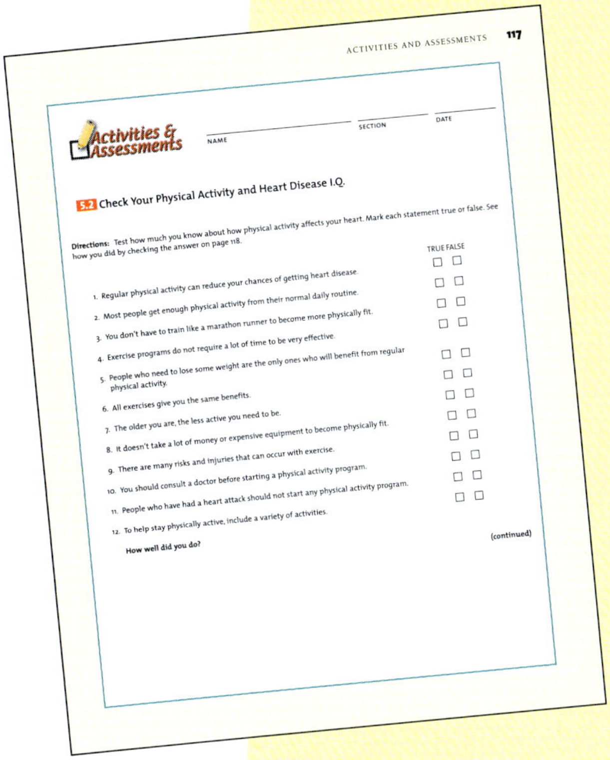

ACTIVITIES AND ASSESSMENTS 117

Activities & Assessments

NAME SECTION DATE

5.2 Check Your Physical Activity and Heart Disease I.Q.

Directions: Test how much you know about how physical activity affects your heart. Mark each statement true or false. See how you did by checking the answer on page 118.

	TRUE	FALSE
1. Regular physical activity can reduce your chances of getting heart disease.	☐	☐
2. Most people get enough physical activity from their normal daily routine.	☐	☐
3. You don't have to train like a marathon runner to become more physically fit.	☐	☐
4. Exercise programs do not require a lot of time to be very effective.	☐	☐
5. People who need to lose some weight are the only ones who will benefit from regular physical activity.	☐	☐
6. All exercises give you the same benefits.	☐	☐
7. The older you are, the less active you need to be.	☐	☐
8. It doesn't take a lot of money or expensive equipment to become physically fit.	☐	☐
9. There are many risks and injuries that can occur with exercise.	☐	☐
10. You should consult a doctor before starting a physical activity program.	☐	☐
11. People who have had a heart attack should not start any physical activity program.	☐	☐
12. To help stay physically active, include a variety of activities.	☐	☐

How well did you do?

(continued)

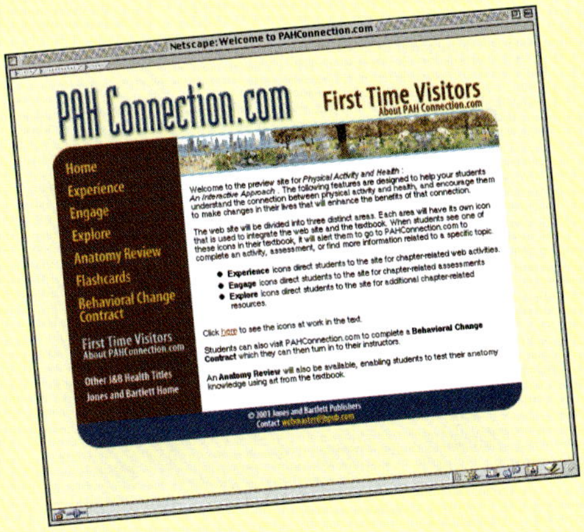

Netscape: Welcome to PAHConnection.com
PAH Connection.com
First Time Visitors
About PAH Connection.com
Home
Experience
Engage
Explore
Anatomy Review
Flashcards
Behavioral Change Contract
First Time Visitors
About PAHConnection.com
Other J&B Health Titles
Jones and Bartlett Home
Welcome to the preview site for Physical Activity and Health: An Interactive Approach. The following features are designed to help your students understand the connection between physical activity and health, and encourage them to make changes in their lives that will enhance the benefits of that connection.
The web site will be divided into three distinct areas. Each area will have its own icon that is used to integrate the web site and the textbook. When students see one of these icons in their textbook, it will alert them to go to PAHConnection.com to complete an activity, assessment, or find more information related to a specific topic.
Experience icons direct students to the site for chapter-related web activities.
Engage icons direct students to the site for chapter-related assessments
Explore icons direct students to the site for additional chapter-related resources.
Click here to see the icons at work in the text.
Students can also visit PAHConnection.com to complete a Behavioral Change Contract which they can then turn in to their instructors.
An Anatomy Review will also be available, enabling students to test their anatomy knowledge using art from the textbook.
© 2001 Jones and Bartlett Publishers

Explore icons indicate that students should visit the web site for a list of links to chapter-relevant sites, such as the American Dietetic Association, American Cancer Society, and more.

Engage icons direct students to the web site for interactive activities and assessments online.

Experience icons lead students to the site for chapter-relevant Web exercises.

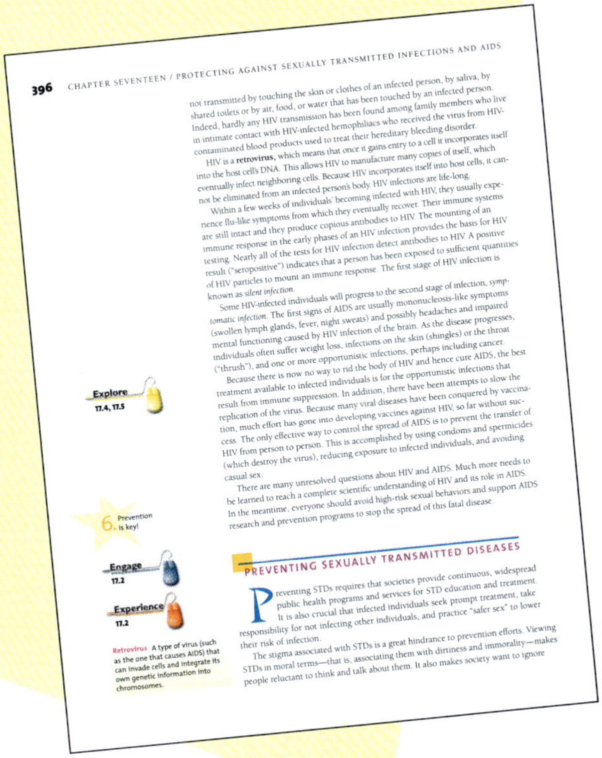

396 CHAPTER SEVENTEEN / PROTECTING AGAINST SEXUALLY TRANSMITTED INFECTIONS AND AIDS

not transmitted by touching the skin or clothes of an infected person, by saliva, by shared toilets or by air, food, or water that has been touched by an infected person. Indeed, hardly any HIV transmission has been found among family members who live in intimate contact with HIV-infected hemophiliacs who received the virus from HIV-contaminated blood products used to treat their hereditary bleeding disorder.

HIV is a **retrovirus,** which means that once it gains entry to a cell it incorporates itself into the host cell's DNA. This allows HIV to manufacture many copies of itself, which eventually infect neighboring cells. Because HIV incorporates itself into host cells, it cannot be eliminated from an infected person's body. HIV infections are life-long.

Within a few weeks of individuals' becoming infected with HIV, they usually experience flu-like symptoms from which they eventually recover. Their immune systems are still intact and they produce copious antibodies to HIV. The mounting of an immune response in the early phases of an HIV infection provides the basis for HIV testing. Nearly all of the tests for HIV infection detect antibodies to HIV. A positive result ("seropositive") indicates that a person has been exposed to sufficient quantities of HIV particles to mount an immune response. The first stage of HIV infection is known as *silent infection.*

Some HIV-infected individuals will progress to the second stage of infection, *symptomatic infection.* The first signs of AIDS are usually mononucleosis-like symptoms (swollen lymph glands, fever, night sweats) and possibly headaches and impaired mental functioning caused by HIV infection of the brain. As the disease progresses, individuals often suffer weight loss, infections on the skin (shingles) or the throat ("thrush"), and one or more opportunistic infections, perhaps including cancer.

Because there is now no way to rid the body of HIV and hence cure AIDS, the best treatment available to infected individuals is for the opportunistic infections that result from immune suppression. In addition, there have been attempts to slow the replication of the virus. Because many viral diseases have been conquered by vaccination, much effort has gone into developing vaccines against HIV, so far without success. The only effective way to control the spread of AIDS is to prevent the transfer of HIV from person to person. This is accomplished by using condoms and spermicides (which destroy the virus), reducing exposure to infected individuals, and avoiding casual sex.

There are many unresolved questions about HIV and AIDS. Much more needs to be learned to reach a complete scientific understanding of HIV and its role in AIDS. In the meantime, everyone should avoid high-risk sexual behaviors and support AIDS research and prevention programs to stop the spread of this fatal disease.

Explore 17.4, 17.5

6. Prevention is key!

Engage 17.2

Experience 17.2

Retrovirus A type of virus (such as the one that causes AIDS) that can invade cells and integrate its own genetic information into chromosomes.

PREVENTING SEXUALLY TRANSMITTED DISEASES

Preventing STDs requires that societies provide continuous, widespread public health programs and services for STD education and treatment. It is also crucial that infected individuals seek prompt treatment, take responsibility for not infecting other individuals, and practice "safer sex" to lower their risk of infection.

The stigma associated with STDs is a great hindrance to prevention efforts. Viewing STDs in moral terms—that is, associating them with dirtiness and immorality—makes people reluctant to think and talk about them. It also makes society want to ignore

SUPPLEMENTS

Instructor's ToolKit CD-ROM Includes lecture outlines, Instructor's Manual, computerized TestBank, PowerPoint presentations, and an image bank. (ISBN: 0-7637-1886-6)

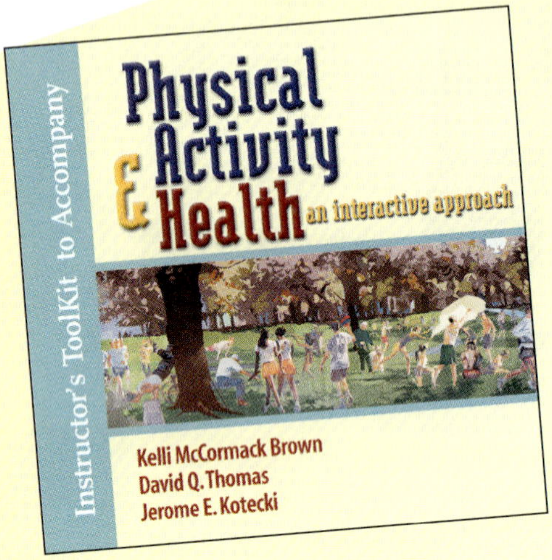

Physical Activity and Health: A Report of the Surgeon General This report is a comprehensive review of the available scientific evidence about the relationship between physical activity and health. (ISBN: 0-7637-0636-1)

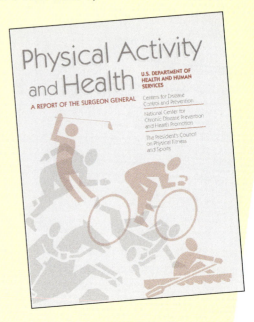

Healthy People 2010 Written by the U.S. Department of Health and Human Services, Healthy People 2010 sets broad public health goals for the next decade. (ISBN: 0-7637-1432-1)

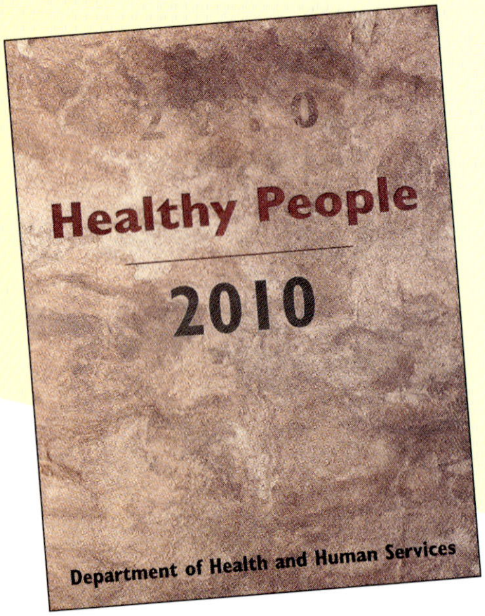

EatRight Analysis Software Developed by ESHA Research, this innovative software, including over 4,000 foods, allows students to analyze their diets by RDAs/DRIs and goal percentages. (ISBN: 0-7637-1692-8)

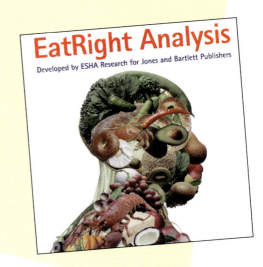

Meet the Authors

The *Physical Activity and Health* author team is comprised of three individuals who bring something very unique to the book.

Kelli McCormack Brown is an Associate Professor in the Department of Community and Family Health at the University of South Florida College of Public Health. She holds a doctorate degree in health education and is a Certified Health Education Specialist (CHES). She is also the 1993 American Alliance for Health, Physical Education, Recreation, and Dance (AAHPERD) Mable Lee Award recipient for excellence in teaching, research and service and is a Fellow of the Research Consortium of AAHPERD. Before coming to the University of South Florida, she taught for seven years at Western Illinois University (1987–1994) and was the chairperson of the Department of Health Sciences at Illinois State University (1994–1996). She is a Co-Principal Investigator at the Prevention Research Center funded by the Centers for Disease Control and Prevention. Today back in the classroom, she uses her educational and practical experiences to facilitate critical thinking and problem-solving skills and encourages the use of technology in obtaining reliable health information to make informed personal health decisions.

David Q. Thomas is an Associate Professor of Exercise Science in the School of Kinesiology and Recreation at Illinois State University. He holds doctorate and master's degrees in physical education (emphasis in exercise science) from Arizona State University. His bachelor's degree is in Health and Physical Education from Penn State University. He is a Fellow of the American College of Sports Medicine (ACSM) and a Fellow of the Research Consortium of the American Alliance for Health, Physical Education, Recreation, and Dance (AAHPERD). His area of expertise is in applied aspects of physical activity and fitness. He has also been on the faculty at the University of Massachusetts/Boston (1985–1990) and Rice University (1990–1995). He has served as the chairperson of the Physical Fitness Council of the Association for Active Lifestyles and Fitness, and as President of both the Massachusetts and Illinois AHPERDs.

Jerome E. Kotecki is an Associate Professor in the Department of Physiology and Health Science at Ball State University. Dr. Kotecki earned his doctorate in health education and his masters degree in exercise science from Indiana University. He is a Certified Health Education Specialist (CHES) and American College of Sports Medicine (ACSM) health fitness instructor. Dr. Kotecki has published numerous articles in professional journals and is co-author of the textbook *An Introduction to Community Health*. His previous experience includes managing a campus-wide fitness program at Indiana State University and serving as a personal trainer for individuals in the entertainment industry in Los Angeles. He is an avid fitness participant and enjoys weight training, running, cycling, tennis, and yoga.

Students and Instructors Ask the Authors

Why is physical activity important for students to understand in relation to their study of overall personal health?

Physical Activity is important to all aspects of health. Physical activity plays a major role in disease prevention and rehabilitation. It helps improve your mood, makes you more attractive, improves your quality of life and makes you live longer. **(Dave)**

How do you integrate physical activity in your daily activities?

I begin each day with some form of physical activity. I alternate between aerobic and anaerobic activities (i.e., running and lifting) and recreational activities (i.e., tennis, basketball, racquetball). Finally, I end each day with 10 to 15 minutes of deep relaxation breathing and stretching exercises. **(Jerome)**

I incorporate physical activity into all aspects of my life. Not only do I instruct others about being physically active, I practice what I preach. I walk, ride my bike, and take the stairs, etc. when practical and possible. I run 4 to 7 miles every other day. On days when I'm not running I lift weights for 45 minutes. I play golf, racquetball, and volleyball. **(Dave)**

Physical activity has been something that I have recently (within the last 5 years) incorporated into my daily routine. *Daily* and *routine* are key words, as before I was an on- and off-again exerciser. Now, I make physical activity part of my day to walk and do little things like park far out in the grocery store parking lot, take the stairs when possible, and participate in both individual and group sports that help keep me active. I have made it a commitment to make physical activity a part of what I do daily and who I am. **(Kelli)**

Behavior change is a key component of this book, why is it so important to begin a healthy lifestyle while I am still in college?

It is increasingly acknowledged that a lifestyle of health-promoting behaviors is largely a matter of personal discipline and will. You can do more for your health than anyone else.

College students are beginning to develop a personal health lifestyle, which, with slight modifications, they will likely follow for the rest of their lives. Research indicates that the earlier one implements a healthy lifestyle, the better the chance for instilling lifelong health habits. Thus, practicing positive health behaviors, with systematic reinforcement and follow-up throughout one's college years, provides the best opportunity for preventing the development of dangerous and health-threatening behaviors, which lead to serious diseases during the middle and later years in life. So it is very important to begin to implement positive health habits early in life and to encourage college students to assume personal responsibility for their own health. **(Jerome)**

What is the most challenging topic you teach in your [physical activity and health] class? How do you meet this challenge?

Overcoming negative images of physical activity. Many people have had negative experiences in physical education or on some youth sport team, and get turned off from physical activity. I teach people that activity must be individualized, I encourage them to explore many different activities to find something they will enjoy, and teach them about the benefits of being active. **(Dave)**

Many college students feel that they are pressed for time and are unable to fit physical activity into their daily routines. I inform them that physical activity should never be disruptive to their daily schedule or to any other aspect of their life. If you are having a hard time finding an extended amount of time to participate in a physical activity, consider spreading out your time throughout the day. For example a 30-minute time block could become a brisk 10-minute walk to class in the morning, a brisk 10-minute walk at lunch, and a brisk 10-minute walk home. During this time make it a mind/body experience, while you stride, introduce a positive mantra—a short meaningful statement—repeated over and over again quietly to yourself. Doing this will keep you fit and clear your head. **(Jerome)**

What topic do you most enjoy teaching? Is this your students' favorite topic?

My favorite topic is well-being and the mind-body connection. A sense of well-being rests on the direct and harmonious relationship between the mind and body. Stress challenges that harmony. There is the short-term stress that excites and inspires us, and the long-term stress that makes us physically and emotionally ill. The key is to recognize and understand our responses to the pressures of modern life and act accordingly. Today, we have access to a huge range of mental and physical therapies, which aim to encourage physical and mental well-being. Once the students understand and have had a chance to practice various forms of these therapies, they realize they have much greater control over their lives. **(Jerome)**

My two favorite classes are exercise physiology and exercise programming. Within those classes, exercise and physical activity consumerism are fun. Exposing products that don't work and taking a comical look at what some people will try is fun for my students and me. **(Dave)**

What advice would you give someone who just started incorporating technology into his/her fitness/health course? What are some good first steps for that person to take?

When beginning to incorporate technology into my health classes, I take a two-part approach. The primary goal of this approach is to reduce the anxiety about use of technology among my students. I first meet with my computer support staff at the university and explain to them what I plan to do with technology in my class. They let me know what computer hardware and software support are available, give me dial-in instructions for students, and tell me what the computer lab hours are. If I believe the class is not aware of the computer lab resources on campus or how to dial in, I ask computer support staff to come into my class at the beginning of the semester to answer questions. The second aspect of this two-part approach is to assure that my technology assignments are meaningful to the students and add value to the course.

If you are going to use the World Wide Web, be sure to take some time to research the websites that you want to use in your course. Universal Resource Locators (URLs) change all the time, so be sure that your addresses are still good before you assign them to students. In the beginning, hold students' hands until they get the hang of doing research on the Web. Be sure to caution them that not all information on the Web is reliable. The website for this book, *Physical Activity and Health: An Interactive Approach* (www.pahconnection.com), helps you find appropriate websites and provides some student exercises that give you ideas on how to write your own exercises. **(Kelli)**

What are the benefits of using technology in the classroom? Have you seen measurable results in your course?

Although I haven't formally measured the use of technology in the classroom, I can say from anecdotal comments and end of class evaluations that the use of technology has been a success. Students who have not had teachers use the Internet to enhance their class (or teach their class solely on the web [web-based]), have indicated that they like using the web to access information that complements what they are learning in class. **(Kelli)**

Acknowledgments

A Note of Thanks

Throughout the preparation of *Physical Activity and Health: An Interactive Approach,* many people have contributed support and guidance. This book has benefited greatly from their comments, opinions, thoughtful critiques, expert knowledge, and constructive suggestions. We are most appreciative for their participation in this project.

Reviewers

Phillip G. Bogle, Ph.D., Eastern Michigan University
L. Jerome Brandon, Ph.D., FACSM, Georgia State University
Cheryl J. Cohen, Ph.D., FACSM, Western Illinois University
Mitchell A. Collins, Ed.D., M.Ed., Kennesaw State University
Anita M. D'Angelo, M.Ed., Florida Atlantic University
Teresa C. Fitts, D.P.E., Westfield State College
Kara I. Gallagher, M.S., Ph.D., Eastern Michigan University
Kathie C. Garbe, Ph.D., CHES, Kennesaw State University
Bernie Goldfine, Ph.D., Kennesaw State University
Walter S. Hamerslough, Ed.D., La Sierra University
Ron Holloway, M.A., Kennesaw State University
Gary Ladd, M.S., MSEd, Southwestern Ilinois College
Kristen M. Lagally, Ph.D., Illinois State University
Kevin Lorson, M.A., B.A., Ohio State University
Susan J. Massad, H.S.D., Framingham State College
Christine M. Miskec, M.A., Minnesota State University–Mankato
Beverly F. Mitchell, Ph.D., M.A., Kennesaw State University
Diana Mozen, Ph.D., Georgia College and State University
David C. Nieman, Appalachian State University
Debra Ann Pace, B.S., M.Ed., Ohio State University
Jane A. Petrillo, Ed.D., M.S., Kennesaw State University
Stephen W. Sansone, Ed.M., Chemeketa Community College
Susan T. Saylor, Ed.D., R.D., Shelton State Community College
Andrew L. Shim, M.A., Southwestern College
Douglas W. Strange, M.A., H.F.I., C.S.C.S., Lehigh University
Patricia A. Sullivan, Ed.D., George Washington University
Frederick C. Surgent, Ed.D, Frostburg State University
Eileen Udry, Ph.D., Indiana University-Purdue University–Indianapolis
Jin Wang, Ph.D., M.Ed., Kennesaw State University
William H. Zimmerli, Ed.D., Fort Valley State University

This book could not have been published without the efforts of the staff at Jones and Bartlett Publishers and the Health team: Judy Hauck, Vice President and Senior Managing Editor; Suzanne Jeans, Acquisitions Editor; Lianne Ames, Senior Production Editor; Amy Austin, Associate Editor; Taryn Wahlquist, Marketing Manager; Amanda Green, Editorial/Production Assistant; Adam Alboyadjian, Web Product Manager; Adam Gould, Programmer; Monica Ohlinger of Ohlinger Publishing Services; and Lorrie Fink of Seventeenth Street Studios. We would also like to thank Berta A. Daniels for the photography in chapters 11 and 12 as well as the models who posed for the photography: Nathan Bressner, Breanne J. Commare, Steve Cotman, Monique Haan, Brett Hickey, Tara L. Holmes, Eric Johnson, Phuong Le, Steve McCarr, Heather Medema, Leslie Miller, Jim Prosser, Michele Rahija, Mike Rettener, Jenny Schmidt, Jeff Seagmiller, Andrew Singleton, Jaima Stowell, Ted Wargo, Prie Woods, Albert Yau, Geoff Young. Thanks also go to Joe Rodgers and Robert Lindsay from Illinois State's Athletic Department, who gave us access to their weight room and helped to make sure the lifts were posed properly.

I want to thank Paul Shepardson for giving me the encouragement to initiate the development of this book, the flexibility in selecting an awesome author team, and for being there as an editor and true friend throughout this process. To Monica Ohlinger, without whom this book would not be what it is today. I thank her for her wisdom, friendship and patience! As with everything we do, nothing is done in isolation; therefore, I want to thank Dave and Jerome for believing in this book and their willingness to join me. Without their individual knowledge, experience, expertise and creative thoughts, this book would not be what it is. I also want to thank my husband, Dennis, who has supported me throughout this endeavor—I love you. *—KRMB*

I would like to thank my parents, Richard and Loretta Thomas, for encouraging me to lead an active lifestyle when I was young, and my wife, Nancy, for keeping me on my toes today. *—Dave Thomas*

I am fortunate to work with administrators who maintain the vision that textbooks represent important learning resources for today's college students and that textbooks reflect faculty contributions that shed favorable light on a college community. I very much appeciate the support of Dr. Ronald L. Johnstone, Dean of the College of Sciences and Humanitities, and Dr. C. Warren Vander Hill, Provost and Vice President for Academic Affairs at Ball State University. Finally, to my colleague and friend, Dr. Budd D. Stalnaker, for his support of my professional life. *—Jerome Kotecki*

Student Guide to Physical Activity and Health

AN INTERACTIVE APPROACH

WHY THIS BOOK?

Our goal in writing this book is to provide you with the information you need to understand the fundamentals of physical activity and implement these basic fundamentals to improve and/or maintain overall health and well-being. This book also provides you with the *connection* between physical activity and health; that physical activity and health are inseparable—you can't have one without the other. As you read this book it should become clear the role physical activity (or physical inactivity) plays in overall health and well-being, as well as quality of life. We have provided the most up-to-date information, integrated learning tools, and critical thinking exercises that reinforce self-responsibility and motivate you toward making healthy decisions that promote positive health and wellness. We believe that the key to overall health and well-being is self-responsibility for one's behaviors (both positive and negative)—being physically active or inactive, eating nutritiously or overeating/undereating, drinking alcohol responsibly or smoking cigarettes.

As authors, we realize that everyone engages in unhealthy behaviors from time to time, but we also realize that these behaviors can be changed. Health and wellness are not static, they are dynamic; they are a lifelong process. We hope that, in your use of this textbook, you will become aware of your unhealthy behaviors, and hope that we can motivate you to change (and/or maintain) and give you some strategies for making change. We want you to achieve lifelong physical activity behaviors that promote lifelong wellness.

This Book's Features

As classroom teachers we are aware of the importance of developing materials and activities that are meaningful to you as a student as well as complementing the materials provided in the textbook. Based on our experiences, and talking with other faculty like your instructor, we have developed a number of features to help you grasp the material and develop lifelong physical activity behaviors that enhance your overall health and well-being.

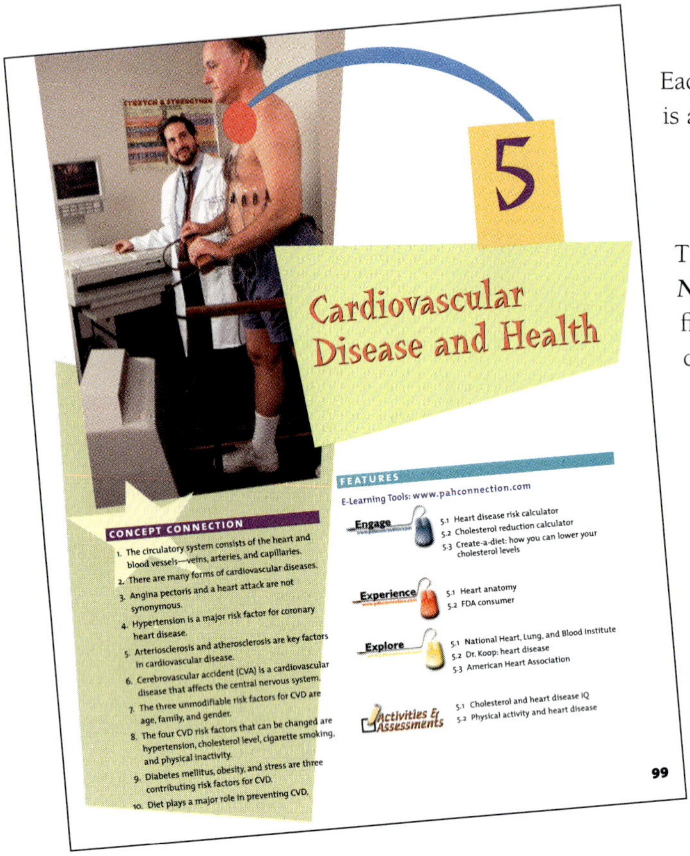
5
Cardiovascular Disease and Health

CONCEPT CONNECTION

1. The circulatory system consists of the heart and blood vessels—veins, arteries, and capillaries.
2. There are many forms of cardiovascular diseases.
3. Angina pectoris and a heart attack are not synonymous.
4. Hypertension is a major risk factor for coronary heart disease.
5. Arteriosclerosis and atherosclerosis are key factors in cardiovascular disease.
6. Cerebrovascular accident (CVA) is a cardiovascular disease that affects the central nervous system.
7. The three unmodifiable risk factors for CVD are age, family, and gender.
8. The four CVD risk factors that can be changed are hypertension, cholesterol level, cigarette smoking, and physical inactivity.
9. Diabetes mellitus, obesity, and stress are three contributing risk factors for CVD.
10. Diet plays a major role in preventing CVD.

FEATURES

E-Learning Tools: www.pahconnection.com

Engage
5.1 Heart disease risk calculator
5.2 Cholesterol reduction calculator
5.3 Create-a-diet: how you can lower your cholesterol levels

Experience
5.1 Heart anatomy
5.2 FDA consumer

Explore
5.1 National Heart, Lung, and Blood Institute
5.2 Dr. Koop: heart disease
5.3 American Heart Association

Activities & Assessments
5.1 Cholesterol and heart disease IQ
5.2 Physical activity and heart disease

99

Each chapter begins with the ***Concept Connection***, which is a numbered list of the chapter's key points.

These key points are referenced in the chapter with a ***Numbered Icon***—this helps you as a student quickly find that information when studying and reviewing the chapter's contents.

1. The circulatory system consists of the heart and blood vessels—veins, arteries, and capillaries.

At the end of each chapter, the concepts are reinforced with a brief narrative following each. This is an excellent tool for chapter review.

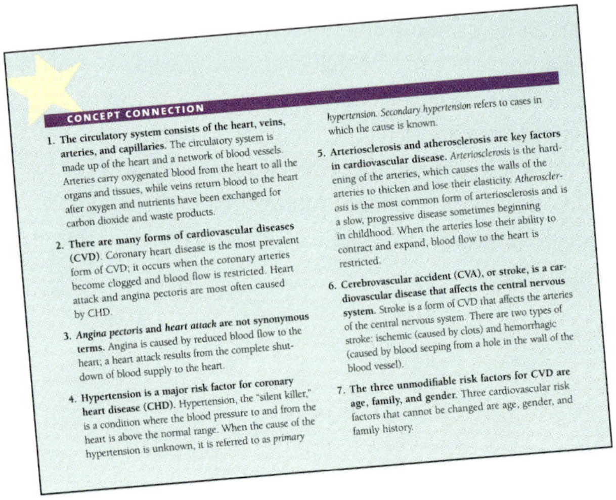
CONCEPT CONNECTION

1. **The circulatory system consists of the heart, veins, arteries, and capillaries.** The circulatory system is made up of the heart and a network of blood vessels. Arteries carry oxygenated blood from the heart to all the organs and tissues, while veins return blood to the heart after oxygen and nutrients have been exchanged for carbon dioxide and waste products.
2. **There are many forms of cardiovascular diseases (CVD).** Coronary heart disease is the most prevalent form of CVD; it occurs when the coronary arteries become clogged and blood flow is restricted. Heart attack and angina pectoris are most often caused by CHD.
3. ***Angina pectoris* and *heart attack* are not synonymous terms.** Angina is caused by reduced blood flow to the heart; a heart attack results from the complete shut-down of blood supply to the heart.
4. **Hypertension is a major risk factor for coronary heart disease (CHD).** Hypertension, the "silent killer," is a condition where the blood pressure to and from the heart is above the normal range. When the cause of the hypertension is unknown, it is referred to as *primary hypertension*. *Secondary hypertension* refers to cases in which the cause is known.
5. **Arteriosclerosis and atherosclerosis are key factors in cardiovascular disease.** *Arteriosclerosis* is the hardening of the arteries, which causes the walls of the arteries to thicken and lose their elasticity. *Atherosclerosis* is the most common form of arteriosclerosis and is a slow, progressive disease sometimes beginning in childhood. When the arteries lose their ability to contract and expand, blood flow to the heart is restricted.
6. **Cerebrovascular accident (CVA), or stroke, is a cardiovascular disease that affects the central nervous system.** Stroke is a form of CVD that affects the arteries of the central nervous system. There are two types of stroke: ischemic (caused by clots) and hemorrhagic (caused by blood seeping from a hole in the wall of the blood vessel).
7. **The three unmodifiable risk factors for CVD are age, family, and gender.** Three cardiovascular risk factors that cannot be changed are age, gender, and family history.

To provide meaningful examples, each chapter starts with ***What's the Connection?*** This short scenario profiles a college student who wants to change a specific behavior that is relevant to that chapter's content. At the end of the chapter, ***Making the Connection*** shows what the student has learned about the behavior they want to change and the action(s) they may take.

WHAT'S THE CONNECTION?

Richard is worried about dying from a heart attack. His father suffered a heart attack at age 45 last year and both of his grandfathers died of cardiovascular disease. Richard does not intend to follow in their footsteps. He knows that his family history and gender put him at risk, so he focuses on things he can control. He doesn't smoke, and he has his blood pressure and cholesterol levels monitored on a regular basis. Richard is convinced that physical activity is unrelated to his risk of developing cardiovascular disease. He thinks he is doing all he can to reduce his risk of cardiovascular disease. Is Richard correct in believing this? Are there any other factors that Richard should be aware of that could reduce his chances of developing cardiovascular disease?

MAKING THE CONNECTION

Richard has learned about the biological mechanisms by which physical activity may contribute to the prevention of coronary heart disease. So, in addition to what he was already doing to prevent cardiovascular disease for the past couple years, he has added a 30-minute walk to his daily routine over the past couple months. Not only does Richard feel better physically as a result of his daily walk, but the internal satisfaction of knowing that he is doing even more to lower his risk of developing coronary heart disease is also very rewarding to him.

Reinforcing the connection between physical activity and health a ***Physical Activity and Health Connection*** icon appears next to the paragraph where information highlights the link between physical activity and health. At the end of each chapter the **Physical Activity and Health Connection** summarizes the connection between physical activity and health.

PHYSICAL ACTIVITY AND HEALTH CONNECTION

Participation in regular physical activity helps to strengthen the function of all components of your cardiovascular system. This is important not only in terms of cardiovascular efficiency but also in terms of disease protection. Many of the chronic diseases of the cardiovascular system result from disuse. Physical activity stresses the cardiovascular system and makes it more fit. The more fit you are, the easier your cardiovascular system adjusts to the stress of physical exertion. Those who have a fit cardiovascular system are less likely to suffer a heart attack, less likely to die if they have a heart attack, and more likely to recover fully after a heart attack.

Regular exposure to physical activity also benefits the pulmonary system, allowing it to coordinate more efficiently the exchange of oxygen and carbon dioxide with the cardiovascular system. Physical activity also plays an important role in the rehabilitation process for those who have developed cardiovascular disease. Cardiac rehabilitation programs allow individuals to return to a normal lifestyle much more rapidly than in the past.

To facilitate the use of the Internet's vast amount of information, as well as provide interactive activities and assessments for you, we have developed a set of ***E-Learning Tools: Explore, Engage,*** and ***Experience*** that are available in each chapter. ***Explore*** icons lead you to a website that provide more in-depth information. These websites are full of good information, and because they are on the Internet the information is updated all the time. ***Engage*** activities direct you to a website for interactive assessments and activities online. These activities are relatively simple and provide immediate feedback to you. Your instructor may assign one or more of these **Engage** activities for you to complete, but if they don't—go ahead, engage yourself and learn! ***Experience*** is just that. Experience icons lead you to a website that has an exercise (developed by the authors) that you complete based on the information from that website. Your instructor may have you complete these exercises and submit them as assignments.

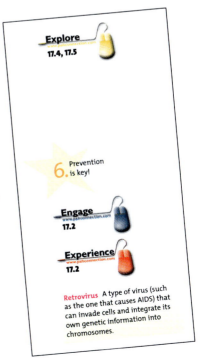

Explore www.pahconnection.com
17.4, 17.5

6. Prevention is key!

Engage www.pahconnection.com
17.2

Experience www.pahconnection.com
17.2

Retrovirus A type of virus (such as the one that causes AIDS) that can invade cells and integrate its own genetic information into chromosomes.

At the end of each chapter are ***Activities and Assessments***. These paper and pencil assessments assist you in better understanding yourself and making health behavior change. Within the chapter appropriate activities and assessments are called out in the margins. Your instructor may assign these for homework, or you can try them on your own. Your answers may surprise you.

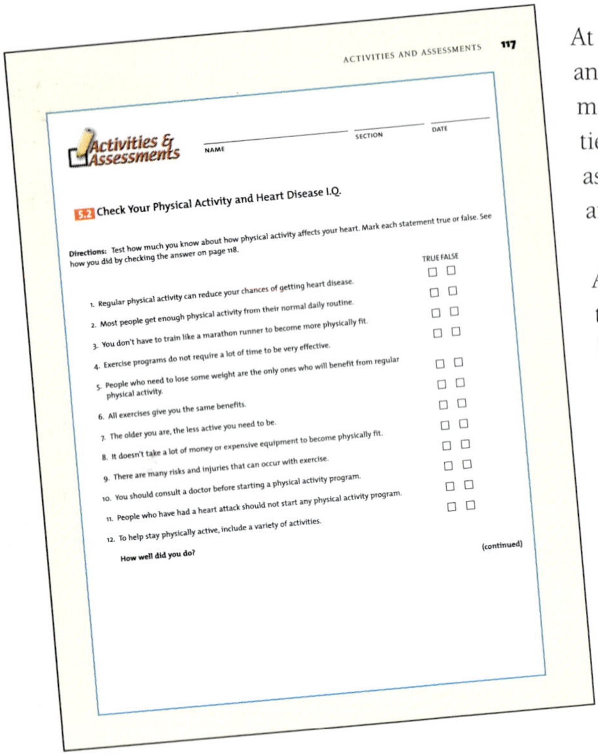
ACTIVITIES AND ASSESSMENTS 117

Activities & Assessments NAME SECTION DATE

5.2 Check Your Physical Activity and Heart Disease I.Q.

Directions: Test how much you know about how physical activity affects your heart. Mark each statement true or false. See how you did by checking the answer on page 118.

	TRUE	FALSE
1. Regular physical activity can reduce your chances of getting heart disease.	☐	☐
2. Most people get enough physical activity from their normal daily routine.	☐	☐
3. You don't have to train like a marathon runner to become more physically fit.	☐	☐
4. Exercise programs do not require a lot of time to be very effective.	☐	☐
5. People who need to lose some weight are the only ones who will benefit from regular physical activity.	☐	☐
6. All exercises give you the same benefits.	☐	☐
7. The older you are, the less active you need to be.	☐	☐
8. It doesn't take a lot of money or expensive equipment to become physically fit.	☐	☐
9. There are many risks and injuries that can occur with exercise.	☐	☐
10. You should consult a doctor before starting a physical activity program.	☐	☐
11. People who have had a heart attack should not start any physical activity program.	☐	☐
12. To help stay physically active, include a variety of activities.	☐	☐

How well did you do?

(continued)

As mentioned previously, self-responsibility is an integral component to this textbook. Also, integral is *behavior change*. So, based on behavior-change theories (Chapter 3) we have developed ***Challenge to Change*** (pages 403–410). This section guides you through the behavior change process for a behavior you would like to change. Your instructor may have you work on this throughout the course, OR you can work on it alone.

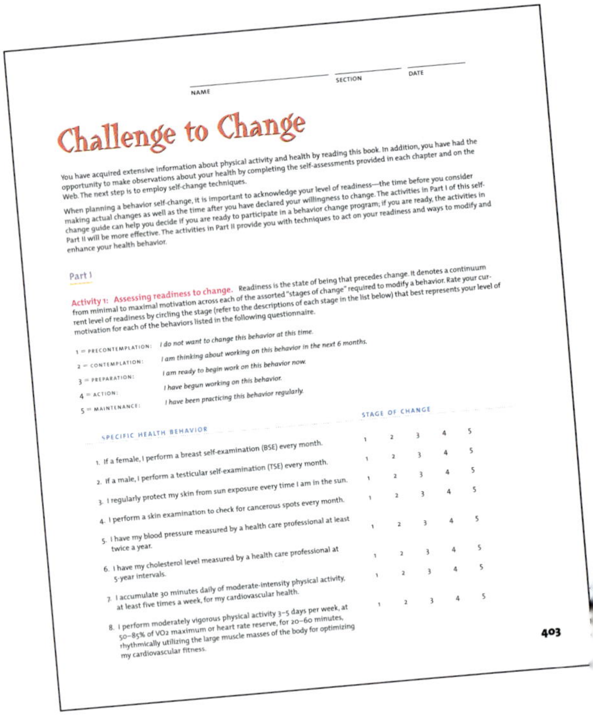
NAME SECTION DATE

Challenge to Change

You have acquired extensive information about physical activity and health by reading this book. In addition, you have had the opportunity to make observations about your health by completing the self-assessments provided in each chapter and on the Web. The next step is to employ self-change techniques.

When planning a behavior self-change, it is important to acknowledge your level of readiness—the time before you consider making actual changes as well as the time after you have declared your willingness to change. The activities in Part I of this self-change guide can help you decide if you are ready to participate in a behavior change program; if you are ready, the activities in Part II will be more effective. The activities in Part II provide you with techniques to act on your readiness and ways to modify and enhance your health behavior.

Part I

Activity 1: Assessing readiness to change. Readiness is the state of being that precedes change. It denotes a continuum from minimal to maximal motivation across each of the assorted "stages of change" required to modify a behavior. Rate your current level of readiness by circling the stage (refer to the descriptions of each stage in the list below) that best represents your level of motivation for each of the behaviors listed in the following questionnaire.

1 = PRECONTEMPLATION: *I do not want to change this behavior at this time.*
2 = CONTEMPLATION: *I am thinking about working on this behavior in the next 6 months.*
3 = PREPARATION: *I am ready to begin work on this behavior now.*
4 = ACTION: *I have begun working on this behavior.*
5 = MAINTENANCE: *I have been practicing this behavior regularly.*

SPECIFIC HEALTH BEHAVIOR	STAGE OF CHANGE				
	1	2	3	4	5
1. If a female, I perform a breast self-examination (BSE) every month.	1	2	3	4	5
2. If a male, I perform a testicular self-examination (TSE) every month.	1	2	3	4	5
3. I regularly protect my skin from sun exposure every time I am in the sun.	1	2	3	4	5
4. I perform a skin examination to check for cancerous spots every month.	1	2	3	4	5
5. I have my blood pressure measured by a health care professional at least twice a year.	1	2	3	4	5
6. I have my cholesterol level measured by a health care professional at 5-year intervals.	1	2	3	4	5
7. I accumulate 30 minutes daily of moderate-intensity physical activity, at least five times a week, for my cardiovascular health.	1	2	3	4	5
8. I perform moderately vigorous physical activity 3–5 days per week, at 50–85% of VO_2 maximum or heart rate reserve, for 20–60 minutes, rhythmically utilizing the large muscle masses of the body for optimizing my cardiovascular fitness.	1	2	3	4	5

403

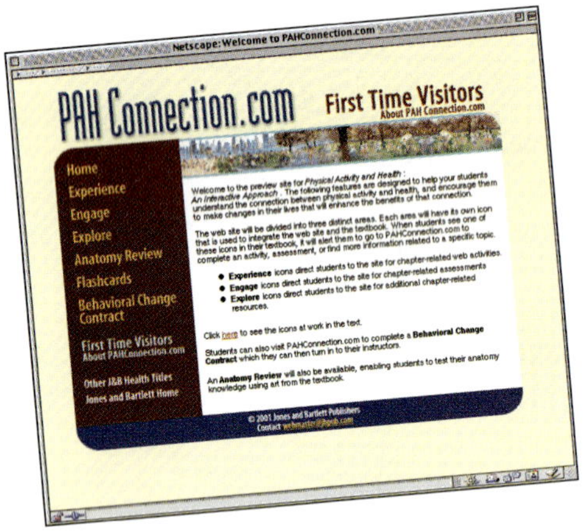

One last note. This book has a website (PAHConnection.com) that has all the ***E-Learning Tool*** webpages, a behavioral change contract, an anatomy review and much more! Bookmark this website for use throughout this course.

As authors we hope that you learn from this textbook and that it makes a positive difference. As lifelong learners we are interested in your feedback. Please feel free to contact Kelli McCormack Brown at kmbrown@jbpub.com.

1

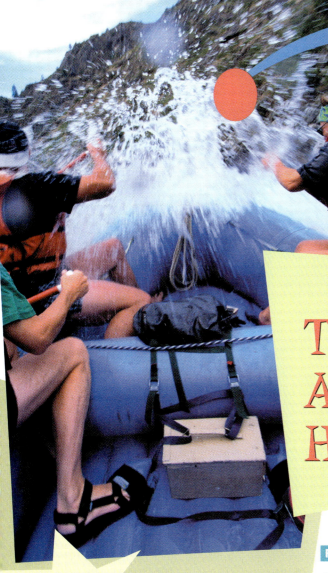

The Physical Activity and Health Connection

CONCEPT CONNECTION

1. Americans do not engage in the recommended amount of physical activity for several reasons.
2. An understanding of what it means to be healthy and well are essential to being responsible for our health behaviors.
3. The six dimensions of wellness are emotional, intellectual, spiritual, occupational, social, and physical.
4. *Healthy People 2010* provides a vision for the nation's health, including physical activity.
5. Physical activity, exercise, and physical fitness refer to different components of an active lifestyle.
6. Everyone should engage daily in physical activity.
7. Regular physical activity reduces many health risks.
8. Self-responsibility is key to achieving health and wellness.

FEATURES

E-Learning Tools: www.pahconnection.com

Engage www.pahconnection.com

1.1 YOU first™ health risk assessment
1.2 National Wellness Institute
1.3 What does it take to be healthy?

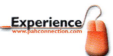

Experience www.pahconnection.com

1.1 College health risk behavior survey—United States, 1995
1.2 Fitness link

Explore www.pahconnection.com

1.1 *Healthy People 2000* midcourse review
1.2 *Healthy People 2010* home page
1.3 The National Institutes of Health consensus statement on physical activity and cardiovascular health

Activities & Assessments

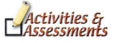

1.1 Defining physical activity and health
1.2 How healthy are you?

WHAT'S THE CONNECTION?

Finding her way to classes. Learning to schedule time for studying. Meeting new people and making friends. These are just a few of Heather's experiences during the first weeks of her freshman year at college. Heather spends lots of time in the library, and when she isn't studying or going to classes she is working as a part-time receptionist at the university bookstore. With all these commitments, Heather is finding it difficult to stay physically active; as a matter of fact, her daily routine requires very little physical activity. In high school, Heather was physically active in club sports and either walked or rode her bike to school every day. As the semester continues, Heather notices that she feels more and more sluggish—she is not as energetic as she used to be. Heather attributes these feelings to being away from home, to the change in environment, and to studying a lot.

INTRODUCTION

The health of millions of Americans suffers as a result of their sedentary lifestyles. Regular physical activity can reduce the risk for developing diabetes, high blood pressure, and colon cancer, reduce feelings of depression and anxiety, and promote psychological well-being. However, more than 60 percent of U.S. adults do not engage in the recommended amount of physical activity, and almost 25 percent are not active at all (CDC, 2001; USDHHS, 1996) (Figure 1.1).

Why are so few people physically active? First, as a society we depend a great deal on the laborsaving devices that have become part of our daily lives. These include washing machines, elevators, riding lawnmowers, and automobiles, to name just a few. These products have made the tasks of daily life easier, but as a result many of us get little physical activity; we have fallen into a sedentary lifestyle. Another possible reason for the lack of physical activity may be that high-intensity exercise is misperceived by health professionals and the general public as the only way to achieve health benefits from physical

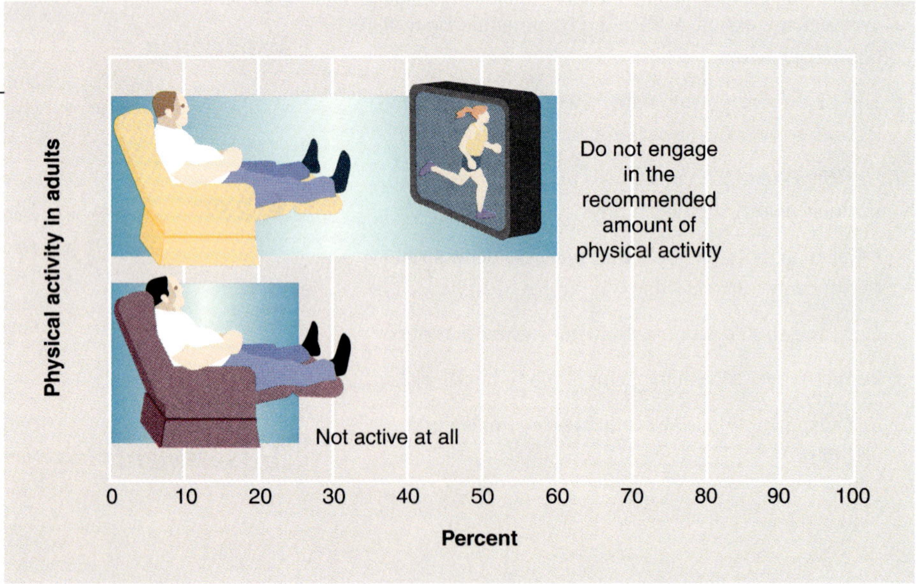

FIGURE 1.1

U.S. Physical Activity Levels. American adults are not as physically active as they could be.

SOURCE: Data compiled from Centers for Disease Control and Prevention. (1992). *Behavior Risk Factor Survey Surveillance (BRFSS).*

activity (Dinger, 1999). A final reason may be the social and environmental barriers that prevent daily physical activity. To promote physical activity, we need safe neighborhoods, with sidewalks, bicycle paths, and recreational facilities (ACSM-CDC, 1993).

Which of the reasons just mentioned (laborsaving devices, perceptions of high-intensity exercise, social and environmental barriers) impact the level of physical activity in your daily life? How does your personal or family health history impact the inclusion of physical activity in your life? As you read this book, think about *why* physical activity is important for you and *how* you can make time to be physically active on a daily basis.

1. Americans do not engage in the recommended amount of physical activity for several reasons.

DEFINING HEALTH, WELLNESS, AND LIFE QUALITY

To be responsible for your health and well-being, you must understand what **health** and **wellness** are. Historically, people wanted to be healthy and well in order to live a long life. That may have made sense in 1900 when the average **life expectancy** was 47 years, but today, with life expectancy almost doubled, we are just as concerned with **quality of life** (Figure 1.2). In the 1940s, the World Health Organization defined health as a "state of complete physical, mental, and social well-being and not merely the absence of disease or infirmity" (World Health Organization, 1947). This definition was significant at the time because it challenged public health officials to see health as something more than the absence of disease.

Today, *health* is defined differently among experts, but for the purposes of this book we consider health multidimensional, involving the whole person's relation to the total environment. Health encompasses the behavioral, social, and physical environments, policies and interventions, and access to quality health care. Wellness is more than simple physical health. We refer to *wellness* as an active process, a lifestyle, that reflects a positive quality of life. This wellness lifestyle emphasizes health-promoting behaviors such as daily physical activity, healthy eating, avoidance of harmful substances, and maintaining of healthy relationships. A wellness lifestyle enhances your overall health and well-being, increases the numbers of years you can expect to live, and provides a superior quality of life.

2. An understanding of what it means to be healthy and well is essential to being responsible for our health behaviors.

Engage www.pahconnection.com 1.1

Health State of complete physical, mental, and social well-being—not merely the absence of disease or infirmity.

Wellness An approach to personal health that emphasizes individual responsibility for well-being through the practice of health-promoting lifestyle behaviors.

Life expectancy The average number of years a person is projected to live.

Quality of life The perception of individuals that their needs are being satisfied and that they are not being denied opportunities to achieve happiness and fulfillment.

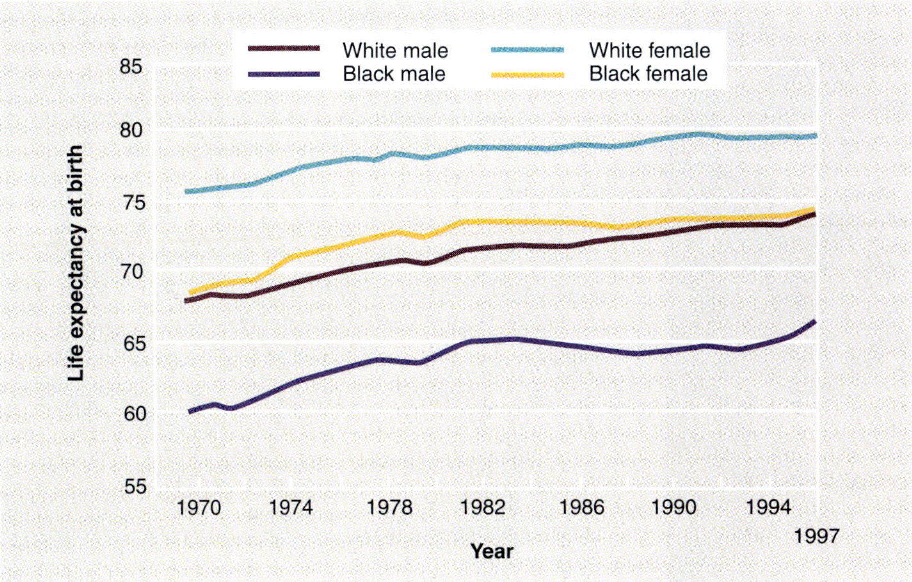

FIGURE 1.2

Life Expectancy at Birth by Race and Gender: 1970–97.

SOURCE: R.N. Anderson. (December 13, 1999). U.S. Life-tables, 1997. *National Vital Statistics Reports*, 47(28), 3.

3. The six dimensions of wellness are emotional, intellectual, spiritual, occupational, social, and physical.

Engage
www.pahconnection.com
1.2

physical activity and health connection

Dimensions of Health and Wellness

Wellness is dynamic and continuous; therefore, no dimension of wellness functions in isolation. When you have a high level of wellness, all dimensions are integrated and functioning harmoniously. Your environment (work, school, family, community) and your physical, emotional, intellectual, occupational, spiritual, and social dimensions of wellness are in harmony with one another. We now look briefly at each of these dimensions:

- *Social wellness* refers to the ability to perform social roles effectively, comfortably, and without harm to others.
- *Physical wellness* is a healthy body maintained by eating right, exercising regularly, avoiding harmful habits, making informed and responsible decisions about health, seeking medical care when needed, and participating in activities that help prevent illness.
- *Emotional wellness* requires understanding emotions and coping with problems that arise in everyday life.
- *Career* or *occupational wellness* lies in being able to enjoy what you do to earn a living and contribute to society, whether by going to college or by working as a receptionist, computer specialist, building contractor, nurse, or accountant. In a job, it means having skills of critical thinking, problem solving, and communicating.
- *Intellectual wellness* involves having a mind open to new ideas and concepts. If you are intellectually healthy, you seek new experiences and challenges.
- *Spiritual wellness* is the state of harmony with oneself and others. It is the ability to balance inner needs with the demands of the rest of the world.

In general, wellness involves (1) being free from symptoms of disease and pain; (2) being active, able to do what you want and what you must at the appropriate times; and (3) being in good spirits most of the time. These characteristics indicate that health is not something suddenly achieved at a specific time, like getting a college degree. Rather, health is a *process,* indeed, a way of life, through which you develop and encourage every aspect of your body, mind, and feelings to interrelate harmoniously as much of the time as possible. Think of wellness as a continuum (Figure 1.3). Most people find themselves in the neutral area of the continuum much of the time. However, many of us can remember times of moving toward disability and times of moving toward optimal health. Thus we know from personal experience that an individual can move from a state of illness or disease back to the neutral point or onward to high-level wellness many times. The wellness continuum also includes prevention, which means taking positive actions to prevent acute and chronic illnesses.

Although this book focuses on the physical dimension of health and wellness, it also recognizes and incorporates, when possible, the other dimensions of health and wellness.

Health is a lifelong endeavor.

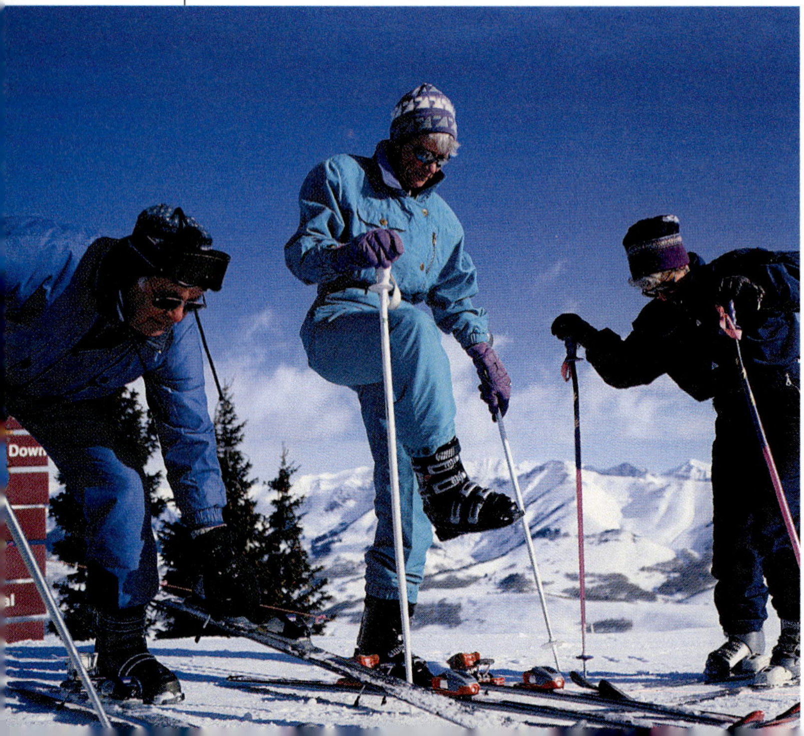

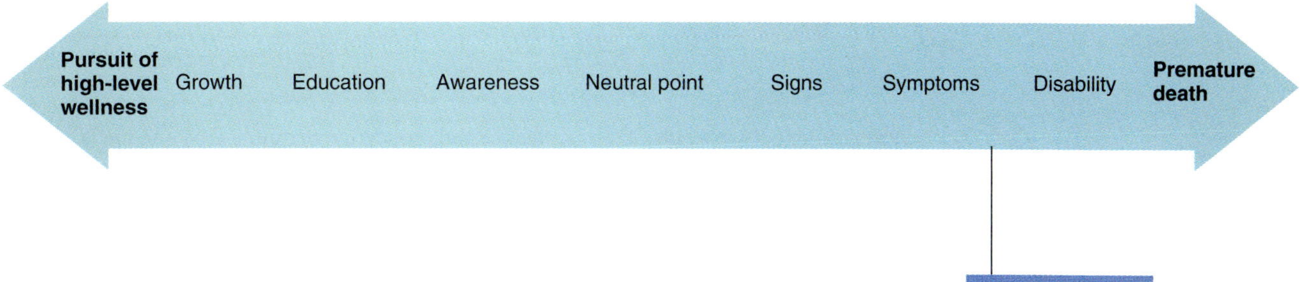

FIGURE 1.3

The Wellness Continuum. The wellness continuum allows you to visualize the difference between wellness and the medical approaches to health.

SETTING THE NATION'S AGENDA: HEALTHY PEOPLE

The *Surgeon General's Report on Health Promotion and Disease Prevention* was first released in 1979. Its purpose was to create a public health revolution by emphasizing prevention of disease and focusing on taking personal responsibility for one's own health by reducing risky habits. The report targeted five groups and one broad health goal: reducing the death rates among infants, children, adolescents and young adults, adults, and older adults.

In 1980, the United States Department of Health and Human Services (USDHHS) published *Promoting Health/Preventing Disease: Objectives for the Nation*. This publication outlined specific objectives for meeting, by 1990, the goals identified in the earlier *Surgeon General's Report*. These objectives were followed by the development of *Healthy People 2000* (USDHHS, 1990), a document setting forth the nation's vision for a new century in which we would be enhancing the quality of life, reducing preventable death and disability, and reducing the disparities in health status of various groups within American society. The purpose of *Healthy People 2000* was "to commit the Nation to the attainment of three broad goals that will help bring us to our full potential" (USDHHS, 1990, p. 6). The goals were:

1. Increase the lifespan of healthy life for Americans
2. Reduce health disparities among Americans
3. Achieve access to preventive services for all Americans

Experience www.pahconnection.com 1.1

4. *Healthy People 2010* provides a vision for the nation's health, including physical activity.

Explore www.pahconnection.com 1.1

Healthy People 2010

Today, *Healthy People 2010* (USDHHS, 2000) is setting the prevention agenda for the United States. It was developed following advances in preventive therapies, vaccines, other pharmaceuticals, assistive technologies, and computerized systems; a heightened awareness and demand for preventive health services and quality healthcare; and changes in demographics, science, technology, and disease spread that will affect public health in the twenty-first century. While the federal government has taken the lead in developing the initial draft objectives, the process is designed to be participatory.

The *2010* physical activity and fitness objectives (Table 1.1) provide opportunities to incorporate physical activity into your daily lifestyle. There are fifteen physical activity and fitness objectives that have the overall goal of improving health, fitness, and quality of life through daily physical activity. The objectives are divided into four areas: physical activity in adults; muscular strength/endurance and flexibility; physical activity in children and adolescents; and access.

TABLE 1.1 *Healthy People 2010* Physical Activity and Fitness Objectives

Physical Activity in Adults	1. Reduce the proportion of adults who engage in no leisure-time physical activity. 2. Increase the proportion of adults who engage regularly, preferably daily, in moderate physical activity for at least 30 minutes per day. 3. Increase the proportion of adults who engage in vigorous physical activity that promotes the development and maintenance of cardiorespiratory fitness 3 or more days per week for 20 or more minutes per occasion.
Muscular Strength/ Endurance and Flexibility	4. Increase the proportion of adults who perform physical activities that enhance and maintain muscular strength and endurance. 5. Increase the proportion of adults who perform physical activities that enhance and maintain flexibility.
Physical Activity in Children and Adolescents	6. Increase the proportion of adolescents who engaged in moderate physical activity for at least 30 minutes on 5 or more of the previous 7 days. 7. Increase the proportion of adolescents who engage in vigorous physical activity that promotes cardiorespiratory fitness 3 or more days per week for 20 or more minutes per occasion. 8. Increase the proportion of the Nation's public and private schools that require daily physical education for all students. 9. Increase the proportion of adolescents who participate in daily school physical education. 10. Increase the proportion of adolescents who spend at least 50 percent of school physical education class time being physically active. 11. Increase the proportion of children and adolescents who view television 2 or fewer hours on a school day.
Access	12. Increase the proportion of the Nation's public and private schools that provide access to their physical activity spaces and facilities for all persons outside normal school hours (that is, before and after the school day, on weekends, and during summer and other vacations). 13. Increase the proportion of work sites offering employer-sponsored physical activity and fitness programs. 14. Increase the proportion of trips made by walking. 15. Increase the proportion of trips made by bicycling.

SOURCE: U.S. Department of Health and Human Services. (2000). *Healthy People 2010.* (PHS 017-001-00550-9). Pittsburgh, PA: U.S. Government Printing Office. Available online: http://health.gov/healthypeople/; accessed 1/30/01).

PHYSICAL ACTIVITY, PHYSICAL FITNESS, EXERCISE AND LEISURE

By defining and contrasting several terms, we can determine the similarities and differences as well as the relationships among physical activity, physical fitness, exercise, and leisure (Table 1.2). **Physical activity** refers to any bodily movement that increases energy expenditure (Caspersen, Powell, & Christenson, 1985). **Exercise,** in contrast, is planned, structured, and repetitive physical activity done to improve or maintain physical fitness (Caspersen et al., 1985). Exercise is a subset of physical activity. **Physical fitness** is a set of attributes that allows individuals to carry out daily tasks without undue fatigue (Caspersen et al., 1985). Exercise and physical activity can lead to physical fitness. **Leisure** applies to physical activities that include the elements of free choice, freedom from constraints, intrinsic motivation, enjoyment, relaxation, personal involvement, and self-expression (Ainsworth & Macera, 1998).

Physical activity Any bodily movement that increases energy expenditure.

Exercise A planned, structured, and repetitive physical activity done to improve or maintain one or more of the components of physical fitness.

Physical fitness A set of attributes that allows individuals to carry out daily tasks without undue fatigue.

Leisure Physical activities that include enjoyment, relaxation, personal involvement, and self-expression.

5. Physical activity, exercise, and physical fitness refer to different components of an active lifestyle.

TABLE 1.2 **Common Definitions**

TERM	DEFINITION
Physical Activity*	Bodily movement produced by skeletal muscles that result in energy expenditure (expressed in kilocalories). Includes a broad range of occupational, leisure-time, and routine daily activities. These activities require either light, moderate, or vigorous effort and can lead to improved health if practiced regularly.
Exercise*	Physical activity that is planned or structured. Involves repetitive bodily movement done to improve or maintain one or more of the components of physical fitness: • Aerobic capacity • Muscular strength • Muscular endurance • Flexibility • Body composition
Physical Fitness*	A measure of a person's ability to perform physical activities that require endurance, strength, or flexibility that is determined by a combination of regular activity and genetically inherited ability.
Leisure**	Activities that include free choice, freedom from constraints, intrinsic motivation, enjoyment, relaxation, personal involvement, and self-expression. **

SOURCE:
*Adapted from U.S. Department of Health and Human Services. Public Health Service, Centers for Disease Control and Prevention, National Center for Chronic Disease Prevention and Health Promotion, Division of Physical Activity and Nutrition. *Promoting physical activity: A guide for community action*. Champaign, IL: Human Kinetics.

**B.E. Ainsworth and C.A. Macera. (1998). Physical inactivity. In R.C. Brownson, P.L. Remington and J.R. Davis (Eds.), *Chronic disease epidemiology and control,* (2nd ed.). Washington, DC: American Public Health Association.

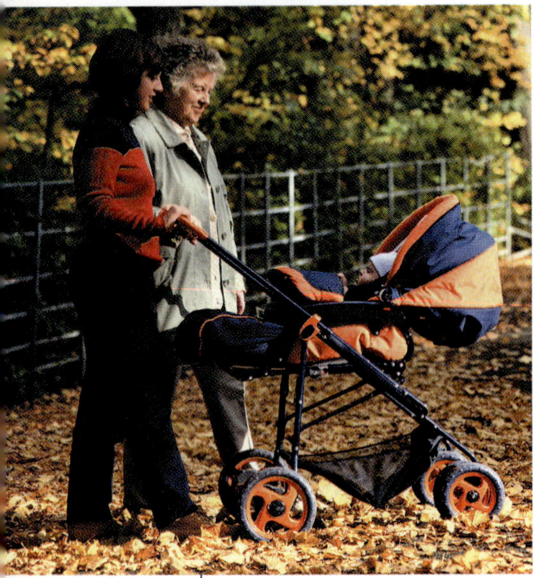

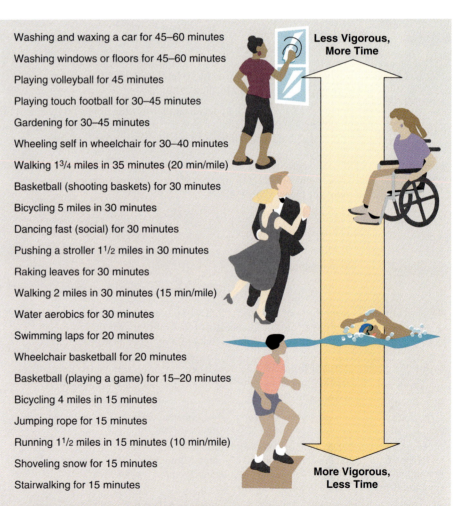

Walks through the park can be relaxing and physically beneficial.

This book focuses on physical activity and on the connection between physical activity and health. We believe that you cannot have health or wellness without physical activity, and that being physically active puts you on the path to becoming healthy and well.

Physical Activity Recommendations

In December 1995, the National Institutes of Health (NIH) convened a panel of professionals and experts representing various fields (NIH Consensus Development Panel, 1996). Based upon scientific evidence indicating that physical inactivity is a major risk factor for cardiovascular disease, that moderate levels of regular physical activity (Figure 1.4) can provide significant health benefits, and that individual and societal factors are critical, the panel recommended the following:

- Development of programs for healthcare providers to communicate to patients the importance of regular physical activity
- Increased community support of regular physical activity with environmental and policy changes at schools, work sites, community centers, and other sites

6. Everyone needs to engage in physical activity daily.

Explore
www.pahconnection.com
1.3

FIGURE 1.4

Examples of Moderate Amounts of Activity.

SOURCE: U.S. Department of Health and Human Services. (1996). *Physical Activity and Health: A Report of the Surgeon General.* Atlanta, GA: USDHHS, Centers for Disease Control and Prevention, National Center for Chronic Disease Prevention and Health Promotion.

Washing and waxing a car for 45–60 minutes
Washing windows or floors for 45–60 minutes
Playing volleyball for 45 minutes
Playing touch football for 30–45 minutes
Gardening for 30–45 minutes
Wheeling self in wheelchair for 30–40 minutes
Walking 1 3/4 miles in 35 minutes (20 min/mile)
Basketball (shooting baskets) for 30 minutes
Bicycling 5 miles in 30 minutes
Dancing fast (social) for 30 minutes
Pushing a stroller 1 1/2 miles in 30 minutes
Raking leaves for 30 minutes
Walking 2 miles in 30 minutes (15 min/mile)
Water aerobics for 30 minutes
Swimming laps for 20 minutes
Wheelchair basketball for 20 minutes
Basketball (playing a game) for 15–20 minutes
Bicycling 4 miles in 15 minutes
Jumping rope for 15 minutes
Running 1 1/2 miles in 15 minutes (10 min/mile)
Shoveling snow for 15 minutes
Stairwalking for 15 minutes

* A moderate amount of physical activity is roughly equivilent to physical activity that uses approximately 150 Calories (kcal) of energy per day, or 1000 Calories per week.
† Some activities can be performed at various intensities; the suggested durations correspond to expected intensity of effort.

- Initiation of a coordinated national campaign involving a consortium of collaborating health organizations to encourage regular physical activity.

These recommendations indicate that we don't have to do as much physical activity to achieve health benefits as was believed in the past. See Chapter 2 for specific recommendations. Table 1.3 illustrates how far we have to go in meeting basic physical activity goals.

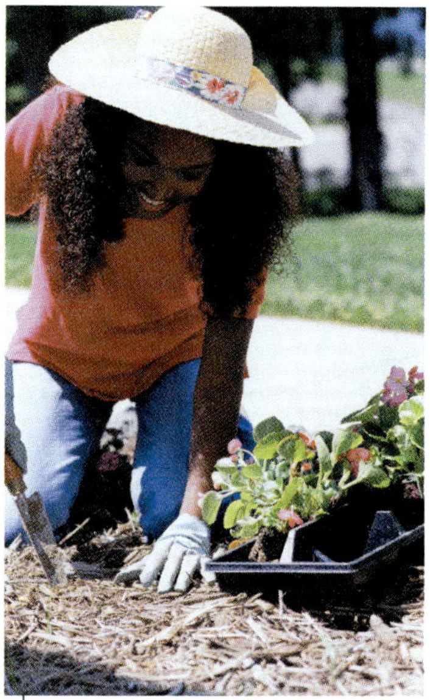

Gardening is enjoyable and expends energy.

Working Definition of Physical Activity

In this book we will often refer to physical activity. We view *physical activity* as any bodily movement that you do daily at a moderate intensity. This means you briskly

TABLE 1.3 Percentage of Americans Who Meet Current Physical Activity Recommendations

U.S. RECOMMENDATION FOR PHYSICAL ACTIVITY	ADULT MEN	ADULT WOMEN	TOTAL AMERICAN ADULTS
Every U.S. adult should accumulate 30 min or more of moderate-intensity activity, on most, preferably all, days of the week. ACSM-CDC Guidelines (Pate et al., 1995)	34.3%	29.8%	32.0%
An amount of physical activity sufficient to burn 150 kilocalories per day (627.6 kj/day) or 1000 kilocalories per week (1484 kj/week). 1996 Surgeon General's Report Guidelines (USDHHS, 1996)	47.7%	29.2%	37.9%

SOURCE: U.S. Department of Health and Human Services, Public Health Service, Centers for Disease Control and Prevention, National Center for Chronic Disease Prevention and Health Promotion, Division of Physical Activity and Nutrition. *Promoting physical activity: A guide for community action* (19). Champaign, IL: Human Kinetics.

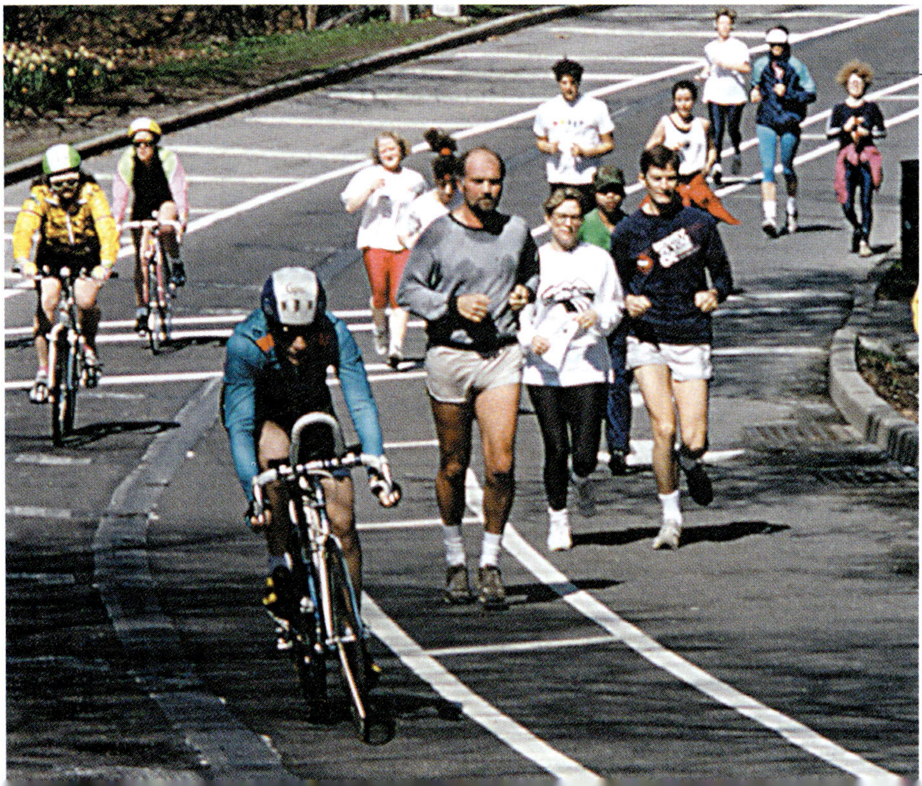

Bicycling, jogging, and walking are fun activities that can lead to better overall physical health and well-being.

walk to school in the morning, walk up three flights of stairs to class, and later wash your car. Before you know it, you are moderately physically active and on your way to leading a healthier lifestyle!

WHY IS PHYSICAL ACTIVITY IMPORTANT TO OVERALL HEALTH?

7. Regular physical activity reduces many health risks.

A survey of the actual causes of death (as opposed to the causes reported on death certificates) revealed that approximately half of all deaths in the United States each year are due to lifestyle factors (McGuiness and Foege, 1993). In 1990, physical inactivity and poor nutrition were responsible for 300,000 deaths, while tobacco was responsible for 400,000 deaths. Other lifestyle risk factors that caused death were alcohol, firearms, motor vehicle accidents, illegal drug use, and unsafe sexual behaviors.

The consequences of physical inactivity are "felt among many dimensions of health including physical, physiological, psychological, and societal" (Ainsworth & Macera, 1998, p. 191). Research tells us that regular physical activity reduces the risk of dying prematurely, dying from coronary heart disease, or developing colon cancer or diabetes; reduces blood pressure among people with hypertension; promotes psychological well-being; and builds and maintains healthy bones, muscles, and joints among older people (Rockhill et al., 2001; Ainsworth & Macera, 1998; USDHHS, 1996; Pate et al., 1995).

These scientific studies should convince us that daily physical activity is important to health both today and tomorrow. All we need to do is take personal responsibility for our health by adopting or maintaining healthy behaviors to achieve health, wellness, and quality of life.

TAKING RESPONSIBILITY FOR YOUR HEALTH

Physical activity is one aspect of self-responsibility.

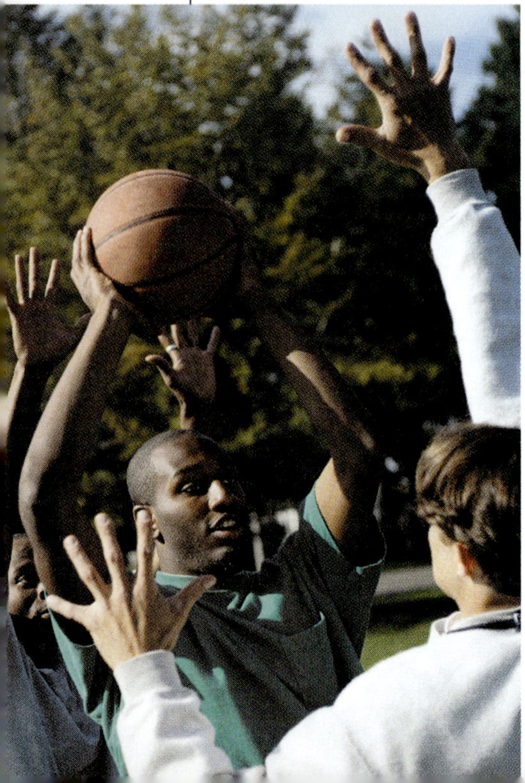

Not so many years ago, people were subject to a variety of diseases over which they had little or no control. In the early part of the twentieth century, infectious diseases caused by micro-organisms were the leading causes of death in the United States (Armstrong, Conn, & Pinner, 1999). Modern public-health methods and modern drugs such as antibiotics were not available. In 1918, millions of people around the world died from influenza, the cause of which was unknown at that time (Table 1.4).

Today, the leading causes of illness and death are not infections, but "lifestyle diseases." These diseases—for example, heart disease and cancer—result from environmental factors and people's chosen behaviors. The idea that lifestyle is a major cause of disease and death in modern societies is not new. A classic study by Belloc and Breslow (1972) demonstrated the importance of individual involvement in achieving health and wellness. Their research findings identified seven personal habits that are the foundation of good health:

- Moderate exercise two to three times a week
- Three meals a day at regular times with no snacking
- Breakfast every day

- Seven to eight hours of sleep every night
- No smoking
- No alcohol (or moderate use)
- Moderate weight

Although we understand more today about health than we did three decades ago, these habits all had one key element in common—they relied on self-responsibility.

Self-responsibility is key to achieving health and wellness. The first step in taking responsibility for your health is recognizing that you make daily choices that impact your total well-being. Sometimes the choices we make allow us to experience positive health and high-level wellness. Sometimes the decisions we make cause us to experience illness. Halbert Dunn (1967) states it simply: "We cannot take high-level wellness like a pill out of a bottle. It will come only to those who work at following its precepts."

This book includes a number of features designed to help you achieve a healthy lifestyle. First, an entire chapter is devoted to behavior change (Chapter 3), the chapter vignettes ("What's the Connection?") focus on behavior change, and the text concludes with *Challenge to Change*. These features are designed to guide you in changing unhealthy behaviors. Next, we have included a number of interactive experiences (Engage, Explore, Experience)—both on our website and at the ends of the chapters (Activities and Assessments). These features will help you assess your levels of health and fitness and present activities you can complete to learn more about physical activity and health. Finally, throughout the text we have pointed out connections between physical activity and health to underscore how important becoming active is to your long-term health.

physical activity and health connection

8. Self-responsibility is key to achieving health and wellness.

Engage www.pahconnection.com 1.3

Experience www.pahconnection.com 1.1

TABLE 1.4 **Health Indicators During the Past Century**

LEADING CAUSES OF DEATH, ALL AGES		10 ACTUAL CAUSES OF DEATH***	10 LEADING CAUSES OF DEATH, AGES 15–24, BOTH SEXES, 1998**
1900*	**1998****		
Pneumonia	Heart disease	Tobacco use	Unintentional injuries
Tuberculosis	Cancer	Dietary practices and physical inactivity	Homicide
Diarrhea and enteritis	Stroke	Alcohol use	Suicide
Diseases of the heart	Chronic obstructive pulmonary disease	Microbial agents	Cancer
Intracranial lesions of vascular origin (stroke)	Unintentional injuries	Toxic agents	Heart diseases
Nephritis (liver disease)	Pneumonia/Influenza	Firearms	Congenital anomalies
All accidents	Diabetes	Consequences of sexual behavior	Chronic obstructive pulmonary disease
Cancer	Suicide	Motor vehicle accidents	Pneumonia/Influenza
Certain diseases of early infancy	Kidney disease	Use of illicit drugs	Human immunodeficiency virus infection
Diphtheria	Chronic liver disease and cirrhosis		Stroke

SOURCES:
*Adapted from Schneider, M.J. (2000). *Introduction to Public Health*. Gaithersburg, MD: Aspen Publishing, Inc.

**National Vital Statistics Report. (2000). U.S. Department of Health and Human Services, Hyattsville, MD. *Deaths: Final Data for 1998*, 48(11), July 24, 2000.

***J.M. McGinnis and W.M. Foege. (1993). Actual Causes of Death in the United States. *JAMA*, 270(18), 2207–2212.

PHYSICAL ACTIVITY AND HEALTH CONNECTION

Physical inactivity is now recognized as having a major impact on your health and longevity. The Centers for Disease Control and Prevention (CDC), the National Institutes of Health (NIH), and the Surgeon General's Office have all issued statements declaring that regular participation in physical activity will make you live longer and improve the quality of your life. *Healthy People 2010* lists physical activity as one of the major factors that can help improve the health of the nation. Physical activity plays an important role in preventing the onset of several degenerative diseases and can also play a role in disease treatment and rehabilitation.

Physical well-being is a key component in the definitions of health and wellness. Health is gained and maintained by exerting self-responsibility for reducing exposure to health risks and maximizing physical activity and good nutrition. Throughout this book, we will show you ways to maximize your health by understanding how your mind and body function, how to develop a physical activity plan, how to make informed decisions about physical activity and health, and how to be responsible for your actions and behaviors. Learning to be responsible while you are young for the degree of health and energy you want helps to ensure lifelong wellness and quality of life.

CONCEPT CONNECTION

1. **Americans do not engage in the recommended amount of physical activity for several reasons.** We depend a great deal on laborsaving devices that have become part of our daily lives; high-intensity exercise is perceived by health professionals and the general public as the only way to achieve health benefits from physical activity; and many social and environmental barriers prevent daily physical activity.

2. **An understanding of what it means to be healthy and well is essential to being responsible for our health behaviors.** *Health* means being responsible for preventing illness and injuries as well as knowing when to seek medical help. *Wellness* is an ongoing, active process, a lifestyle that emphasizes health-promoting behaviors.

3. **The six dimensions of wellness are emotional, intellectual, spiritual, occupational, social, and physical.** The commonly stated dimensions of wellness are *emotional* (understanding emotions and coping with problems), *intellectual* (having a mind open to new ideas and concepts), *spiritual* (being in a state of harmony with oneself and others), *occupational* (contributing to society), *social* (performing social roles effectively), and *physical* (having a healthy body maintained by making informed and responsible decisions about health).

4. ***Healthy People 2010* provides a vision for the nation's health.** *Healthy People 2010*, the prevention agenda for the United States, is based on scientific knowledge and can be used by states, communities, and professional organizations for decision making and action.

5. **Physical activity, exercise, and physical fitness refer to different components of an active lifestyle.** *Physical activity* is any bodily movement that increases energy expenditure; *exercise* is a planned, structured, and repetitive physical activity done to improve or maintain one or more of the physical fitness components; and *physical fitness* is a set of attributes that

allows individuals to carry out daily tasks without undue fatigue.

6. **Everyone should engage in physical activity daily at a moderate intensity.** We all can benefit from moderately intense physical activity, and we can accumulate those minutes throughout the day.

7. **Regular physical activity reduces many health risks.** Regular physical activity reduces the risk of premature death, coronary heart disease, colon cancer, and diabetes. It also reduces blood pressure, promotes psychological well-being, and builds and maintains healthy bones, muscles, and joints.

8. **Self-responsibility is key to achieving health and wellness.** The leading causes of illness and death in the United States are lifestyle diseases that result from environmental factors and people's behaviors.

TERMS

Health, 3
Wellness, 3
Life expectancy, 3
Quality of life, 3
Physical activity, 7
Exercise, 7
Physical fitness, 7
Leisure, 7

MAKING THE CONNECTION

Heather realizes that she is in college to learn and do well academically. Her mid-term grades are fine, but she doesn't like feeling tired all the time. After reading Chapter 1, Heather realizes that she must take more responsibility for how she is feeling. She surmises that the lack of physical activity in her life may be contributing to her worn-out feeling and begins to think of ways she can find time to become more physically active while still maintaining other positive aspects of college life.

CRITICAL THINKING

1. Are you feeling lethargic and tired, like Heather? Could it be because of lack of physical activity? If so, what physical activity are you currently doing? If not, what can you do to increase your physical activity? Develop a list of campus events or organizations that involve physical activity (hiking club, co-ed intramural volleyball, walking club, kick boxing). Investigate several of them to see which one best fits your needs and schedule. Begin adding this activity into your daily or weekly college routine.

2. Using the six dimensions of wellness, identify two behaviors you do that would be an example of each dimension.

3. Morning newspaper headline: "Scientific studies indicate physical activity is important to health and quality of life." The article mentions studies from the "Prestigious International Health & Medicine Journal." Later that day you hear a local radio report suggesting that too much physical activity can lead to a instant heart attack, maybe even death. We are bombarded with health messages daily. What is your major source of health information? Television? If so, which shows in particular? Magazines? School? Friends? How carefully do you analyze health information? Do you believe most of what you read about health, or does it depend on the source?

REFERENCES

Ainsworth, B.E., & Macera, C.A. (1998). Physical inactivity. In Brownson, R.C., Remington, P.L., & Davis, J.R., eds., *Chronic Disease Epidemiology and Control*, 2nd ed. Washington, DC: American Public Health Association.

American College of Sports Medicine and U.S. Centers for Disease Control and Prevention (1993). Summary statement: Workshop on physical activity and public health. *Sports Medicine Bulletin 28*(4): 7.

Armstrong, G.L., Conn, L.A., & Pinner, R.W. (1999). Trends in infectious disease mortality in the United States during the 20th century. *Journal of the American Medical Association 281*(1): 61–66.

Belloc, N., & Breslow, L. (1972). Relationship of physical health and health practices. *Preventive Medicine 1*:409–421.

Caspersen, C.J., Powell, K.E., & Christenson, G.M. (1985). Physical activity, exercise, and physical fitness: Definitions and distinctions for health-related research. *Public Health Reports 100*(2):126–31.

Centers for Disease Control and Prevention (2001). Physical activity trends—United States, 1990–98. *MMWR, 50*(9), 166–169.

Dinger, M.K. (1999). Physical activity: An update for health educators. *The International Journal of Health Education 2*(2):81–83.

Dunn, H. (1967). *High Level Wellness*. Arlington, VA: Charles B. Slack.

McGuiness, J. M., & Foege, W. H. (1993). Actual causes of death in the United States. *Journal of the American Medical Association 270*(18):2207–2212.

NIH Consensus Development Panel on Physical Activity and Cardiovascular Health. (1996). *Journal of the American Medical Association 276*(3):241–46.

Pate, R.R., et al. (1995). Physical activity and public health: A recommendation from the Centers for Disease Control and Prevention and the American College of Sports Medicine. *Journal of the American Medical Association 273*(5):402–407.

Rockhill, B., Willett, W.C., Mason, J.E., Leitzmann, M.F., Stampfer, M.J., Hunter, D.J., & Colditz, G.A. (2001). Physical activity and mortality: A prospective study among women. *American Journal of Public Health, 91*(4): 578–583.

United States Department of Health and Human Services (1979). *Healthy people: The Surgeon General's report on health promotion and disease prevention*. (PHS 79-55071). Washington, DC.

United States Department of Health and Human Services (1980). *Promoting health/preventing disease: Objectives for the nation*. (PHS 84-19046). Washington, DC.

United States Department of Health and Human Services (1990). *Healthy people 2000: National health promotion and disease prevention objectives*. (PHS 91-50212). Washington, DC.

United States Department of Health and Human Services (1996). *Physical activity and health: A report of the Surgeon General*. Atlanta, GA.

United States Department of Health and Human Services (2000). *Healthy people 2010: Understanding & Improving Health*. 2nd ed. Washington, DC: US Government Printing Office.

World Health Organization (1947). *Constitution of the World Health Organization*. Geneva, Switzerland.

Activities & Assessments

NAME ____________ SECTION ____________ DATE ____________

1.1 Defining Physical Activity and Health

You have had the opportunity to review several definitions regarding physical activity and health. Each person, however, defines physical activity and health according to his or her own values, goals, interests, and other factors that make that person unique. Respond to the following questions based on your personal definition of physical activity and health.

1. What is your personal definition of physical activity?

2. What is your personal definition of health?

3. Are there any similarities in these two definitions?

4. What aspects of your lifestyle reflect your definition of physical activity?

5. What aspects of your lifestyle reflect your definition of health?

6. What aspects of your lifestyle conflict with your definition of physical activity?

7. What aspects of your lifestyle conflict with your definition of health?

8. Describe three actions you plan to take that support your personal definition of physical activity and health.

SOURCE: Adapted from D.A. Birch and M.J. Cleary. (1996). *Managing Your Health: Assessment and Action.* Boston: Jones and Bartlett.

Activities & Assessments

NAME ____________ SECTION ____________ DATE ____________

1.2 How Healthy Are You?

Directions: The following questionnaire is designed to increase your knowledge and awareness of your overall health, and to highlight potential areas of concern. It doesn't pinpoint how you compare to the rest of the population, but the scoring chart at the end will show you areas where you're making healthy choices and others where there's room for improvement. Keep in mind that, although health risks associated with age, sex, and heredity are beyond your control, you can modify a range of other factors such as blood pressure, smoking, blood cholesterol levels, exercise, diet, stress, and excess body weight.

SECTION A: PHYSICAL FITNESS

	YES	NO
1. Do you exercise or play a sport for at least 30 min three or more times a week?	☐	☐
2. Do you warm up and cool down by stretching before and after exercising?	☐	☐
3. Do you fall into the appropriate weight category for someone of your height and gender?	☐	☐
4. In general, are you pleased with the condition of your body?	☐	☐
5. Are you satisfied with your current level of energy?	☐	☐
6. Do you use stairs rather than escalators or elevators whenever possible?	☐	☐
Number of answers in each column:	___	___

SECTION B: FAMILY HISTORY

Do you have a grandparent, parent, aunt, uncle, brother, or sister who

	YES	NO
1. Had a heart attack before age 40?	☐	☐
2. Had high blood pressure requiring treatment?	☐	☐
3. Developed diabetes?	☐	☐
4. Developed glaucoma?	☐	☐
5. Developed gout?	☐	☐
6. Developed breast cancer?	☐	☐
Number of answers in each column:	___	___

SECTION C: SELF-CARE AND MEDICAL CARE

	YES	NO
1. Do you floss your teeth daily?	☐	☐
2. Do you have a dental checkup at least once a year?	☐	☐
3. Do you use sunscreen regularly and avoid extensive exposure to the sun?	☐	☐
4. For women: Do you examine your breasts for unusual changes or lumps at least once a month?		
5. For men: Do you examine your testicles for unusual changes or lumps at least once a month?	☐	☐

	YES	NO
6. Do you usually know what to do in case of illness or injury?	☐	☐
7. Do you avoid unnecessary X rays?	☐	☐
8. Do you normally get an adequate amount of sleep?	☐	☐
9. Have you had your blood pressure checked in the past year?	☐	☐
10. For women: Have you had a Pap smear within the last 2 years?	☐	☐
11. If you are over 40: Have you had a test for glaucoma within the last 4 years?	☐	☐
12. If you are over 40: Have you had a test for hidden blood in your stool within the last 2 years? If you are over 50: within the last year?	☐	☐
13. If you are over 50: Have you had a least one endoscopic exam of the lower bowel?	☐	☐
Number of answers in each column:	___	___

SECTION D: EATING HABITS

	YES	NO
1. Do you drink enough fluids so that your urine is pale yellow?	☐	☐
2. Do you avoid special or fad diets?	☐	☐
3. Do you minimize the salt you add to foods during cooking and at the table?	☐	☐
4. Do you minimize your intake of sweets, especially candy and soft drinks, and avoid adding sugar to foods?	☐	☐
5. Is your diet well balanced (including vegetables, fruits, breads, cereals, dairy products, and adequate sources of protein)?	☐	☐
6. Do you limit your intake of saturated fats (butter, cheese, cream, fatty meats)?		
7. Do you limit your intake of cholesterol (eggs, liver, meats)?	☐	☐
8. Do you eat fish and poultry more often than red meats?	☐	☐
9. Do you eat high-fiber foods (vegetables, fruits, whole grains) several times a day?	☐	☐
Number of answers in each column:	___	___

SECTION E: ALCOHOL, TOBACCO, AND OTHER DRUG USE

	YES	NO
1. Do you choose not to smoke cigarettes, cigars, or a pipe, chew tobacco, or use other drugs?	☐	☐
2. Do you limit yourself to no more than 2 drinks a day?	☐	☐
3. Are you able to stop drinking when you want to?	☐	☐
4. If you drink, do you rely on someone else to drive?	☐	☐
5. Are you able to drink responsibly when you are under a lot of stress or pressure?	☐	☐
6. Do you read and follow the label directions when using prescribed and over-the-counter drugs?	☐	☐
Number of answers in each column:	___	___

(continued)

1.2 How Healthy Are You? (cont.)

SECTION F: ACCIDENTS	YES	NO
1. Do you use a designated driver after drinking or using other drugs?	☐	☐
2.. Do you obey traffic laws?	☐	☐
3. As a driver and passenger, do you wear a seatbelt at all times?	☐	☐
4. Are the vehicles you drive well maintained?	☐	☐
5. When you drive, do you stay within the speed limit?	☐	☐
6. Are you informed and careful when using potentially harmful products or substances, such as household cleaners, poisons, flammables, solvents, and electrical devices?	☐	☐
7. If you own a gun, do you store it in a secure place?	☐	☐
Number of answers in each column:	___	___

SECTION G: INTELLECTUAL LIFE, VALUES, AND SPIRITUALITY	YES	NO
1. Are you interested in, and do you keep up-to-date on, social and political issues?	☐	☐
2. Are you satisfied with what you do for entertainment?	☐	☐
3. Do you engage in creative and stimulating activities as often as you would like?	☐	☐
4. Are you satisfied with the degree to which your work is consistent with your values?	☐	☐
5. Are you satisfied with the degree to which your leisure activities are consistent with your values?	☐	☐
6. Do you accept the values and lifestyles of others when they are different from your own?	☐	☐
7. Are you satisfied with your spiritual life?	☐	☐
Number of answers in each column:	___	___

SECTION H: STRESS AND SOCIAL SUPPORT	YES	NO
1. Are you satisfied with the amount of excitement in your life?	☐	☐
2. Do you find it easy to laugh?	☐	☐
3. Are you able to express your feelings of anger constructively?	☐	☐
4. Do you make decisions with minimal stress and worry?	☐	☐
5. Do you include relaxation time as part of your daily routine?	☐	☐
6. Do you anticipate and prepare for events or situations likely to be stressful?	☐	☐
7. Are you able to make the appropriate adjustments in your life following stressful events?	☐	☐

	YES	NO
8. If a close friend or family member were to die, be seriously injured, or become seriously ill, do you have adequate social support you can rely on to help you cope?	☐	☐
9. Are you able to express your feelings to others?	☐	☐
10. Do you maintain positive health habits (i.e., eating, physical activity) during stressful life events?	☐	☐
11. Are you able to fall asleep when you are ready and to sleep through the night uninterrupted?	☐	☐
12. Do you wake up feeling rested?	☐	☐
13. Do you have one or more persons with whom you can discuss personal concerns, worries, or problems?	☐	☐
14. Do those persons make you feel respected and/or admired?	☐	☐
15. Is there someone you can turn to if you need help, such as to lend you money?	☐	☐
16. Are you satisfied with the support you provide to others?	☐	☐
Number of answers in each column:	___	___

SECTION I: ENVIRONMENT

	YES	NO
1. Are you able to protect yourself from significant air and/or noise pollution?	☐	☐
2. Are you able to protect yourself from environmental hazards such as asbestos, vinyl chloride, formaldehyde, or other toxins?	☐	☐
3. Do you seldom miss days at work due to illness or just not feeling up to it? (Work here refers to daily activities, including school or work in the home.)	☐	☐
4. Are you able to get up and move around several times during the work day?	☐	☐
5. Are you satisfied with your ability to plan your workload?	☐	☐
6. Do you receive adequate feedback to judge your performance?	☐	☐
7. Are you satisfied with your balance between work and leisure time?	☐	☐
Number of answers in each column:	___	___

SECTION J: SEXUALITY

	YES	NO
1. Are you satisfied with your level of sexual activity?	☐	☐
2. Are you satisfied with your sexual relationships?	☐	☐
3. Are you satisfied with your use (or nonuse) of contraceptives?	☐	☐
4. Are you satisfied with your use (or nonuse) of' "safer-sex" practices?	☐	☐
Number of answers in each column:	___	___

(continued)

1.2 How Healthy Are You? (cont.)

SCORING

For each section of the questionnaire, write the number of answers you marked in the *lefthand* column in the blanks below.

Sections: A_____ B_____ C_____ D_____ E_____ F_____ G_____ H_____ I_____ J_____

In the circle graph below, shade the number of subsections that correspond with the numbers you wrote above. Start with the innermost section. For example, if there are four answers marked in the lefthand answer column of Section D, that portion of the circle graph should look like the one that follows.

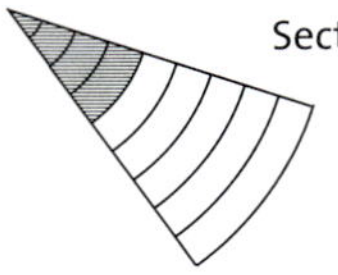

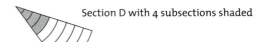

Section D with 4 subsections shaded

Sections that are *completely shaded* indicate that you're making healthy behavior and lifestyle choices in these areas. Keep up the good work.

Sections that are *partially shaded* indicate room for improvement. With a little more awareness and effort in these areas, you could improve the quality of your life—and live longer.

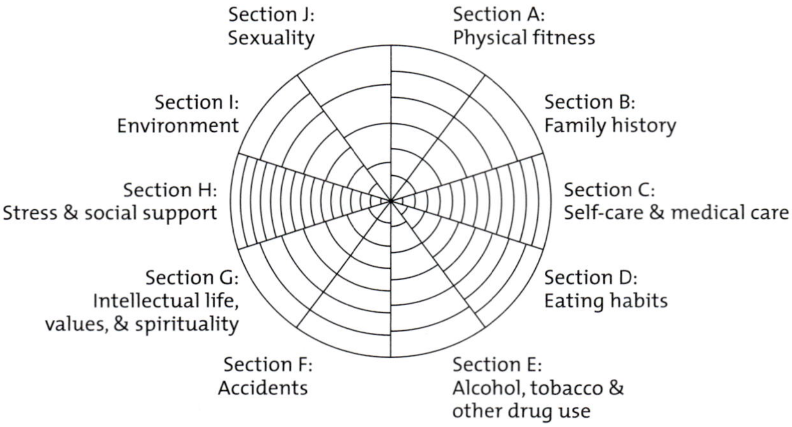

Sections that are *barely shaded* or not shaded at all indicate that there is significant room for increasing your health and satisfaction in these areas. Work first on those areas in which you are most likely to be successful, then tackle the tougher sections.

NOTE: This grading system doesn't apply to Section B, because you have no control over your family history. If you answered yes to several questions about family history, try to compensate by concentrating on the areas over which you do have control.

SOURCE: Adapted from *The Wellness Encyclopedia* (pp 12–15), © Health Letter Associates, New York (1991).

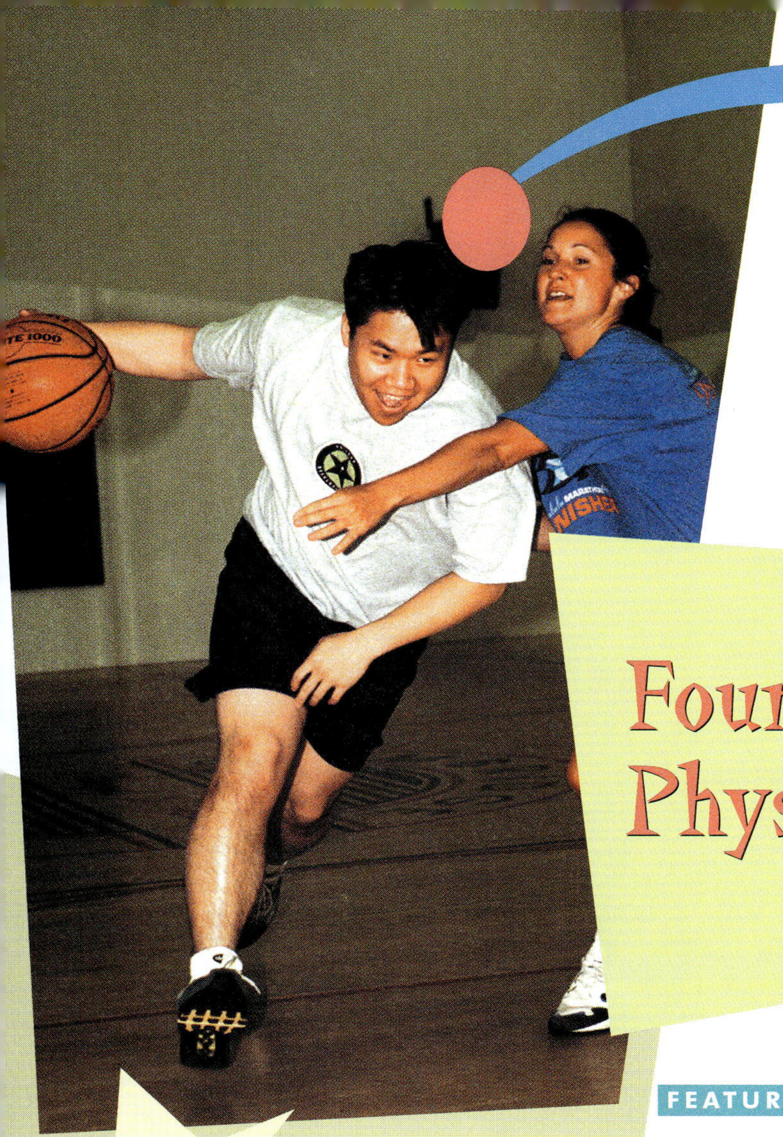

2

Foundations of Physical Activity

CONCEPT CONNECTION

1. Being physically active provides many health benefits.
2. A safe and effective physical activity program requires proper preparation.
3. How much activity you need is dependent on your goals, interests, and fitness level.
4. Optimize your benefits by individualizing your program.
5. A flexible approach is important in overcoming obstacles to physical activity.
6. Adhering to your program ensures an active lifestyle.

FEATURES

E-Learning Tools: www.pahconnection.com

Engage www.pahconnection.com

- 2.1 Physical Activity Readiness Questionnaire (PAR-Q)
- 2.2 Your medical history
- 2.3 Determining your activity status
- 2.4 Calculating your target training zone

Experience www.pahconnection.com

- 2.1 Try something new!
- 2.2 Common reasons for physical activity

Explore www.pahconnection.com

- 2.1 Signs and symptoms of disease
- 2.2 Risk factors for cardiovascular disease
- 2.3 Disease risk classification
- 2.4 Table of physical activities
- 2.5 Physical activity pyramid
- 2.6 Alternative activities
- 2.7 Professional organizations
- 2.8 Information on physical activities

Activities & Assessments

- 2.1 PAR-Q
- 2.2 Medical history questionnaire
- 2.3 Determining your activity status
- 2.4 Calculating your target training zone

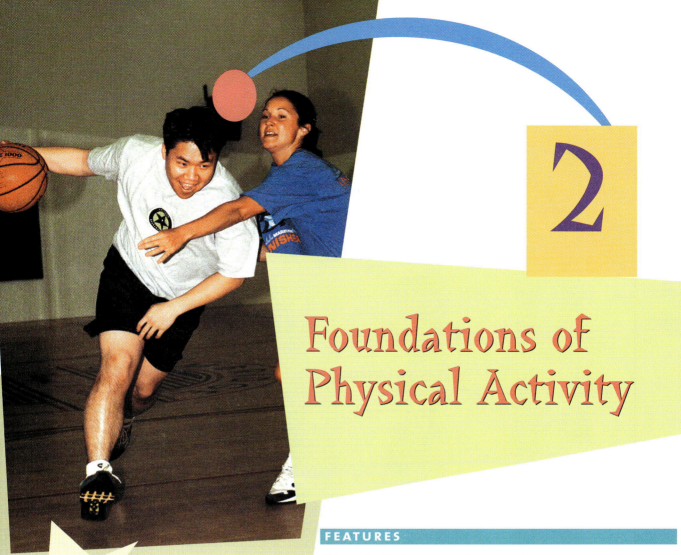

WHAT'S THE CONNECTION?

Bob is planning to start a regular physical activity program. He has never participated in one before. He is not pleased that he feels out-of-shape and has gained nearly 10 pounds over the last year. His time schedule has been hectic, with classes most of the day and a part-time job in the evenings. However, Bob's grandfather had a heart attack last month and the doctor attributed some of its origin to a sedentary lifestyle. This experience made Bob realize that maybe he should begin taking better care of himself, especially when it comes to being physically active. Bob is not altogether sure about the benefits of physical activity, and even less sure about how to get started and exactly which activities would be best for him.

INTRODUCTION

1. Being physically active provides many health benefits.

Why should people be concerned about their physical activity patterns? What benefits are there to being physically active? What is the difference between physical activity and exercise? How does someone begin a physical activity program? If you have ever asked yourself any of these questions, then this chapter is designed for you. We start off with a discussion of the importance and benefits associated with being physically active. We then present the basic principles that underlie a regular physical activity program. Then we will help you determine if your body is ready for physical activity and explain how to select appropriate activities based on your needs and objectives. Overall, we show you how to establish a regular physical activity routine and how to achieve positive results while ensuring safety and effectiveness.

YOUR BODY WAS MEANT TO MOVE

physical activity and health connection

The human body was built for movement. Our skeletal system provides us with a lightweight framework on which our muscles can act to produce motion. The structure of our skeleton is designed to provide stability and shock absorption, while remaining light enough to allow for rapid movement. We can withstand daily compressive forces many times our body weight, yet still move gracefully. As further proof that our bodies need movement, our bones actually become stronger over time when we are active (Figure 2.1).

However, it's not just our skeletal system that benefits from regular movement. Our cardiorespiratory system provides us with an efficient means of delivering needed fuels and oxygen, while simultaneously removing waste products. The functional capacity of our cardiorespiratory system can be enhanced through regular physical activity (see Chapter 6). By making the heart and blood vessels function under the physical stress of being active, the cardiac and smooth muscles found in these systems become stronger. In fact, all systems of the body respond best to regular exposure to moderate levels of physiological stress.

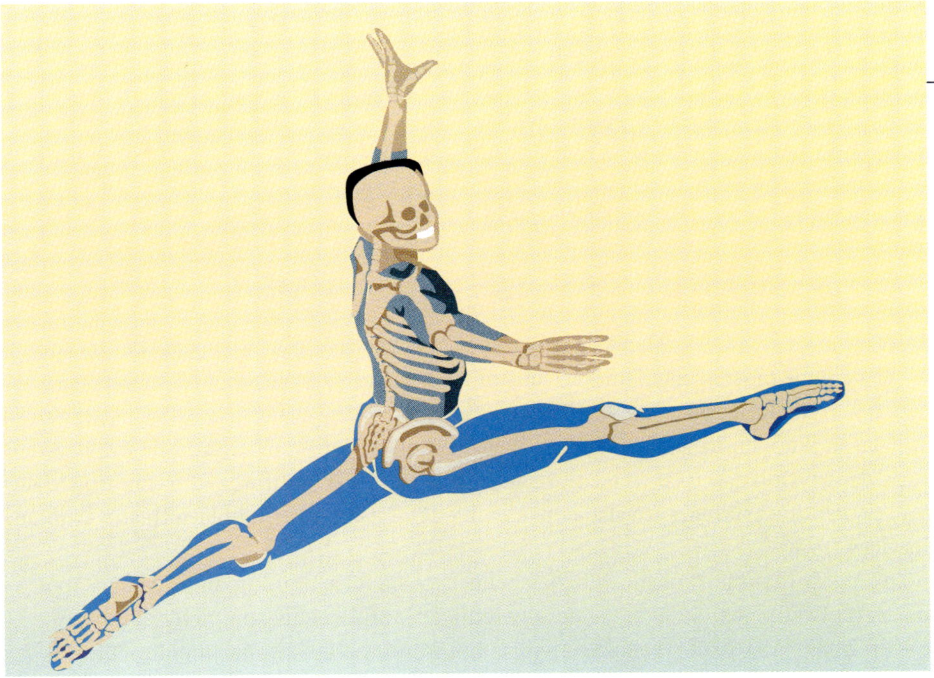

FIGURE 2.1

Function of the Skeleton. Even though the skeleton is built for support, it also allows for rapid and graceful movement.

We also know that an inactive body shows symptoms of **degeneration.** Inactive muscle **atrophies,** becoming weak and flabby. We put on extra fat (e.g., the old beer bicep, spare tire, or saddle bags) when we expend fewer calories than we consume. Sores may even result when inactivity leads to being in one position for an extended period of time.

We need to remember to pay attention to our bodies; they will remind us of the need to move. If we resist being physically active, we will feel tired and lack energy. We may feel weak and stiff, our joints may ache, and we may start getting soft and flabby. This chapter offers tips on how you can get started and achieve the most from your physical activity program.

Degeneration A gradual decrease in function.

Atrophies Decreases in cell size, usually in reference to muscle or fat.

Organ system A collection of specialized tissues that provide an important body function (musculoskeletal, cardiovascular).

Response A short-term change in reaction to a stimulus (increased breathing rate after moving from inactive to active state).

Adaptation A long-term change in reaction to regular exposure to a stimulus (lower resting heart rate with increased fitness).

Response and Adaptation to Physical Activity

Physical activity acts as a stimulus on the human body. Applied in appropriate doses, it can bring about positive changes in the way your body functions. A short-term change in an **organ system** is termed a **response.** A long-term change is termed an **adaptation.** With respect to physical activity, organ system response and adaptation typically determine the fitness level of the body. For example, when you first start to move, there is almost an immediate change in your heart rate. With increasing workloads, the heart rate increases rapidly. Such a change would be an example of a response of the cardiovascular system to the body's increasing demand for greater blood flow. If the body is regularly exposed to a stimulus that brings about this response, an adaptation will occur. For example, regular exposure to physical activity will result in a lowering of the resting heart rate. The change in resting heart rate is due to an adaptation in the cardiac muscle. This adaptation takes place in reaction to being regularly stressed by physical activity. The heart muscle becomes capable of contracting with greater force, thereby increasing the stroke volume, or the amount of blood forced out of the heart, with each contraction. If more blood can be ejected with each contraction, the heart does not have to beat as often to circulate the same amount of blood.

All systems of the body that are affected by the stress of physical activity will undergo response and adaptation. It should be noted that these changes are not always positive. For instance, if a joint is exposed to physical stress far beyond its normal functional capacity, the response may be swelling and pain to prevent further activity from potentially damaging the joint. With this in mind, the need to apply the correct amount of physical stress to the organ systems of the body becomes evident. Too much can cause damage, while just the right amount results in positive adaptation.

Benefits Associated with Regular Physical Activity

We know that physical activity has numerous beneficial physiological effects. The organ systems most affected are the cardiovascular and musculoskeletal systems, but benefits in the function of metabolic (including increasing your metabolic or energy utilization rate), endocrine (including the secretion of hormones that cause improved bone density, increased fat utilization, and greater muscle building), and immune (disease prevention) systems are also considerable (U.S. Department of Health and Human Services, 1996a).

We know that many of the beneficial effects of exercise training diminish within 2 weeks if physical activity is substantially reduced, and benefits completely disappear within 2 to 8 months if physical activity is not resumed (U.S. Department. of Health and Human Services, 1996a).

Physical Activity and Women's Health

As more and more women become physically active, it is important to take a look at what is currently known about women and physical activity. More than 60 percent of U.S. women do not engage in the recommended amount of physical activity (U.S. Department. of Health and Human Services, 1996ba), with more than 25 percent of U.S. women not active at all. As a group, girls and women are less active than boys and men are, with women of color the least active (Wells, 1996).

There is strong observational and experimental evidence that physical inactivity plays a significant role in the development of cardiovascular disease in women, and that habitual physical activity and at least a moderate level of cardiorespiratory fitness offers protection from these diseases in women as well as in men (Wells, 1996). Although there is less research available, it seems clear that regular physical activity reduces the risk of hypertension in women and is a primary preventive measure against stroke (Wells, 1996). Physical activity may also enhance the effect of estrogen replacement therapy and help decrease bone loss after menopause (U.S. Department. of Health and Human Services, 1996b). Research shows that lifetime physical activity appears to reduce the risk of colon cancer and breast cancer in white women, but not enough studies have been performed involving minority women to allow us to draw the same conclusions (Wells, 1996).

Physical activity plays an important role in women's health.

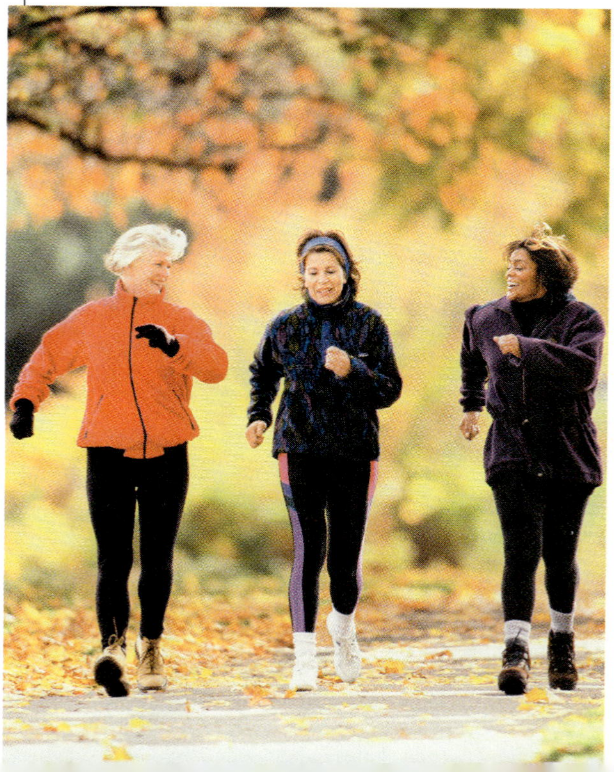

Title IX has helped women and girls gain more opportunity for participation in sport and physical activity. Social support from family and friends has been consistently and positively related to regular physical activity (U.S. Depart-

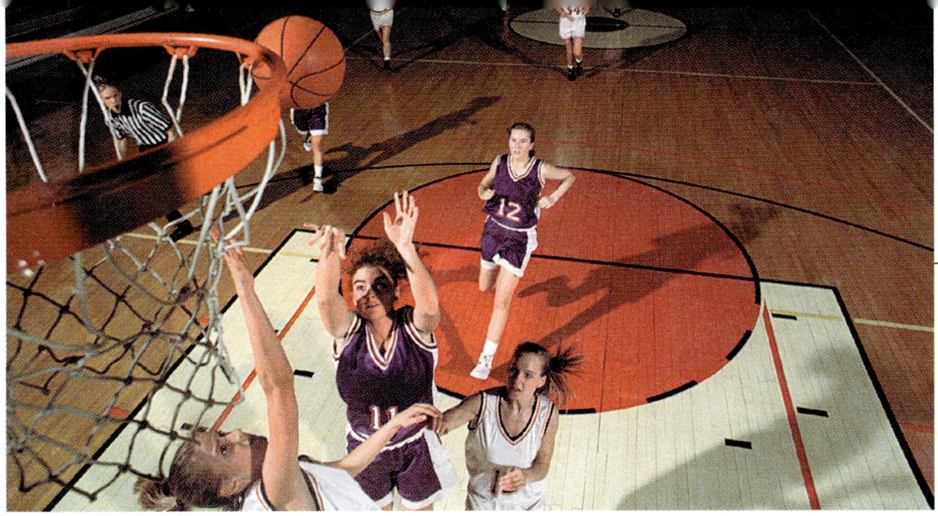

Title IX has increased opportunities for women and girls.

ment of Health and Human Services, 1996b), There is no physiologic reason for a healthy woman not to be physically active.

PRESCREENING, MEDICAL HISTORY, AND SELF-ASSESSMENT

It is very important to make sure that your body is ready for physical activity before starting any activity program, and prescreening is the first step in ensuring safety and effectiveness. Several parts of the prescreening process can be completed on your own. Others require a visit to your physician.

2. A safe and effective physical activity program requires proper preparation.

The United States Public Health Service (USPHS) and the Surgeon General's Office suggest that all individuals consult with a physician, regardless of their age, before beginning a new physical activity program (USDHHS, 1996a). Consulting with a physician is especially important for people with chronic diseases, such as cardiovascular disease and diabetes mellitus, or for those who are at high risk for these diseases. Men over 40 years of age and women over age 50 are advised to consult a physician before beginning a vigorous activity program.

Prescreening and Medical History

According to Heyward (1998), the key components of a comprehensive pre-exercise health evaluation include the use of:

1. A physical activity readiness questionnaire (PAR-Q) to determine one's readiness for physical activity.
2. A determination of any signs or symptoms of disease to identify an individual in need of medical referral.
3. A coronary risk factor analysis to determine the number of coronary heart disease risk factors.
4. A disease risk classification to categorize yourself as apparently healthy, at increased risk, or with known disease.

   You should check with your physician to review the following important pieces of information.

5. Obtain a medical history to review your past and present personal and family health histories, focusing on conditions requiring medical referral and clearance.

Engage www.pahconnection.com 2.1, 2.2, 2.3

Activities & Assessments 2.1, 2.2

Explore www.pahconnection.com 2.1, 2.2, 2.3

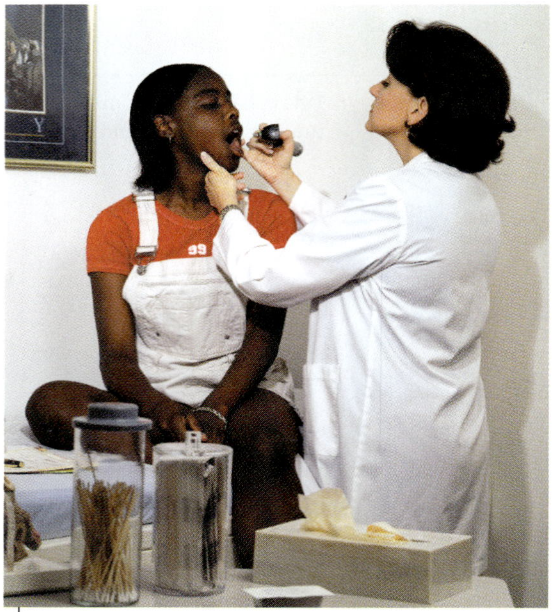

Check with your physician before starting a physical activity program.

6. Schedule a physical examination to detect signs and symptoms of disease.
7. Obtain medical clearance indicating physician approval for exercise testing and participation.
8. Consider laboratory tests to provide a more thorough assessment of your health status, particularly if you have known disease.
9. Request cholesterol and lipoprotein (HDL, LDL, and VLDL) profiling to determine if you have hyperlipidemia (high blood lipids or fats) and to aid in determining coronary risk status. High HDL levels protect you against heart disease. High LDL or VLDL levels place you at greater risk for heart disease.
10. Have your blood pressure assessed to determine if you are hypertensive (have high blood pressure) and to aid in determining coronary risk status.
11. Request measurement of your resting heart rate and a 12-lead ECG (an electrocardiogram that traces the electrical activity of your heart) to help evaluate cardiac function and detect cardiac abnormalities that would exclude you from participating in an exercise program.
12. Consider a graded exercise test to assess aerobic fitness capacity and to detect cardiac abnormalities due to exercise stress.

3. How much activity you need depends on your goals, interests, and fitness level.

Self-Assessment

Self-assessment plays an important role in allowing you to take responsibility for your own physical activity program. By testing yourself, you learn how much progress you are making, gain a better understanding of the aspect of fitness you are working on, and understand when to make adjustments to your physical activity program.

People can be classified as belonging to one of three physical activity categories. The first includes those individuals who are predominantly sedentary. Participation in physical activity is not a regular component of their lifestyles. In the U.S., these individuals comprise the largest segment of our society. They are at the greatest risk for developing **hypokinetic diseases.** Examples of hypokinetic diseases include cardiovascular disease, obesity, diabetes, stroke, and some forms of cancer.

Hypokinetic diseases Diseases associated with an inactive lifestyle (cardiovascular disease, obesity, diabetes).

Engage www.pahconnection.com 2.3

Activities & Assessments 2.3

The second group includes those individuals who are moderately active, on most if not all days of the week. They may be participating in a wide variety of physical activities such as walking, yard work, or recreational sport. We now know that moving from the first category to the second provides a great deal of protection against hypokinetic disease.

The smallest segment of our society falls into the category of those who are vigorously active on a regular basis. This category would include athletes in training and individuals seeking maximal fitness and health benefits. These individuals receive the highest degree of protection from hypokinetic disease (Figure 2.2).

FIGURE 2.2

Health Benefits and Activity Levels.
Moving from the sedentary category to the moderately active category provides the greatest improvement in health benefits, although additional gains may be achieved by becoming vigorously active.

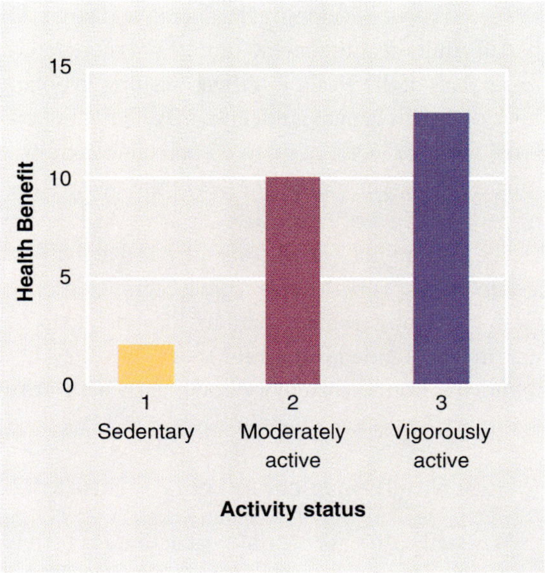

physical activity and health connection

HEALTH BENEFITS AND OPTIMAL FITNESS

While we have known for some time that an active body is a healthy body, evidence supporting this fact has gained increasing attention in the last decade. Where it was once thought that activity had to be extremely stressful to bring about improvements in fitness, it is now recognized that physical activity of lower intensities is also beneficial. In fact, we now know that recreational and leisure activities of low-to-moderate intensity offer significant improvements in health status (USDHHS, 1996a).

However, because we can obtain some benefit from low-to-moderate intensity activity, we should not take this to mean that more intensive exercise is not beneficial. For those who are already active, and for those wishing to achieve optimal health and fitness benefits, vigorous exercise offers benefits beyond those available through moderate-intensity physical activity (USDHHS, 1996a). It is wise for previously sedentary people who are embarking on a physical activity program to start with short-duration, low-to-moderate intensity activity and gradually increase the duration and/or intensity until their goals are reached (USDHHS, 1996a).

One of the keys to achieving health benefits from physical activity is consistency. Physical activity should be performed on most, if not all, days of the week. It is the regularity of physical activity that is responsible for the long-term adaptations that bring about protection from hypokinetic diseases (USDHHS, 1996a).

Different Guidelines for Different Outcomes

The American College of Sports Medicine (ACSM) has established guidelines for physical activity programs that are designed to meet the diverse needs of the general public (ACSM, 1998). Based on the best research available to date, the ACSM recognizes that there are at least two sets of guidelines that you might follow depending on desired outcomes. For those interested solely in obtaining basic health benefits

Physical activity includes many forms of movement.

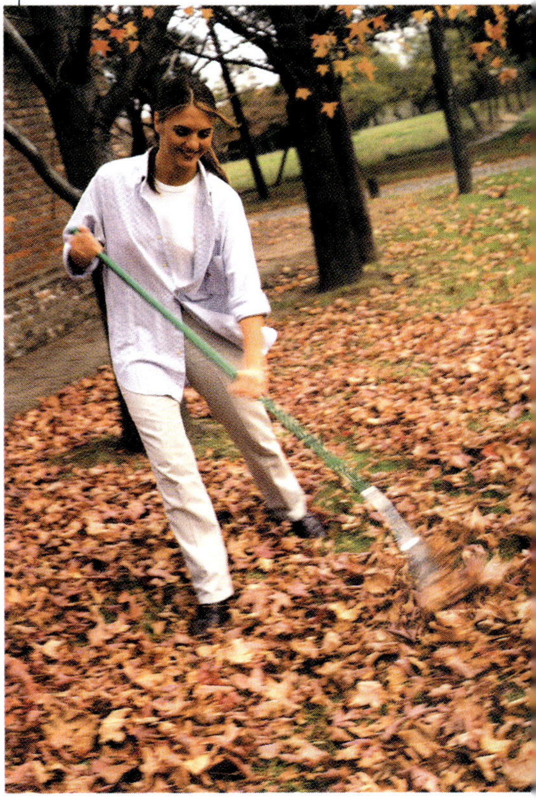

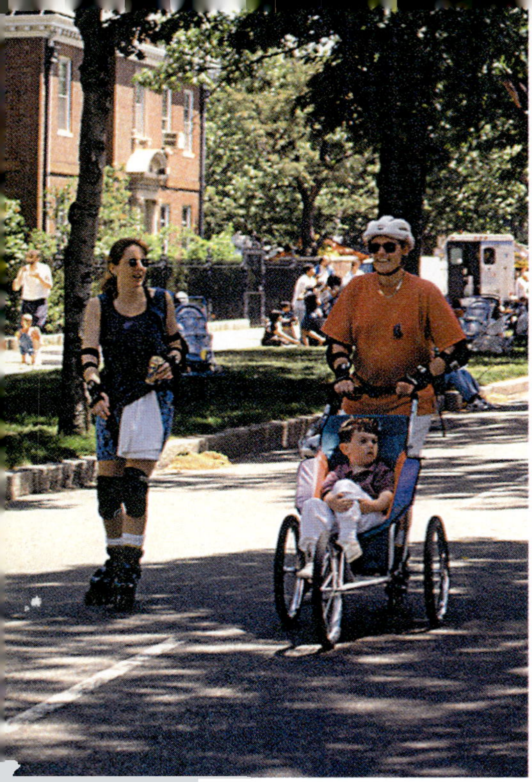

Make physical activity a family affair.

(lowered risk of developing degenerative disease, for example), the guidelines suggest that all adults accumulate 30 minutes of moderately vigorous physical activity on most if not all days of the week. For those wishing to obtain optimal fitness and health benefits, the basic health benefit guidelines may be built upon to include exercise that is performed 3 to 5 days per week, at 50 to 85 percent of aerobic capacity, for 20 to 60 minutes, while utilizing the larger muscle masses of the body. The last recommendation means performing activities that primarily use the arms, legs, and trunk muscles.

The bottom line is that some physical activity is better than none, while more (to a certain extent) is better than some. Significant improvements in fitness and health will result in moving from a sedentary lifestyle into a regularly active lifestyle. These benefits can be extended further for those interested in the attainment of optimal function, by moving from the category of regularly active to a category that includes exposure to vigorous exercise on a regular basis.

How Much Physical Activity Is Enough?

As stated earlier, some physical activity is better than none. However, based on the most current research, to obtain basic health benefits, 30 minutes of moderately vigorous physical activity should be achieved on most if not all days of the week (ACSM, 1998). These guidelines allow for flexibility in the types of activities you may select and even allow you to break your activity session into multiple segments. For instance, activities such as yard work, walking, or cycling will meet the basic health benefit goal, and you may break a 30-minute session down into two 15-minute segments or three 10-minute sessions.

There is, however, a minimal level of activity that must be consistently maintained. Being active fewer than 2 days per week, at less than 40 to 50 percent of aerobic capacity, and for less than 10 minutes, is generally not a sufficient stimulus for developing and maintaining fitness in healthy adults (ACSM, 1998).

For those interested in more health benefit, and who wish to obtain higher levels of fitness, more vigorous guidelines are suggested. The following section contains a spectrum of activity recommendations that may be followed based upon your desired outcomes.

PERSONALIZING YOUR PHYSICAL ACTIVITY PROGRAM

4. Optimize your benefits by individualizing your program.

Physical activity programs must be tailored to meet the needs of the individual. Choose activities that are fun for you and that you think you would like to continue for some time. Be aware that, by alternating activities, you are less likely to become bored and more likely to make physical activity a regular part of your lifestyle. Table 2.1 presents suggested activities that you may find enjoyable.

Explore www.pahconnection.com 2.4

Experience www.pahconnection.com 2.1

Choosing Activities

Your activity program needs to relate specifically to the outcomes you wish to obtain. Franks (1997), recommends activities based on your current activity status and your goals and objectives:

TABLE 2.1 **Physical Activities**

Backpacking	Cricket	Kayaking	Snowboarding
Baseball	Equestrian Sports	Racquetball	Soccer
Basketball	Fishing	Roller Blading	Squash
Bicycling	Football	Rowing	Swimming
Boating	Golf	Rugby	Tennis
Bowling	Handball	Skating	Walking
Bungee Jumping	Hang Gliding	Skateboarding	Water Skiing
Camping	Hiking	Skiing	Windsurfing
Canoeing	Jogging	Snorkling	

1. **Activities everyone should do as part of their daily routine.** Activities should be of the type that can be done as part of an individual's routine at home, work, and during leisure. To increase physical activity as part of your daily life, you need to walk rather than ride when possible; climb stairs rather than take the elevator or escalator; park farther away from the store, school, or office for a short walk to and from the car; get off the bus or train one stop earlier and walk the rest of the way to the office, store, school, or home. You need to emphasize weight-bearing activities to use more energy and enhance bone health. Include a daily routine of stretching to prevent low-back problems.

2. **Advice for sedentary individuals starting a physical activity program.** Sedentary (inactive) individuals should strive to incorporate activity in their daily routine, starting with at least 30 minutes of moderate-intensity activity daily. *Sedentary* individuals may be defined as those who currently do no regular physical activity, or who cannot walk for 30 minutes continuously without discomfort or pain.

   Recommended activities for sedentary individuals include walking, yard work, cycling, slow dancing, and low-impact exercise to music. The activity can be broken into 2 to 4 segments: for example, take two 10-minute exercise breaks during the work day, add another exercise break in the morning or at night during the week, and add a 30-minute walk on the weekend. You also need to include weight-bearing activities, without being overly concerned with trying to maintain a moderate-to-high intensity level.

3. **Activities for moderately active people focusing on health goals.** Individuals who have specific health goals should perform all of the previous recommendations plus the activities in Table 2.2 based on the health goal desired.

4. **Activities for moderately active people with fitness goals.** Individuals seeking fitness goals should perform all of the previous recommendations and consult Table 2.3 to achieve the desired fitness goal.

5. **Activities for vigorously active individuals with performance goals.** People interested in vigorous activity, or those who have performance goals, should fulfill all of the previous recommendations and check Table 2.4 for additional suggestions.

Determining Activity Status

It is important to remember that activity recommendations should be based on an individual's activity status. The goal is to get each person involved in a daily routine that is active in nature and to supplement that routine with 30 minutes of moderate-intensity activity. After an individual is engaging in the daily activities on a regular basis and not experiencing any problems, discomfort, or fatigue, activities for the development of greater health and fitness goals may be included. After daily physical activity

TABLE 2.2 Physical Activity for Specific Health Goals

HEALTH GOAL	RECOMMENDATIONS
Cardiovascular health	• Do at least 30 minutes of daily moderate-intensity physical activity. • Include longer-duration and/or higher-intensity activities, as you become accustomed to being active.
Bone health	• Choose weight-bearing activities like walking. • Perform resistance exercises such as weight lifting.
Low-back health	• Perform static stretching in the mid-trunk and thigh regions. • Include abdominal curl-ups.
Psychological health	• Select enjoyable activities performed in a fun environment.

TABLE 2.3 Physical Activity for Fitness Goals

FITNESS GOAL	RECOMMENDATIONS
Aerobic fitness	• Perform 20–60 minutes of vigorous-intensity activity, 3–5 days per week.
Relative leanness	
Too little fat	• Eat more calories, especially carbohydrates. • Include resistance exercise to build muscle.
Too much fat	• Reduce caloric consumption, especially fat. • Increase duration of aerobic activity to increase caloric expenditure. • Include resistance exercise to maintain muscle.
Muscular strength/endurance	• Include resistance exercise, 8–10 exercises, 1–2 sets, 10–15 repetitions involving each major muscle group, 2–3 days per week.
Flexibility	• Perform daily static stretching. Hold each stretch for 10–30 sec and perform each stretch 2–3 times.

TABLE 2.4 Physical Activity for Performance Goals

PERFORMANCE GOAL	RECOMMENDATIONS
Sport or physical task	• Develop and/or maintain fitness levels. • Perform interval training (high-intensity activity interspersed with low-to-moderate-intensity activity). • Practice motor tasks related to performance. • Target specific skills related to performance. • Prepare strategy and become mentally ready.

and fitness activities have been included as part of a person's lifestyle, then a variety of performance goals, based on personal interests, can be considered (Franks, 1997). There are numerous ways to calculate the appropriate intensity level for optimal fitness.

More detailed information on calculating exercise intensity is found in Chapter 6.

Guidelines for Those Seeking Optimal Fitness

The following guidelines (ACSM, 1998) are designed for the middle-to-higher end of the physical activity continuum. They particularly target those seeking optimal fitness and maximal health benefit. For optimal cardiorespiratory fitness and body composition, it is recommended that you:

1. Exercise at a frequency (F) of 3–5 days per week. Exercising less than 3 days per week will not bring about maximal fitness benefit. Exercising more than 5 days per week at these higher intensities will bring about marginal fitness improvements and increase the risk of injury dramatically. It is recommended that you remain active on the two "off" days by performing activities of low-to-moderate intensity.
2. Depending on the method selected to determine aerobic capacity, the intensity (I) should fall between 50 and 85 percent of your aerobic capacity. Exercising at an intensity beyond the recommended levels shifts you from **aerobic** exercise into **anaerobic** exercise. Aerobic exercise is best for improvements in cardiovascular fitness (Figure 2.3).

Aerobic Metabolic process that relies on oxygen. For aerobic metabolism to take place, exercise intensity must be low to moderate.

Anaerobic Metabolic process that does not rely on oxygen. Anaerobic metabolism occurs at start of physical activity and when intensity is high.

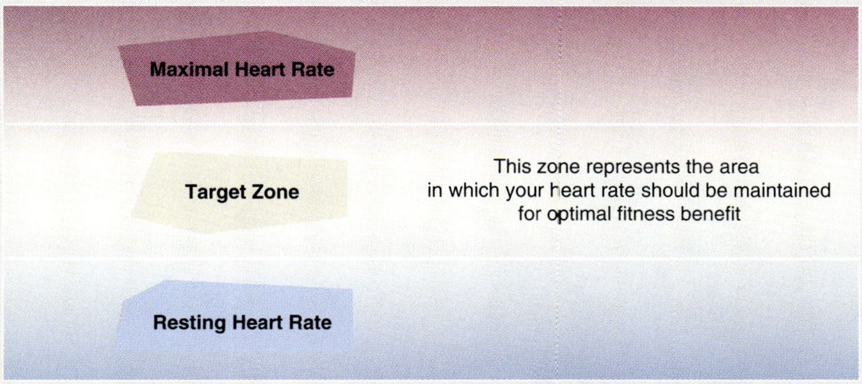
Maximal Heart Rate
Target Zone
This zone represents the area in which your heart rate should be maintained for optimal fitness benefit
Resting Heart Rate

To calculate target heart rate zone:

1. Subtract your age from 220. This gives you your estimated maximum heart rate (MHR).
   Example: 220 − 20 = 200
2. Subtract your resting heart rate from your MHR. This gives you your heart rate reserve (HRR).
   Example: 200 − 65 = 135
3. Multiply your HRR by 50%. This gives you your lower limit factor (LLF).
   Example: 135 × .50 = 67.5 or 68
4. Multiply your HRR by 85%. This gives you your upper limit factor (ULF).
   Example: 135 ×. 85 = 114.75 or 115
5. Add your LLF plus your resting heart rate to get the lower limit of your target zone.
   Example: 68 + 65 = 133
6. Add your ULF plus your resting heart rate to get the upper limit of target zone.
   Example: 115 + 65 = 180
7. You should exercise at a heart rate that falls between 133 and 180 for optimal fitness.

FIGURE 2.3

Calculating Your Target Heart Rate Zone.
To improve your fitness, try to keep your heart rate in your target zone.

Engage
www.pahconnection.com
2.4

Activities & Assessments
2.4

3. The duration (T) of each exercise session should be established at 20–60 minutes of continuous or intermittent (minimum of 10-minute bouts accumulated throughout the day) aerobic activity. The duration is dependent on the intensity of the activity. Thus lower-intensity activity should be conducted over a longer period of time (30 minutes or more).

   Moderate-intensity activity of longer duration is recommended for adults not training for athletic competition. This recommendation is made because of the importance of "total fitness," which is more readily attained with exercise sessions of longer duration, and because of the potential health and adherence hazards associated with high-intensity activity.

Explore
www.pahconnection.com
2.5

4. For the mode (S), or type of activity, you can select any activity that uses the large-muscle groups, which can be maintained continuously and is rhythmical and aerobic in nature. Examples would include walking-hiking, running-jogging, cycling-bicycling, cross-country skiing, aerobic dance/group exercise, rope skipping, rowing, stair climbing, swimming, skating, and various endurance game activities or some combination thereof.

   An additional source of information on how much activity to perform is the physical activity pyramid (Figure 2.4).

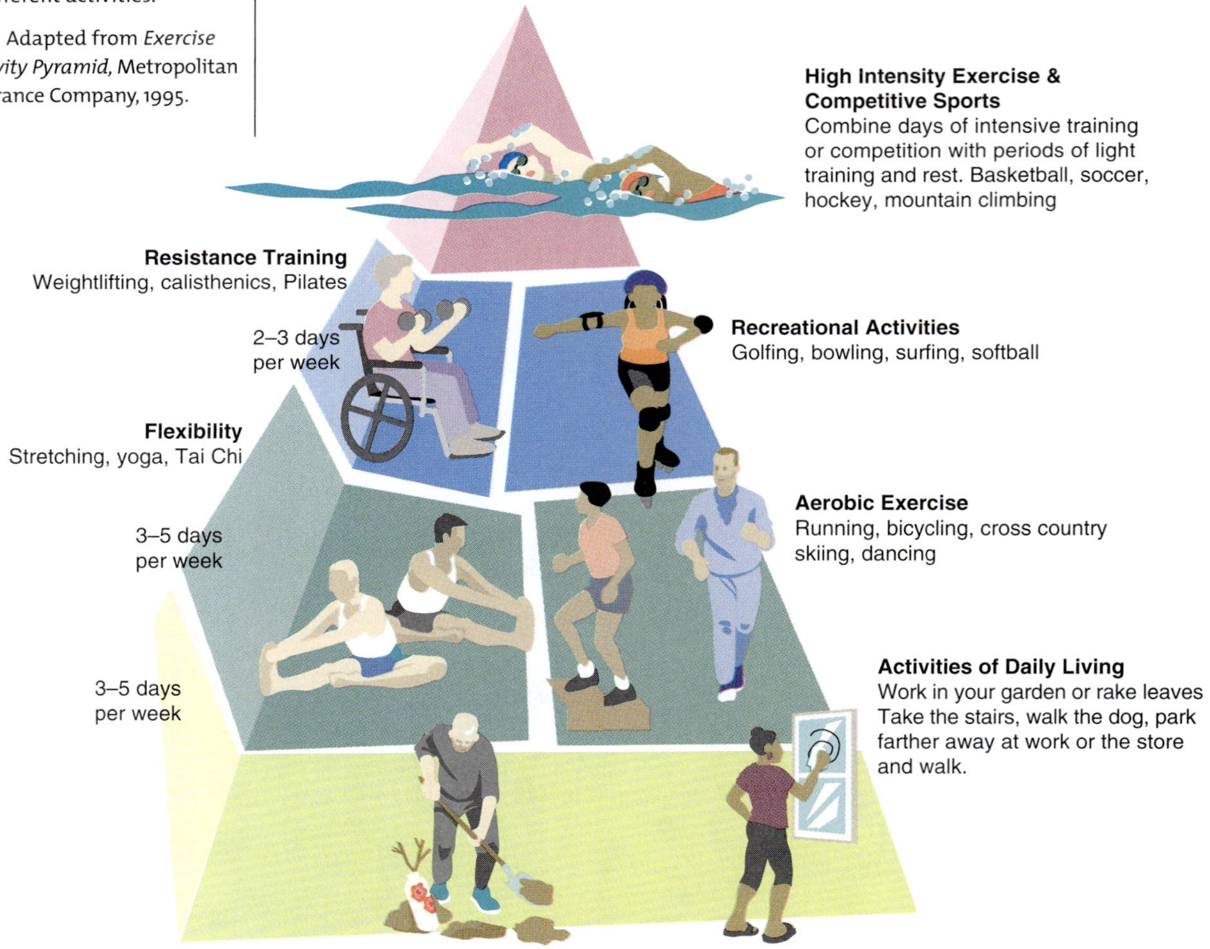

High Intensity Exercise & Competitive Sports
Combine days of intensive training or competition with periods of light training and rest. Basketball, soccer, hockey, mountain climbing
Resistance Training
Weightlifting, calisthenics, Pilates
2–3 days per week
Recreational Activities
Golfing, bowling, surfing, softball
Flexibility
Stretching, yoga, Tai Chi
3–5 days per week
Aerobic Exercise
Running, bicycling, cross country skiing, dancing
3–5 days per week
Activities of Daily Living
Work in your garden or rake leaves Take the stairs, walk the dog, park farther away at work or the store and walk.

FIGURE 2.4

The Exercise and Physical Activity Pyramid.
An active lifestyle can involve many different activities.

SOURCE: Adapted from *Exercise and Activity Pyramid,* Metropolitan Life Insurance Company, 1995.

HOW DO I GET STARTED?

When starting a physical activity program, the first step should always be to determine your goals and objectives. People are active for a variety of reasons. To optimize the benefits associated with being regularly active, you must have a clear idea of what you wish to obtain from your activity program. Some people start activity programs to obtain health benefits; others are interested in improving their overall fitness levels; still others are simply interested in looking and feeling better.

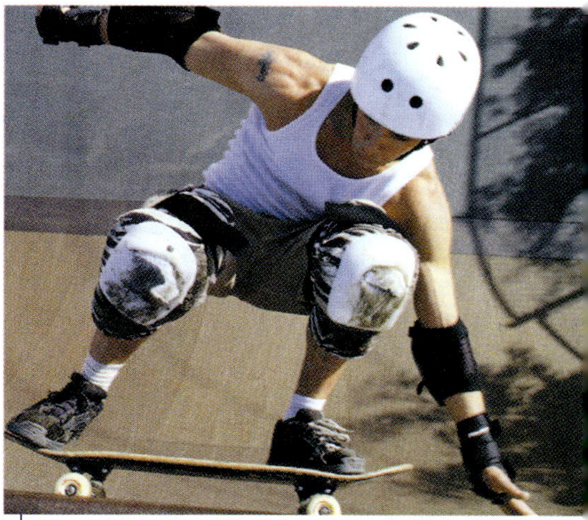

Safety is an important factor to consider when participating in physical activity.

Setting Goals

Whatever your reasons for wanting to start a physical activity program, you need to develop a clear idea of where you are going in order to get there efficiently. In contemplating your reasons for becoming active, remember to be realistic when you define your goals and objectives. Goals and objectives should be attainable, adjustable, and allow for individual need. Remember that the overriding factors that must be incorporated in any physical activity program are *safety* and *effectiveness*. You want to make sure that you don't injure yourself, and you want to make sure that your goals are achieved. Planning a safe and effective program should influence your goal-setting by encouraging you to think in terms of both short-term and long-term goals.

We are all born with different genetic blueprints. In terms of our responses and adaptations to physical activity, this difference means that we all will respond and adapt at different physiological rates and magnitudes. Some people will see rapid changes in response to exercise, while others will see measurable change only over an extended period of time. Certain individuals will see their body function improve to an extent not achievable by other individuals, who might be working just as hard or harder. Taking the variation in improvement rate into consideration, programs must be **individualized** to bring about optimal benefit based on individual need and response. Not everyone should be performing the same activities at the same intensities for the same period of time. You need to find the activities that are best suited to meet your individual needs.

Individualized Based on differing needs of different people.

Confirming Your Health Status

All individuals should consult with their physician before starting or making major adjustments to any physical activity program. For most healthy individuals, this step may only reinforce what appears to be obvious: you are healthy. However, many underlying health conditions do not have overt signs and symptoms and are only detectable through a medical exam. Activity, though safe in almost all instances, can trigger life-threatening events if performed improperly and without knowledge of underlying disease.

Building Slowly

When beginning an activity program it is wise to start gradually, build slowly, and maintain consistency. A common mistake made by beginners is to try to do too much, too soon. Relying on what others are doing to determine how much you should do is not wise. Remember that fitness is individual in nature. What may appear to be a low-intensity warm-up for one person may be an exhaustive workout for another. It is

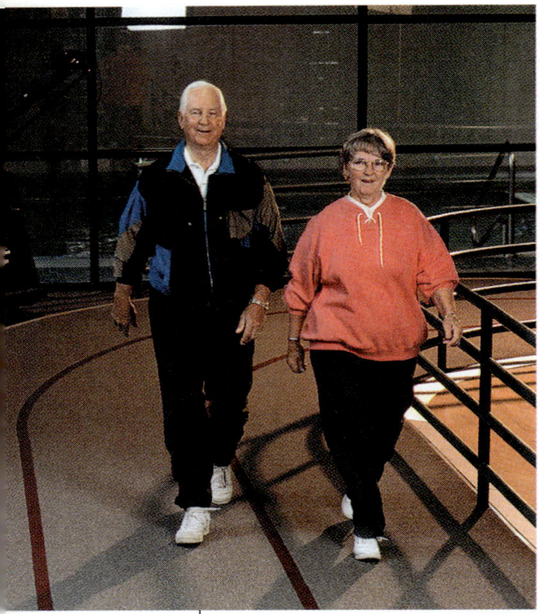

Genetic variation impacts our response and adaptation to physical activity.

far better to delay the acquisition of benefits to some degree rather than to do too much, become sore or injured, and set your program back significantly—or, worse, stop completely. Chapter 3 will provide more information on strategies to use when changing your behavior.

Heredity and Health-Related Fitness

We know that our genetics will impact the extent and rate at which we will benefit in response to being physically active. The best estimates tell us that genetics accounts for about 25 percent of the **variability** we see in people's body fatness levels (Bouchard, 1993). Approximately 20 to 40 percent of the variability for muscle fitness, and 10 to 25 percent for cardiovascular fitness, is inherited (Bouchard, 1993). For example, the **heritability** for body fatness (25 percent) tells us that factors (environment, diet, activity status) other than genetics account for 75 percent of the variability we see when we compare different people. Twenty-five percent is due directly to our genetics.

Not only do people differ in fitness based on heredity, but people of different genetic backgrounds respond differently to training. In other words, two people of different genetic backgrounds could do the exact same exercise program and get quite different benefits. Some people may get as much as ten times the benefit from activity as others who do the same program (Bouchard, 1993).

The genetic influence on how we respond to being physically active makes recognizing individual differences even more important. Assumptions about a person's fitness are not always good indicators of their current activity levels. Bouchard (1993) also suggests that different people respond differently to each component of fitness. So, while some people may respond well to strength training, they may not respond as well to cardiovascular training. Typically, we see a three- to ten-fold difference between low responders (people who don't show much change) and high responders (people who show a good deal of change) on the same standardized physical activity regimen if performed for a period of 15–20 weeks (Bouchard, 1993). The magnitude of the difference is somewhat dependent on the component of fitness considered.

PROGRAM DESIGN

There are several factors that must be considered when developing a physical activity program. The amount of time you are willing to set aside for activity, your access to exercise equipment, your motivation, the activities you enjoy, and your current state of conditioning will all play important roles in designing a regular physical activity program.

The Three Stages of Conditioning

There are three recognized stages of conditioning programs (Heyward, 1998). The **initial stage** defines the early portion of a program, in which you become accustomed to making physical activity a regular portion of your life. During this phase, you should be exposed to a wide variety of activities, learn the proper techniques of various activities, experience the fastest rate of improvement, and determine a schedule to accommodate physical activity in your lifestyle.

Variability The differences among people.

Heritability The amount genetics determines the differences between people.

Initial stage Early portion of a program in which you become accustomed to making physical activity a regular part of your life.

In the second stage, the **progression stage**, you continue to apply the principles of conditioning to develop greater levels of fitness and more health benefit. This stage is usually short in duration because of the high level of stress it can apply to the body. It is, however, during this stage that optimal levels of fitness and health are obtained.

The **maintenance stage** is the stage in which most active people spend the majority of their time. During the maintenance stage, you have established a regular physical activity routine and participate frequently to maintain your current level of fitness and health. This stage allows for the consolidation of gains and for recovery from the progression stage. Occasionally, people in the maintenance stage shift back into the progression stage to move their fitness and health to a higher level. They then shift back to the maintenance stage to hold onto the gains they have just achieved.

Progression stage Stage in which you stress your body so as to develop greater levels of conditioning and fitness. This stage is short due to high levels of stress on the body. Optimal levels of fitness are obtained.

Maintenance stage Stage of established regular physical activity designed to maintain current levels of fitness and health. Consolidation of gains and recovery from the progression stage.

Components of an Activity Session

All exercise and physical activity sessions should follow a similar format. This format allows you to optimize gains while minimizing the risk of injury. Depending on the type of physical activity you are going to perform, you may need to modify these instructions slightly.

Preparation The first stage is to prepare the body for physical activity. Make sure you are in appropriate attire and using safe equipment that is designed for the activity to follow (see Chapter 15). If you are preparing for a walking program, make sure you are in comfortable clothes and have good walking shoes; if you are about to perform yard work, make sure you have on clothes suited for the activity and the weather.

Preparing your body is best accomplished by gradually shifting the body from an inactive state to an active state. Low-intensity aerobic activity (slow walking) and slow stretching usually characterize this portion of an exercise routine. The purpose of this is to increase blood flow to the muscles, increase the temperature of the muscles, and ease into the cardio and respiratory adjustments required for the more intensive activity to follow. Though you may be performing an activity that is not traditionally "exercise," you still need to warm up. Muscle strains and low-back injuries can occur when a person performs a sudden movement for which the body is not prepared. You don't have to be "exercising" for this to happen.

Transition The second phase is one of transition, in which you move gradually into the focal point of the activity you will be performing. It is necessary to move gradually during this phase, increasing intensity as the body indicates that it has adjusted to the physiological demands of the activity. You will begin to loosen up and your body temperature will start to increase. You may also notice that you start to perspire during this transitional phase.

Activity The third phase is that in which you focus on the activity in which you are participating for its health benefit or for improvement of fitness. The intensity and duration of activity will be determined by your goals, fitness level, access to facilities and equipment, and allotted time.

Cool Down The fourth and final phase is a combination cool-down/flexibility enhancement phase. During this portion of an activity routine, you gradually bring the intensity down toward resting values. Reducing the intensity is important in keeping blood from pooling in the legs and aiding the flow of blood back to the heart for recirculation. Breathing rate, heart rate, and temperature are all brought back to baseline

Stretching exercises help to improve flexibility.

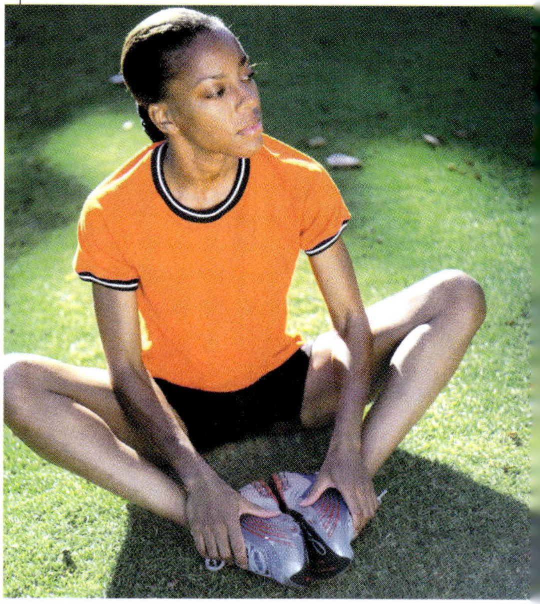

levels. The speed with which you return to pre-activity levels can be a good indicator of your fitness level. Fit people return to resting levels more rapidly than people who are less fit. It is important to perform stretching exercises during the cooldown because it is during the cooldown that the muscles are their warmest. Warm muscles are more pliable muscles, so the stretching exercises will have their greatest impact on improving your flexibility or range of motion.

Variety of Experiences and Cross Training

Exposure to a wide range of activities is important for individuals starting physical activity programs. Boredom can be one of the major obstacles to being regularly active. We all know that variety is the spice of life, and if we have a range of activities to select from we are more likely to find something we like and to adhere to our activity program. Figure 2.5 shows several combinations of activities that one may choose.

Explore 2.6

Cross training involves the incorporation of different activities into your program. Cross training serves the purpose of adding variety to an activity program and making sure that various body systems and muscle groups are included. By using cross training effectively, you also allow one system to recover on what would be an "off" day while stressing another system. Stressing one system while another recovers allows you to meet the Surgeon General's suggestion that we are active on most if not all days of the week.

Monitoring Your Progress

It is important to check regularly to see if your program is working and if adjustments need to be made. Monitoring is accomplished by performing self-assessment on a regular basis. Another important aspect of monitoring your progress is that it will provide positive motivation as you see that what you are doing is actually producing

FIGURE 2.5

Cross Training Combinations. It's best to vary your activity program by combining different types of activities.

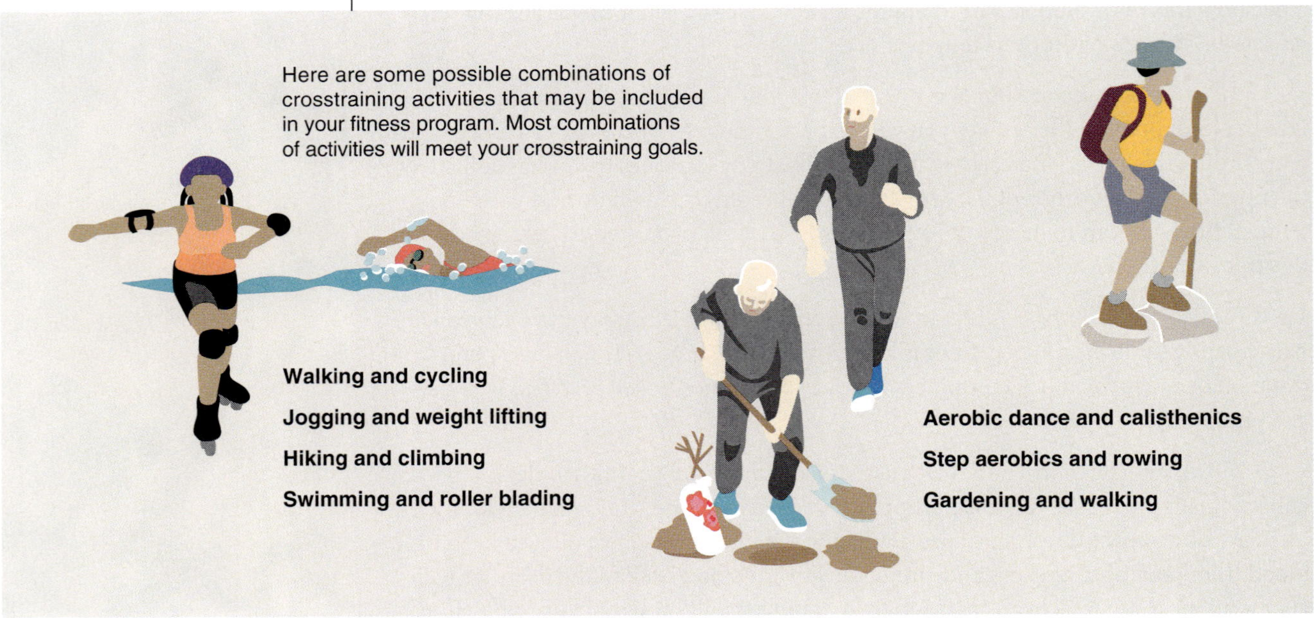
Here are some possible combinations of crosstraining activities that may be included in your fitness program. Most combinations of activities will meet your crosstraining goals.
Walking and cycling
Jogging and weight lifting
Hiking and climbing
Swimming and roller blading
Aerobic dance and calisthenics
Step aerobics and rowing
Gardening and walking

benefit and moving you closer to the attainment of your goals and objectives. It also allows you to update your objectives so that new ones may be set after initial ones have been achieved.

COMPONENTS OF HEALTH-RELATED FITNESS

Physical activity is a process that produces improvement in health and fitness. Several aspects of fitness directly relate to health and are considered to be components of health-related fitness.

Cardiovascular function refers to the ability of the heart and vascular network to deliver key nutrients, such as oxygen and fuel, while simultaneously removing waste products (see Chapters 5 and 6). A related component of physiology is cardiorespiratory function, which involves the integration of the pulmonary and cardiovascular systems. We must be able to breathe in oxygen, transfer it into the blood, circulate the blood to our muscles, exchange the oxygen and other nutrients at the muscle, and remove carbon dioxide and other waste products, if we are to function physically at optimal levels.

Body composition refers to the major chemical components of the body. The main components under consideration are fat mass, muscle mass, bone density, and water volume (see Chapter 9). If we have too much of one component, or not enough of another, our health will suffer.

Muscular strength is the ability of the muscles to generate force. The larger the cross sectional area of the muscle, the greater the amount of force it can produce (see Chapter 11). Stronger muscles allow us to do more work, protect our joints from injury, and help to make our bones stronger.

Muscular endurance is the muscle's ability to generate force repeatedly. Improved endurance allows us to repeat a physical activity for a greater number of repetitions or for a longer period of time (see Chapter 11). Good muscular endurance is important in carrying out the activities of daily living and in protecting the back against chronic pain.

Flexibility describes the range of motion available at a joint (see Chapter 12). Several factors impact flexibility, including muscle elasticity, muscle temperature, bony structure, connective tissue integrity, and the points of origin and insertion of the muscles. In physical activity programs, flexibility is enhanced through stretching exercises. When stretching, one attempts to improve muscle elasticity and compliance. Good flexibility helps prevent injury and low-back pain and provides greater mobility.

THE PRINCIPLES OF TRAINING

There are certain principles that govern how your body will respond to the physical stress of physical activity. Following these principles will ensure the safety and effectiveness of your activity program.

The **overload principle** states that a body system (muscular, skeletal) must be exposed to physical stress beyond the ordinary in order to adapt and improve function. For

Cardiovascular function The heart and vascular network deliver key nutrients while removing waste products.

Body composition The major chemical components of the body: fat mass, muscle mass, bone density, and water volume.

Muscular strength The ability of the muscles to generate force.

Muscular endurance The muscle's ability to generate force repeatedly.

Flexibility The range of motion available at a joint.

Overload principle A body system (muscular, skeletal, cardiovascular) must be exposed to physical stress beyond that which is ordinary in order to adapt and improve function.

Principle of progression The logical and systematic application of the overload principle.

Principle of specificity You must target activities to specific systems to improve their particular function.

Principle of reversibility All benefits gained through participation in a physical activity program will be lost if the activity is not continued.

Principle of individuality All people are different genetically and have different levels of potential physical development.

Principle of recovery An adequate rest period must be allowed for your body to adapt and become stronger.

example, to build stronger muscles you must work against resistance that pushes your muscles to their limits. Over a period of time, your muscles adapt to this new workload and become stronger.

The **principle of progression** states that, to ensure safety and effectiveness, the overload must be applied in a systematic and logical fashion. If too much physical stress is applied too soon, the system will not have time to adapt properly and benefits may be delayed or injury may occur. You need to overload your body gradually so it has time to adjust and improve. If you are sore after exercising, you are doing more than your current level of fitness allows. You should reduce the intensity of your activity and progress more gradually.

The **principle of specificity** states that particular activities must be performed to bring about particular adaptations. For instance, if the goal is to build muscular strength, you need to undertake an activity that overloads the muscles. For example, you must do exercises that physically stress the biceps muscles of the upper arm if strength gain in the biceps is desirable. Stressing the quadriceps muscles of the thigh will not develop strength in the biceps of the arm.

The **principle of reversibility** tells us that any gains we may get through regular physical activity will disappear if we do not continue to be active—thus the maxim, use it or lose it. If we decrease our activity levels, we will experience some loss in fitness in as little as 2 weeks (Coyle, 1990). This is why it is important to continue our activity program for life (Figure 2.6).

The **principle of individuality** reinforces the concept that all people have different genetic blueprints, and activity programs must be designed with this in mind. Determine what you wish to achieve, find activities that will bring about those results, and set out to obtain your desired outcomes.

The **principle of recovery** reminds us that our bodies take time to adjust to the physical stress of being active. We must allow adequate time for adaptation to take place. It is generally recommended that we allow 48 to 72 hours between exhaustive activity sessions that are similar in nature. This doesn't mean that we shouldn't be active at all for this period of time. It does mean that we should vary our activities so that one system is allowed time to adjust before it is stressed again.

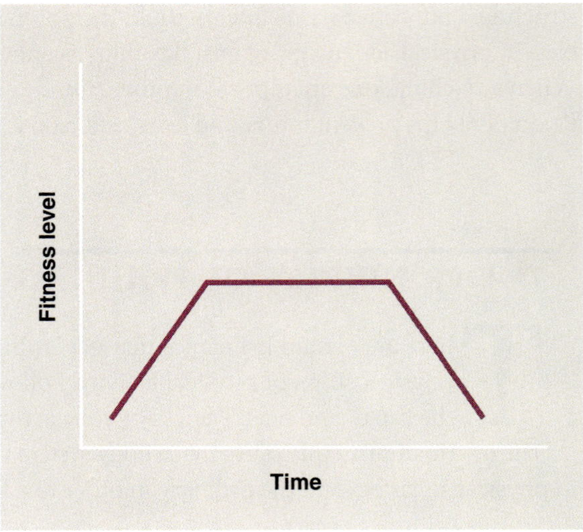

FIGURE 2.6

Principle of Reversibility. If you don't continue to do the things that drive up your fitness level, it will degrade and return to previous levels.

BECOMING INDEPENDENTLY ACTIVE

To maintain an active lifestyle successfully, you must learn the knowledge and skills associated with becoming independently active. A lifestyle of physical activity requires that you select activities that are enjoyable, me ingful, and designed with your needs in mind. The most effective way to increase adherence to an activity program is to make sure the program meets your goals and objectives. Responsibility for this lies with the person developing and executing the activity program. You must learn to gather information on how to become physically active, discern what is of use for your particular needs, and develop a program structured to meet those needs. Dependence on someone else for your activity program limits your ability to obtain optimal benefit and satisfaction.

5. A flexible approach is important in overcoming obstacles to physical activity.

OVERCOMING BARRIERS TO PHYSICAL ACTIVITY

Barriers to physical activity may be psychological or physical. The number and strength of these perceived barriers are consistently related to participation rates in physical activity for both adults and adolescents. The more barriers you perceive, or the stronger those barriers, the less likely it is that you will continue to participate in a physical activity program (Sallis, 1994).

Experience www.pahconnection.com 2.2

Time

The most common barrier is a perceived lack of time. When this explanation is presented as the reason for being inactive, it usually means that participation in physical activity is not high enough on your priority list. Physical activity must be considered as important to your body as eating, sleeping, and breathing. Physical activity does not take long intervals of time, and the benefits you receive will bring you a longer life that is of a higher quality. By preventing many of the diseases that rob us of a healthy life, physical activity actually provides us with additional free time. Once you have determined that physical activity is important to you, you can begin to overcome potential barriers to activity.

If limited time is a concern, recent information demonstrates that we can benefit from activity without having to participate in exercise of long duration. We now know that activity sessions broken down into multiple intervals over the course of a day provide significant health benefits. In other words, instead of having to schedule a continuous 30-minute exercise period into your day, you can obtain similar benefits by accumulating the 30 minutes in three 10-minute sessions. You could take 10-minute walks in the morning, at lunch, and in the evening to achieve this goal.

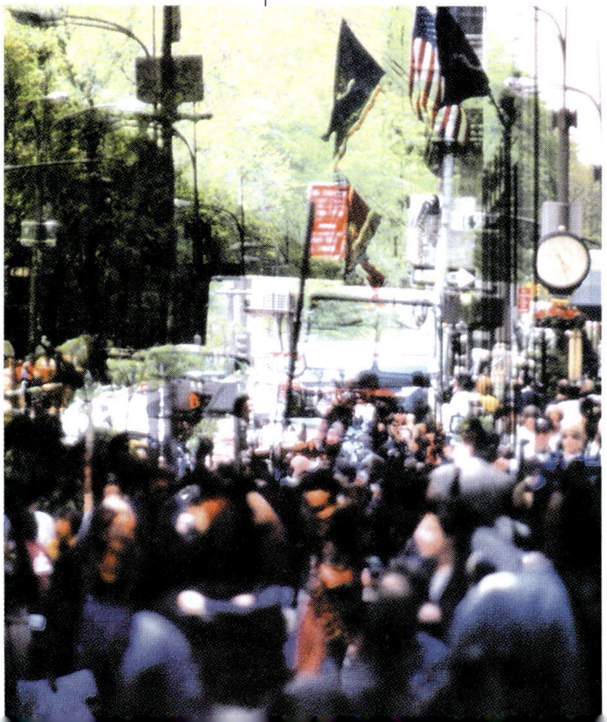

Physical activity can be performed in three 10-minute segments to fit a busy schedule.

No Pain, No Gain

A second barrier to being regularly active involves thinking that activity has to be unpleasant to be effective. The perception that activity must be unpleasant usually derives from previous

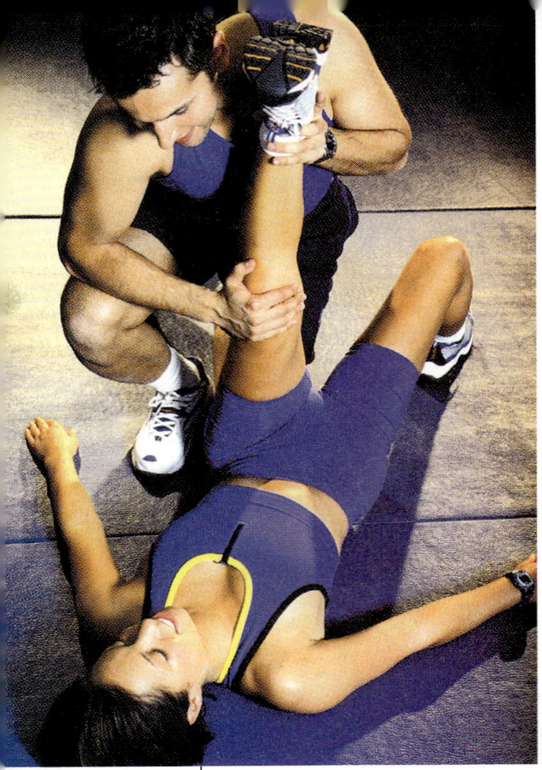

Qualified instruction can enhance your physical activity experience.

Explore
www.panconnection.com
2.7, 2.8

negative experiences with physical activity. Unfortunately, some physical educators and coaches have used exercise and activity as punishment. Using exercise as punishment teaches us to avoid exercise. Being active should be an enjoyable experience. Don't let past negative experiences prevent you from finding activities that you may enjoy.

If we perform activities improperly, or try to perform beyond our level of competence and fitness, any resultant soreness and injury could develop into another barrier to physical activity. We need to realize that if we hurt while being active, our body is telling us that we are doing something wrong. Forget the old adage "No pain, no gain." Pain brought on by physical activity is equivalent to injury. *There will be no gain without effort or without fatiguing your muscles, but we shouldn't look to hurt ourselves in an attempt to improve our fitness or health.*

Skill

To make physical activity a part of your lifestyle, you must choose activities that you find enjoyable and interesting. However, confidence in your ability to perform the activity increases the likelihood that you will enjoy what you are doing. To increase your skill in various activities, it is recommended that you receive instruction from an expert and then practice the activity on a regular basis. See the websites on professional organizations and sources of information on physical activity for more on finding expert advice.

Psychological Factors

A number of psychological factors appear to influence participation in physical activity among adults (Sallis, 1994). Your personal beliefs about your physical abilities are usually related to your participation in physical activity. If you have a strong self-image and confidence regarding your ability to be regularly active, you are more likely to continue participating in physical activity. We know that both adults and children must enjoy physical activity if they are to continue it. One of the main determinants of whether a person enjoys an activity is the degree of exertion required by that activity (Sallis, 1994). Not surprisingly, children and adults usually prefer activities with lower levels of exertion. Dropout rates are significantly higher from vigorous activities than from moderate-intensity activities. Examples of lower-intensity activities would include walking and gardening. More vigorous activities include running, heavy weight lifting, or rock climbing. Chapter 3 contains more information on psychological barriers to physical activity.

Social and Environmental Factors

The social and physical environment in which you live may also supply barriers to physical activity. These barriers could be community-based, or they may be individual in nature. If you live in a community that does not provide adequate outlets for being physically active, this may be a barrier to your participation. Some communities have developed centers to provide facilities for recreational sport and exercise options; others have built walking, cycling, or roller blading trails to provide another outlet for being physically active.

Support from friends, coworkers, or family members impacts individual adherence to activity programs (Sallis, 1994). Another societal factor, important to some parents, is the availability of childcare. For adolescents, the influence of peers is extremely important. The younger the child, the more influential parents are. Parents can be supportive by being a role model, providing encouragement, and directly helping children to be active through participating in activities with them, organizing activities, or transporting children to places where they can be active.

Climate and weather, sedentary leisure activities, and the availability of labor saving devices may also prove to be barriers to physical activity (Sallis, 1994). We must counter these barriers by providing safe and attractive space for outdoor activities, and access to exercise equipment, facilities, and programs.

Other Barriers

Other barriers to physical activity include age, gender, previous injury, genetics, educational level, and economic status (Sallis, 1994). Activity tends to decrease across the age span, with the decline starting with entry into school. Women and girls have been traditionally less active than men and boys at virtually all ages. A partial explanation for this may relate to the different socialization processes boys and girls experience. Another factor that may prove to be a barrier to physical activity is a previous history of injury. Once a person has been injured, the likelihood of continuing to be active diminishes. We also know that people with higher educational levels and a more secure financial status participate in physical activity programs at higher rates than others, so educational and socioeconomic barriers must be considered. Individuals who understand the benefits of being active, who can afford the time, and who have greater opportunity for exposure to a variety of activities are more active.

Contrary to popular belief, activity levels in childhood are not always reliable predictors of becoming a physically active adult (Sallis, 1994). One potential explanation for this might be that many children are taught activities like team sports that are difficult to carry over to adulthood (Sallis, 1994). We must ensure that children are exposed to individual activities if we wish to have a carryover effect into adulthood.

EXERCISE PROGRAM ADHERENCE

Many factors affect program adherence. Perhaps the most important is establishing regular physical activity as a priority in your life. Once activity becomes self-motivated, adherence is no longer a problem. Several categories of factors are related to exercise program adherence (Heyward, 1998). The first category includes **biological factors** such as being overweight. Sometimes people who are overweight, or who have a high proportion of fat to muscle, find activity difficult to perform because of the mechanical stresses placed upon the body. They may also feel uncomfortable exercising around others, or be dissatisfied with their own appearance when dressed in exercise attire.

The second category includes **psychological factors** such as self-motivation, self-efficacy, the attainment of exercise goals, and depression/anxiety/introversion. These factors all relate to how your perceive yourself. You need to ask yourself, are you confident in your ability to perform certain activities properly? Do you feel good about yourself?

The third category includes **social factors** such as family support, family problems, exercise/job conflicts, and income and education levels. Are the social aspects of your life conducive to your participation in a physical activity program?

The fourth category includes **behavioral factors** such as smoking, leisure time availability and use, and Type A behavior. Do negative lifestyle behaviors interfere with your ability to get the most out of yourself physically?

The final category includes **program factors** such as social support (group vs. individual exercise), location and convenience of an activity facility, activity leadership and supervision, initial activity intensity, variety of activity options, and program costs. Is it easy for you to be active?

6. Adhering to your program insures an active lifestyle.

Biological factors Factors related to your biology that impact your adherence to an activity program.

Psychological factors Factors related to your state of mind that impact your adherence to an activity program.

Social factors Factors from your social environment that impact your adherence to an activity program.

Behavioral factors Factors related to your behavior patterns that impact your adherence to an activity program.

Program factors Factors related to your physical activity program that impact your adherence to that program.

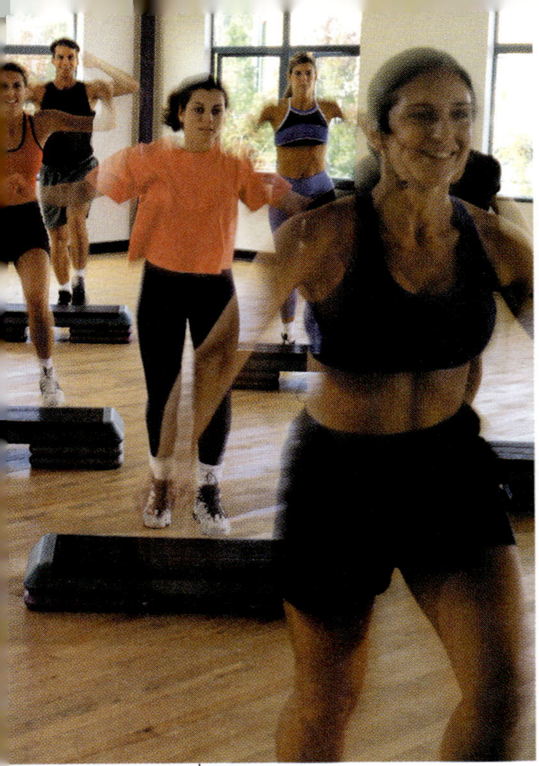

Group activities are preferred by some people.

STRATEGIES TO INCREASE ADHERENCE

The best strategies for increasing adherence include individualizing your program, finding activities you like, and scheduling the activities into your lifestyle. The importance of scheduling the activity is that you ensure having the time to be physically active (make it a priority), you develop a sense of consistency, and you reinforce its importance in your life.

Exercising with others has been shown to be effective for some people. Knowing that someone else is depending on them to show up for an exercise session will make some people show up those days even when they don't feel like exercising for themselves. Others prefer to exercise alone.

The following strategies can increase physical activity program adherence (Heyward, 1998). In developing your activity program: incorporate both group and individual activities; select times and locations that are convenient for you; select a variety of exercise and fitness activities; monitor your progress toward your goals; set realistic short-term and long-term goals; educate yourself about exercise, physical fitness, and health benefits; reward yourself for maintaining a regular activity program; and encourage social support.

If you prefer to exercise under the direction of an exercise leader, choose one who is a positive role model, shows interest in participants (follow-up phone calls when you have several unexplained absences, for example), exhibits enthusiasm, develops good rapport with program participants (learns their names), rewards accomplishments of participants, motivates and encourages participants to make a long-term commitment to exercise, and attends to orthopedic and musculoskeletal problems of participants.

According to the National Institutes of Health (1995), physical activity is more likely to be initiated and maintained if the individual perceives a net benefit, chooses an enjoyable activity, feels competent doing the activity, feels safe doing the activity, can easily access the activity on a regular basis, can fit the activity into the daily schedule, feels that the activity does not generate undue financial or social costs, experiences a minimum of negative consequences (injury, loss of time, negative peer pressure, problems with self-identity), is able to address issues of competing time demands, and recognizes the need to balance the use of laborsaving devices and sedentary activities with activities that involve a higher level of physical exertion.

PHYSICAL ACTIVITY AND INTRINSIC MOTIVATION

To enhance **intrinsic motivation,** Whitehead (1993) suggests that we: do emphasize individual mastery; don't over-emphasize peer comparisons of performance; do promote perceptions of choice; don't undermine an intrinsic focus by misusing extrinsic rewards; do promote the intrinsic fun and excitement of exercise; don't turn exercise into a bore or a chore; do promote a sense of purpose by teaching the value of physical activity to health, optimal function, and quality of life; and don't create a motivation by spreading fitness misinformation. Rather than relying on a bland repetitive "diet" of a physical activity, we should think of a "menu" in which taste is enhanced by new "recipes," and the "sugar and spice" of fun, excitement, and thrills are added in (Whitehead, 1993).

Intrinsic motivation Performing a behavior (being active) because you want to rather than because some outside influence is motivating you to do it.

SAFETY AND EFFECTIVENESS

The cornerstones of any physical activity program are safety and effectiveness. If you get hurt when physically active, the point of the activity is lost. Remember that we are physically active to improve our health, to look better, and to feel better. Injury is counter-productive to these outcomes. Many people make physical activity unsafe by trying to rush results. Patience is crucial to reducing the risk of injury.

An effective activity program is one that allows you to reach your goals and objectives and one that makes you wish to continue to be physically active. By following the suggestions outlined in this book, an effective program is ensured.

Overtraining and Overuse Syndrome

Physical activity can provide wonderful benefits to those who participate regularly. However, too much physical activity can be harmful. Remember that what constitutes too much activity for one may be nothing more than a warm-up for another. In other words, too much exercise is relative to your state of fitness.

If you exercise at a level well beyond your current state of fitness (over-train), you may develop a condition called **over-use syndrome.** Over-use syndrome may be caused by a variety of factors including an inadequate warm-up, poor conditioning, ill-fitting or worn-out shoes, biomechanical abnormalities, rushing results, or differences in activity surfaces. The best way to prevent over-use syndrome is to plan carefully, follow the plan, progress gradually, and listen to your body. If you start to feel that your body is not responding the way it should be, you need to reassess what you are doing.

Over-use syndrome Condition in which too much exercise or physical activity causes the body to start to break down (symptoms: increased risk of injury, lethargy, loss of appetite, irritability, decreased motivation).

Injuries

The *Surgeon General's Report on Physical Activity and Health* (USDHHS, 1996a), suggests that being active may increase your risk for getting injured. However, most musculoskeletal injuries related to physical activity are believed to be preventable if you gradually work up to a desired level of activity and avoid excess. Serious cardiovascular events can occur with physical exertion, but the net effect of regular physical activity is a lower risk of mortality from cardiovascular disease. Shephard (1994) explains that a big fear is that an activity program will provoke a fatal heart attack. However, the risk that vigorous physical activity will provoke a cardiac emergency is low—about one death per 400,000 hours of jogging—and this risk is even lower in those who are regularly active (Shephard, 1994).

Too much activity for your level of fitness can lead to injury.

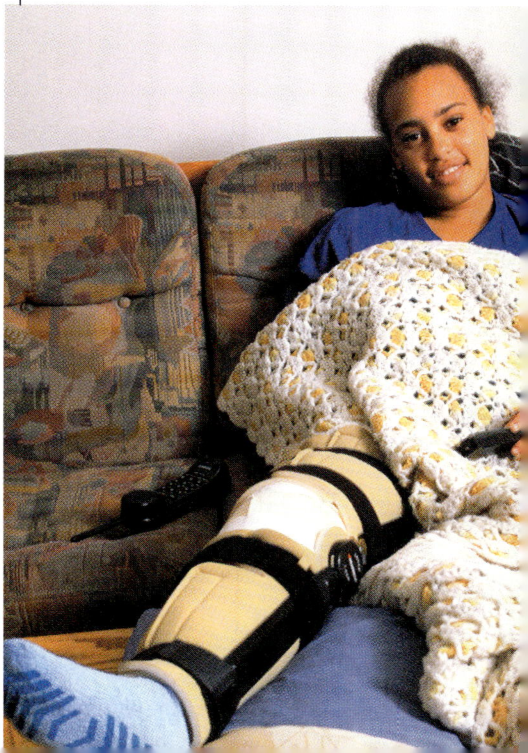

Proper prescreening will further lower this risk. Shephard (1994) outlines factors to be considered in prescreening subjects, including the age of the subject (males over 40, females over 50), the proposed intensity of effort, and associated symptoms or major cardiac risk factors. A common rule to follow in beginning an activity program is that it is better to progress slowly and possibly delay benefits than to rush into activities for which your body is not prepared and risk injury.

A variety of injuries may be related to improper exercise. These include muscular strains, ligamentous sprains, and more serious injuries such as heart attack or stroke. By planning carefully and following directions properly, we know that the risk of injury is lessened. If an injury occurs, it is best to seek professional medical advice.

For more information on injuries, see Appendix B.

Being active can also play an important role in the recovery from an injury. Injured muscles lose strength and fitness. Being active is the best way to regain these lost attributes. Remember that, just because you have an injury in one part of your body, you should not neglect using other parts of your body. Water based-activity is a therapeutic modality that allows you to stress healthy portions of your body while protecting injured areas. It is best to seek your physician's advice on what you can and cannot do when injured.

PHYSICAL ACTIVITY AND HEALTH CONNECTION

Regular participation in a physical activity program provides many health benefits, including the prevention of hypokinetic diseases. Physical activity improves the function of the heart, lungs, muscles, and bones, leading to better health and lowered risk for injury. Being active has also been shown to improve immune function, decreasing the likelihood of catching colds, and allowing you to recover faster. Recent evidence indicates that physical activity is an important factor in the health of women. Activity increases bone mass and reduces the risk for osteoporosis. We now know that we don't have to torture ourselves with exhaustive exercise to obtain health benefits. In fact, regular participation in low-to-moderate-intensity physical activity for 30 minutes on most days of the week provides significant health benefit. Physical activity and health are interconnected. You cannot have good health without being physically active.

CONCEPT CONNECTION

1. **Being physically active provides many health benefits.** An active lifestyle has been shown to provide physical and mental health benefits. You do not need to exercise vigorously to obtain these benefits. Simple daily activity can help you to live longer and with a higher quality of life.

2. **A safe and effective physical activity program requires proper preparation.** To obtain optimal benefit from a physical activity program: you need to make sure you are prepared to be active; you need to know if there are any medical limitations to your being active; you need to be aware of how much activity you can handle safely; and you need to make sure that your body is prepared to participate in the activity you have selected.

3. **How much activity you need is dependent on your goals, interests, and fitness level.** There are two recommended guidelines for physical activity. The first focuses solely on health benefit. These goals require that you accumulate 30 minutes of moderate-intensity physical activity on most if not all days of the week. The second set of goals is for the attainment of the optimal health and fitness benefit. These guidelines require that you exercise at moderate-to-vigorous intensities, 3–5 days per week, for 20–60 minutes. These guidelines should be met in addition to the first set of guidelines.

4. **Optimize your benefits by individualizing your program.** To achieve optimal health and fitness benefits and to make sure that the physical activity program you start is one that you will adhere to, be certain the program is developed with your particular likes and dislikes taken into consideration. The program must be enjoyable and help lead you to meet your individual goals and objectives. Your physical activity program should reflect your personality and lifestyle.

5. **A flexible approach is important in overcoming obstacles to physical activity.** There are many factors that may interfere with your desires to be more active. You need to deal with these factors by developing a physical activity program that meets your needs within the limitations of your lifestyle. Being flexible in developing your program will allow you to find activities that you can fit into your daily routine and provide the health benefits you desire. An important first step is to give being active a higher priority. Second, make sure you are active because you desire to be active and not because someone else is forcing you to be active.

6. **Adhering to your program ensures an active lifestyle.** The benefits of being physically active are transient in nature. Any benefits you achieve will disappear over a period of time if you do not continue to be active. Adhering to a physical activity program is therefore crucial if you wish to live a life that is both long and of high quality.

TERMS

Degeneration, 23
Atrophies, 23
Organ system, 23
Response, 23
Adaptation, 23
Hypokinetic diseases, 26
Aerobic, 31
Anaerobic, 31
Individualized, 33
Variability, 34
Heritability, 34
Initial stage, 34
Progression stage, 35
Maintenance stage, 35
Cardiovascular function, 37
Body composition, 37
Muscular strength, 37
Muscular endurance, 37
Flexibility, 37
Overload principle, 37
Principle of progression, 38
Principle of specificity, 38
Principle of reversibility, 38
Principle of individuality, 38
Principle of recovery, 38
Biological factors, 41
Psychological factors, 41
Social factors, 41
Behavioral factors, 41
Program factors, 41
Intrinsic motivation, 42
Over-use syndrome, 43

MAKING THE CONNECTION

Bob has learned that regular physical activity has numerous beneficial physiological effects, especially when it comes to the cardiovascular and musculoskeletal systems. He has also learned that participating in a prescreening program is an essential step toward ensuring safety and effectiveness. Finally, he has learned the basic principles that govern how your body responds to the physical stress of physical activity.

CRITICAL THINKING

1. Unfortunately, sometimes it takes an incident (Bob's grandfather having a heart attack) to motivate our change of behavior. However, based on what Bob has learned, he is beginning to make a physical activity plan for himself. You can do the same. One step in the planning process is overcoming barriers to physical activity (page 39). Identify the barriers *you* have for participating in regular physical activity. Make sure you consider time and skill, as well as psychological, social, and environmental factors. Review the barriers you have listed, ask yourself *why* they are barriers, and list several ways you might begin overcoming each one.

2. Physical activities, like your nutrition habits, need to have variety. To maintain a physically active lifestyle you will want to have a variety of activities

to participate in; otherwise, you will get bored doing the same activity all the time. List five activities in which you would enjoy participating (hiking, basketball, jogging, biking). For each activity, find someone (social support) who also likes to do the activity, or find a university/college/community club that supports the activity. Begin making plans to participate in different activities, to add spice to your life!

3. "I just don't have time!" This is commonly heard when referring to physical activity. What you need to do is examine *how* you spend your time and determine how you can make time for physical activity. Keep a diary of what you do daily. Include when you get up, classes you attend, breakfast, lunch, dinner, work schedule, study time, time spent with friends, and time spent watching TV. Look at your daily patterns. When can you make time for physical activity? If there isn't an hour block of time, do you have two 30-minute blocks? Can't find 30 minutes, how about 15 minutes? As your daily diary builds, you will be able to see when you can fit physical activity in your daily routine, and soon you'll be saying "I make time to be physically active!"

REFERENCES

American College of Sports Medicine (1995). *ACSM's Guidelines for Exercise Testing and Prescription,* 5th ed. Baltimore: Williams & Wilkins.

American College of Sports Medicine (1998). Position stand: The recommended quantity and quality of exercise for developing and maintaining cardiorespiratory and muscular fitness, and flexibility in healthy adults. *Medicine and Science in Sports and Exercise 30*(6):975–91.

Astrand, P-O. (1992). J.B. Wolfe Memorial Lecture: Why exercise? *Medicine and Science in Sports and Exercise 24*(2):153–62.

Bouchard, C. (1993). Heredity and health-related fitness. In Corbin, C., Pangrazi, R., eds., *The President's Council on Physical Fitness and Sports Research Digest,* Series 1, No. 4. Washington, DC: Department of Health and Human Services.

Coyle, E.F. (1990). Detraining and retention of training-induced adaptations. Sports Science Exchange 2(23). Chicago: Gatorade Sports Science Institute.

Franks, B.D. (1997). Personalizing physical activity prescription. In Corbin, C., Pangrazi, R., eds., *The President's Council on Physical Fitness and Sports Research Digest,* Series 2, No. 9. Washington, DC: Department of Health and Human Services.

Heyward, V.H. (1998). *Advanced Fitness Assessment and Exercise Prescription,* 3rd ed. Champaign, IL: Human Kinetics.

National Institutes of Health. (1995). *NIH Consensus Statement: Physical Activity and Cardiovascular Health 13*(3). Bethesda, MD.

Sallis, J.F. (1994). Influences on physical activity of children, adolescents, and adults, or determinants of active living. In Corbin, C., Pangrazi, R., eds., *The President's Council on Physical Fitness and Sports Research Digest,* Series 1, No. 7. Washington, DC: Department of Health and Human Services.

Shephard, R.J. (1994). Readiness for physical activity. In Corbin, C., Pangrazi, R., eds., *The President's Council on Physical Fitness and Sports Research Digest,* Series 1, No. 5. Washington, DC: Department of Health and Human Services.

U.S. Department of Health and Human Services (1996a). *Physical Activity and Health: A Report of the Surgeon General, Executive Summary.* Washington, DC.

U.S. Department of Health and Human Services. (1996b). *A Report of the Surgeon General: Physical Activity and Health, Women.* Washington, DC.

Wells, C.L. (1996). Physical activity and women's health. In Corbin, C., Pangrazi, R., eds., *The President's Council on Physical Fitness and Sports Research Digest,* Series 2, No. 5. Washington, DC: Department of Health and Human Services.

Whitehead, J.R. (1993). Physical activity and intrinsic motivation. In Corbin, C., Pangrazi, R., eds., *The President's Council on Physical Fitness and Sports Research Digest,* Series 1, No. 2. Washington, DC: Department of Health and Human Services.

Activities & Assessments

NAME ______ SECTION ______ DATE ______

2.1 PAR-Q & You: A Questionnaire for people aged 15 to 69

Regular physical activity is fun and healthy, and more people are starting to become more active every day. Being more active is safe for most people. However, some people should check with their doctor before they start becoming much more physically active.

If you are planning to become much more physically active, start by answering the seven questions below.

If you are between the ages of 15 and 69, the PAR-Q will tell you if you should check with your doctor before you start. If you are over 69 years of age, and you are not used to being very active, check with your doctor. Common sense is your best guide when you answer these questions. Please read the questions carefully and answer each one honestly: check YES or NO.

YES	NO	
☐	☐	1. Has your doctor ever said that you have a heart condition *and* that you should only do physical activity recommended by a doctor?
☐	☐	2. Do you feel pain in your chest when you do physical activity?
☐	☐	3. In the past month. have you had chest pain when you were not doing physical activity?
☐	☐	4. Do you lose your balance because of dizziness or do you ever lose consciousness?
☐	☐	5. Do you have a bone or joint problem that could be made worse by a change in your physical activity?
☐	☐	6. Is your doctor currently prescribing drugs (for example, water pills) for your blood pressure or heart condition?
☐	☐	7. Do you know of *any other reason* why you should not do physical activity?

(continued)

2.1: How Healthy Are You? (cont.)

IF YOU ANSWERED YES TO ONE OR MORE QUESTIONS → DELAY BECOMING MUCH MORE ACTIVE

Talk with your doctor by phone or in person *before* you start becoming much more physically active or *before* you have a fitness appraisal. Tell your doctor about the PAR-Q and which questions you answered YES.

- You may be able to do any activity you want—as long as you start slowly and build up gradually. Or, you may need to restrict your activities to those that are safe for you. Talk with your doctor about the kinds of activities in which you wish to participate and follow the doctor's advice.
- Find out which community programs are safe and helpful for you.

DELAY BECOMING MUCH MORE ACTIVE

- If you are not feeling well because of a temporary illness such as a cold or a fever—wait until you feel better; or
- If you are or may be pregnant—talk to your doctor before you start becoming more active.

IF YOU ANSWERED NO TO ALL QUESTIONS

If you answered NO honestly to *all* PAR-Q questions, you can be reasonably sure that you can:

- Start becoming much more physically active—begin slowly and build up gradually. This is the safest and easiest way to go.
- Take part in a fitness appraisal—this is an excellent way to determine your basic fitness so that you can plan the best way for you to live actively.

Informed Use of the PAR-Q: The Canadian Society for Exercise Physiology, Health Canada, and their agents assume no liability for persons who undertake physical activity, and, if in doubt after completing this questionnaire, consult your doctor prior to physical activity.

You are encouraged to copy the PAR-Q but only if you use the entire form.

Note: If the PAR-Q is being given to a person before he or she participates in a physical activity program or a fitness appraisal, this section may be used for legal or administrative purposes.

I have read, understood and completed this questionnaire. Any questions I had were answered to my full satisfaction.

NAME ______________________________

SIGNATURE ______________________ DATE ______________________

SIGNATURE OR PARENT OR GUARDIAN (for participants under the age of majority) ______________________ WITNESS ______________________

Activities & Assessments

NAME ______ SECTION ______ DATE ______

2.2 Medical History Questionnaire

Directions: This questionnaire is designed to provide your exercise and physical activity professional with information necessary to assist you in the development of a physical activity program. It is not designed as a medical screening device. It is strongly suggested that you check with your physician before making any significant changes in your physical activity status.

Name: ______
LAST NAME FIRST NAME MI

Address: ______

______

______

Phone number: ______
HOME WORK EXT:

Sex: ______ Date of birth: ______ Height: ______ Weight: ______

Name of physician: ______

Physician's address: ______

______

Physician's phone number: ______

Person to contact in case of emergency: ______

Contact's address: ______

______

Contact's phone number: ______

Any medications, foods, or other substances to which you are allergic:

______

______

When was the last time you had a physical examination? ______

(continued)

2.2 Medical History Questionnaire (cont.)

Please list any chronic or serious illnesses you have as diagnosed by your physician.

____

____

____

____

Please list any operations you may have had.

____

____

____

Please list any hospitalizations lasting more than one day you may have had (other than normal pregnancies for women).

____

____

____

Please list any prescription medications you are currently taking.

____

____

____

Please list any over-the-counter medications you are currently taking.

____

____

____

Have you experienced any of the following symptoms in the past 12 months?	YES	NO
Fainting, light-headedness, or blackouts	☐	☐
Dyspnea or trouble breathing	☐	☐
Unusual difficulty sleeping	☐	☐
Blurred vision	☐	☐
Severe headaches or migraines	☐	☐
Chronic coughing	☐	☐
Slurring or loss of speech	☐	☐

	YES	NO
Unusual nervousness or anxiety	☐	☐
Unusual heartbeats, skipped beats, or palpitations	☐	☐
Sudden tingling, numbness, or loss of sensation	☐	☐
Cold feet and hands in warm weather	☐	☐
Swelling of the feet and/or ankles	☐	☐
Pains or cramps in the legs	☐	☐
Pain or discomfort in the chest	☐	☐
Pressure or heaviness in your chest	☐	☐

Has a physician ever told you that you have any of the following conditions?	YES	NO
High blood pressure	☐	☐
Diabetes	☐	☐
High cholesterol	☐	☐
High triglycerides	☐	☐
Heart attack	☐	☐
Stroke	☐	☐
Arteriosclerosis	☐	☐
Heart murmur	☐	☐
Angina	☐	☐
Rheumatic fever	☐	☐
Aneurysm	☐	☐
Cancer	☐	☐
Abnormal ECG	☐	☐
Emphysema	☐	☐
Epilepsy	☐	☐
Arthritis	☐	☐

Has any member of your immediate family (parents, brothers, sisters, children, grandparents) ever been treated for, or died from, any of the following conditions?	YES	NO
Diabetes	☐	☐
Heart disease	☐	☐
Stroke	☐	☐
High blood pressure	☐	☐
Do you smoke tobacco products? If yes, how many per day? ____________	☐	☐

Activities & Assessments

NAME SECTION DATE

2.3 Determining Your Activity Status

You can classify your activity status by selecting the category below that best describes your activity habits.

Predominantly sedentary	I do not participate in physical activity on a regular basis (less than once a week).
Occasionally active	I participate in physical activity on an intermittent basis (once or twice a week).
Moderately active	I accumulate 30 minutes of moderate-intensity physical activity on most if not all days of the week.
Vigorously active	I participate in vigorous physical activity 3 to 5 days a week.

Activities & Assessments

NAME ______ SECTION ______ DATE ______

2.4 Calculating Appropriate Physical Activity Intensity Levels

Step 1:
Select desired variable to calculate intensity from (this will be determined by what data are available to you).

HEART RATE (Go to step 2)
METS (Go to step 15)
VO_2 RESERVE (Go to step 20)

HEART RATE

Step 2:
Select desired intensity level: moderate (Proceed to step 3), or vigorous (Go to step 9)

Step 3:
Subtract your age from 220.

220 − age ______ = ______

Step 4:
Subtract your resting heart rate from your answer to step 3.

Step 3 ______ − resting heart rate ______ = ______

Step 5:
Multiply your answer to step 4 by 40%.

Step 4 ______ × 0.40 = ______

Step 6:
Add your resting heart rate to your answer from step 5. This represents the minimum heart rate you should try to achieve when active.

Resting heart rate ______ + Step 5 ______ = ______

Step 7:
Multiple your answer to step 4 by 55%.

Step 4 ______ × 0.55 = ______

Step 8:
Add your resting heart rate to your answer from step 7. This represents the maximum heart rate you should try to achieve when active.

Resting heart rate _____ + Step 7 ______ = ______

This ends the steps for calculating moderate physical activity intensity from heart rate.

Step 9:
Subtract your age from 220.

220 − age ______ = ______

Step 10:
Subtract your resting heart rate from your answer to Step 9.

Step 9 ______ − resting heart rate ______ = ______

Step 11:
Multiply your answer to step 10 by 50%.

Step 10 ______ × 0.50 = ______

Step 12:
Add your resting heart rate to your answer from step 11. This represents the minimum heart rate you should try to achieve when active.

Resting heart rate ______ + Step 11 ______ = ______

Step 13:
Multiple your answer to step 10 by 85%.

Step 10 ______ × 0.85 = ______

Step 14:
Add your resting heart rate to your answer from Step 13. This represents the maximum heart rate you should try to achieve when active.

Resting heart rate _____ + Step 13 ______ = ______

This ends the steps for calculating vigorous physical activity intensity from heart rate.

(continued)

2.4 Calculating Appropriate Physical Activity Intensity Levels (cont.)

METS

Step 15:
Select desired intensity level: moderate (Go to Step 16), or vigorous (Go to step 18)

Step 16:
To calculate intensity based on METS, you need to assess your functional aerobic capacity through a graded exercise test.

Step 17:
Take 40% and 55% of your maximal MET capacity as determined through a graded exercise test to find the limits for moderate physical activity. For example: if your MET capacity is 10 METS, you should be active at a level of 4 to 5.5 METS.

This ends the steps for calculating moderate physical activity intensity from METS.

Step 18:
To calculate intensity based on METS, you need to assess your functional aerobic capacity through a graded exercise test.

Step 19:
Take 50% and 85% of your maximal MET capacity as determined through a graded exercise test to find the limits for vigorous physical activity. For example: if your MET capacity is 10 METS, you should be active at a level of 5 to 8.5 METS.

This ends the steps for calculating vigorous physical activity intensity from METS.

VO_2 RESERVE

Step 20:
To calculate moderate intensity based on VO_2 reserve, you need to assess your functional aerobic capacity through a graded exercise test. For vigorous intensity calculations, go to step 26.

Step 21:
Subtract your resting VO_2 (3.5 ml · kg^{-1} · min^{-1}) from your VO_2 max score as determined through a graded exercise test to obtain your VO_2 reserve.

Step 22:
Multiply your VO_2 reserve by 40%. For example: if your VO_2 reserve is 40 ml · kg^{-1} · min^{-1}, when this figure is multiplied by 40% you get 16 ml · kg^{-1} · min^{-1}.

Step 23:
Add your resting VO_2 to your answer from Step 22. This represents the minimum VO_2 you should try to achieve when active.

3.5 ml · kg^{-1} · min^{-1} + Step 22 ______ = ______

Step 24:
Multiply your VO_2 reserve by 50%. For example: if your VO_2 reserve is 40 ml · kg^{-1} · min^{-1}, when this figure is multiplied by 50% you get 20 ml · kg^{-1} · min^{-1}.

Step 25:
Add your resting VO2 to your answer from Step 24. This represents the maximum VO_2 you should try to achieve when active.

This ends the steps for calculating moderate physical activity intensity from VO_2 reserve.

Step 26:
To calculate vigorous intensity based on VO_2 reserve, you need to assess your functional aerobic capacity through a graded exercise test.

Step 27:
Subtract your resting VO_2 (3.5 ml · kg^{-1} · min^{-1}) from your VO_2 max score as determined through a graded exercise test to obtain your VO_2 reserve.

Step 28:
Multiply your VO_2 reserve by 50%. For example: if your VO_2 reserve is 40 ml · kg^{-1} · min^{-1} when this figure is multiplied by 50% you get 20 ml · kg^{-1} · min^{-1}.

Step 29:
Add your resting VO_2 to your answer from Step 28. This represents the minimum VO_2 you should try to achieve when active.

3.5 ml · kg^{-1} · min^{-1} + Step 28 ______ = ______

Step 30:
Multiply your VO_2 reserve by 85%. For example: if your VO_2 reserve is 40 ml · kg^{-1} · min^{-1}, when this figure is multiplied by 85% you get 34 ml · kg^{-1} · min^{-1}.

Step 31:
Add your resting VO_2 to your answer from Step 29. This represents the maximum VO_2 you should try to achieve when active.

This ends the steps for calculating vigorous physical activity intensity from VO_2 reserve.

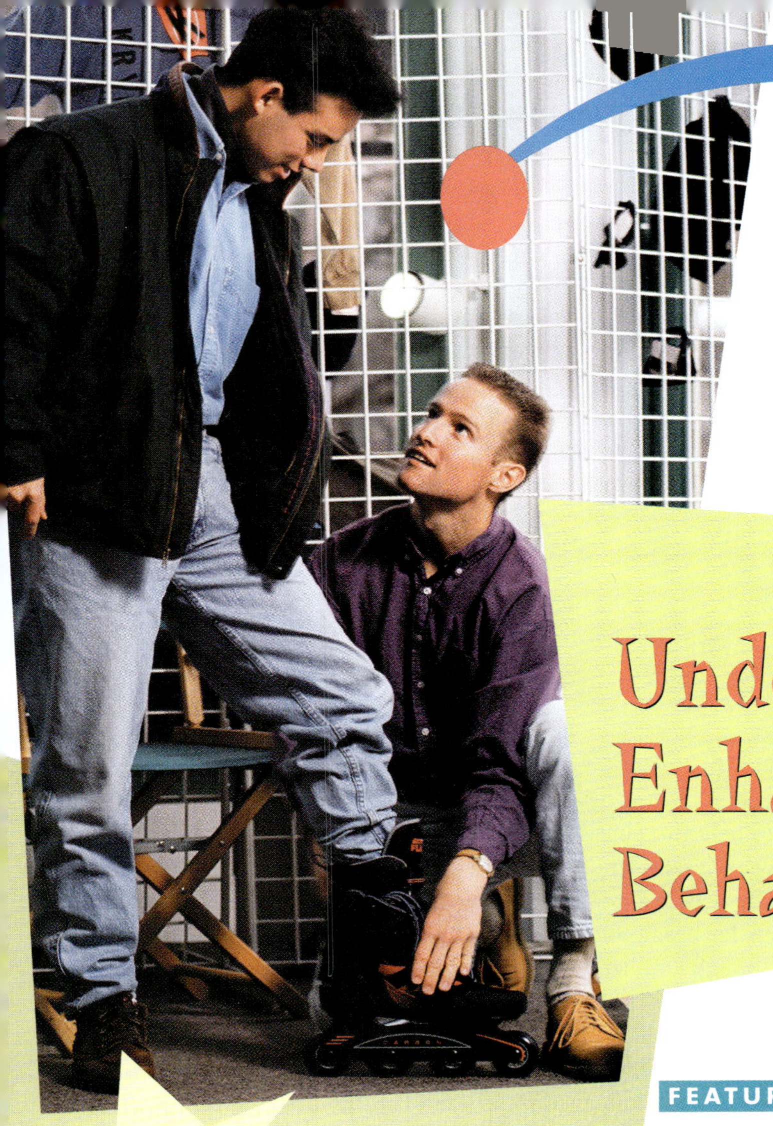

3

Understanding and Enhancing Health Behaviors

CONCEPT CONNECTION

1. Lifestyle plays an important role in determining your quality of life.
2. Health behaviors can be categorized as symptomatic or asymptomatic responses.
3. Three universal learning principles—true learning, empowerment, envisioning—can help us to be self-responsible for our health and are precursors to implementing self-change related to our health behaviors.
4. Reciprocal determinism, self-efficacy, and readiness are important concepts in understanding health behavior.
5. The stages of change represent a continuum of an individual's motivational readiness to modify health behaviors.
6. In progressing through the stages of change, we can utilize a variety of behavior change techniques.

FEATURES

E-Learning Tools: www.pahconnection.com

Engage www.pahconnection.com

3.1 Self-Esteem general inventory
3.2 Locus of control general inventory
3.3 Stages of change—exercise measure
3.4 Exercise self-efficacy

Experience www.pahconnection.com

3.1 Personal growth and self improvement
3.2 Information on self-efficacy
3.3 Identify, plan and achieve your goals

Explore www.pahconnection.com

3.1 Think your way to an excellent life
3.2 Daily inner guidance inspirations
3.3 Self-help
3.4 Transtheoretical model and processes of change

Activities & Assessments

3.1 Stages of change—continuous measure
3.2 Self-efficacy toward physical activity
3.3 Pros and cons of physical activity

WHAT'S THE CONNECTION?

John is 20 years old, a college sophomore majoring in telecommunications and earning mostly A's. John is well liked by his classmates and is socially active in his fraternity. When he experienced low-back pain and visited the college health center, the attending physician noted that he was overweight with slightly elevated blood pressure. Questioned about physical activity, John said he doesn't exercise at all. "Exercise involves a lot of discomfort and requires too much effort. The idea of participating in an activity whose mantra is 'No pain, no gain' just doesn't appeal to me," he explained. "Besides," he continued, "I'm way too busy and don't have time to exercise. I'm here to receive treatment for low-back pain, not to start a physical activity program."

INTRODUCTION

Our goal is to help promote physical activity and exercise as a regular part of your life. Behavioral scientists have made significant progress in understanding why people choose to be physically active and identifying the most effective methods for promoting physical activity. This research has shown that people generally go through a rather orderly decision-making process when changing their physical activity and other health-related behaviors.

The practical value of increasing your knowledge about, and understanding of, research in health behavior changes is that it can help you have a healthy life. We believe that the methods used to influence your health behaviors should be based on good-quality research because that increases your chances of success. Current research information provides many valuable cues to the appropriate means for initiating, maintaining, or resuming physical activity.

To support your efforts to improve your own health, we begin with a discussion of the role lifestyle plays in your quality of life. We then present three universal learning principles that are important as you act responsibly in moving toward your chosen lifestyle; being self-responsible for your lifestyle is fundamental to implementing changes in your health behaviors. Next, we proceed with a discussion of underlying factors that influence health behaviors and then introduce a pattern of changing health behavior that takes place over time. Finally, we present factors that impact your physical activity and exercise behavior and ways that you can use them to improve your chances of changing. While this chapter focuses on changing and enhancing your physical activity behavior, the fundamentals presented here are encouraged throughout this book.

QUALITY OF LIFE: OUR MOTIVATION TO BE HEALTHY

1. Lifestyle plays an important role in determining your quality of life.

The concept of quality of life has been used in a number of programs for managing and treating illnesses such as heart disease and cancer. Here, we expand the concept to include times when a person is not suffering from illness (Chapter 1). We use quality of life in the broad sense to exemplify an indi-

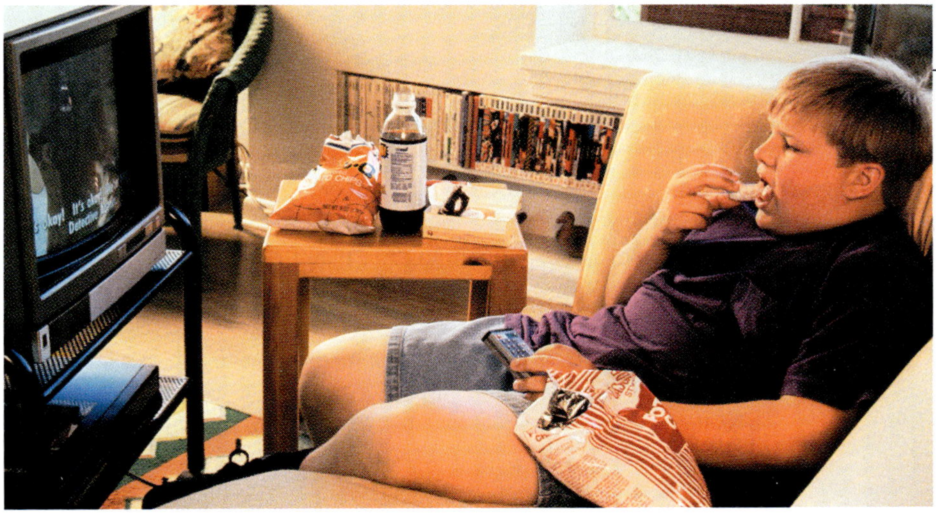

Many young Americans are following sedentary lifestyles that place them at greater health risks.

vidual's capacity to function, carry out, and derive satisfaction from each of the six dimensions of wellness.

Our lifestyle is the single most important and modifiable factor influencing our health and wellness today. **Lifestyle,** with its relationship to health, comprises an enduring pattern of behaviors. The persistence of these behaviors as they relate to disease prevention has become increasingly important. Seemingly innocent acts—like avoiding regular physical activity or consuming high-fat foods—account for much of the disease, disability, and premature deaths in our society. We believe that the individual must and can take an active role in the implementation of health behavior change.

Lifestyle An enduring pattern of behaviors related to one's health.

The answer to the question "Why be healthy?" seems obvious. Nationwide polls indicate that Americans place great value on their health as a source of happiness. However, the actions of many Americans do not produce the good health they desire. In fact, public surveys reveal declining satisfaction among many regarding their personal health (Barsky, 1988). Americans now report higher rates of symptoms, disability, and general dissatisfaction with their health. To obtain a higher level of wellness, most people still turn to the medical care system. While heroic efforts are being made in medicine, two trends must be understood: (1) Most of today's major killers—for example, lung cancer and chronic obstructive lung disease—are largely preventable through proper health behavior, and (2) in spite of the remarkable strides in basic medical research and technology, most lung cancers and chronic obstructive lung disease cases are not curable. As it is revealed in the *Book of Common Prayer:*

> We have left undone those things we ought to have done
> and done those things we ought not to have done
> and there is no health in us.

One of the stated goals of the medical health care system is to treat diseases and prolong life. However, while advances in medical care have lowered the mortality rate, this decline in deaths has led to an increased incidence of chronic and degenerative disorders. This has been termed the "failure of medical care success." We may live longer, but a greater proportion of our life is spent in ill health.

Health educators, physicians, researchers, and others have suggested that the next major step in improving the general health of the U.S. population will be behavioral rather

Participation by this man in physical activity increases his likelihood of enjoying a more satisfying life.

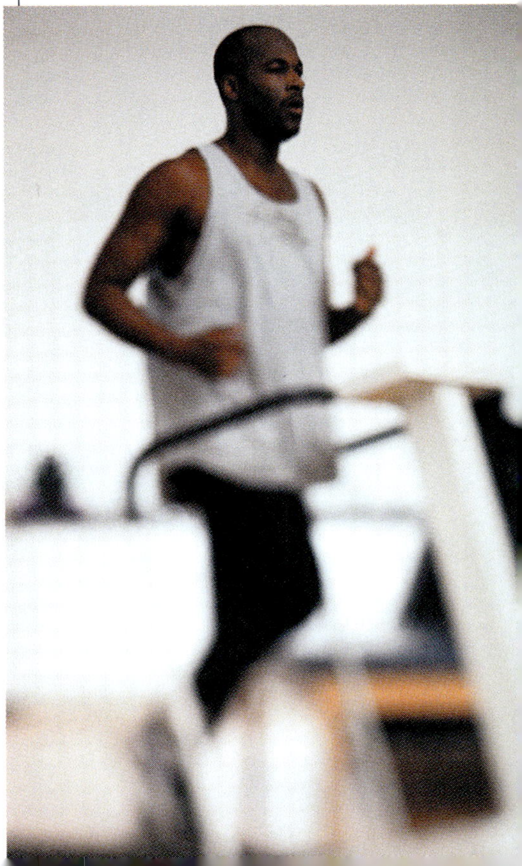

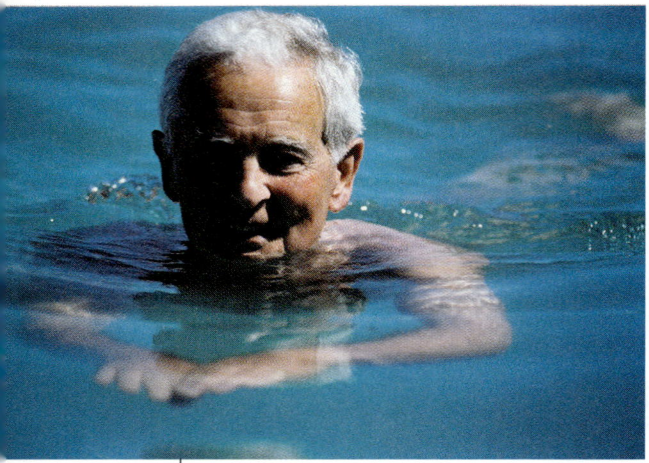

Physically active people are likely to be healthier and more vigorous later in life.

than solely medical (Healthy People 2010, 2000). For example, *Healthy People 2010* examined the leading causes of death in the United States and concluded that most are largely behavioral in origin. They could be substantially reduced if people were to modify their diet, stop smoking, drink only in moderation, and increase physical activity. The potential control of these major health risks lies at the heart of health behavior change efforts.

People must also recognize the need to participate and be responsible for their own behaviors in obtaining and maintaining a high quality of life. Very few people are motivated to be healthy for health's sake. Jesse Feiring Williams, progressive thinker in the 1930s, observed that "Health as freedom from disease is a standard of mediocrity; health as a quality of life is a standard of inspiration and increasing achievement." We believe that wellness is what so many people want, yet it is an elusive dream for many because obtaining wellness is misunderstood. We call for more and more medical care, expecting unrealistic therapeutic outcomes, and continue to be frustrated and dissatisfied. Over time we have gradually lost the art of personal responsibility and self-discipline and have confused what we want with what we need regarding our health.

physical activity and health connection

Experience www.pahconnection.com 3.1

The wisdom we need is within us. When you think of it, there is something truly remarkable in the fact that practically all human beings want to be better than they are. Life continually presents us with opportunities for achieving what we desire. Most of us strive to be **self-changers.** A *self-change* approach assumes that we can manage and control our own lives. Self-change means that our behavior is under our control—that when it is necessary to change, we can do it. We want to be able to control our behavior so that we can change in a desired way, increasing physical activity if we are sedentary and managing stress more effectively if we are feeling overwhelmed. Self-change means recognizing the changes you want and being able to actualize your own values.

2. Health behaviors can be categorized as symptomatic or asymptomatic responses.

Categories of Health Behavior

The path to a high quality of life, or wellness lifestyle, lies in our behaviors. Our choices and subsequent actions make our lives what they are. John Seffrin, Executive Director of the American Cancer Society, has said that "The need to choose is the most constant aspect of human life. It constitutes our greatest asset and our heaviest burden." How many times have you asked yourself "Why do I do what I do?" or "Why is it so difficult for me to change?" The behavioral sciences and the field of psychology offer helpful theories and methods for improving our strategies for health behavior change (Roberts, Banspach, & Peacock, 1997). Psychologists have long been interested in why people choose certain behaviors. In fact, psychologists have become increasingly involved in understanding behavioral health, the study of the maintenance of health and prevention of illness and dysfunction in currently healthy persons.

Health researchers distinguish a number of behaviors related to health and disease (Kolbe, 1988). These distinctions are consistent with our definition of health behavior and the wellness continuum in Chapter 1 (see especially Figure 1.3). Kolbe proposed nine categories of **health behavior** (Table 3.1). The health behaviors are responses in *symptomatic* disease conditions (illness, self-care, sick-role behavior) as well as in *asymptomatic* situations (wellness, preventive, at-risk behavior). Kolbe's first six behaviors are related directly to an individual's personal health and the last three are related to the way an individual's behavior directly influences another person's health. For convenience, we will refer to all nine of them simply as health behaviors.

Self-changers An approach that assumes that we can manage and control our own lives.

Health behavior Behaviors that can be symptomatic responses (as in illness, self-care, or sick-role behavior) as well as asymptomatic responses (as in wellness, preventive, or at-risk behavior).

The Nature and Complexity of Health Behaviors

Health behaviors are important not only in disease prevention and health promotion but also because they often represent habits. Every action we choose sets into motion a behavior that may become habit. A *health habit* is a health-related behavior that is firmly established and often performed automatically, without thought. Although the habit may have developed because it was reinforced by specific positive outcomes, eventually it becomes independent of the reinforcement process and is maintained by the environmental factors with which it is customarily associated (Hunt et al., 1979). As such, the habit

TABLE 3.1 A Typology of Health Behavior

Wellness Behavior	any activity undertaken by an individual who believes himself/herself to be healthy, for the purpose of attaining an even greater level of health
Preventive Health Behavior	any activity undertaken by an individual who believes himself/herself to be healthy, for the purpose of preventing illness or detecting it in an asymptomatic state (Kasl & Cobb, 1966)
At-Risk Behavior	any activity undertaken by an individual who believes himself/herself to be healthy but at greater risk than normal of developing a specific health condition, for the purpose of preventing that condition or detecting it in an asymptomatic state (Baric, 1969)
Illness Behavior	any activity undertaken by an individual who believes himself/herself to be ill, to define the state of his/her health and to discover a suitable remedy (Kasl & Cobb, 1966)
Self-Care Behavior	any activity undertaken by an individual who believes himself/herself to be ill, for the purpose of getting well; includes minimal reliance on appropriate therapists, involves few dependent behaviors, and leads to little neglect of one's usual duties
Sick-Role Behavior	any activity undertaken by an individual who believes himself/herself to be ill, for the purpose of getting well; includes receiving treatment from appropriate therapists, generally involves a whole range of dependent behaviors, and leads to some degree of neglect of one's usual duties (Kasl & Cobb, 1966)
Reproductive Behavior	any activity undertaken by an individual to influence the occurrence or normal continuation of pregnancy
Parenting Health Behavior	any wellness, preventive, at-risk, illness, self-care, or sick-role behavior performed by an individual for the purposes of ensuring, maintaining, or improving the health of a conceptus or child for whom the individual has responsibility
Health-Related Social Action	any activity undertaken by an individual singularly or in concert with others (i.e., collectively) through organizational, legal, or economic means, to influence the provision of medical services, the effects of the environment, the effects of various products, or the effects of social regulations that influence the health of populations

SOURCE: L.J. Kolbe. (1988). The application of health behavior research: Health education and health promotion. In D. Gochman (Ed.), *Health behavior: Emerging research perspectives*. New York: Plenum Publishing, 382.

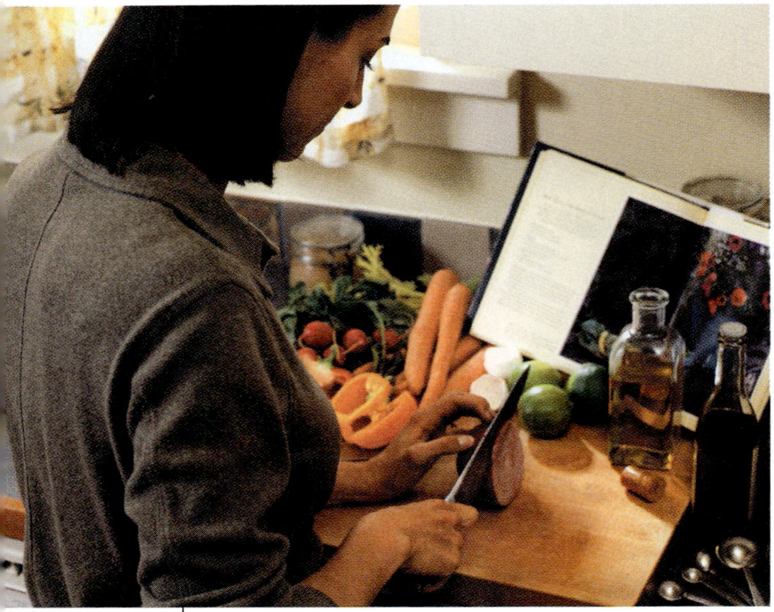

Good nutrition is an important aspect of a healthy lifestyle.

can be highly resistant to change. Obviously, it is important to establish good health behaviors and eliminate bad ones as early as possible—but it is also important to realize that even deeply rooted negative behaviors can be changed in time. Changing negative behavior patterns or adopting health-enhancing ones, however, is usually a time-consuming process that requires a number of learning attempts. Mark Twain probably best summed it up: "Habit is habit, and not to be flung out the window by anyone, but coaxed downstairs a step at a time."

Additional factors that may amplify the difficulty in changing health behaviors include:

1. **Firmly established habits.** Many health habits developed early in life are well established and difficult to change by the time a person enters adulthood. Over 90 percent of adult cigarette smokers began smoking before age 18. The overwhelming majority of adult smokers want to quit but have significant difficulty in doing so.
2. **Delayed gratification.** People prefer instant gratification and resist changing behaviors that provide immediate pleasure. When people are faced with a short-term gain—the pleasure of eating a high-fat diet, for example—it can be difficult to choose differently for the sake of the long term.
3. **Too much scientific information.** Changing present behaviors to reduce the probability of an undesirable outcome down the road is difficult for many people to understand. It can be challenging to relate risk factors to future health.
4. **Fear of failure.** Some people have a history of failure in attempts to change a specific health behavior. These individuals may become demoralized and pessimistic about their future chances of success.
5. **"It won't happen to me" attitude.** Some people tend to be unrealistic in judging their personal risk for developing certain health problems. People hear so much contradictory evidence that many decide "it won't happen to me" and take no preventive action.
6. **Too many choices.** Providing too many health choices can make a person decide not to take any of them. Some people can feel overwhelmed by too many choices and remain at status quo.
7. **Low internal locus of control.** People feel they do not have control over their lives or the things that are going to happen to them (Dejoy, Wilson, & Huddy, 1995).

In summary, a healthy lifestyle is more than just eliminating harmful habits—it is a way of living. Your lifestyle can significantly decrease the risk of disease, while significantly *increasing* your chances of living healthfully throughout your lifespan. A healthy lifestyle is predicated on the idea that our chances for self-fulfillment are directly increased or decreased by our level of wellness. A healthy lifestyle includes almost every decision we make, from when we get up in the morning to when we go to bed at night. It involves our choices related to social, physical, emotional, career, intellectual, environmental, and spiritual dimensions. The choice, at every moment, is ours. We have the personal power, with every decision we make, to act in ways that promote our wellness.

Virtually every decision we make involves some degree of health risk or health benefit. People with healthy lifestyles make intelligent decisions about their health and well-being without stripping life of all excitement and enjoyment. When an activity involves some inherent risk to health, these persons minimize the risk by proceeding with care. For example, a person who wants to begin a weight-lifting program will thoroughly understand the appropriate technique before attempting any lift. The person with a healthy lifestyle makes every reasonable effort to compare the risks and benefits of any behavior before engaging in it. More and more, these individuals take responsibility for their own health.

Your lifestyle is the single most important and modifiable factor influencing your health and wellness today. Choosing to participate in a healthy lifestyle reduces your risk for developing chronic disease and significantly increases your chances for a high quality of life. Most of us strive to be self-changers. A self-change approach assumes that we can manage and control our own lives. Self-change means that our behavior is under our control—that when it is necessary to change, we can. To establish a pattern of behaviors that lowers your risk of disease and improves your quality of life requires self-responsibility. To develop one's self-responsibility requires a person to be a true learner, feel empowered, and be able to envision a quality of life. We now turn attention to these learning principles.

UNIVERSAL LEARNING PRINCIPLES

3. Three universal learning principles—true learning, empowerment, envisioning—can help us to be self-responsible for our health and are precursors to implementing self-change related to our health behaviors.

The development of a high quality of life in each of the six dimensions of health discussed in Chapter 1 involves true learning, empowerment, and envisioning by the individual (Girdano & Dusek, 1988) (Figure 3.1). These three universal learning principles support our being self-responsible and are precursors to implementing a self-change approach to health behavior. Self-change is a personal phenomenon. In order to accomplish it, you'll need to have firm notions about how you can create change rather than relying on others to do it for you.

Explore www.pahconnection.com **3.1**

True Learning

True learning Actively taking control of your learning and subsequent actions.

True learning occurs when you actively take control of your learning and subsequent actions. Many of our failures to change health behavior are rooted in the belief that we are not in control of our behavior. Sometimes we passively make decisions based on what others think in order to gain their acceptance. It is all too easy to blame

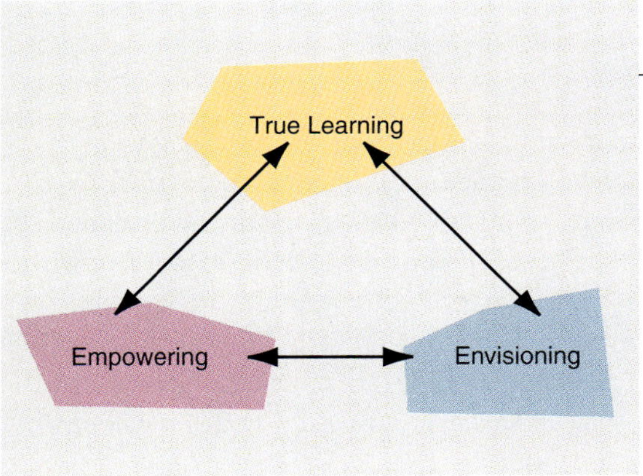

FIGURE 3.1

Universal Learning Principles. True learning, empowering, and envisioning must be integrated into the process of health behavior change, and together they provide a never-ending circle.

our friends, spouses, or co-workers for our actions. Our self-acceptance should not be dependent on the perceptions or the actions of someone else, nor is it dependent on attention, or lack of it, from friends.

True learning activities give meaning to your internal and external experiences in a way that empowers you. Every experience teaches us something if we agree to learn, and everything we learn enhances our life. True learning experiences allow you to set your own goals and strategies, an essential process of participating in health behavior change (Greenburg, 1978).

Be willing to participate in internal learning regarding your feelings, beliefs, and behaviors. Belief in yourself precedes achievement. Your successes are always within your control if you understand your responsibility to your feelings and beliefs about yourself. Positive self-talk is powerful. Assigning meaning to each experience can help you develop a healthy ego. Negative self-talk, on the other hand, can lead to a low self-image. Rather than developing a healthy ego, you may doubt your experiences and question your self-worth. Your growth is dependent upon the removal of irrational beliefs about yourself and your experiences. Your positive internal resources enhance self-concept and need to be cultivated. Surrounding yourself with others who are in a similar true learning mode can enhance these internal resources. All of the aspects of true learning lead to the outcome of self-empowerment.

Explore
www.pahconnection.com
3.2, 3.3

Empowerment

Empowerment means the giving of power or authority. In our context of life quality, empowerment is the process that promotes self-actualization among individuals. In his book *The Farthest Reaches of Human Nature,* Abraham Maslow described self-actualization as the highest level of personality growth. According to Maslow, self-actualized individuals have fulfilled their human potential by utilizing their particular personal strengths. This process includes understanding who you are and what you are capable of doing. You cannot empower someone else, and others cannot empower you. Components of self-actualization include self-awareness, self-understanding, self-efficacy, self-esteem, self-regard, self-love, self-respect, and self-worth (Girdano & Dusek, 1988).

Engage
www.pahconnection.com
3.1, 3.2

In health psychology, empowerment is referred to as **internal locus of control.** In fact, one of the first social learning theories applied to health behavior was "internal vs. external locus of control" (Rotter, 1966). Individuals with internal locus of control believe that their own behaviors determine their health; conversely, individuals with external locus of control believe their health is determined by chance, luck, or fate. Research has found that having an internal locus of control is a significant predictor of healthy behavior. You can determine your own locus of control related to your health by completing Engage 3.2, "Health Locus of Control," on the website.

Envisioning

Envisioning involves imagining what is possible and desirable regarding your health. These potentials arise from our own experiences, intuitions, and desires. Our desires can be realized through intent, but we must generate the picture in our mind before action will follow. Envisioning sets the target for quality of life. We are all moving along some health pathway at every moment, and each of us needs to accept responsibility for our course. Having a target inspires concrete action. It fosters planned movement; it facilitates decision making. For example, deciding that you would like to increase the number of vegetables you eat each day will make it more likely that you will purchase them the next time you go grocery shopping.

Empowerment To give power or authority.

Internal locus of control An attitude that one's own behavior determines one's health.

Envisioning Imagining what is possible and desirable regarding your health.

Living without targets means missing out on the joy of successfully confronting the obstacles on the health behavior path we have chosen. Envisioning the attainment of our goals through our chosen health behaviors is essential to the change process. For example, you are much more likely to succeed in eating more vegetables if you are not always focusing on the behavior (eating vegetables) but are reminding yourself how your life will be enhanced when your outcome (better control of your weight) has been reached.

True learning, empowerment, and envisioning must be integrated into a health behavior change program (Girdano & Dusek, 1988). We can only recognize where we are going when we have command of our direction through some degree of empowerment. Similarly, empowerment must come through true learning activities and experiences. Picture this process as a never-ending circle (Figure 3.1). One of our goals for you is that you will develop the principles that allow you to be self-responsible about your health. This responsibility will lead you to take an active role in implementing the behaviors that produce a fulfilling life.

Choosing to participate in a healthy lifestyle requires self-responsibility and a self-change approach. Self-responsible individuals participate in true learning experiences, feel empowered, and are able to imagine what is possible and desirable regarding their health. These three universal learning principles are important precursors for implementing change successfully.

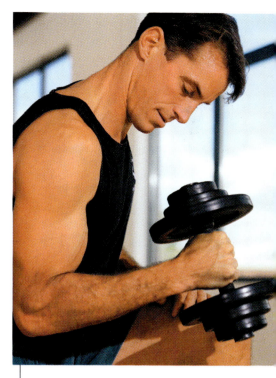

Weight lifting is an excellent form of physical activity.

UNDERSTANDING YOUR HEALTH BEHAVIOR

It has been said that practice without theory is like exploration without a map: we do not know where we are and cannot figure out where we are going. Using a conceptual background provides you with means for organizing your knowledge so that you can more clearly understand how and why your change efforts are effective or ineffective. On the other hand, theory without practice is like reading a map without ever leaving home. You will be encouraged through various exercises in this book to travel a path to health, to participate actively in your journey, and to learn from your experiences as you work on changing or enhancing your health behaviors. A self-change guide to enhanced health behavior is found in Appendix A. The next section presents a sound method that is both empirical and theoretical to help you understand health behavior based on learning theory and the readiness to change.

As we have discussed, many health habits are difficult to change because they are deeply embedded within the person. Even when this is so, they can be changed into more positive behaviors through education. We discussed earlier the importance of universal learning principles—true learning, empowerment, envisioning—to developing self-responsibility. Learning theory is an appropriate tool for health behavior modification because the behaviors important to good health must be learned and incorporated into a person's lifestyle, and undesirable behaviors that lead to ill health must be recognized and changed. This is why research has focused on the principles of learning theory to modify unhealthy and destructive health behaviors.

Albert Bandura of Stanford University, a leading social psychologist, is a strong advocate of using the principles of learning to influence health behavior change. Bandura has spent his life researching individual health behaviors. His highly comprehensive model for explaining the factors influencing individual health behavior is called the **social cognitive theory (SCT)** (Bandura, 1986). The social cognitive theory is a

Social cognitive theory A scholarly method for understanding human social behavior that provides justification for both organizational and individual approaches to health behavior change.

scholarly method for understanding human social behavior that undergirds both organizational and individual approaches to changes in health behavior. Three key concepts that are especially useful in understanding health behavior are reciprocal determinism, self-efficacy, and readiness to change. Understanding these concepts will significantly assist you in your self-change efforts.

Reciprocal Determinism

4. Reciprocal determinism, self-efficacy, and readiness are important concepts in understanding health behavior.

The organizing principle of SCT theory is that of **reciprocal determinism**, the constant, dynamic interaction that takes place among a person's cognitions, behavior, and environment. Figure 3.2 illustrates reciprocal determinism among the person, the behavior, and the environment. The SCT perspective is that individual behavior change can be achieved by modifying people's personal factors and altering their environmental factors. This view is a balanced and optimistic view of health behavior change. People shape their environments through their behaviors, and their behaviors are shaped by the environment. The concept of reciprocal determinism suggests that influencing any one factor will influence all the others, providing a profound change. Behavioral scientists and health educators have used many of the SCT ideas and principles to help people succeed in changing many different types of health behavior (Baranowski, Perry, & Parcel, 1997).

Self-Efficacy

One of the most important ideas proposed by Bandura was that of a person's behavior expectancies. He termed these **self-efficacy** beliefs. Self-efficacy is defined as "a judgement of one's capability to accomplish a certain level of performance" (Bandura, 1986, p. 391). Earlier, we discussed the importance of outcome expectancies as they relate to your locus of control. A high internal locus of control indicates that you believe your actions are responsible for your health status. Self-efficacy goes even further and assesses your belief that you can perform the specific behavior to meet your desired outcome. Thus, self-efficacy beliefs represent judgments of your personal competence.

Self-efficacy is the confidence you have in yourself about performing a specific behavior or activity in a variety of situations. Self-efficacy assesses your belief that you can do the behavior in order to achieve your desired outcome; it is your perceived confidence that you can change and maintain your health behavior across a variety of difficult situations.

Reciprocal determinism The constant, dynamic interaction that takes place among a person's cognitions, behavior, and environment.

Self-efficacy A judgment of your own capability to achieve a certain level of performance.

FIGURE 3.2

Reciprocal Determinism. This concept suggests that influencing any one factor will influence all the others.

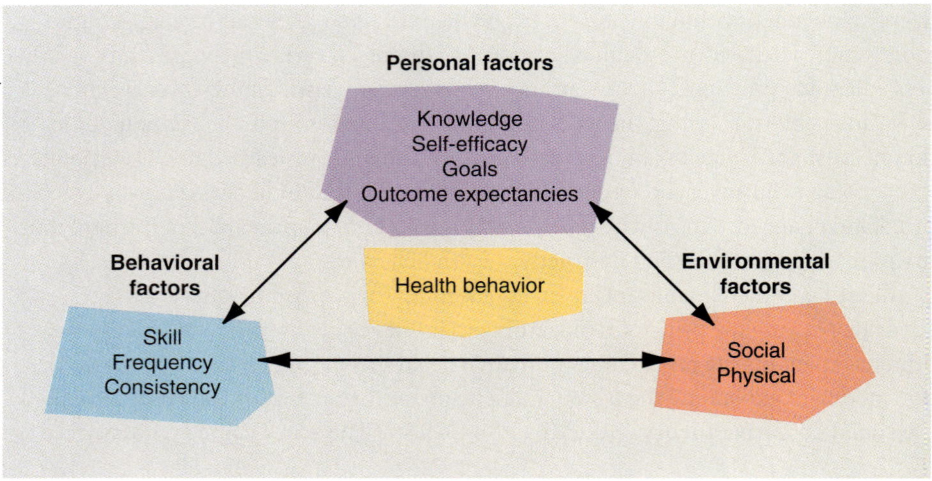

Many factors are influential in decisions regarding behavior change, but self-efficacy is considered the strongest predictor for physical activity (McAuley, 1993). Numerous studies have substantiated what most people knew all along: people who strongly believe they can initiate and adhere to a physical activity program, do. What's more, they exert an elevated level of effort to accomplish this goal, persisting in the face of the difficulties that inevitably rise. Similarly, people who believe they will fail, usually do. In other words, there is truth to the adage "Whether you believe you can, or whether you believe you can't, you are probably right."

Enhancing Self-Efficacy According to Bandura (1986) there are four important ways that you can enhance self-efficacy: performance attainment, vicarious experience, verbal persuasion, and physiological states. *Performance attainments* are the most convincing because they are based on personal success experiences. Having swum on the high school swimming team will no doubt enhance your belief that you can choose swimming as part of your college physical activity program. *Vicarious experience* increases self-efficacy through observing the effective or ineffective performances of others. If you are a nonswimmer, watching other swimmers may convince you that you can learn to swim. *Verbal persuasion* or counseling is thought be less effective than vicarious experience, but it can be useful nevertheless to have a good friend talk you through your experience. Finally, *physiological states* may inform individuals (correctly or not) as to whether they are capable of performing a given action. You may feel a bit anxious about getting into the pool but your friend reminds you that this is normal.

physical activity and health connection

Readiness and Motivation to Change

When planning a behavior change, most people ask how, but it is also important to ask why, when, and what now? These questions are especially important when planning a modification of exercise behavior.

Physical activity is a unique health behavior that encompasses a complex and dynamic range of behavioral demands. Moreover, physical activity is perceived as requiring more time and effort than other health behaviors (Turk, Rudy, & Salovey, 1984). Planning for physical activity, adopting your plan, and maintaining it can involve a number of behavioral techniques (Dishman, 1990).

An important first step is to assess your **readiness.** Readiness can be defined as motivation. Readiness can be seen as a continuum from minimal to maximal motivation across each of the steps required to change a behavior. Janis (1983) describes three periods where individuals need motivating capacity: the first period is that of becoming aware of the problem behavior; the second period includes a commitment to change; and the third period is the actual process of change. Readiness is the possession of cognitions, skills, and resources that make it possible for individuals to incorporate positive health behavior into a permanent lifestyle and make negative health behavior extinct. Each of these learning experiences requires motivation. The next section will discusses your level of readiness and motivation as a series of stages.

We have realized that our behaviors strongly influence our health outcomes. We have decided we want to better understand why we do the things we do, or fail to do. The principles of learning theory can now provide ways to modify unhealthy and destructive health behaviors through powerful cognitive concepts. Recall that the concepts were *reciprocal determinism,* the constant, dynamic interaction among our cognitions, behavior, and environment; *self-efficacy,* our belief that we can perform the specific behavior to meet a desired health outcome; and, *readiness,* our level of motivation to change. Now we provide you with a behavioral road map that successful self-changers have followed in their course of altering their health behaviors.

Readiness A continuum from minimal to maximal motivation across each of the assorted steps required to change a habit or deeply ingrained behavior.

5. The stages of change represent a continuum of an individual's motivational readiness to modify health behaviors.

Stages of change Process of health behavior change that can best be represented as a series of stages.

Precontemplation Stage of change during which the individual does not intend to take action within 6 months.

Contemplation Stage of change begins when the person starts to think seriously about changing in the near future (within 6 months).

Preparation Stage of change in which the individual intends to take action within the next 30 days.

Action Stage of change in which the individual has made significant effort to change and, more important, has achieved some degree of success with that change.

Maintenance Stage of change in which the individual continues to implement behavior strategies in an attempt to avoid relapses regarding their health behavior.

Termination Stage of change in which the former problem behavior presents no threat or temptation.

Cycle of change Cyclical concept of behavior change within the first five-stage process, related to a person's readiness to change over a period of time.

Engage www.pahconnection.com 3.3

Activities & Assessments 3.1

STAGES OF CHANGE

Since the early 1980s, three clinical psychologists have been observing how people intentionally change their health behaviors (Prochaska, Norcross, & DiClemente, 1994). By observing self-changers, they have conceived a powerful model for understanding how people change their health behaviors. Their novel approach to change focuses on what they call stages of change. They found that successful self-changing individuals follow a controllable and predictable course of change, avoiding the all-or-nothing approach. The stages of change represent a continuum of motivational readiness to modify health behaviors. Earlier, we discussed readiness and motivation as they apply to developing your program for health behavior change. The creators of the stages of change model have conceptualized readiness in stages:

1. Precontemplation
2. Contemplation
3. Preparation
4. Action
5. Maintenance
6. Termination

Precontemplation is the stage during which the individual intends to take no action within 6 months (Reed et al., 1997); this is the *I won't* stage. The **contemplation** stage begins when the person starts to think seriously about changing in the near future (within 6 months); this is the *I might* stage. The **preparation** stage is one in which the individual intends to take action within 30 days; this is the *I will* stage. Preparation is a stage in which a person makes an actual effort to change a behavior. There is a plan for action and small or preliminary behavior changes are already being made. Thus, the preparation stage includes intentional and behavioral dimensions. In the **action** stage, the individual has made significant effort to change and, more important, has achieved some degree of success with that change; this is the *I am* stage. The action stage is described as a 6-month period following the actual behavior change. Once the behavioral practice becomes routine, the person is said to be in the **maintenance** stage; this is the *I Have* stage. Here, the individual continues to implement behavior strategies in an attempt to avoid relapses. The authors estimate that maintenance generally lasts from 6 months to about 5 years for many health behaviors. As the maintenance of the desired health behavior becomes protracted, and heightened resistance to relapse develops, the person could enter the **termination** stage. Prochaska defines *termination* as the stage where your former problem behavior presents no threat or temptation to you. You have complete confidence that you can cope without fear of relapse. You are no longer in the stages of change as it relates to the problem behavior. At this point, your intent is not to return to the old unhealthy habit no matter what. According to Prochaska, you have exited the cycle of change, an important concept we will discuss next. Termination is not a practical reality for most health behaviors, and is alluded to here to denote the concept of exiting the cycle of change.

The Cycle of Change

The **cycle of change** operates within the stages of change and is related to readiness. People progress through the stages of change at varying rates. Typically, they move back and forth along the continuum a number of times before attaining the goal of maintenance. Regression or relapse may occur at any part of the change sequence. Thus the stages of change are better conceptualized as *spiraling* rather than linear (Prochaska et al., 1994) (Figure 3.3). This way of looking at relapse carries a positive connotation because relapse is viewed as a true learning experience rather than a failure. Successfully completing the journey from precontemplation to maintenance requires continuing application of the appropriate processes of change (Prochaska et al., 1994) and needs to include a relapse prevention plan.

Despite our best efforts, relapses remain the rule rather than the exception when it comes to solving most of our health behavior problems. We make mistakes because we are human; we are imperfect. It is normal at the time of our relapse to be conscious of our incompetencies while lacking awareness of our abilities. The feelings and beliefs evoked by relapses are not pleasant. You may feel as though you have completely failed, which may lead to guilt or embarrassment. You may begin to believe that all of your efforts were wasted. A couple of setbacks in succession may trigger your wanting to give up completely on changing the problem behavior, so you slide from the action or maintenance stage back to contemplation or precontemplation and decide that you have gained nothing from your attempts. This is where you are incorrect.

In the spiral model, the good news is that all of your setbacks are positive because the path you are taking is always spiraling upward. We can always rechart our steps

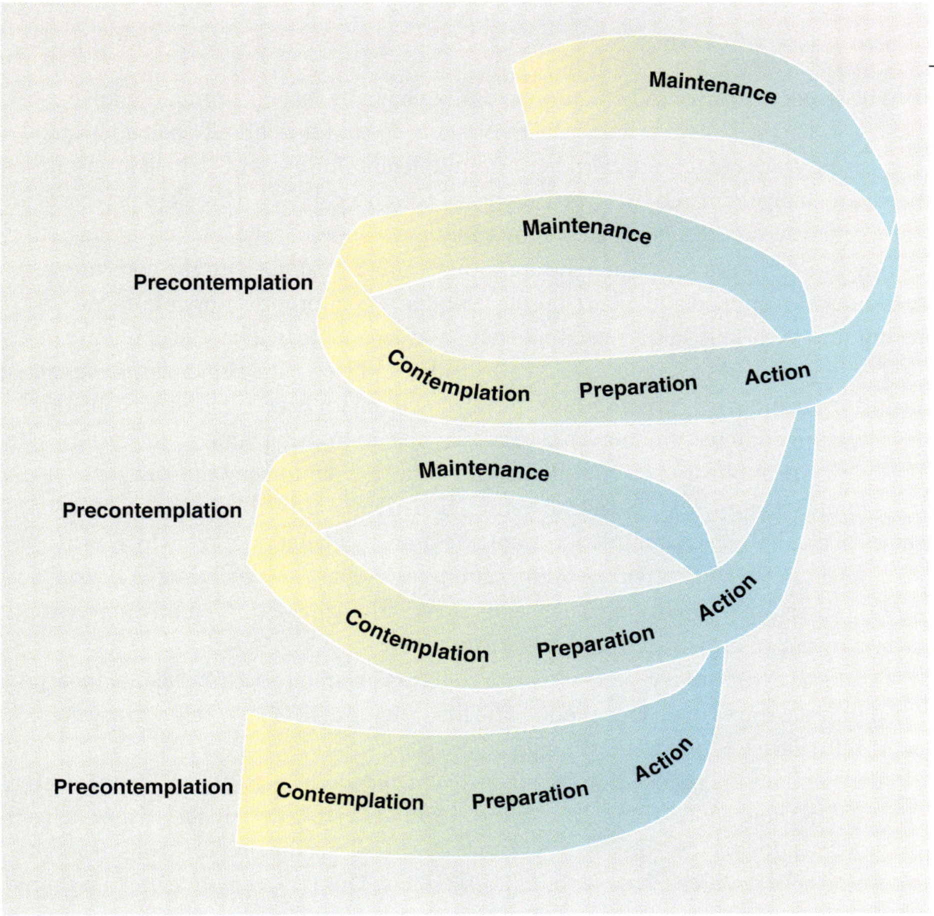

FIGURE 3.3

The Spiral of Change.
A spiral model of the stages of change.

SOURCE: J.O. Prochaska, C.O. DiClemente, and J.C. Norcross. (1992). In search of how people change: applications to addictive behaviors. *American Psychologist*, 47, 1102–1114. Copyright © 1992 by the American Psychological Association. Reprinted by permission.

and, armed with experience, make some corrections (see true learning–empowerment–envisioning concepts). Corrections triggered by our relapses lead to increased learning and can be responsible for improved outcomes. Never is a task completed without some modifications along the way. In fact, relapses may be thought of as necessary to keeping focused on our health behavior change. We need to dwell, not on the relapse, but on the remedy.

Prochaska and his colleagues found the majority of people they studied struggled for years to find effective solutions to their problems. They also found that the majority of relapsers do not go back all the way to precontemplation, but return to the contemplation stage—and, because they have learned from their recent efforts, soon begin to plan their next action attempt. Relapsing or, more appropriately, *recycling* on the spiral model of change provides many learning opportunities. Corrections triggered by our recycling may often be responsible for better outcomes. In fact, the researchers found that people who took action, then recycled or regressed in the next month, were twice as likely to succeed over the next 6 months than those who did not take action at all.

The stages of change model proposes behavior change as a process related to a person's readiness to change over a period of time. The stages are precontemplation, contemplation, preparation, action, maintenance, and termination. People progress through the stages at varying rates and frequently relapse to previous stages. Relapse is not a reprehensible thing. Never is a task completed without some modifications along the way. Our corrections of relapses are responsible for increased learning and can be responsible for improved future outcomes. In fact, relapses may be thought of as necessary to focusing on our health behavior change.

Processes of Change

Explore www.pahconnection.com 3.4

The stages of change call attention to particular shifts that occur in intention and behavior. This section describes how these shifts occur. Efficient self-change through the various stages requires incorporating ten different processes of change from various behavior change research theories (Prochaska & Velicer, 1997). These ten processes are comprehensive approaches that employ countless techniques. People move more efficiently through the stages when the appropriate process (along with the coinciding techniques) is applied at the correct stage. Similarly, inappropriate use of process and techniques at various stages may limit change or even increase chances of relapse.

The ten processes are grouped into *experiential* and *behavioral* principles. Experiential processes include: (1) consciousness raising, (2) dramatic relief, (3) self-reevaluation, (4) environmental reevaluation, and (5) social liberation; behavioral principles include: (1) helping relationships, (2) counterconditioning, (3) reinforcement management, (4) stimulus control, and (5) self-liberation. Experiential principles relate to the early stages of change (precontemplation, contemplation, preparation); behavioral principles are applied in later stages (preparation, action, maintenance) (Prochaska & Velicer, 1997). These processes of change are consistent with many of the cognitive-behavioral factors from Bandura's social cognitive theory.

In addition to these ten processes, two concepts you read about earlier are incorporated into the stages of change model. The first is Bandura's (1986) self-efficacy concept. Self-efficacy is important through all the stage transitions.

Engage www.pahconnection.com 3.4

Activities & Assessments 3.2, 3.3

Another measure included in the stages of change model is Janis and Mann's decision-making concept (O'Connell & Velicer, 1988). Creating decisional balance helps predict transitions across the stages of change by examining the pros and cons of adopting the behavior (Marcus, Rakowski, & Rossi, 1992). This approach measures a person's readiness to change.

During the precontemplation stage the cons tend to outweigh the pros. If this is true for you when you look at increasing your physical activity, then we must get you to a better understanding of its benefits to move you into the contemplation stage. If the gap between the pros and cons can be narrowed, you will be more likely to contemplate physical activity—and, when you begin to rate the pros higher than the cons, you will be much more likely to participate in physical activity and maintain your commitment to it.

CHANGING YOUR HEALTH BEHAVIOR

6. In progressing through the stages of change, we can utilize a variety of behavior change techniques.

Engage
www.pahconnection.com
3.2

We know that your level of readiness, or motivation related to modifying a specific behavior, is important to your success. The higher your level of readiness, the more likely you are to be successful in your efforts to change behavior. What stage of change did you relate to in the exercise (Engage 3.1)? If you rated yourself in the precontemplation or contemplation stage, your level of readiness is probably not yet sufficient to begin a physical activity program. The techniques we encourage you to use are increase your knowledge, acknowledge your feelings, and self-talk.

If you rated yourself in the preparation stage, your level of readiness is higher, and you are ready to make a detailed plan for developing your physical activity program. Adopting a physical activity program involves incorporating different techniques. The techniques recommended at this stage include *self-monitor, self-contract, plan of attack,* and *shaping.*

If you rated yourself in the action stage, you are already participating in some form of exercise. This stage is visible to others. You would most likely benefit from *self-reinforcement, social support,* and *reminder systems.* Finally, if you rated yourself in the maintenance stage, you want to retain the gains you have made through each of the stages (that is, prevent relapse) and we encourage you to apply the techniques used in the action stage.

Behavioral Change Techniques

It is important to recognize that each of the techniques mentioned here is aimed at modifying one or more of the factors that influence your current stage. By changing the influencing factor, you prompt changes in your readiness level. A technique that changes confirmed factors may not always be as effective as we would like. However, it will always be more effective than trying to change behavior with unsupported techniques. We now look at each technique.

Increase Your Knowledge Take time to further increase your knowledge about the benefits of physical activity (consciousness raising). You may want to explore the next few chapters of this book to check out the various types of physical activity and the benefits they provide. In addition, you can obtain further fitness information from your instructor as well as other health educators and fitness professionals, the World Wide Web, the mass media, and family and friends. Your college probably has health professionals to assist you, and you can also check with local hospitals, community agencies, and corporations that employ health professionals. A tremendous amount of health information is available in books, in magazine articles, and on the Internet.

A daily planner is a helpful behavior change tool.

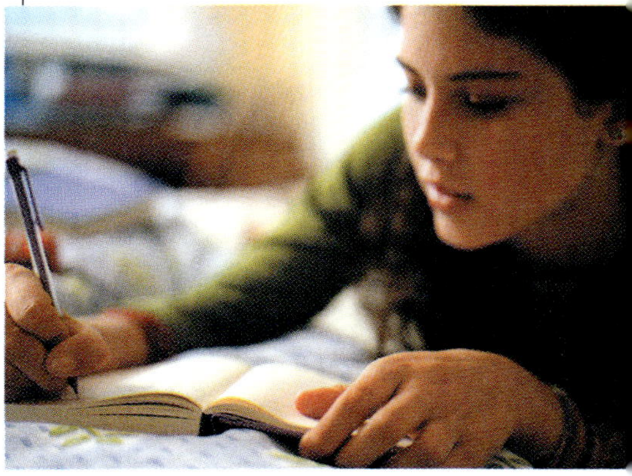

Acknowledge Your Feelings You may want to record how you feel about not intending to become physically active on a regular basis. To express your emotions about it (dramatic relief), try the following *rational emotive technique* recommended by Ellis and Harper (1971). Using a journal:

1. Record the events as they occurred at the time you felt emotionally uneasy about becoming physically active. Be objective and avoid judgments.
2. Next, write down your subjective assumptions, worries, and beliefs related to your emotions about becoming physically active.
3. Then, write down your emotions about physical activity, stating both appropriate and inappropriate emotions.
4. Finally, list your beliefs about why you had the right to be upset by the events and to respond the way you did. Is there support or truth for any of your beliefs? Last, explore appropriate alternative thoughts, emotions, and actions.

Self-Talk Use positive affirmations related to physical activity. An *affirmation* is a statement that claims the characteristics of the ideal self. This will help you examine your self-image related to physical activity. Do you say things such as "I don't like to exercise" or "I have to exercise" or "I should exercise"? These are all self-limiting statements. If you use them, it is important that you change your self-talk to the content of goal obtainment (self-reevaluation). Self-talk phrased in the negative regarding something positive is processed by the mind as a punishment and wastes valuable energy. Focusing on a more positive statement such as "I will find some type of physical activity I like," allows you to use your energy in a positive search for ways that will eventually lead to your goal. Continually increase the number of positive affirmations you make about physical activity. Such statements may include "I am confident that I can be physically active" or "I see myself as being physically active." Self-talk, when positive, cultivates a healthy self-image—one that offers security. Taking charge of the messages we send ourselves is an option that is always available to us.

Self-Monitor This technique involves behavior record keeping. Make a written record of the times you were physically active or inactive during the past two weeks. Next to each, write down the surrounding circumstances and whether or not you felt it was your choice. The act of simply monitoring and recording your behavior comprises a very powerful form for setting up specific objectives to reach your physical activity goals.

Experience 3.3
www.pahconnection.com

Self-Contract Make a physical activity self-contract with yourself (self-liberation). This interpersonal agreement to act should be consistent with your physically active self-image. You must understand what motivates you to be physically active and write it down. Research shows that goals are more likely to be accomplished when they are written down. Don't just think it, ink it! Be as specific as possible in detailing your goal of physical activity (Figure 3.4). Eliciting this type of personal commitment has been shown to be one of the most important aspects of health behavior change. When you commit in writing what you want to accomplish, you increase the likelihood that you will act accordingly within a certain period of time.

Plan of Attack Objectives are the steps you must take to achieve your goal (Figure 3.4). A carefully planned strategy is especially useful for physical activity because this health behavior ranges over a wide array of dynamic behavioral conditions (see Chapter 2). Therefore, it generally requires that more objectives be met compared to

Self-Contract

I ______________________ commit to begin a physical activity program.

Goal Type (Circle one) Short-term Mid-term Long-term

Goal: ______________________

Date goal set: ______________________

Date you'd like to accomplish goal: ______________________

Date goal accomplished: ______________________

Plan of attack for accomplishing my goal: ______________________

____

____

Goal re-evaluation and change from first writing: ______________________

____

____

FIGURE 3.4

Self-Contract.
When you commit in writing what you want to accomplish, you increase the likelihood that you will act accordingly within a certain period of time.

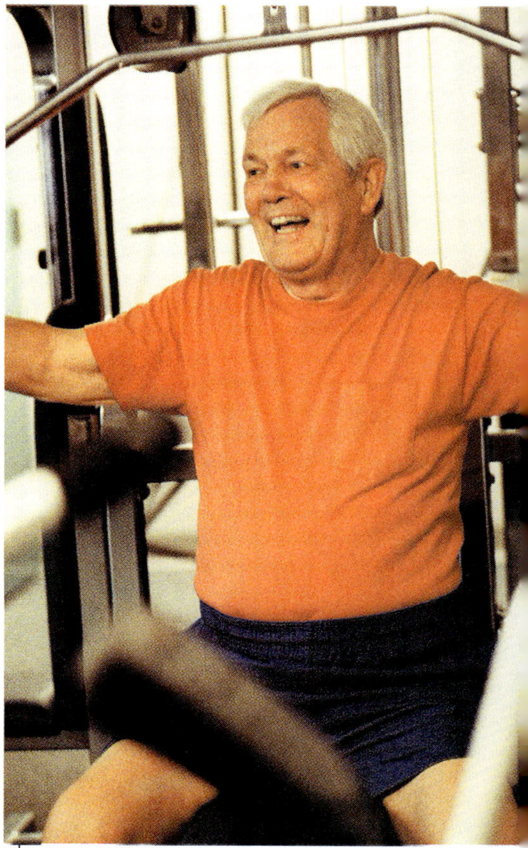

Repeated successful performances increase your confidence in your ability to perform the desired activity.

other health behaviors. We recommend orientating yourself to a variety of physical activities, which will help when it comes to developing different types of fitness—as well as avoiding boredom and over-use injuries.

Shaping Your Physical Activity Behavior Gradual increases make it easier to implement the desired behavior and significantly reduce your chances of becoming injured. Slowly and gradually work on increasing the frequency, intensity, and time of your specific activity.

Another important benefit derived from starting slowly is that through repeated successful performances of small tasks you will increase your confidence (self-efficacy) in your ability to perform your desired physical activity. As you gain self-confidence with each step, you will eventually build your self-efficacy for the entire task.

Social Support It is much easier to maintain your habit of regular physical activity if you are encouraged by others (helping relationships). Share your goals with your friends and family. Obtaining encouragement and support from significant people in your life is a powerful reinforcement for keeping you on your physical activity program. Social support can also be obtained by enrolling in classes and joining others who are physically active. Signing up for an exercise class at your college or university (social liberation) or organizing your own physical activity group that meets regularly are excellent ways to obtain social support.

Reminder Systems Place reminders throughout your environment to prompt you to be physically active (stimulus control). These reminders can take the form of notes left in places where you will see them, like your daily planner or the front of your refrigerator or television. Schedule specific daily times that you are going to be physically active. Another way to remember to be physically active is to keep your activity clothes in a highly visible location.

Self-Reinforcement Periodically check your goals and reward yourself for your progress toward specific goals (contingency management). Internal reinforcements are generally better than external ones. However, we recommend both. An internal reinforcement occurs when your own experience or perception of an event has value. For example, when you finish your run for the day you feel a sense of enjoyment or accomplishment. Relive your positive experiences by stating out loud to yourself and others that you are proud of your recent accomplishments: "I feel good about myself after running two miles." Remember, positive self-talk allows a flow of positive energy that not only makes a goal obtainable but can also significantly assist in maintaining it. An external reinforcement would be providing yourself with a special treat (for example, the purchase of a special item).

PHYSICAL ACTIVITY AND HEALTH CONNECTION

The path toward obtaining a high quality of life, or a wellness lifestyle, lies in our behaviors. Our choices and subsequent actions make our lives what they are. They *do* make a difference. Physical activity is one important health behavior choice. Planning for physical activity, its initial adoption, and your continued participation and maintenance can involve different factors and justify different behavioral techniques.

The stages of change model complements what is known about your readiness related to physical activity. You may be in *precontemplation,* not thinking about being physically active; *contemplation,* thinking about being physically active; *preparation,* seriously planning physical activity; *action,* doing some physical activity on a regular basis; or *maintenance,* maintaining regular physical activity. The methods you use to initiate and maintain a physical activity program may vary with whether you are trying to start or to maintain a physical activity program. Believing we can make positive health behavior changes is important in bringing about lasting health benefits. If we value physical activity as an important health behavior, we are more likely to participate in it and more likely to achieve the health benefits associated with being active. Behavioral skill building must be incorporated into your physical activity program if you are to become more physically active.

CONCEPT CONNECTION

1. **Lifestyle plays an important role in determining your quality of life.** Lifestyle, with its relationship to health, is considered an enduring pattern of behaviors. The persistence of these behaviors, as they relate to disease prevention, has become increasingly important. Seeming innocent acts, like not participating in regular physical activity or consuming foods high in fat content, account for the majority of disease, disability, and premature death in our society.
2. **Health behavior can be categorized by symptomatic and asymptomatic responses.** Some health researchers distinguish between behaviors related to health and to disease. The health behaviors where one responds to symptoms (disease conditions) include, illness, self-care, and sick-role. The health behaviors where one is acting in asymptomatic situations include wellness, preventive, and at-risk.
3. **Three universal learning principles—true learning, empowerment, envisioning—relate to our self-responsibility for health.** True learning occurs when you actively take control of your learning and subsequent actions. Many of our failures are rooted in the belief that we are not in control of our behavior. Empowerment means to give power or authority. In our context of life quality, empowerment is the process that promotes self-actualization among individuals. Finally, envisioning involves imagining what is possible and desirable regarding your health. These possibilities evolve from our own experiences, intuition, and desires.
4. **Reciprocal determinism, self-efficacy, and readiness are concepts important to understanding health behavior.** Reciprocal determinism is the constant, dynamic interaction that takes place among a person's cognitions, behavior, and environment. Self-efficacy is a judgment of one's capability to accomplish a certain level of performance, and readiness falls on a continuum from minimal to maximal motivation across each of the assorted steps required to change a habit or deeply ingrained behavior.
5. **The stages of change are a process of health behavior change.** The six stages of change are precontemplation, contemplation, preparation, action, maintenance, and termination.
6. **Progressing through the stages of change requires using various behavior change techniques.** These include increasing your knowledge, acknowledging your feelings, self-talk, self-contracting, self-monitoring, deciding on a plan of attack, shaping behavior, eliciting social support, using reminder systems, and providing self-reinforcement.

TERMS

Lifestyle, 57
Self-changers, 58
Health behavior, 58
True learning, 61
Empowerment, 62
Internal locus of control, 62
Envisioning, 62
Social cognitive theory, 63.
Reciprocal determinism, 64
Self-efficacy, 64
Readiness, 65
Stages of change, 66
Precontemplation, 66
Contemplation, 66
Preparation, 66
Action, 66
Maintenance, 66
Termination, 66
Cycle of change, 66

MAKING THE CONNECTION

Based on what you have read in this chapter about the stages of change, John would be considered to be in the precontemplation stage. John is not "ready" to begin a physical activity program at this time. He may need to increase his knowledge about the benefits of participating in a regular physical activity program. In addition, John may want to acknowledge his feelings related to participating in regular physical activity by using the rational emotive technique (page 70) described in this chapter.

CRITICAL THINKING

1. Often, like John, we are not ready to make a health behavior change, especially if we think our effort will be greater than the benefit of the behavior. List 10 reasons people begin a physical activity program (benefits) and 10 reasons people do not begin a physical activity program (barriers). Put an "L" next to the benefits that are long-term, and a "B" next to those that are short-term. Turning to the barriers, indicate which you have control over and which you do not. Do the barriers seem to outweigh the benefits? This time focus on short-term benefits and on barriers over which you have control. Does this change the picture?
2. As a friend, housemate, fraternity brother, or sorority sister, what role(s) can you play in supporting someone who is beginning a physical activity program? In analyzing your role, be aware of things you might do that would deter your friend from beginning or maintaining a physical activity program. Avoid those behaviors.

REFERENCES

Bandura, A. (1986). *Social Foundations of Thought and Action: A Social Cognitive Theory.* Englewood Cliffs, NJ: Prentice Hall.

Barsky , A.J. (1988). The paradox of health. *New England Journal of Medicine 318*:414–18.

DeJoy, D.M., Wilson, M.G., & Huddy, D.G. (1995). Health behavior change in the workplace. In Dejoy, D.M., Wilson, M.G., eds., *Critical Issues in Worksite Health Promotion.* Boston, MA: Allyn & Bacon.

Dishman, R.K. (1990). Determinants of participation in physical activity. In Bouchard, R.J. et al., eds., *Exercise, Fitness, and Health.* Champaign, IL: Human Kinetics.

Ellis, A., & Harper, R. (1971). *A Guide to Rational Living.* Hollywood, CA: Wilshire.

Girdano, D.A., & Dusuk, D.E. (1988). *Changing Health Behavior.* Scottsdale, AZ: Gorsuch Scarisbrick.

Greenburg, J.S. (1978). Health education as freeing. *Health Education* 9(2):20–21.

Hunt, W.A., Matarazzo, J.D., Weiss, S.M., & Gentry, W.D. (1979). Associative learning, habit, and health behavior. *Journal of Behavioral Medicine* 2:111–15.

Janis, I.L. (1983). *Short-Term Counseling: Guidelines Based on Recent Research.* New Haven: Yale University Press.

Kolbe, L.J. (1988). The application of health behavior research: Health education and health promotion. In Gochman, D., ed., *Health Behavior: Emerging Research Perspectives.* New York: Plenum.

Marcus, B., Rakowski, W., & Rossi J. (1992). Assessing motivational readiness and decision-making for exercise. *Health Psychology 22*:257–61.

Maslow, A.H. (1983). *The Farthest Reaches of Human Nature.* Magnolia, MA: Peter Smith.

McAuley, E. (1992). The role of efficacy cognitions in the prediction of exercise behavior in middle-aged adults. *Journal of Behavioral Medicine 15*:65–88.

O'Connell, D., & Velicer, W. (1988). A decisional balance measure and the stages of change model. *International Journal of the Additions 23*:729–50.

Roberts, G.W., Banspach, S.W., & Peacock, N. (1997). Behavioral scientists at the Centers for Disease Control and Prevention: Evolving and integrated roles. *American Psychologist 52*(2):143–46.

Perry, C.L., Baranowski, T., & Parcel, G. (1997). How individuals, environments, and health behavior interact: Social cognitive theory. In Glanz, K., Lewis, F.M., Rimer, B.K., eds., *Health Behavior and Health Education: Theory, Research, and Practice,* 2nd ed. San Francisco: Jossey-Bass.

Prochaska, J.O., & Velicer, W.F. (1997). The transtheoretical model of health behavior change. *American Journal of Health Promotion 12*(1):38–48.

Prochaska, J.O., Norcross, J.C., & DiClemente, C.C. (1994). *Changing for Good.* New York: Avon.

Reed, G.R., Velicer, W.F., Prochaska, J.O., Rossi, J.S., & Marcus, B.H. (1997). What makes a good staging algorithm? Examples from regular exercise. *American Journal of Health Promotion 12*(1):57–66.

Rotter, J.B. (1966). Generalized expectancies for internal versus external control of reinforcement. *Psychological Monographs 80*: 1–28.

Turk, D.C., Rudy, T.E., & Salovey, P. (1984). Health protection: Attitudes and behaviors of LPNs, teachers, and college students. *Health Psychology 3*:189–210.

United States Department of Health and Human Services (January 2000). *Healthy People 2010* (Conference Edition in Two Volumes). Washington, DC.

Activities & Assessments

NAME ____________ SECTION ____________ DATE ____________

3.1 Stages of Change—Continuous Measure

DIRECTIONS

Please use the following definition of exercise when answering these questions:

Regular exercise is any planned physical activity (brisk walking, aerobics, jogging, bicycling, swimming, rowing) performed to increase physical fitness. Such activity should be performed 3 to 5 times per week for 20–60 min per session. Exercise does not have to be painful to be effective but should be done at a level that increases your breathing rate and causes you to break a sweat.

Please circle the number that indicates how strongly you agree or disagree with the following statements.
1 = Strongly disagree 2 = Disagree 3 = Undecided 4 = Agree 5 = Strongly agree

1. As far as I'm concerned, I don't need to exercise regularly.	1	2	3	4	5
2. I have been exercising regularly for a long time and I plan to continue.	1	2	3	4	5
3. I don't exercise, and right now I don't care.	1	2	3	4	5
4. I am finally exercising regularly.	1	2	3	4	5
5. I have been successful at exercising regularly and I plan to continue.	1	2	3	4	5
6. I am satisfied with being a sedentary person.	1	2	3	4	5
7. I have been thinking that I might want to start exercising regularly.	1	2	3	4	5
8. I have started exercising regularly within the last 6 months.	1	2	3	4	5
9. I could exercise regularly, but I don't plan to.	1	2	3	4	5
10. Recently, I have started to exercise regularly.	1	2	3	4	5
11. I don't have the time or energy to exercise regularly right now.	1	2	3	4	5
12. I have started to exercise regularly, and I plan to continue.	1	2	3	4	5
13. I have been thinking about whether I will be able to exercise regularly.	1	2	3	4	5
14. I have set up a day and a time to start exercising regularly within the next few weeks.	1	2	3	4	5
15. I have managed to keep exercising regularly through the last 6 months.	1	2	3	4	5

(continued)

3.1 Stages of Change—Continuous Measure (cont.)

16. I have been thinking that I may want to begin exercising regularly.	1	2	3	4	5
17. I have arranged with a friend to start exercising regularly within the next few weeks.	1	2	3	4	5
18. I have completed 6 months of regular exercise.	1	2	3	4	5
19. I know that regular exercise is worthwhile, but I don't have time for it in the near future.	1	2	3	4	5
20. I have been calling friends to find someone to start exercising with in the next few weeks.	1	2	3	4	5
21. I think regular exercise is good, but I can't figure it into my schedule right now.	1	2	3	4	5
22. I really think I should work on getting started with a regular exercise program in the next 6 months.	1	2	3	4	5
23. I am preparing to start a regular exercise group in the next few weeks.	1	2	3	4	5
24. I am aware of the importance of regular exercise but I can't do it right now.	1	2	3	4	5

SCORING:

Precontemplation (nonbelievers in exercise) items: 1, 3, 6, 9

Precontemplation (believers in exercise) items: 11, 19, 21, 24

Contemplation items: 7, 13, 16, 22

Preparation items: 14, 17, 20, 23

Action items: 4, 8, 10, 12

Maintenance items: 2, 5, 15, 18

SOURCE: Cancer Prevention Research Center (CPRC). Measures. Exercise: Stages of change—Continuous measure [On-line]. Available: http://www.uri.edu/research/cprc/Measures/Exercise01.htm; accessed 2/6/01.

Activities & Assessments

NAME ____________ SECTION ____________ DATE ____________

3.2 Self-Efficacy toward Physical Activity

Directions: Please circle the number that indicates your response to these statements:

1 = Not confident 2 = Slightly confident 3 = Moderately confident 4 = Very confident 5 = Extremely confident

I am confident that I can participate in regular exercise when:

Negative Affect					
1. I am under a lot stress.	1	2	3	4	5
2. I am depressed.	1	2	3	4	5
3. I am anxious.	1	2	3	4	5
Excuse Making					
1. I feel I don't have time.	1	2	3	4	5
2. I don't feel like it.	1	2	3	4	5
3. I am busy.	1	2	3	4	5
Must Exercise Alone					
1. I am alone.	1	2	3	4	5
2. I have to exercise alone.	1	2	3	4	5
3. My exercise partner decides not to exercise today.	1	2	3	4	5
Inconvenient to Exercise					
1. I don't have access to exercise equipment.	1	2	3	4	5
2. I am traveling.	1	2	3	4	5
3. My gym is closed.	1	2	3	4	5
Resistance from Others					
1. My friends don't want me to exercise.	1	2	3	4	5
2. My significant other does not want me to exercise.	1	2	3	4	5
3. I am spending time with friends or family who do not exercise.	1	2	3	4	5
Bad Weather					
1. It's raining or snowing.	1	2	3	4	5
2. It's cold outside.	1	2	3	4	5
3. The roads or sidewalks are snowy.	1	2	3	4	5

SOURCE: Cancer Prevention Research Center (CPRC). Measures. Exercise: Self-efficacy [On-line]. Available: http://www.uri.edu/research/cprc/Measures/Exercise04.htm; accessed 2/6/01.

REFERENCES: Benisovich, S.V., Rossi, J.S., Norman, G.J., and Nigg, C.R. "A multidimensional approach to exercise self-efficacy: Relationship with exercise behavior and attitudes towards exercise." Paper presented at the annual meeting of the New England Psychological Association, Boston, March 1998; Benisovich, S.V., Rossi, J.S., Norman, G.J. & Nigg, C.R. "Development of a multi-dimensional measure of exercise self-efficacy." Poster presented at the Society of Behavioral Medicine (SBM), New Orleans, March 1998; Marcus, B.H., Selby, V.C., Niaura, R.S., & Rossi, J.S. (1992). "Self-efficacy and the stages of exercise behavior change." *Research Quarterly for Exercise and Sport* 63:60–66.

Activities & Assessments

NAME ____________ SECTION ____________ DATE ____________

3.3 Pros and Cons of Physical Activity

Directions: Please circle the number that indicates your response to these statements:

1 = Not Important 2 = Slightly Important 3 = Modernly Important 4 = Very Important 5 = Extremely Important

1. I would have more energy for my family and friends if I exercised regularly.	1	2	3	4	5
2. Regular exercise would help me relieve tension.	1	2	3	4	5
3. I would feel more confident if I exercised more.	1	2	3	4	5
4. I would sleep more soundly if I exercised regularly.	1	2	3	4	5
5. I would feel good about myself if I kept my commitment to exercise regularly.	1	2	3	4	5
6. I would like my body better if I exercised regularly.	1	2	3	4	5
7. It would be easier for me to perform routine physical tasks if I exercised regularly.	1	2	3	4	5
8. I would feel more comfortable with my body if I exercised regularly.	1	2	3	4	5
9. I would feel less stressed if I exercised regularly.	1	2	3	4	5
10. Regular exercise would help me have a more positive outlook on life.	1	2	3	4	5
11. I think I would be too tired to do my daily work after exercising.	1	2	3	4	5
12. I would find it difficult to find an exercise activity that I enjoy that is not affected by bad weather.	1	2	3	4	5
13. I feel uncomfortable when I exercise because I get out of breath and my heart beats very fast.	1	2	3	4	5
14. Regular exercise would take too much of my time.	1	2	3	4	5
15. I would have less time for my family and friends if I exercised regularly.	1	2	3	4	5
16. At the end of the day, I am too exhausted to exercise.	1	2	3	4	5

SOURCE: B.H. Marcus, W. Rakowski, and J.S. Rossi. (1992). Assessing motivational readiness and decision making for exercise. *Health Psychology*, 11(4):257–261.

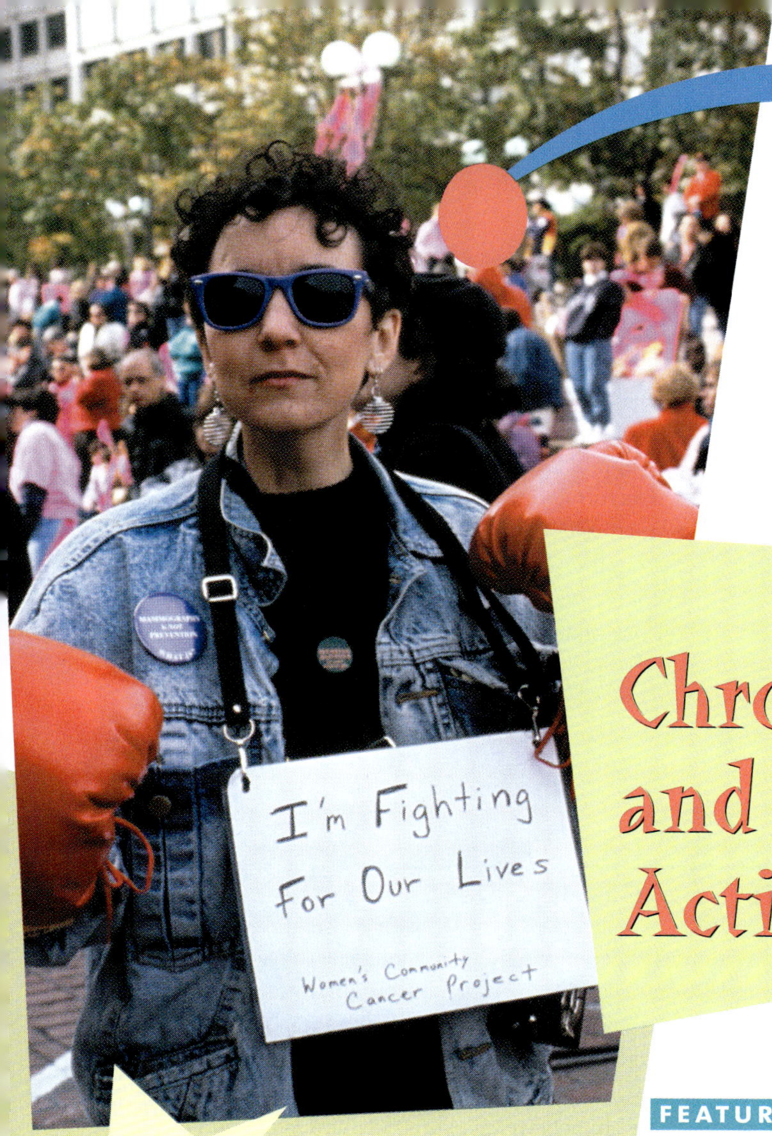

4

Chronic Diseases and Physical Activity

CONCEPT CONNECTION

1. The incidence of chronic diseases is steadily increasing.
2. Cancer is a group of diseases characterized by the uncontrollable growth and spread of abnormal cells.
3. Cancer is the second leading cause of death in the United States.
4. Lung cancer is the single largest cause of cancer deaths in the United States.
5. Breast cancer is prevalent among women, and physical activity is thought to be a protective factor.
6. Prostate cancer is the most prevalent cancer among men.
7. Colorectal cancer and physical activity is the most thoroughly investigated cancer–physical activity relationship.
8. Skin cancer is one of the most common forms of cancer.
9. Diabetes mellitus is a condition in which the body is unable to produce and/or properly use insulin.

FEATURES

E-Learning Tools: www.pahconnection.com

Engage www.pahconnection.com

- 4.1 Your cancer risk
- 4.2 Diabetes risk test
- 4.3 Diabetes quiz

Experience www.pahconnection.com

- 4.1 Health Oasis: Mayo Clinic cancer center
- 4.2 Ask NOAH about: cancer
- 4.3 FDA consumer

Explore www.pahconnection.com

- 4.1 About chronic disease
- 4.2 Chronic diseases and their risk factors
- 4.3 CancerSource
- 4.4 National Cancer Institute
- 4.5 American Cancer Society
- 4.6 Cancer Information Service
- 4.7 National Institute of Diabetes and Digestive and Kidney Diseases
- 4.8 American Diabetes Association

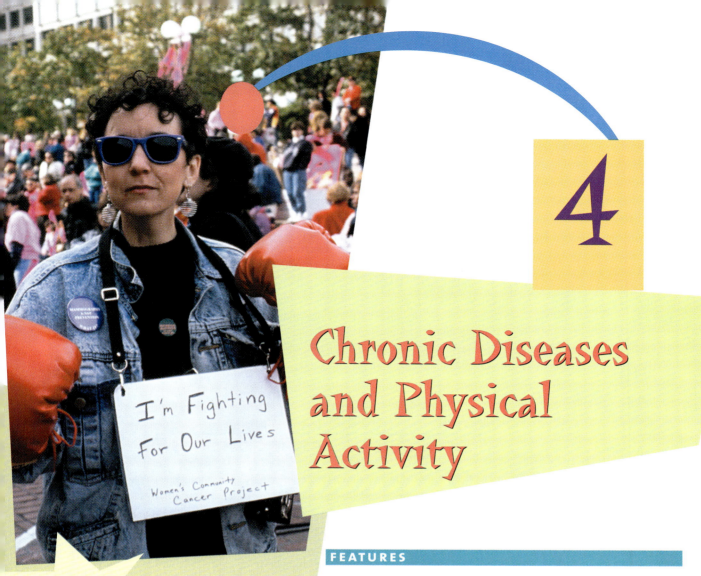

WHAT'S THE CONNECTION?

Monica has been smoking cigarettes for the past couple of years. She is aware that cigarettes are bad for your health, but savors the instant pleasure that comes from smoking. Besides, she believes she will be able to quit smoking once she graduates from college. Despite the large number of Americans who die annually from this disease, Monica had never thought that cancer would impact her—it was something that happens to others. This attitude changed abruptly in the past month. Last week Monica's uncle was diagnosed with lung cancer. His diagnosis came just weeks after her mother's best friend was diagnosed with colon cancer. Monica is understandably upset and concerned by these diagnoses of cancer. In an attempt to understand why these cancers occurred in people close to her, she begins to examine the causes of cancer.

Monica learns that, according to the National Cancer Institute, approximately 80 percent of all cancers are due to identified factors and thus are potentially preventable. Furthermore, as much as 35 to 50 percent of all cancers are due to our diet and another 30 percent are due to tobacco use. Monica begins to contemplate the role of her cigarette smoking as it relates to her risk of developing cancer.

> We as a nation must give chronic diseases the attention they demand. These diseases are the nation's leading killers, responsible for more than 70% of all deaths. The real tragedy is that many of the 1.7 million deaths among Americans from chronic diseases each year are in large part preventable.
>
> F.E. Thompson, Jr., MD, MPH
> State Health Officer and
> Chief Executive, Mississippi State
> Department of Health

1. The incidence of chronic diseases is steadily increasing.

> *Epidemiology* is the study of disease in the human population.

See Table 1.4, Ten Leading Causes of Death, 1900, 1998

Explore 4.1

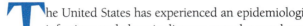

INFECTIOUS VS. CHRONIC DISEASES

The United States has experienced an epidemiological transition regarding infectious and chronic diseases over the past hundred years (Omran, 1977; 1971). There has been a dramatic decrease in infectious diseases (influenza, diarrhea) and an increase in chronic diseases (cancer, cardiovascular disease, diabetes). The decrease in infectious diseases is due in part to medical advances such as antibiotics and vaccines, as well as public health achievements that include safer and healthier foods, motor-vehicle safety, and healthier mothers and babies (Centers for Disease Control and Prevention [CDC], 2000a).

Until recently, bacteria, viruses, and other infectious organisms have caused millions of people to become ill and die. Improvements in sanitation, personal hygiene, nutrition, and immunization have drastically reduced deaths from infectious diseases in the United States. In many developing countries, however, infectious diseases (cholera, malaria) still cause millions of deaths per year. Although we have seen a decline in infectious disease mortality overall (Armstrong, Conn, & Pinner, 1999), today in the United States infectious diseases such as tuberculosis, hantavirus, and strep are increasing in number and frequency (Patlak, 1996).

Because many infectious diseases are caused by specific pathogenic organisms, the *etiology*, or cause of the disease, is often known. For instance, the etiology of tuberculosis is *Mycobacterium tuberculosis*. While infectious diseases are usually ascribed to a specific etiologic agent (tuberculosis, for example), in reality most infectious diseases do not have a single cause.

There are four methods to counter infectious diseases: sanitation, treatment with antibiotics and other drugs, vaccinations, and healthful living. Unlike infectious diseases, chronic diseases have a prolonged course that does not resolve spontaneously, and a complete cure is often not achieved. Chronic diseases are not treated with antibiotics, and to date we have no vaccination for cancer or heart disease. Chronic diseases are characterized by uncertain etiology, multiple risk factors, a long *latency period* (when you are infected but not showing signs or symptoms of the disease), a prolonged course of illness, and a noncontagious origin (Brownson, Remington, & Davis, 1998a).

The incidence of chronic diseases has seen a steady increase over the past century. The major chronic disease killers—cardiovascular disease, cancer, diabetes, and chronic obstructive pulmonary disease (COPD)—are basically caused by what people *do* or *do not do;* this is why they are sometimes referred to as "lifestyle diseases." Approximately 7 out of every 10 deaths in the United States result from a chronic disease (CDC, 1999). Not only are the costs in lives overwhelming but the medical costs due to chronic diseases are also staggering; over $400 billion annually, or more than 60 percent of the total medical care expenditures in the United States, is spent on treating chronic diseases.

Incidence refers to the frequency of occurrence of a particular disease, the number of new cases of a disease. *Prevalence* is the predominance of a disease, the number of people who have the disease at one given point in time.

Although chronic diseases are often referred to as lifestyle diseases, the environment we live in and our access to preventive services and medical care are also important. An example of a lifestyle choice would be choosing not to smoke, but if your parents and co-workers smoked, you would be exposed to secondhand smoke (environmental tobacco smoke [ETS]), which increases your risk of cardiovascular disease and/or cancer. Often as individuals we do not have access to primary, secondary, or tertiary prevention programs and services. *Primary prevention* reduces disease incidence (immunizations). *Secondary prevention* decreases the duration and severity of the disease through early detection and treatment before signs and symptoms occur (mammograms). *Tertiary prevention* reduces the complications of the existing disease (someone who has had a heart attack joins a cardiac rehabilitation exercise program). "Although individuals have a choice in these matters [personal health choices], as early as 1952 the President's Commission on Health Needs of the Nation noted that individual responsibility for health can be fully effective only if society ensures access to necessary education and professional services" (Breslow, 1999, p. 1030).

Explore www.pahconnection.com
4.2, 4.3

physical activity and health connection

However, chronic diseases do not have to decrease our quality of life or cause an early death because we know that *how we live* can significantly decrease our risk of getting such a disease (Hahn, Teutsch, Rothenberg, & Marks, 1990). Three risk behaviors in particular—lack of physical activity, tobacco use, and poor nutrition—are major contributors to both cardiovascular disease and cancer, our nation's number one and number two causes of death. After reviewing the leading causes of death among all ages, and among those 15–24 years of age, and taking into consideration the role physical activity plays in decreasing the morbidity and mortality among these illnesses, we decided to focus here on three chronic diseases: cardiovascular disease, cancer, and diabetes. This chapter will review cancer and diabetes with emphasis on the importance of self-responsibility in maintaining a positive lifestyle *early in life*. Both Chapters 5 and 6 address cardiovascular disease.

2. Cancer is a group of diseases characterized by an uncontrollable growth and spread of abnormal cells.

WHAT IS CANCER?

Cancer is actually a group of more than one hundred diseases characterized by the uncontrollable growth and spread of abnormal cells. In normal body cells the rate of cell division is controlled; however, when cancer is present, the cells divide rapidly, assuming irregular shapes, and tumors develop and invade normal tissue. The two types of **tumors** are benign and malignant. **Benign** tumors grow slowly and remain localized, but a **malignant** tumor grows rapidly and infiltrates surrounding tissues, frequently infiltrating the bloodstream and lymphatic system. When cancer spreads from its primary site to another site, the process is called **metastasis.** The term *cancer* is used to indicate any type of malignant tumor.

Tumors are named according to the type of tissues and cells from which they originate. There are many types of malignant tumors but they all can be classified into three groups: carcinoma, sarcoma, and leukemia. Like most classification systems, there are exceptions. Although they do not fall into one of the three groups just mentioned, lymphomas and skin tumors have their own separate classifications (Table 4.1).

Cancer A term for diseases in which abnormal cells divide without control. Cancer cells can invade nearby tissues and spread through the bloodstream and lymphatic system to other parts of the body.

Tumor An abnormal mass of tissue that results from excessive cell division. Tumors perform no useful body function and can be benign or malignant.

Benign Not cancerous; does not invade nearby tissue or spread to other parts of the body.

Malignant Cancerous; a growth with a tendency to invade and destroy nearby tissue and spread to other parts of the body.

Metastasis The spread of cancer from one part of the body to another. Cells in the metastatic (secondary) tumor are the same as those in their original (primary) tumor.

Experience www.pahconnection.com
4.1

TABLE 4.1 Classification of Malignant Tumors

CLASSIFICATION	DEFINITION	EXAMPLE(S)
Carcinoma	Any malignant tumor arising from surface, glandular, or parenchymal epithelium.	Squamous cell carcinoma of the esophagus Adenocarcinoma of the pancreas
Sarcoma	A general term referring to a malignant tumor arising from primary tissues other than the surface, glandular, or parenchymal epithelium. Prefixing the term by designating the cell of origin identifies the exact type of sarcoma.	Chondrosarcoma (cartilage) Fibrosarcoma (fibrous tissue) Myosarcoma (muscle) Osteosarcoma (bone)
Leukemia Lymphomas	Any neoplasm of blood-forming tissues. All tumors of lymphoid tissue are lymphomas. Lymphomas are malignant, with rare exception.	Hodgkin's disease
Melanomas	Skin tumors that arise from the keratin-forming cells or pigment-producing cells of the epidermis	Basal cell carcinoma Squamous cell carcinoma (a more aggressive tumor)

SOURCE: Adapted from L.V. Crowley. (2001). *Introduction to Human Disease* (5th ed.). Sudbury, MA: Jones and Bartlett .

UNDERSTANDING CANCER

3. Cancer is the second leading cause of death in the United States.

Mortality refers to the death rate, generally per 100,000 population. *Morbidity* refers to illness rate.

Cancer is the second leading cause of death in the United States. Approximately 1 out of every 2 American males and 1 out of every 3 American females will develop some type of cancer during their lifetimes, and about 1 person in 4 will die from cancer. Since 1990 alone, approximately 13 million new cases of cancer have been diagnosed.

Between 1970 and 1994, 10.6 million Americans died from cancer (National Cancer Institute [NCI], 1999a). Approximately 60 percent of all cancer deaths among men were due to four primary sites of cancer: lung, prostate, colon, and pancreas. Among women, almost 60 percent of all cancer deaths were due to cancers of the breast, lung, colon, ovary, and pancreas. For both men and women, four major cancers (lung, colorectal, breast, and prostate) account for 55 percent of the deaths from cancer (Ames, Gold & Willett, 1995). In addition to the human toll of cancer, the financial costs are staggering, with an estimated $107 billion for medical costs (United States Department of Health and Human Services [USDHHS], 2000a). The good news is that, overall, we are seeing trends that suggest certain cancer deaths are decreasing (stomach, uterine, and colorectal cancers in women; stomach, prostate, and colorectal cancers in men) (Figure 4.1).

Explore 4.4

Despite this rather dismal outlook, most cancers can be prevented. Several researchers have estimated overall cancer deaths due to various causes/factors (Table 4.2). Brownson, Reif, Alavanja, and Bal (1998b, p. 340) suggest "priority must be given to eliminating tobacco use, becoming more physically active, and adopting diets that contain less fat and more fresh fruits and vegetables." The data presented in Table 4.2

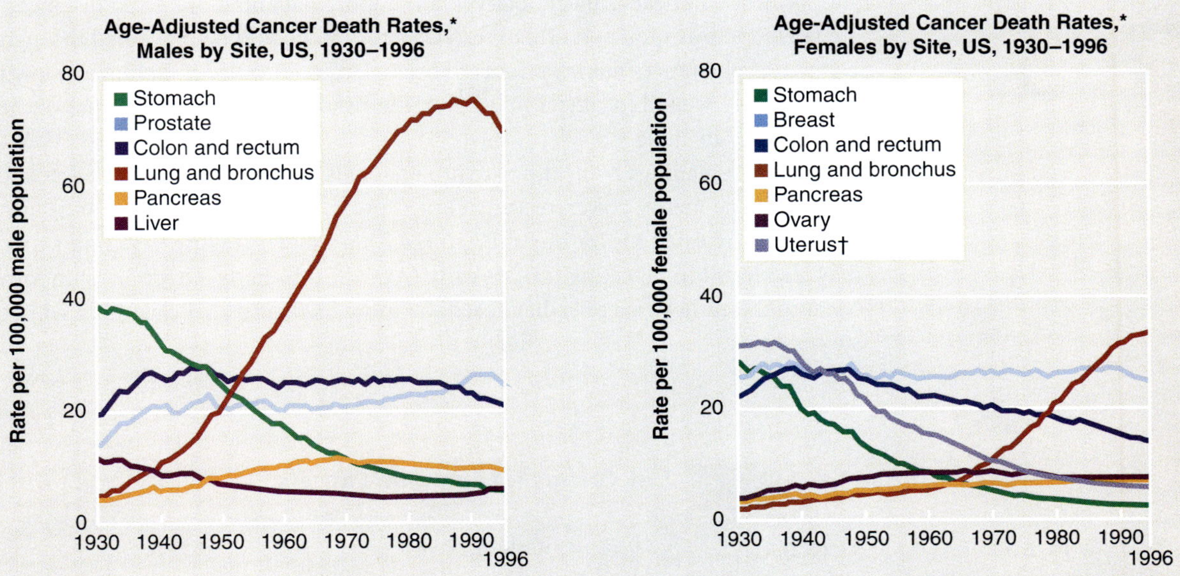

*Per 100,000, age-adjusted to the 1970 US standard population.
Note: Due to changes in ICD coding, numerator information has changed over time. Rates for cancers of the liver, lung and bronchus, and colon and rectum are affected by these coding changes.

*Per 100,000, age-adjusted to the 1970 US standard population.
†Uterus cancer death rates are for uterine cervix and uterine corpus combined.
Note: Due to changes in ICD coding, numerator information has changed over time. Rates for cancers of the uterus, ovary, lung and bronchus, and colon and rectum are affected by these coding changes.

FIGURE 4.1

Age-Adjusted Cancer Deaths, Males and Females by Site, United States, 1930–1996.

SOURCE: Reprinted by permission of the American Cancer Society, Inc.

TABLE 4.2 Estimates of the Proportion of Cancer Deaths Attributed to Various Factors

FACTOR ESTMATE (%)	DOLL & PETO ESTIMATE (%)	HARVARD ESTIMATE (%)	MILLER ESTIMATE (%)
Tobacco	30	29	30
Diet	35	20	30
Infective processes	10	—	5[a]
Occupation	4	9	5
Family history	—	8	5
Reproductive and sexual history	7	7[b]	3
Sedentary lifestyle	—	—	5
Perinatal factors/growth[c]	—	—	5
Geophysical[d]	3	1	2
Alcohol[e]	3	6	3
Socioeconomic status	—	—	3
Pollution	2	—	2
Medication and medical procedures	1	2[f]	1
Industrial and consumer products	<1	—	
Salt/other food additives/ contaminants	—	—	1

a. Viruses and other biologic agents.
b. Attributed to parity (4%) and sexual activity (3%).
c. Excess energy intake early in life and/or larger birth weight.
d. Mainly natural background radiation and sunlight.
e. With the exception of liver cancer, most alcohol-related cancers result from the combination of alcohol consumption and cigarette smoking.
f. Attributed to drugs (1%) and radiation (1%).

SOURCE: R.C. Brownson, J.S. Reif, M.C.R. Alavanja and D.G. Bal. (1998). Cancer. In R.C. Brownson, P.L. Remington and J.R. Davis (Eds.), *Chronic disease epidemiology and control*, 2nd ed. Washington, DC: American Public Health Association.

Explore 4.5

support the American Cancer Society's contention that about one-third of cancer deaths are related to nutrition and other lifestyle factors and could be prevented through behavioral changes (American Cancer Society [ACS], 2000). Although we know many of the factors related to cancer in general, the risk factors for specific types of cancer are provided in Table 4.3.

Regular screenings by health care professionals can result in the early detection of cancers of the breast, colon, rectum, cervix, prostate, testis, oral cavity, and skin (Table 4.4). Self-examinations for breast (Figure 4.2), testicular (Figure 4.3), and skin cancer may also result in detecting tumors early (ACS, 2000). Early detection is important, because the earlier cancer is diagnosed the more likely it is that treatment will be successful.

TABLE 4.3 Risk Factors for Common Cancers

CANCER	RISK FACTORS
Lung cancer	• Cigarette smoking is the greatest risk factor • Others include exposure to industrial substances, some organic chemicals, radon and asbestos, air pollution, tuberculosis, and environmental tobacco smoke in nonsmokers
Breast cancer	• Age • Personal or family history • A long menstrual history (menstrual periods starting early in life and ending late in life) • Recent use of oral contraceptives or postmenopausal estrogen • Never had children or had their first child after age 30 • Consume 2 or more drinks of alcohol daily • Higher education and socioeconomic status • New research is looking into susceptibility genes for breast cancer (BRCA1 and BRCA2)
Prostate cancer	• Age (more than 75% of all prostate cancers are diagnosed in men over age 65) • Black Americans have the highest prostate cancer incidence rates in the world • Strong familial disposition • Dietary fat may also be a factor
Colorectal cancer	• Personal or family history of colorectal cancer or polyps • Low-fat and/or high-fiber diet • Physical inactivity
Skin cancer	• Excessive exposure to ultraviolet radiation • Fair complexion • Occupational exposure to coal tar, pitch, creosote, arsenic compounds, or radium • Family history • Multiple moles (nevi) or atypical mole

TABLE 4.4 **Summary of ACS Recommendations for Early Detection of Cancer in Asymptomatic People**

SITE	RECOMMENDATION
Cancer-related checkup	A cancer-related checkup is recommended every 3 years for people aged 20–40 and every year for people age 40 and older. This exam should include health counseling and, depending on a person's age, might include examinations for cancers of the thyroid, oral cavity, skin, lymph nodes, testes, and ovaries, as well as for some nonmalignant diseases.
Breast	Women 40 and older should have an annual mammogram, an annual clinical breast examination (CBE) by a health-care professional, and should perform monthly breast self-examination. The CBE should be conducted close to the scheduled mammogram. Women ages 20–39 should have a clinical breast examination by a health care professional every 3 years and should perform monthly breast self-examination.
Colon and rectum	Beginning at age 50, men and women should follow *one* of the examination schedules below: A fecal occult blood test every year and a flexible sigmoidoscopy every 5 years.* A colonoscopy every 10 years.* A double-contrast barium enema every 5 to 10 years.* *A digital rectal exam should be done at the same time as the sigmoidoscopy, colonoscopy, or double-contrast barium enema. People who are at moderate or high risk for colorectal cancer should talk with a doctor about a different testing schedule.
Prostate	The ACS recommends that both the prostate-specific antigen (PSA) blood test and the digital rectal examination be offered annually, beginning at age 50, to men who have a life expectancy of at least 10 years and to younger men who are at high risk. Men in high-risk groups, such as those with a strong familial predisposition (i.e., two or more affected first-degree relatives), or blacks may begin at a younger age (i.e., 45 years).
Uterus	**Cervix.** All women who are or have been sexually active or who are 18 and older should have an annual Pap test and pelvic examination. After three or more consecutive satisfactory examinations with normal findings, the Pap test may be performed less frequently. Discuss the matter with your physician. **Endometrium.** Women at high risk for cancer of the uterus should have a sample of endometrial tissue examined when menopause begins.

SOURCE: Reprinted by permission of the American Cancer Society, Inc.

BREAST SELF-EXAMINATION (BSE)

By regularly examining her own breasts, a woman is likely to notice any changes that occur. The best time for breast self examination (BSE) is about a week after your period ends, when your breasts are not tender or swollen. If you are not having regular periods, do BSE on the same day every month.

- Lie down with a pillow under your right shoulder and place your right arm behind your head.
- Use the finger pads of the three middle fingers on your left hand to feel for lumps in the right breast.
- Press firmly enough to know how your breast feels. A firm ridge in the lower curve of each breast is normal. If you're not sure how hard to press, talk with your doctor or nurse.
- Move around the breast in a circular (a), up and down line (b), or wedge pattern (c). Be sure to do it the same way every time, check the entire breast area, and remember how your breast feels from month to month.
- Repeat the exam on your left breast, using the finger pads of the right hand. (Move the pillow to a position under your left shoulder.)
- If you find any changes, see your doctor right away.

Repeat the examination of both breasts while standing, with one arm behind your head. The upright position makes it easier to check the upper and outer part of the breasts (toward your armpit). This is where about half of breast cancers are found. You may want to do the standing part of the BSE while you are in the shower. Some breast changes can be felt more easily when your skin is wet and soapy.

For added safety, you can check your breasts for any dimpling of the skin, changes in the nipple, redness, or swelling, while standing in front of a mirror right after your BSE each month.

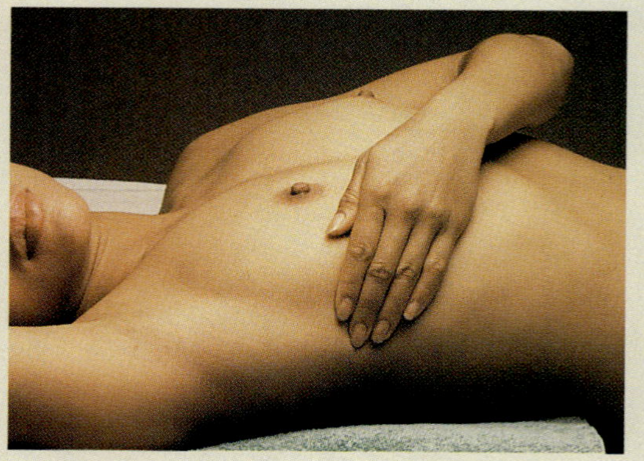

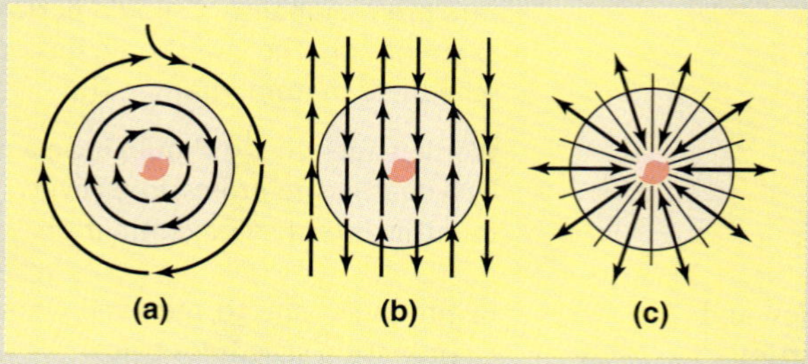

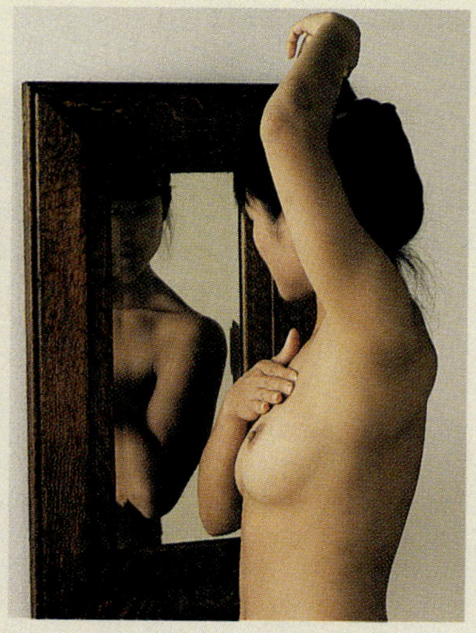

FIGURE 4.2

Breast Self-Examination (BSE). A monthly breast self-examination is recommended.

SOURCE: Reprinted by permission of the American Cancer Society, Inc.

The *Healthy People 2010* goal for cancer reduction is 158.7 cancer deaths per 100,000 population (USDHHS, 2000a), compared to over 200 cancer deaths per 100,000 population currently. In 1985, the National Cancer Institute set a goal of reducing cancer deaths by 50 percent by the year 2000 (Greenwald & Sondik, 1986); unfortunately, this goal was not met. However, we are seeing a decline in cancer deaths, in part due to systematic cancer control efforts. These efforts have six key elements: (1) reduce the prevalence of smoking, (2) reduce the percentage of total calories in the

TESTICULAR SELF-EXAMINATION (TSE)

You should examine your testicles regularly to check for changes or irregularities. Make sure to examine each testicle separately. See a doctor if you notice any of the following symptoms:

- A painless lump or swelling in either testicle;
- Any enlargement of a testicle or change in the way it feels;
- A feeling of heaviness in the scrotum;
- A dull ache in the lower abdomen or the groin (the area where the thigh meets the abdomen);
- A sudden collection of fluid in the scrotum;
- Pain of discomfort in a testicle or in the scrotum.

These symptoms can be caused by cancer or by other conditions. It is important to see a doctor to determine the cause of any symptoms.

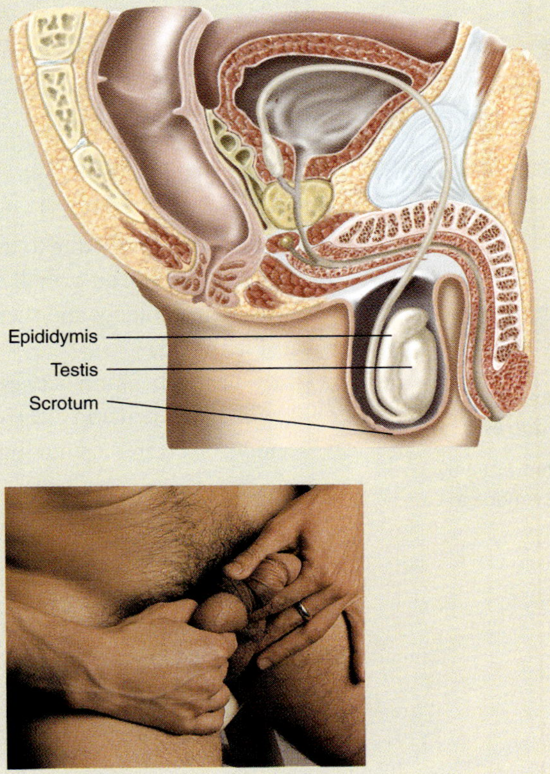

FIGURE 4.3

Testicular Self-Examination (TSE). A regular testicular self-examination is recommended.

SOURCE: Adapted from National Cancer Institute. (2000). *Cancer facts: Questions and answers about testicular cancer.* Available online: http://cis.nci.nih.gov/fact/6_34.htm.

diet from fat, (3) increase the average daily consumption of fiber, (4) increase the percentage of women who undergo annual breast cancer screening, (5) increase the percentage of women who have annual Pap tests, and (6) increase adoption of state-of-the-art cancer treatments. The majority of these efforts require the individual to take action—to quit smoking, to eat a nutritionally balanced diet, and to receive annual cancer screening.

Because many of the causes of cancer are known, it is possible to reduce cancer incidence rates. Ames et al. (1985) stated: "Decreases in physical activity and increases in smoking, obesity, and recreational sun exposure have contributed importantly to increases in some cancers in the modern industrial world, whereas improvements in hygiene have reduced cancers related to infection."

physical activity and health connection

COMMON CANCERS

Cancer can strike virtually any part of the body; however, it occurs more commonly in certain areas. Some cancers of particular concern include lung cancer, breast cancer, prostate cancer, colon and rectum cancer, and skin cancer.

4. Lung cancer is the single largest cause of cancer deaths in the United States.

Experience www.pahconnection.com 4.2

Explore
4.6

Anything that increases your chances of developing a disease is called a risk factor.

Lung Cancer

Lung cancer is the largest single cause of cancer deaths in the United States and is responsible for approximately 1 in 3 (28 percent) cancer deaths in this country (NCI, 1998a) (Figure 4.4). Lung cancer is the leading cause of cancer death among both men and women; however, since the early 1980s we have seen a decrease in lung cancer in men, and since the beginning of the 1990s the increase of lung cancer in women has slowed (ACS, 2000) (Figure 4.1). The decrease in lung cancer incidence and mortality rates is primarily due to the decrease in smoking rates over the past 30 years. Although there has been an overall decrease in smoking, we are still seeing a high percentage of women smoking, and there is an increase of tobacco use among youth (CDC, 2000b) (Figure 4.5).

The association between lung cancer and cigarette smoking is one of the most widely studied and clearly defined in cancer research. Based on numerous studies and reports, cigarette smoking is the strongest risk factor for lung cancer (Brownson et al.,

FIGURE 4.4

Leading Sites of Cancer Cases and Deaths—2000 Estimates.

SOURCE: Reprinted by permission of the American Cancer Society, Inc.

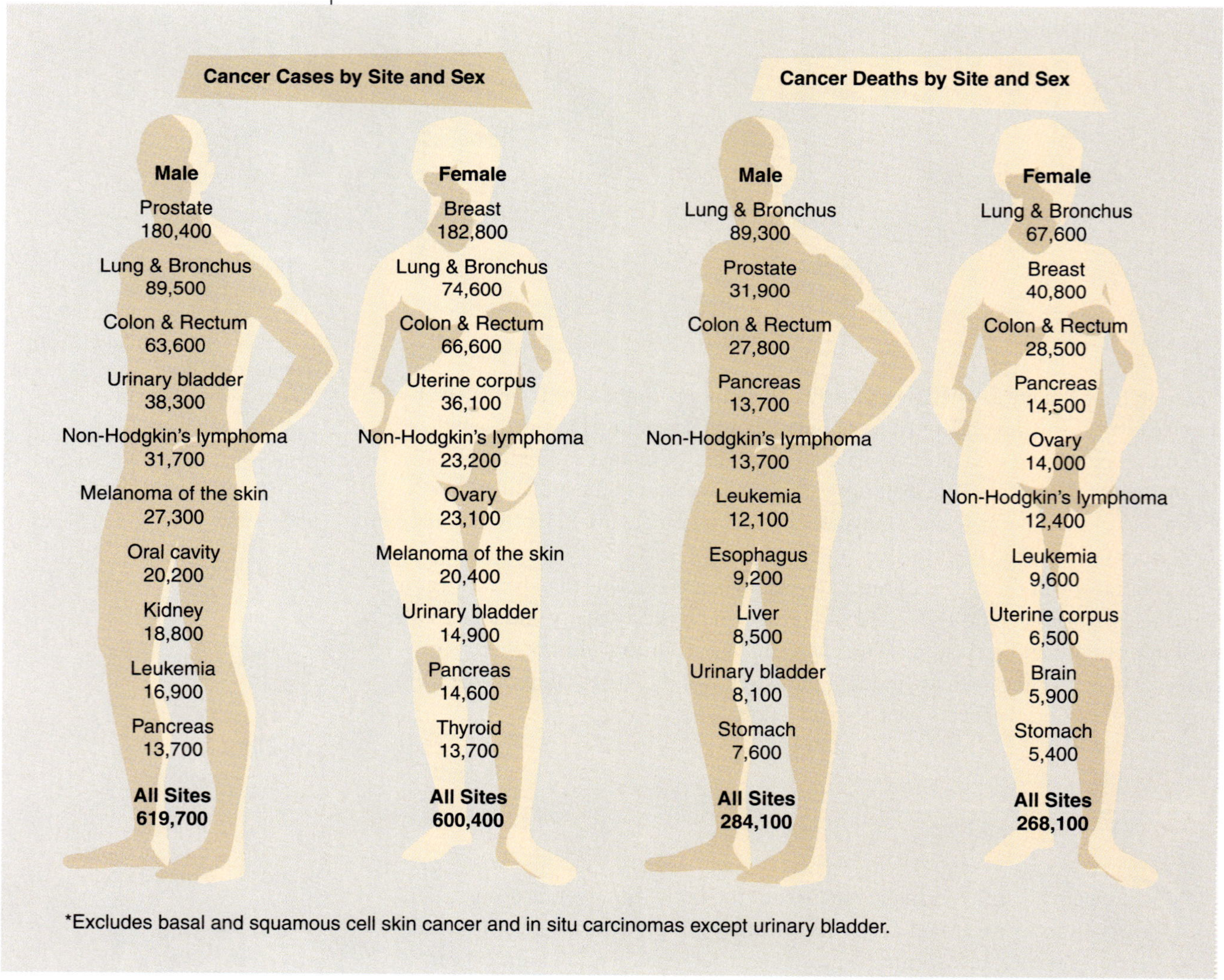
Cancer Cases by Site and Sex
Male
Prostate 180,400
Lung & Bronchus 89,500
Colon & Rectum 63,600
Urinary bladder 38,300
Non-Hodgkin's lymphoma 31,700
Melanoma of the skin 27,300
Oral cavity 20,200
Kidney 18,800
Leukemia 16,900
Pancreas 13,700
All Sites 619,700
Female
Breast 182,800
Lung & Bronchus 74,600
Colon & Rectum 66,600
Uterine corpus 36,100
Non-Hodgkin's lymphoma 23,200
Ovary 23,100
Melanoma of the skin 20,400
Urinary bladder 14,900
Pancreas 14,600
Thyroid 13,700
All Sites 600,400
Cancer Deaths by Site and Sex
Male
Lung & Bronchus 89,300
Prostate 31,900
Colon & Rectum 27,800
Pancreas 13,700
Non-Hodgkin's lymphoma 13,700
Leukemia 12,100
Esophagus 9,200
Liver 8,500
Urinary bladder 8,100
Stomach 7,600
All Sites 284,100
Female
Lung & Bronchus 67,600
Breast 40,800
Colon & Rectum 28,500
Pancreas 14,500
Ovary 14,000
Non-Hodgkin's lymphoma 12,400
Leukemia 9,600
Uterine corpus 6,500
Brain 5,900
Stomach 5,400
All Sites 268,100
*Excludes basal and squamous cell skin cancer and in situ carcinomas except urinary bladder.

1998b). Although physical activity may not directly impact your risk for lung cancer, smoking can affect your capacity to participate in sustained physical activity. Tobacco contains 43 known carcinogens plus nicotine, which is the substance that causes tobacco to be addictive. When tobacco is smoked, nicotine is rapidly absorbed through the lung's membranes and small airways. This absorption decreases the flexibility of the membranes and airways, thus decreasing the amount of oxygen available for sustained physical activity.

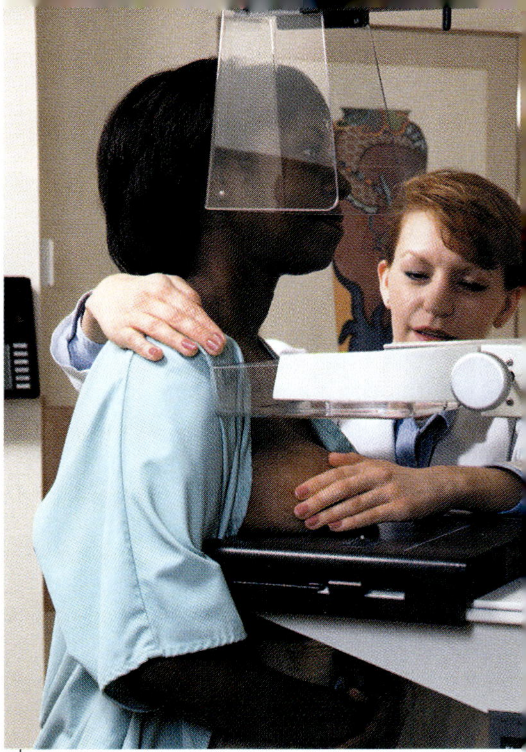

Mammograms are one means of detecting breast cancer early.

Breast Cancer

Breast cancer is the most commonly diagnosed cancer and the second leading cause of cancer deaths among women in the United States (ACS, 2000) (Figure 4.4). Breast cancer is the leading cause of cancer deaths among women aged 40 to 55 (ACS, 2000). The incidence rate of breast cancer increases with age, with approximately 77 percent of new cases of breast cancer occurring in women over the age of 50.

At the present, early detection through the use of mammography is the most effective method for detecting breast cancer early and before it spreads (CDC, 1999). Current estimates indicate that breast cancer mortality can be reduced by from 19 to 30 percent through routine clinical breast examinations and mammography screening for women 50 through 74 years of age (U.S. Preventive Services Task Force, 1996).

Healthy People 2010 set a goal to have 70 percent of women aged 40 years and older screened for breast cancer within the past 2 years (USDHHS, 2000a). Despite efforts to reach these goals, breast cancer screening services are still under-utilized.

5. Breast cancer is prevalent among women and physical activity is thought to be a protective factor.

Breast Cancer and Physical Activity There has been no abundance of research studies looking at the effects of physical activity on breast cancer. However, as reported in *Physical Activity and Health: A Report to the Surgeon General* (USDHHS, 1996), nine studies had been published to date. These studies were inconclusive in showing a statistically significant relationship between physical activity and breast cancer. However, since the release of the 1996 report, several studies have been published suggesting physical activity as a protective factor against breast cancer. Kavanagh, Singletary, Einhorn, and Depetrillo (1999) reported that women who spent 1 to 3 hours in physical activity per week reduced their risk of breast cancer by 30 percent as compared to

Engage
www.pahconnection.com
4.1

physical activity and health connection

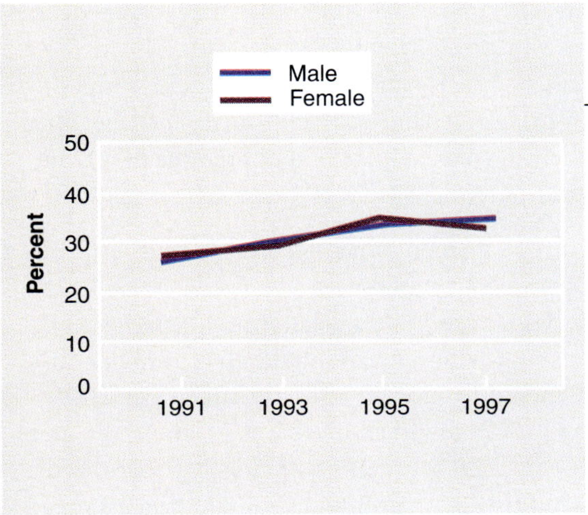

FIGURE 4.5

Percentage of High School Students who Smoked a Cigarette in the Past Month, by Gender.

SOURCE: Centers for Disease Control and Prevention, Division of Adolescent and School Health. (2000). *Assessing health risk behaviors among young people: Youth Risk Surveillance System At-a-Glance, 2000.* Atlanta, GA: Centers for Disease Control and Prevention. Available: http://www.cdc.gov/nccdphp/dash/yrbs/yrbsaag.htm; accessed 1/29/01.

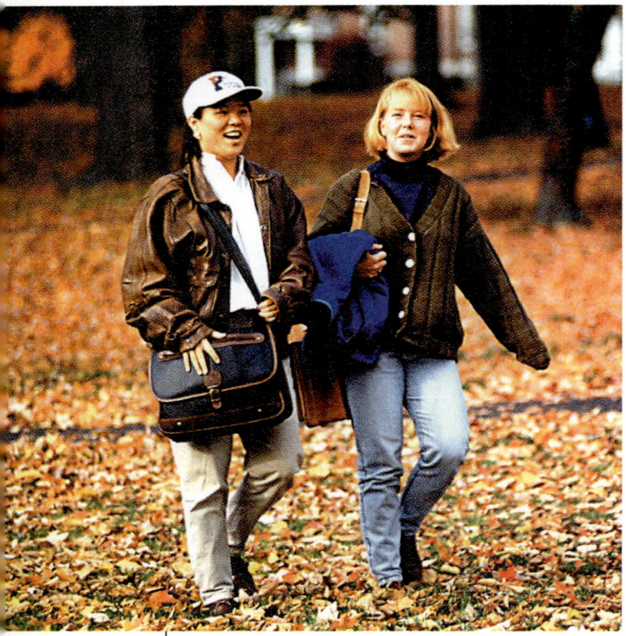

Physical activity may reduce breast cancer risk.

inactive women. They also noted that women who exercised at least 4 hours per week reduced their breast cancer risk by 50 percent. Another study evaluated the influence of physical activity, both work and leisure-time activity, on the risk of breast cancer in a group of 25,624 pre- and post-menopausal women (Thune, Brenn, Lund, & Gaard, 1997). The researchers concluded that physical activity during leisure time and at work is associated with a reduced risk of breast cancer.

A study conducted by the researchers at the Netherlands Cancer Institute compared the physical activity histories of 918 women aged 20 to 54 who had been diagnosed with invasive breast cancer to 918 women who did not have cancer (ACS News Today, 2000a). The researchers found that active women had a 30 percent lower risk of breast cancer than those who were inactive.

Despite knowing that physical activity in women reduces overall mortality, diabetes, stroke, osteoporosis, obesity, and disability (Powell, Caspersen, Koplan, & Ford, 1989), we still do not know the effects of physical activity on breast cancer. McTiernan (1997, p. 1131) states: "With respect to whether exercise reduces the risk of breast cancer, too many questions remain for women and their doctors to make informed decisions on whether, how, and how much to exercise." The verdict is still out as the researchers continue to ask "Does physical activity reduce one's risk of breast cancer?" and "If so, how and why?" Although the jury may still be out on the positive effects of physical activity on breast cancer, physical activity has not been shown to increase your risk—so go ahead and exercise!

An association between two factors compares the risk or incidence of disease among people within the population who have a certain characteristic (such as smoking) to those who do not have the characteristic.

6. Prostate cancer is the most prevalent cancer among men.

The PSA measures a specific protein in the prostate cells and is measured in nanograms per milliliter (ng/ml). Between 4 and 10 ng/ml is considered borderline and represents a higher likelihood of the presence of cancer.

Prostate Cancer

Prostate cancer is a major health problem worldwide and has been described as an epidemiological enigma (Mettlin, 1997), with many different suspected risk factors but few showing consistent or strong associations with the disease. Dramatic increases in prostate cancer occurred in the late 1980s and early 1990s in the United States, with peak incidence in 1992 (Mettlin, 1997; NCI, 1998b).

Prostate cancer is the most prevalent cancer among men and the second leading to cancer death among men (ACS, 2000) (Figure 4.4), with approximately 1 of every 11 men developing prostate cancer (Brownson et al., 1998b). Between 1989 and 1992 the prostate cancer *incidence* rates increased dramatically; however, between 1992 and 1996, prostate cancer *mortality* rates declined significantly (ACS, 2000). The increase in incidence rates could be due in part to earlier diagnosis in men without symptoms, increased use of prostate-specific antigens (PSA) blood test screenings, and digital rectal exams (DRE). Prostate cancer is rarely diagnosed in men under the age of 50, but the incidence rises faster for every decade after that (NCI, 1999b).

Prostate Cancer and Physical Activity Second to colorectal cancer, the effects of physical activity on prostate cancer are most commonly studied (USDHHS, 1996). Data to date reveal inconsistent results with regard to the relationship between physical activity and prostate cancer. Brownson, Chang, Davis, and Smith (1991) investigated the risk of various cancer types, including prostate and testicular cancer, in relation to occupational physical activity. They found an inverse association (the more physical activity on the job, the greater the risk) between occupational physical activity and prostate and testicular cancer, noting that their findings should be considered preliminary and require confirmation from other studies.

Colon and Rectum Cancer

Cancer of the colon and rectum, or *colorectal* cancer, is the second leading cause of cancer-related deaths in the United States (CDC, 2000c), and is the third leading cancer and cause of cancer deaths in both men and women (ACS, 2000a) (Figure 4.4). Colorectal cancer mortality is greater for men than women, and higher among blacks than whites (Brownson et al., 1998b). Two-thirds of the people who get colorectal cancer are over the age of 50. However, there are people under the age of 50 who get colorectal cancer (for example, Darryl Strawberry of the New York Yankees).

7. The relationship between colorectal cancer and physical activity is the most thoroughly investigated.

Colorectal Cancer and Physical Activity The relationship between physical activity and colorectal cancer has been the most thoroughly investigated cancer–physical activity relationship (USDHHS, 1996). Because some studies suggest that the relationship between physical activity and the risk of colon cancer may differ from the risk for rectal cancer, we will review the studies individually. Many studies have measured occupational physical activity and the risk of colon cancer (USDHHS, 1996; Brownson et al., 1991; Brownson, Zahm, Chang, & Blair, 1989). These studies have shown an inverse relationship between occupational physical activity and risk of colon cancer—meaning the less active one is on the job, the greater the risk of colon cancer. However, some researchers did not find a direct relationship between occupational physical activity and the risk of colon cancer (Arbman, et al., 1993; Vetter et al., 1992). Despite some conflicting results, the *Surgeon Generals' Report on Physical Activity* states: "Together, the research on occupational and leisure-time physical activity strongly suggests that physical activity has a protective effect against the risk of developing colon cancer" (USDHHS, 1996, p. 116).

Many of the same studies that investigated the relationship between physical activity and the risk of colon cancer also studied rectal cancer as a separate outcome. The overall conclusion from these studies suggests that occupational or leisure-time physical activity, or total physical activity, is unrelated to the risk of rectal cancer (USDHHS, 1996).

Skin Cancer

Incidence of one of the most common forms of cancer, skin cancer, has rapidly increased during the past three decades in the United States (Graffunder et al., 1999). The most serious form of skin cancer is melanoma; squamous cell and basal cell cancer are less serious types of skin cancer (NCI, 1999c). The number of new cases

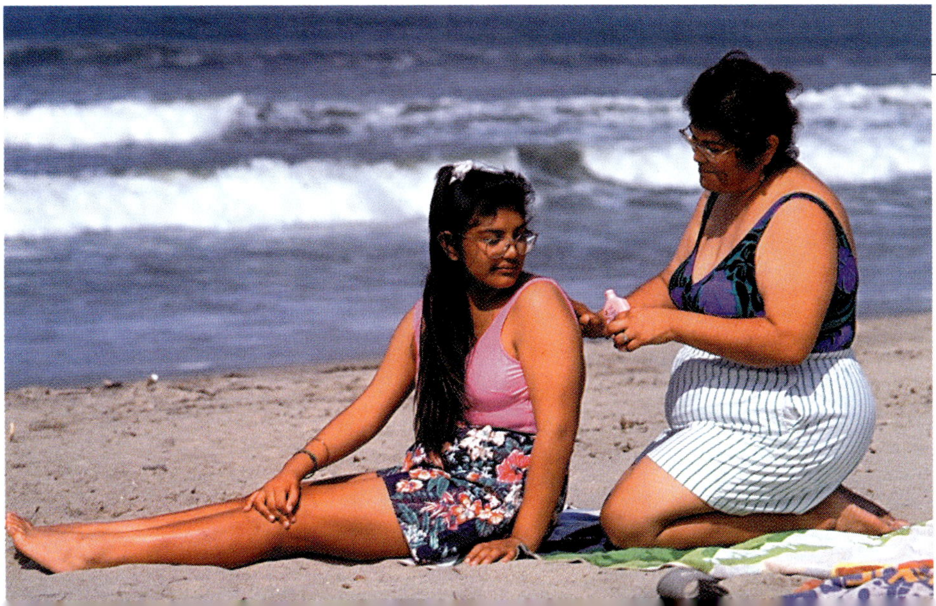

Using sunscreen can help prevent melanoma.

8. Skin cancer is one of the most common forms of cancer.

Experience www.pahconnection.com 4.3

Solar Protection Factor (SPF) A scale for rating the level of sunburn protection in sunscreen products. The higher the SPF, the more protection provided.

of melanoma has more than doubled in the past 20 years in the United States. Although melanomas account only for 4 percent of all skin cancers, they account for 79 percent of skin cancer deaths (ACS News Today, 2000b). Melanoma occurs when pigment cells (melanocytes) become malignant; it can occur on any surface of the skin.

Primary prevention is key to melanoma skin cancer. The sun's ultraviolet rays are strongest during midday (from the hours of 10 AM to 4 PM) and we should avoid or limit our sun exposure during these times. If you have to be outside, it is best to keep as much skin covered as possible, and use a sunscreen with an SPF **(solar protection factor)** of 15 or higher. The ACS suggests that you do a skin self-exam at least once a month (Figure 4.6). During your skin self-exam you need to look for changes in size, texture, shape, and color of blemishes or a sore that does not heal. The ABCD rule is a helpful guide to the signs of melanoma (Figure 4.7). When detected early, melanoma can be cured.

HOW TO DO A SKIN SELF-EXAM

Your doctor or nurse may recommend that you do a regular skin self-exam. If your doctor has taken photos of your skin, you can use these pictures when looking for changes.

The best time to do a skin self-exam is after a shower or bath. You should check your skin in a well-lighted room using a full-length mirror and a hand-held mirror. It's best to begin by learning where your birthmarks, moles, and blemishes are and what they usually look and feel like. Check for anything new, especially a change in the size, shape, texture, or color of a mole or a sore that does not heal.

Check yourself from head to toe. Don't forget to check *all* areas of the skin, including the back, the scalp, between the buttocks, and the genital area.

1. Look at the front and back of your body in the mirror, then raise your arms and look at your left and right sides.
2. Bend your elbows and look carefully at your fingernails, palms, forearms (including the undersides), and upper arms.
3. Examine the back, front, and sides of your legs. Also look between the buttocks and around the genital area.
4. Sit and closely examine your feet, including the toenails, the soles, and the spaces between the toes.
5. Look at your face, neck, ears, and scalp. You may want to use a comb or a blow dryer to move hair so that you can see better. You also may want to have a relative or friend check through your hair because this is difficult to do yourself.

By checking your skin regularly, you will become familiar with what is normal for you. It may be helpful to record the dates of your skin exams and to write notes about the way your skin looks. If you find anything unusual, see your doctor right away.

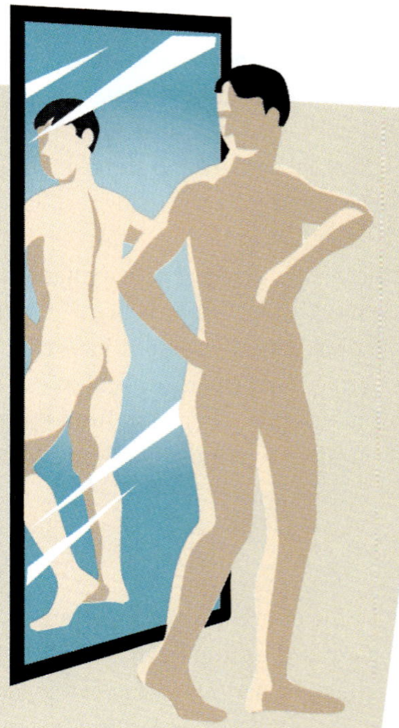

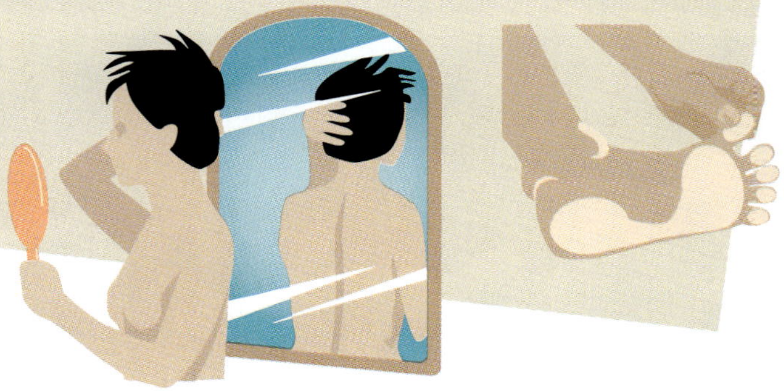

FIGURE 4.6

How to Do a Skin Self-Exam.

SOURCE: National Cancer Institute. (1999). *What you need to know about melanoma.* (NIH Publication No. 99-1563). Bethesda, MD: National Cancer Institute.

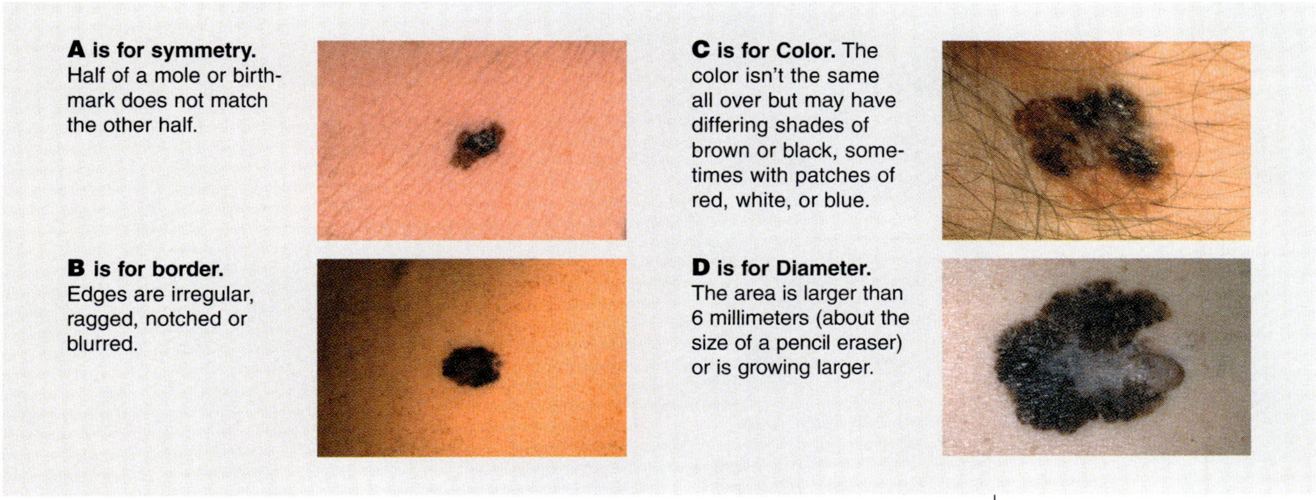
A is for symmetry. Half of a mole or birthmark does not match the other half.
B is for border. Edges are irregular, ragged, notched or blurred.
C is for Color. The color isn't the same all over but may have differing shades of brown or black, sometimes with patches of red, white, or blue.
D is for Diameter. The area is larger than 6 millimeters (about the size of a pencil eraser) or is growing larger.

FIGURE 4.7

ABCD Rule for Skin Cancer Detection.

UNDERSTANDING DIABETES MELLITUS

Diabetes mellitus affects approximately 16 million people in the United States, and over 5 million of these people do not know they have the disease (CDC, 1999). Diabetes has been ranked among the top ten leading causes of death in the United States since 1932 (Bishop, Zimmerman, & Roesler, 1998), and during the last decade it has been the seventh leading cause of death in the United States (USDHHS, 2000b) (Figure 4.8). Despite the fact that diabetes has been known for centuries, and is epidemic in many countries, our knowledge of the nature of diabetes is still incomplete (Zimmet, 1999).

Diabetes mellitus is a group of diseases in which the body is unable to produce and/or properly utilize insulin. Insulin, a hormone secreted by the pancreas, is needed by muscle, fat, and the liver to metabolize glucose. Diabetes is diagnosed by identifying high levels of blood glucose. There are four types of diabetes: Type 1, Type 2, gestational, and other. Type 1, or what used to be referred to as insulin-dependent diabetes mellitus (IDDM), is simply defined as diabetes caused by an inability to produce enough insulin. Five to 10 percent of the U.S. population has Type 1 diabetes. Diabetes is a serious, lifelong condition that can cause heart disease, kidney failure, and blindness.

9. Diabetes mellitus is a condition in which the body is unable to produce and/or properly use insulin.

Engage www.pahconnection.com **4.2, 4.3**

Explore www.pahconnection.com **4.7, 4.8**

Activities & Assessments **4.1**

Type 2 diabetes, or what was once called non-insulin-dependent diabetes mellitus (NIDDM), accounts for 90 to 95 percent of all diagnosed cases of diabetes. Type 2 diabetes is often associated with obesity and physical inactivity, which may account for recent occurrences of Type 2 diabetes among younger people. This type of diabetes allows sufficient production of insulin, but the body is unable to use it effectively. You have heard the term **hyperglycemia** used to describe a condition where there is too much glucose in the blood. Hyperglycemia means that your pancreas is not producing enough insulin or your body cannot use its own insulin well; both result in an increased amount of glucose in the blood. This is the opposite of **hypoglycemia**, which indicates insufficient glucose in the blood.

Gestational diabetes develops in 2 to 5 percent of all pregnancies and usually disappears when the pregnancy is over. Other type of diabetes result from specific genetic syndromes, drugs, malnutrition, infection, and other illnesses. This type of diabetes accounts for 1 to 2 percent of all diagnosed cases of diabetes.

Hypergylcemia Too much blood sugar.

Hypoglycemia Not enough blood sugar.

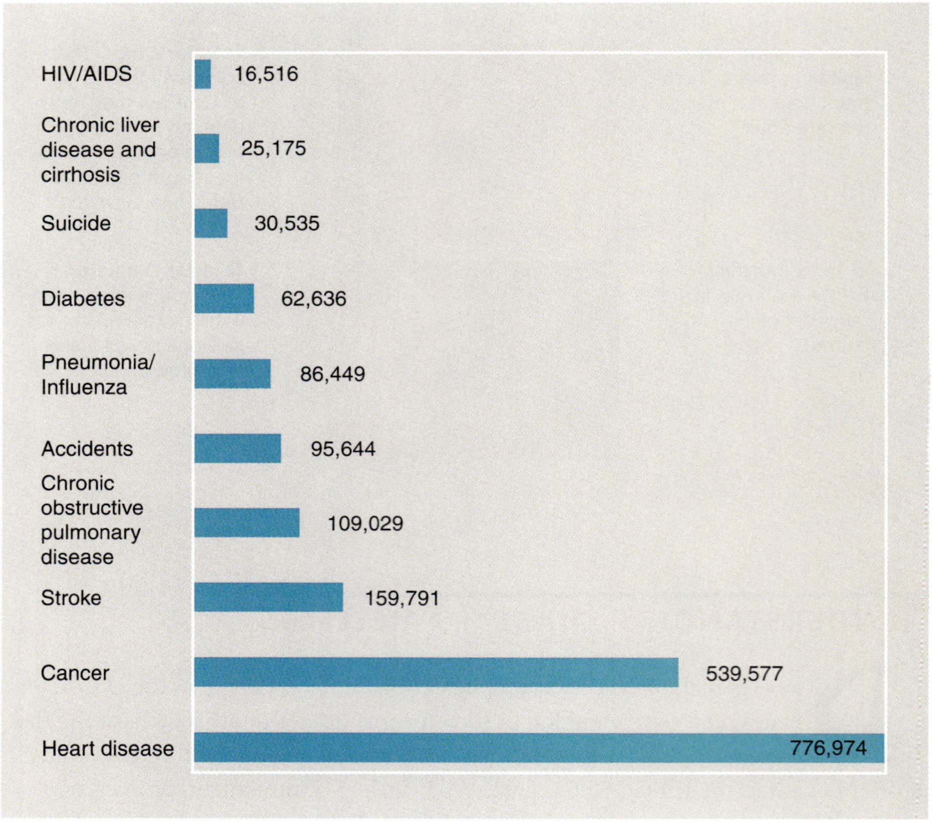

FIGURE 4.8

Chronic Disease Mortality.

SOURCE: National Center for Health Statistics, Centers for Disease Control and Prevention. (1999). Chronic disease mortality. *National Vital Statistics Report,* 47(19).

Type 2 Diabetes and Physical Activity

There is considerable research supporting the relationship between physical inactivity and type 2 diabetes (USDHHS, 1996). Studies suggest that exercise burns calories, which in turn helps with weight reduction, in turn improving the body's response to insulin (Health and Administration Development Group [HADG], 1999). Physical activity has been shown to play a role in the prevention of type 2 diabetes (Colberg & Swain, 2000). Frisch et al. (1986) found a significantly lower prevalence of diabetes among female athletes as compared to female nonathletes. In conclusion, the research literature suggests a strong relationship between physical activity and Type 2 diabetes: the more physical activity, the less the likelihood of developing Type 2 diabetes.

People with diabetes need to balance their diet and insulin (Type 1) with their physical activity regimen. Whether you have Type 1 or Type 2 diabetes, physical activity is a cornerstone in diabetes therapy.

TAKING RESPONSIBILITY FOR YOUR HEALTH

Although you may not be thinking about chronic diseases because you are young and healthy, at some point in your life it is likely that you or someone you care about will be diagnosed with a chronic disease. We now know what we can do today to decrease the chances of getting a chronic disease tomorrow. All the data to date suggest that risk factors for most chronic diseases are factors over which you have control—physical activity, cigarette smoking, and dietary habits. You have the ability to begin to make changes in your lifestyle today that can make a difference for you in the future, especially when you consider that physical activity is a protective factor for breast cancer, colon cancer, and diabetes.

PHYSICAL ACTIVITY AND HEALTH CONNECTION

During the last century, our society experienced a decline in the rate of infectious disease; at the same time, there was an increase in the rate of chronic disease. Chronic diseases are commonly related to lifestyle and their symptoms may take many years to surface. A lack of physical activity is a major contributor to the increased incidence of such chronic diseases as cardiovascular disease, diabetes, and several forms of cancer. Evidence now demonstrates that, by leading a physically active lifestyle, you can reduce your risk for developing hypertension, stroke, heart attack, breast cancer, colorectal cancer, and Type 2 diabetes. Physical activity plays its most important role in the prevention of chronic diseases, but in certain circumstances (cardiovascular disease, diabetes), it can also play an important role in the rehabilitation process. The amount of research supporting the preventive role of physical activity and chronic disease varies by disease. Compelling evidence exists regarding the role of physical activity in the prevention of cardiovascular disease, type II diabetes, and colorectal cancer. More limited evidence suggests physical activity may also play an important role in the prevention of breast cancer. This chapter has illustrated the integral role between physical activity and health.

CONCEPT CONNECTION

1. **Chronic diseases are steadily increasing.** The United States is currently in an epidemiological transition with regard to infectious and chronic diseases. Three risk behaviors in particular—lack of physical activity, tobacco use, and poor nutrition—are major contributors to both cardiovascular disease and cancer, our nation's number one and number two chronic diseases and causes of death.

2. **Cancer is a group of diseases characterized by an uncontrollable growth and spread of abnormal cells.** Two types of tumors are *benign* and *malignant.* Cancer is the second leading cause of death in the United States. The term *cancer* is used to indicate any type of malignant tumor.

3. **Lung cancer is the single largest cause of cancer deaths in the United States.** Lung cancer is the leading cause of cancer death among both men and women. The strongest risk factor for lung cancer is cigarette smoking.

4. **Breast cancer is prevalent among women, and physical activity is thought to be a protective factor.** Breast cancer is the most commonly diagnosed cancer and the second leading cause of cancer deaths among women in the United States. Several recent studies have suggested physical activity as a protective factor against breast cancer.

5. **Prostate cancer is the most prevalent cancer among men.** Prostate cancer is the most prevalent cancer among men and the second leading cancer death among men. Increase in incidence rates could be due in part to earlier diagnosis.

6. **Colorectal cancer and physical activity is the most thoroughly investigated cancer–physical activity relationship.** Colorectal cancer is the second leading cause of cancer-related deaths in the United States. Many studies have measured occupational physical activity and the risk of colon cancer that strongly suggest physical activity has a protective effect against colon cancer.
7. **Skin cancer is one of the most common forms of cancer.** The most serious form of skin cancer is *melanoma. Prevention* is key. Avoid or limit sun exposure but if you have to be outside keep as much skin covered as possible and use a sunscreen with an SPF of 15 or higher.
8. **Diabetes mellitus is a serious lifelong condition.** Diabetes has been ranked among the top ten leading causes of death in the United States since 1932. Diabetes mellitus is a group of diseases in which the body is unable to produce and/or properly use insulin. Types of diabetes include Type 1 (insulin dependent) and Type 2 (non-insulin dependent). The more physical activity you participate in, the less likely it is that you will develop Type 2 diabetes.

TERMS

Cancer, 81
Tumor, 81
Benign, 81
Malignant, 81
Metastasis, 81
Solar Protection Factor (SPF), 92
Hypergylcemia, 93
Hypoglycemia, 93

MAKING THE CONNECTION

Monica has learned much about the causes of cancer. In so doing, she has gained an appreciation for the ways in which behavioral changes could help her lessen her own risk of developing cancer. She understands that she needs to eliminate her smoking habit. In addition, eating a wide variety of fruits and vegetables will supply her with nutrients that will not only help her obtain optimal health now but also pave the way for years of health in the future. Monica decides to stop smoking first. She prepares for quitting by beginning to self-monitor her smoking habit. She records the number of cigarettes she smokes a day, when she smokes them, and signs up for a smoking cessation class to begin in 2 weeks.

CRITICAL THINKING

1. Monica is not unlike many college-age adults—she is addicted to nicotine and wishes to stop smoking. Go to the American Cancer Society website (www.acs.org) and search for ways to stop smoking. Outline the American Cancer Society suggestions to stop smoking.
2. A risk factor of cancer is family history. Family history of cancer does not "guarantee" that you will get the disease, nor does it cancel out the importance of a healthy lifestyle (good nutritional balance, regular physical activity, and no smoking). A family history of cancer does predispose you to the disease; therefore, it is important for you to determine your family cancer history. Construct a family tree by listing your biological parents, siblings, grandparents (maternal and paternal), and aunts and uncles (paternal and maternal). Next to each name list the type of cancer and the age at which it was discovered. Your family may be helpful with this activity. After completing your tree, you may want to share it with your family and discuss prevention efforts.
3. Make a list of all the factors that increase your chance of getting cancer (review Table 4.3). Order the list from the highest to lowest risk. Which risk factors pertain to you? How can you modify or change any of these risk factors?

REFERENCES

Ames, B.N., Gold, L.S., & Willett, W.C. (1995). The causes and prevention of cancer. *Proc National Academy of Science, USA 92*:5258–65.

ACS News Today (February 23, 2000a). *Regular exercise may lower breast cancer risk.* Atlanta: American Cancer Society.

ACS News Today (May 2, 2000b). *Skin self-exams: Tips on spotting cancers early.* Atlanta: American Cancer Society.

American Cancer Society (2000). *Cancer Facts and Figures, 2000.* Atlanta.

Arbman, G., Axelson, O., Fredriksson, M., Nilsson, E., & Sjodahl, R. (1993). Do occupational factors influence the risk of colon and rectal cancer in different ways? *Cancer 72*: 2543–49.

Armstrong, G.L., Conn, L.A., & Pinner, R.W. (1999). Trends in infectious disease mortality in the United States during the 20th century. *Journal of the American Medical Association 281*(1):61–66.

Bishop, D.B., Zimmerman, B.R., & Roesler, J.S. (1998). Diabetes. In Brownson, R.C., Remington, P.L., & Davis, J.R., eds., *Chronic Disease Epidemiology and Control,* 2nd ed. Washington, DC: American Public Health Association.

Breslow, L. (1999). From disease prevention to health promotion. *Journal of the American Medical Association 281*(11):1030–33.

Brownson, R.C., Remington, P.L., & Davis, J.R. (1998a). *Chronic Disease Epidemiology and Control,* 2nd ed. Washington, DC: American Public Health Association.

Brownson, R.C., Reif, J.S., Alavanja, M.R.R., & Bal, D.G. (1998b). Cancer. In Brownson, R.C., Remington, P.L., & Davis, J.R., eds., *Chronic Disease Epidemiology and Control,*2nd ed. Washington, DC: American Public Health Association.

Brownson, R.C., Chang, J.C., Davis, J.R., & Smith, C. (1991). Physical activity on the job and cancer in Missouri. *American Journal of Public Health 81*(5): 639–42.

Brownson, R.C., Zahm, S.H., Chang, J.C., & Blair, A. (1989). Occupational risk of colon cancer: An analysis by anatomic subsite. *American Journal of Epidemiology 130*(4):675–86.

Centers for Disease Control and Prevention (2000a). *Ten Great Public Health Achievements—United States—1900–1999.* Atlanta. Online: http://www.cdc.gov/phtn/tenachievements/ [accessed August 22, 2000].

Centers for Disease Control and Prevention (2000b). *Assessing Health Risk Behaviors among Young People: Youth Risk Behavior Surveillance System. At -a-Glance, 2000.* Atlanta: CDC, Division of Adolescent and School Health. Online: http://www.cdc.gov/nccdphp/dash/yrbs/yrbsaag.htm [accessed January 29, 2001].

Centers for Disease Control and Prevention (2000c). *Colorectal Cancer: The Importance of Prevention and Early Detection. At-a -Glance, 2000.* Atlanta: CDC, National Center for Chronic Disease Prevention and Health Promotion. Online: http://www.cdc.gov/cancer/colorctl/colorect.htm [accessed May 8, 2000].

Centers for Disease Control and Prevention (1999). *Chronic Diseases and Their Risk Factors: The Nation's Leading Causes of Death.* Atlanta.

Colberg, S.R., & Swain, D.P. (2000). Exercise and diabetes control. *The Physician and Sports Medicine 28*(4):63ff.

Frisch, R.E., Wyshak, G., Albright, N.L., Albright, T.E., & Schiff, I. (1986). Lower prevalence of diabetes in female former college athletes compared with nonathletes. *Diabetes 35*:1101–1105.

Graffunder, C.M., et al. (1999). Skin cancer prevention: The problem, responses, and lessons learned. *Health Education and Behavior 26*(3):308–316.

Greenwald, P., & Sondik, E.J. (eds.). (1986). *Cancer Control Objectives for the Nation: 1985–2000.* National Cancer Institute Monographs, No. 2. USDHHS Pub. No. 86-2880. Washington, DC: U.S. Government Printing Office.

Hahn, R.A., Teutsch, S.M., Rothenberg, R.B., & Marks, J.S. (1990). Excess deaths from nine chronic diseases in the United States, 1986. *Journal of the American Medical Association 264*(20):2654–59.

Health Administration Development Group (1999). *Diabetes Management: Clinical Pathways, Guidelines, and Patient Education.* Gaithersburg, MD: Aspen.

Kavangh, J.J., Singletary, S.E., Einhorn, N., & Depetrillo, A.D. (1999). *Breast Cancer.* New York: Blackwell Science.

McTiernan, A. (1997). Breast cancer: Time to get moving? *New England Journal of Medicine 336*(18):1311–12.

Mettlin, C. (1997). Recent developments in the epidemiology of prostate cancer. *European Journal of Cancer 33*(3):340–47.

National Cancer Institute (1999a). *Atlas of Cancer Mortality in the United States, 1950–1994.* NIH Pub. No. 99-4564. Bethesda.

National Cancer Institute (1999b). *Screening for Prostate Cancer. PDQ Screenings and Prevention: Health Professional.* Online: http://www.cancernet.nci.nih.gov/clinpdq/screening/Screening_for_Prostate_Cancer.html [accessed May 8, 2000].

National Cancer Institute (1999c). *What You Need to Know about Melanoma.* NIH Pub. No. 99-1563. Bethesda.

National Cancer Institute (1998a). *Lung Cancer Backgrounder.* Bethesda.

National Cancer Institute (1998b). *Cancer Facts—Screening. Questions and Answers about Early Prostate Cancer.* Online: http://cancernet.nci.nih.gov/Cancer_Types/Prostate_Cancer.shtml. [Accessed: February 7, 2001].

Omran, A.R. (1971). The epidemiologic transition: A theory of the epidemiology of population change. *Milbank Quarterly 49*:509–538.

Omran, A.R. (1977). A century of epidemiologic transition in the United States. *Preventive Medicine 6*:30–51.

Patlak, M. (1996). Book reopened on infectious diseases. *FDA Consumer* 30(4): 19–26.

Powell, K.E., Caspersen, C.J., Koplan, J.P., & Ford, E.S. (1989). Physical activity and chronic diseases. *American Journal of Clinical Nutrition* [suppl] 49:999–1004.

Thune, I., Brenn, T., Lund, E., & Gaard, M. (1997). Physical activity and the risk of breast cancer. *New England Journal of Medicine 336*(18):1269–75.

United States Department of Health and Human Services (2000a). *Healthy People 2010: Conference Edition—Cancer.* CD-ROM. Washington, DC.

United States Department of Health and Human Services (2000b). *Healthy People 2010: Conference Edition—Diabetes.* CD-ROM. Washington, DC.

United States Department of Health and Human Services (1996). *Physical Activity and Health: A Report of the Surgeon General.* Atlanta.

United States Preventive Services Task Force (1996). Screening for breast cancer. In *U.S. Preventive Services Task Force. Guide to Clinical Preventive Services,* 2nd ed., pp. 73–87. Baltimore: Williams & Wilkins.

Vetter, R., et al.(1992). Occupational physical activity and colon cancer risk in Turkey. *European Journal of Epidemiology 8*: 845–50.

Zimmet, P.Z. (1999). Diabetes epidemiology as a tool to trigger diabetes research and care. *Diabetologia 42*: 499–518.

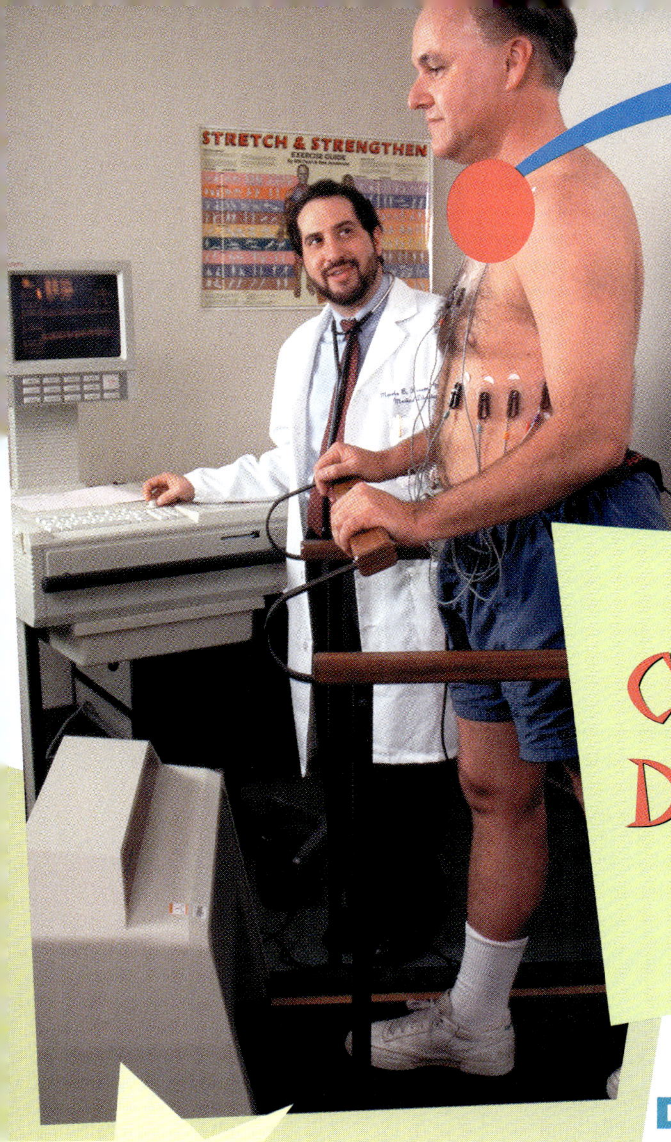

5 Cardiovascular Disease and Health

CONCEPT CONNECTION

1. The circulatory system consists of the heart and blood vessels—veins, arteries, and capillaries.
2. There are many forms of cardiovascular diseases.
3. Angina pectoris and a heart attack are not synonymous.
4. Hypertension is a major risk factor for coronary heart disease.
5. Arteriosclerosis and atherosclerosis are key factors in cardiovascular disease.
6. Cerebrovascular accident (CVA) is a cardiovascular disease that affects the central nervous system.
7. The three unmodifiable risk factors for CVD are age, family, and gender.
8. The four CVD risk factors that can be changed are hypertension, cholesterol level, cigarette smoking, and physical inactivity.
9. Diabetes mellitus, obesity, and stress are three contributing risk factors for CVD.
10. Diet plays a major role in preventing CVD.

FEATURES

E-Learning Tools: www.pahconnection.com

Engage www.pahconnection.com

- 5.1 Heart disease risk calculator
- 5.2 Cholesterol reduction calculator
- 5.3 Create-a-diet: how you can lower your cholesterol levels

Experience www.pahconnection.com

- 5.1 Heart anatomy
- 5.2 FDA consumer

Explore www.pahconnection.com

- 5.1 National Heart, Lung, and Blood Institute
- 5.2 Dr. Koop: heart disease
- 5.3 American Heart Association

Activities & Assessments

- 5.1 Cholesterol and heart disease IQ
- 5.2 Physical activity and heart disease

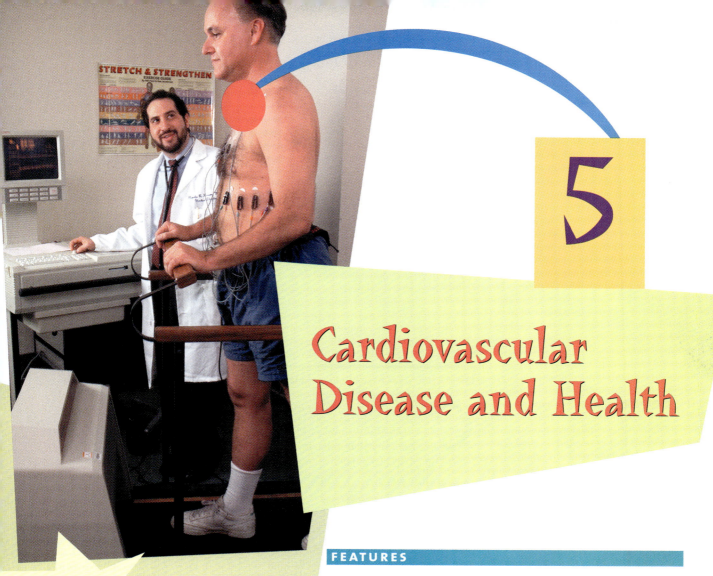

WHAT'S THE CONNECTION?

Richard is worried about dying from a heart attack. His father suffered a heart attack at age 45 last year and both of his grandfathers died of cardiovascular disease. Richard does not intend to follow in their footsteps. He knows that his family history and gender put him at risk, so he focuses on things he can control. He doesn't smoke, and he has his blood pressure and cholesterol levels monitored on a regular basis. Richard is convinced that physical activity is unrelated to his risk of developing cardiovascular disease. He thinks he is doing all he can to reduce his risk of cardiovascular disease. Is Richard correct in believing this? Are there any other factors that Richard should be aware of that could reduce his chances of developing cardiovascular disease?

UNDERSTANDING THE CARDIOVASCULAR SYSTEM

Explore 5.1

1. The circulatory system consists of the heart and blood vessels—veins, arteries, and capillaries.

Pericardium Thin, closed outer sac that surrounds the heart.

Myocardium Muscular middle layer that surrounds the heart.

Endocardium Thin, inner layer that lines the heart.

Cardiovascular disease (CVD) is the leading cause of death in the United States, accounting for approximately 4 in 10 deaths. Although gender, age, and heredity play roles in cardiovascular disease, CVD is primarily a lifestyle disease. This chapter focuses on an overview of the heart's functions, cardiovascular diseases, cardiovascular health risk factors, and the role of diet in preventing cardiovascular disease.

To understand how physical activity can lower your risk for CVD, you must first understand how the cardiovascular system works. The cardiovascular system is both simple and complex. A marvel of engineering, this system is comprised of a high-pressure output center and low-pressure return network. The blood in the arterial system moves from the heart, which generates a great deal of pressure, into smaller and smaller vessels, which help to maintain a high-pressure outflow. This pressure is referred to as *blood pressure*. Maintaining adequate blood flow is important in the delivery of oxygen and the removal of carbon dioxide. If the blood pressure drops rapidly (for example, if you stand up too quickly), you feel dizzy. This dizziness is caused by diminished blood flow to the brain.

The Heart

Physical activity increases cardiovascular function.

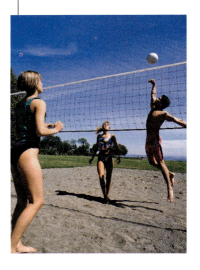

The cardiovascular system consists of the heart (the pump) and a network of blood vessels that transport the blood throughout the body (Figure 5.1). The heart's primary function is to pump blood containing oxygen and nutrients throughout the body. The heart also receives blood filled with waste products (such as carbon dioxide) that need to be eliminated from the body. The heart is a highly specialized muscle about the size of an adult fist that pumps blood throughout the body. The heart pumps slightly more than a gallon of blood per minute through the approximately 50,000 miles of blood vessels in the body. Each day the heart expands and contracts 100,000 times, pumping about 2000 gallons of blood. In a 70-year lifetime, an average human heart beats more than 2.5 billion times. Maintaining a healthy heart and blood vessels is essential for survival. The walls of the heart are composed of three layers: the pericardium, the myocardium, and the endocardium. The **pericardium** is a thin, closed sac that surrounds the heart. The middle layer is the thickest, consists of muscle cells, and is called the **myocardium.** The **endocardium** is the inner layer that lines the heart chambers.

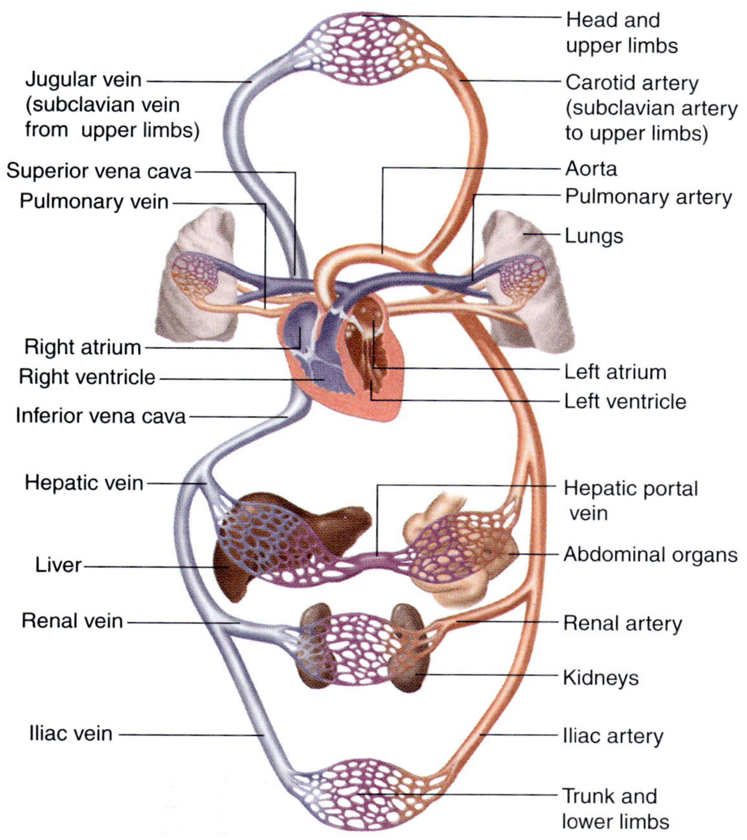

FIGURE 5.1

The Circulatory System.
The circulatory system includes the heart, arteries, and veins. The heart receives oxygenated blood from the lungs and pumps it to all tissues in the body.

The heart contains four separate chambers: the upper two chambers are the left and right atrium; the lower two chambers are the right and left ventricle (Figure 5.2). The heart also has four valves: the tricuspid valve (located between the right atrium and right ventricle), the pulmonary valve (between the right ventricle and pulmonary artery), the mitral valve (between the left atrium and left ventricle), and the aortic valve (between the left ventricle and aorta). To maintain uniform blood flow in one direction through arteries and veins, the cardiovascular system is equipped with one-way valves, both in the chambers of the heart and in blood vessels. With every heartbeat, the valves in the heart open and close to allow blood to circulate in just one direction.

Experience www.pahconnection.com **5.1**

Blood that is depleted of oxygen returns to the heart via the right atrium and then flows to the right ventricle. From there blood is pumped to the lungs, where it is reoxygenated and returned via the pulmonary artery to the left atrium. Finally, the fresh blood is pumped throughout the body's tissues from the left ventricle through the large artery called the **aorta.** The atria receive blood entering the heart: the right atrium receives **deoxygenated blood** returning from the various cells and muscles of the body, and the left atrium receives **oxygenated blood** from the lungs. The right ventricle pumps deoxygenated blood out to the lungs, while the left ventricle pumps oxygenated blood out to the cells and muscles of the body.

A healthy heart beats rhythmically at a pace initiated by the heart itself. In the right atrium, a region called the **sinoatrial node** (pacemaker) generates an electric signal that causes the heart to contract and pump blood. The pace of the heartbeat is also influenced by electrical signals from the brain, which explains how emotions, excitement, or stress can suddenly change the rhythm of the heartbeat.

Aorta Large artery that receives blood from the heart's left ventricle and distributes it to the body.

Deoxygenated blood Blood returned to the heart, to be replenished with oxygen in the lungs.

Oxygenated blood Blood leaving the heart that is oxygen-rich.

Sinoatrial node The natural pacemaker of the heart.

FIGURE 5.2

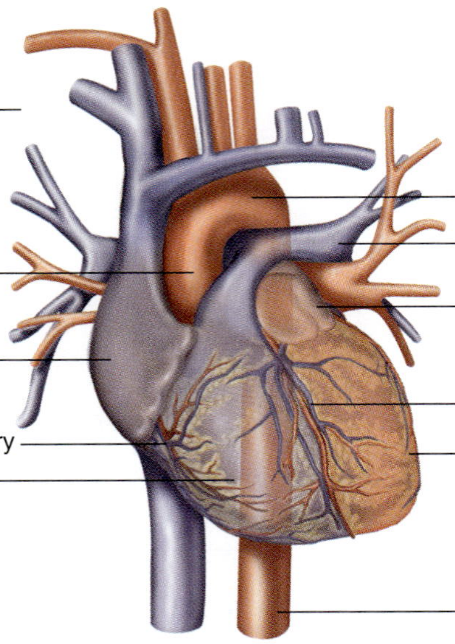

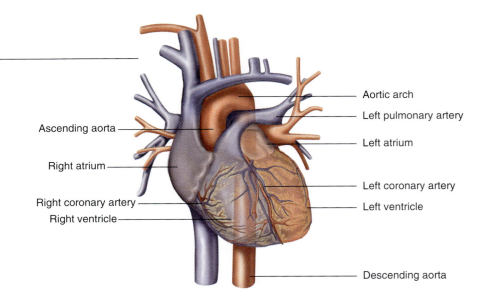

The Heart.
Oxygenated blood is pumped through the arteries (red) and oxygen-depleted blood is returned to the heart via veins (blue).

Arteries Blood vessels that carry oxygenated blood from the heart to the body.

Arterioles Small, muscular branches of arteries; when they contract, they increase resistance to blood flow, and blood pressure increases.

Veins Blood vessels that return deoxygenated blood to the heart.

Capillaries Tiny blood vessels that circulate blood to all the body's cells.

Blood pressure The force blood applies to the walls of the blood vessels.

Blood pressure cuff (sphygmomanometer); instrument that measures blood pressure.

Systolic pressure The highest blood pressure measured in the arteries; occurs as the heart contracts with each heartbeat.

The Blood Vessels

There are many different types of blood vessels that carry blood through the body. **Arteries** carry oxygenated blood from the heart to all organs and tissues in the body. The arteries closest to the heart are large; as they move further from the heart they divide into smaller vessels called **arterioles.** Arterioles lead to **capillaries**, tiny blood vessels that branch out from arteries and veins and circulate blood to all the cells in the body. **Veins** return blood to the heart after oxygen and nutrients have been exchanged for carbon dioxide and waste products. Blood vessels can be damaged by injury or by disease; this damage may obstruct the flow of blood carrying oxygen and nutrients. Veins and arteries for the most part run side by side throughout the body.

Measuring Blood Pressure **Blood pressure** is the force that blood applies to the walls of a blood vessel. Blood pressure varies from time to time, based on our physical activity or stress levels. Blood pressure is measured using a **blood pressure cuff,** or **sphygmomanometer.** The blood pressure cuff is wrapped around the upper part of the arm and a stethoscope is placed over the artery just below the cuff. Air is pumped into the cuff until pressure stops the flow of blood through the artery. The pressure in the cuff is gradually reduced as the air is released. The measure of the blood's pressure as it starts flowing through the vessel again is known as **systolic pressure;** this is the higher of the two numbers stated in a blood pressure reading. The air continues to be released from the cuff until no pulse is audible, indicating that the blood is flowing normally through the artery; this is known as the **diastolic pressure.** A typical reading for a healthy, young adult is 130/85, although readings may vary from individual to individual.

Knowing your blood pressure is vital to your overall health and well-being.

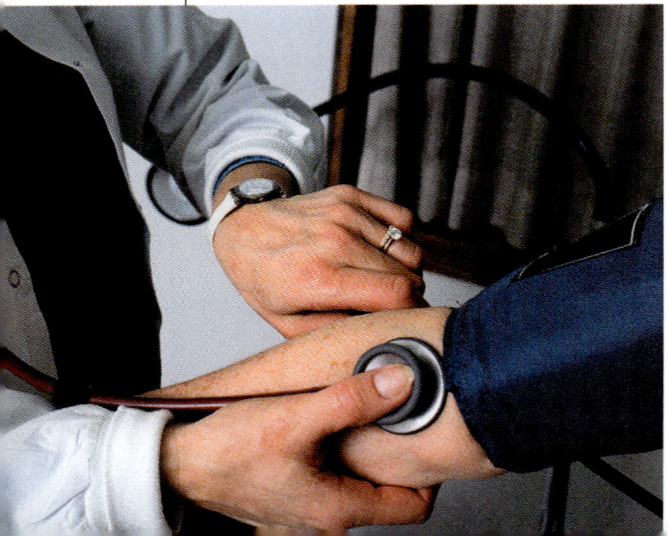

The Circulation of Blood

When returning to the heart, blood moves from one-cell-thick capillaries into larger *venules* and then even larger veins. This movement from small vessels into larger vessels accounts for the low-pressure return system of our vascular network. One of the benefits of moving during the cool-down phase of a workout is that muscle contraction aids in **venous return,** making it easier for blood to return to the heart and helping you recover from exercise more rapidly. It will also prevent you from fainting and keeling over from rapid blood-pressure fluctuations.

The Function of Blood

The heart (a muscle) is responsible for circulating the blood that nourishes our cells and maintains life. Blood (the fluid circulated by the heart) plays an important role in removing waste products, assisting in *thermoregulation* (temperature control), and delivering hormones. A fluid portion of the blood, called *plasma,* consists primarily of water and thus makes circulation possible. The blood also contains **hemoglobin,** which is responsible for the transportation of oxygen. Oxygen binds to the hemoglobin found in red blood cells. Carbon dioxide is also carried in the blood, primarily in the form of **bicarbonate ions.** The circulatory system functions to deliver oxygen to working muscles and remove carbon dioxide.

This closed system maintains blood pressure and flow. When you start to move, your heart must respond by beating more forcefully and rapidly to deliver the blood that the muscles need. The more fit you are, the easier your heart adjusts to the stress of physical activity.

Neural Control

The heart has its own electrical conduction network, which is regulated by the sinoatrial (SA) node. The SA node is a collection of specialized tissue that sets the neural rhythm regulating cardiac function. This **auto-regulation** allows the cardiac muscle to maintain a regular rhythm, or rate of beating, without the brain having to become consciously involved in setting the pace of the heart. The heart also responds to chemical and neural impulses that can alter the force or rate of contraction. When our skeletal muscles send signals that they need more oxygen, the heart responds by beating faster or harder. The electrical activity within the heart can be measured through the use of an electrocardiograph (ECG).

The Pulmonary/Respiratory Link

The **pulmonary system,** like the circulatory system, is important to the delivery of oxygen and the removal of carbon dioxide. In fact, the integration of the circulatory and pulmonary systems is crucial for survival and activity. In terms of physical activity, movements that stress (and improve) the circulatory system also stress (and improve) the functioning of the pulmonary system. We need to be aware that the environment in which we exercise has an impact on pulmonary function. We need to choose locations for physical activity where air quality is optimal. In most instances, unless an individual has a chronic obstructive pulmonary disease (bronchitis, emphysema, asthma), pulmonary function will not be a major limiting factor to activity performance.

Diastolic pressure The lowest blood pressure measured in the arteries; occurs when the heart muscle is relaxed between beats.

Venous return Blood returning through the veins to the heart.

Hemoglobin The oxygen-carrying pigment of the red blood cells.

Bicarbonate ion HCO_3 As a buffer, it prevents a change in blood pH.

Auto-regulation Self-regulation.

Pulmonary system Pertaining to the lungs; includes pulmonary arteries and veins.

UNDERSTANDING CARDIOVASCULAR DISEASES

Cardiovascular diseases (CVD) include a variety of diseases of the heart and blood vessels, coronary heart disease, stroke, hypertension, congestive heart failure, and peripheral artery disease. Cardiovascular diseases claimed 949,000 lives in the United States in 1998 (National Heart, Lung, and Blood Institute [NHLBI], 2000) (Figure 5.3). This is 41 percent of all deaths, or 1 of every 2.4 deaths. In 1997,

2. There are many forms of cardiovascular diseases.

Explore 5.2

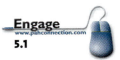

Engage
www.pahconnection.com
5.1

3. Angina pectoris and a heart attack are not synonymous.

the total cost of CVD was estimated at $259 billion (Newschaffer, Brownson, & Dusenbury, 1998). In fact, CVD claims more lives each year than the next seven leading causes of death combined. We will review several types of CVD: coronary heart disease (CHD), hypertension, arteriosclerosis, and stroke.

Coronary Heart Disease

Coronary heart disease (CHD) is the most prevalent form of heart disease in the United States (NHLBI, 1998) (Figure 5.4). Coronary heart disease occurs when the coronary arteries become occluded with blood fats and other substances that collect on their walls, narrowing the opening through which blood can flow through. When the coronary arteries become clogged or narrowed, they cannot supply enough blood to the heart. Coronary heart disease, or coronary artery disease, most often is implicated in causing angina and heart attack.

Coronary heart disease Disease of the heart caused by atherosclerotic narrowing of the coronary arteries.

Angina pectoris Chest pain due to coronary heart disease.

Ischemia Decreased blood flow to an organ, usually due to constriction or obstruction of an artery.

Myocardial infarction Heart attack.

Heart attack Death of, or damage to part of, the heart muscle due to insufficient blood supply.

Angina Pectoris If not enough oxygen-carrying blood reaches the heart, the heart may respond with pain called **angina pectoris,** or simply **angina.** This pain is usually felt on the left side of the chest or sometimes in the left arm to shoulder. Lack of blood supply is called **ischemia.** Angina can occur when blood circulation to the heart is not sufficient to meet the heart's increased needs during physical activity or emotional excitement. Running up several flight of stairs to class or to a meeting could trigger an angina attack. Angina may be a warning sign for a heart attack.

Heart Attack When the blood supply to the heart is completely cut off, the result is a **myocardial infarction (MI),** or what is commonly referred to as a **heart attack** (Table 5.1). The part of the heart that does not receive oxygen (via the blood) begins to die, and this sometimes causes permanent damage to the heart muscle.

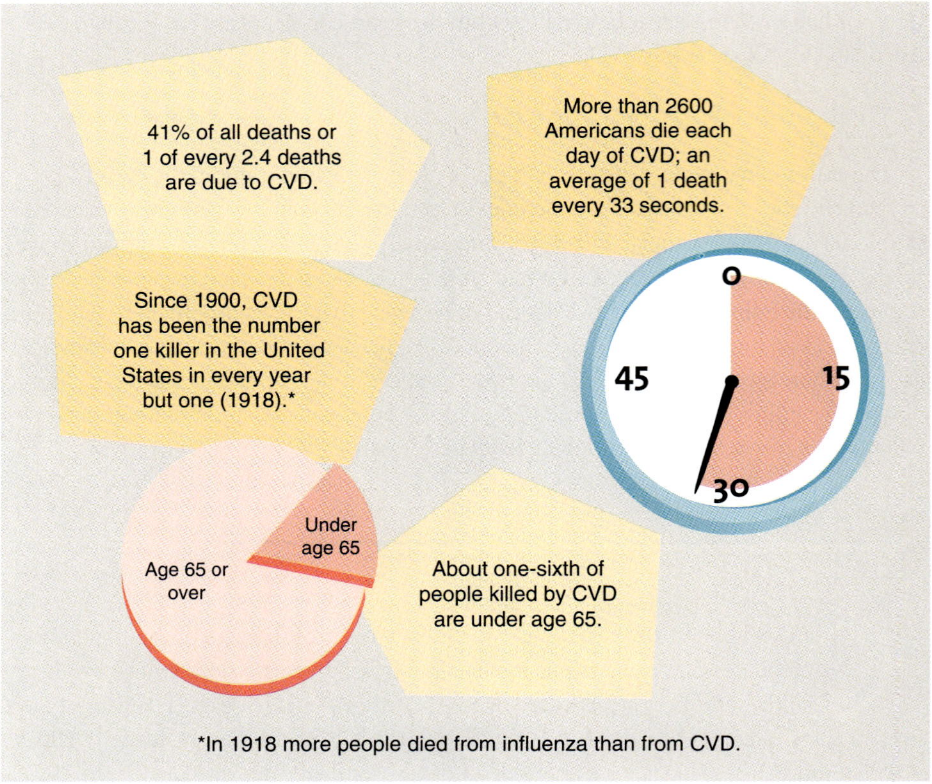
41% of all deaths or 1 of every 2.4 deaths are due to CVD.
More than 2600 Americans die each day of CVD; an average of 1 death every 33 seconds.
Since 1900, CVD has been the number one killer in the United States in every year but one (1918).*
0
15
30
45
Under age 65
Age 65 or over
About one-sixth of people killed by CVD are under age 65.
*In 1918 more people died from influenza than from CVD.

FIGURE 5.3

Some Facts about Cardiovascular Disease (CVD).

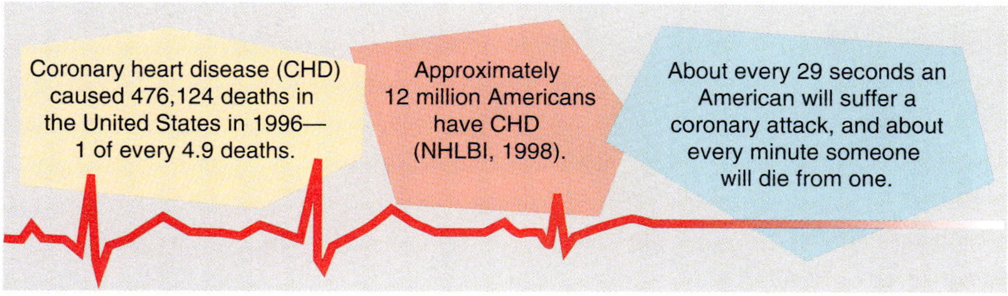

FIGURE 5.4

Some Facts about Coronary Heart Disease (CHD).

TABLE 5.1 Heart Attack: Signals and Action

Know the warning signals of a heart attack:

- Uncomfortable pressure, fullness, squeezing, or pain in the center of the chest that lasts more than a few minutes, or goes away and comes back.
- Pain that spreads to the shoulders, neck, or arms.
- Chest discomfort with lightheadedness, fainting, sweating, nausea, or shortness of breath.

Not all these warning signs occur in every heart attack. But if some start to occur, don't wait. Get medical help immediately. Delay can be deadly!

Know what to do in an emergency:

- Find out which area hospitals have 24-hour emergency cardiac care.
- Know in advance which hospital or medical facility is nearest your home and office, and tell your family and friends to call this facility in an emergency.
- Keep a list of emergency rescue service numbers next to the telephone and in your pocket, wallet, or purse.
- If you have chest discomfort that lasts more than a few minutes, call the emergency rescue service.
- If you can get to a hospital faster by going yourself and not waiting for an ambulance, have someone drive you there.

SOURCE: American Heart Association. (1996). *Heart and stroke facts.* Dallas, TX: American Heart Association

Hypertension

Hypertension, or high blood pressure (HBP), is known as the "silent killer" and remains a major risk factor for CHD and stroke. Approximately 50 million adult Americans have HBP, but almost three-forths of them are unaware of it (Sixth Report, 1997; Burt, Culter, & Higgins, 1995). An acceptable blood pressure for an adult is less than 140/90 mm Hg (Table 5.2). If an adult's systolic pressure is equal to or greater than 140 mm Hg and/or the diastolic pressure is equal to or greater than 90 mm Hg, and these readings occur for an extended period of time, that person is said to have hypertension. With high blood pressure, the heart is working harder, resulting in an increased risk of heart attack, stroke, heart failure, kidney and eye problems, and peripheral vascular disease.

The two types of hypertension are primary (or essential) hypertension and secondary hypertension. **Primary hypertension** accounts for more than 90 percent of all hypertension cases. The cause of primary hypertension is unknown. Although the cause is unknown, we know that arteriosclerosis contributes to the elevation of blood pressure. **Secondary hypertension** refers to cases for which a cause is known, such as a kidney abnormality, tumor of the adrenal gland, or a congenital defect of the aorta.

4. Hypertension is a major risk factor for coronary heart disease.

Hypertension A chronic increase in blood pressure above its normal range.

Primary hypertension Hypertension where the cause is unknown.

Secondary hypertension Hypertension arising from another physical condition, such as kidney disease.

TABLE 5.2 **Categories for Blood Pressure Levels in Adults***

	BLOOD PRESSURE LEVEL (MM HG)	
CATEGORY	SYSTOLIC	DIASTOLIC
Normal	Below 130	Below 85
High normal	130 – 139	85 – 89
High blood pressure		
• Stage 1	140 – 159	90 – 99
• Stage 2	160 – 179	100 –109
• Stage 3	180 or above	110 or above

* For those not taking medicine for high blood pressure and not having a short-term illness. These categories are from the National High Blood Pressure Education Program. Adults are those age 18 years and older.

SOURCE: National Heart, Lung, and Blood Institute. *How to Prevent High Blood Pressure.* Online: http://www.nhlbi.nih.gov/health/hbp/prevhbp/index.htm

5. Arteriosclerosis and atherosclerosis are key factors in cardiovascular disease.

Experience 5.2 www.pahconnection.com

Arteriosclerosis "Hardening of the arteries;" arterial walls thicken and lose elasticity.

Atherosclerosis A form of arteriosclerosis in which the inner layers of the artery become thick and irregular due to fatty deposits called plaque.

Plaque A fatty deposit on the inner lining of the artery wall.

Stroke Loss of muscle function, vision, or speech resulting from brain-cell damage caused by insufficient blood supply.

Atherosclerosis

Arteriosclerosis, hardening and thickening of the arteries, includes several conditions that cause the walls of the arteries to thicken and lose their elasticity. The most common form of arteriosclerosis is **atherosclerosis,** which can begin as early as childhood (Ross, 1993). Atherosclerosis is a slow, progressive process that begins with damage to the heart's arteries and leads to formation of fibrous, fatty deposits called **plaque**. These plaque deposits accumulate on the artery walls, causing the arteries to lose their elasticity (ability to expand and contract), and eventually restricting blood flow (Figure 5.5). The restriction of blood flow also makes the blood more susceptible to forming blood clots. Restriction or obstruction of blood flow to an artery is very serious because heart cells die when deprived of oxygenated blood.

Stroke

When considered separately from other cardiovascular diseases, stroke ranks as the third leading cause of death in the United States, behind diseases of the heart and cancer. **Stroke,** or **cerebrovascular accident (CVA),** is a form of cardiovascular disease

FIGURE 5.5

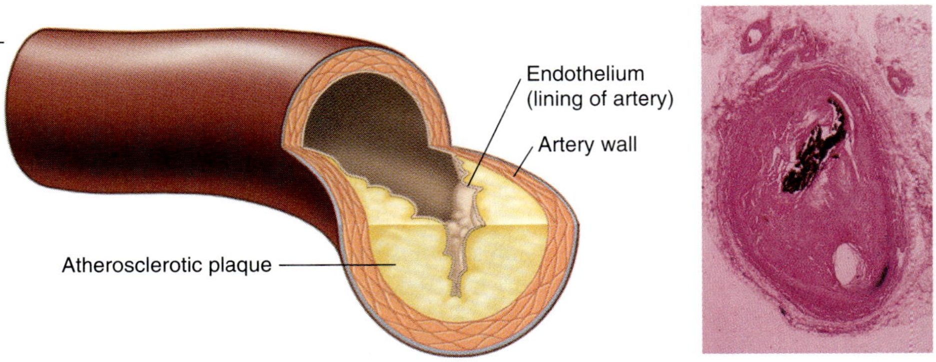

Plaque in an Artery.
Plaque is the buildup of fatty material on the artery wall. The illustration (left) shows the interior of an artery narrowed by plaque. The photo (right) shows an occluded blood vessel that has been entirely blocked by plaque and a blood clot (dark area).

that affects the arteries of the central nervous system. A stroke results when the brain doesn't get enough oxygen because the arteries supplying blood to the brain are blocked or damaged. Brain cells die within minutes without oxygen.

There are two broad categories of stroke: ischemic and hemorrhage. **Ischemic strokes** are caused by clots and account for approximately three-fourths of all strokes. The two types of ischemic strokes are cerebral thrombosis and cerebral embolism. **Cerebral thrombosis** is the most common type of stroke; it occurs when a thrombus (blood clot) forms and blocks flow in an artery bringing blood to the brain. A **cerebral embolism** occurs when a wandering clot (embolus) occurs in a blood vessel away from the heart. The embolus is carried through the bloodstream until it lodges in an artery, blocking blood flow to the brain. Arteries damaged by arteriosclerosis are generally present in both types of ischemic strokes.

Hemorrhagic strokes occur when blood seeps from a hole in the wall of a blood vessel. There are two types of hemorrhagic strokes: cerebral hemorrhage and subarachnoid hemorrhage. **Cerebral hemorrhage** occurs when a defective artery in the brain ruptures, flooding the surrounding tissue with blood. A **subarachnoid hemorrhage** occurs when a blood vessel on the surface of the brain ruptures and bleeds into the space between the brain and the skull.

The effects of a stroke vary from person to person, depending on the type of stroke and the area of the brain affected (Figure 5.6). A stroke can cause paralysis and affect sight, touch, movement, and cognitive abilities.

6. Cerebrovascular accident (CVA), or stroke, is a cardiovascular disease that affects the central nervous system.

Ischemic strokes Strokes caused by clots.

Cerebral thrombosis Blood clot in an artery that supplies the brain.

Cerebral embolism Blood clot formed in one part of the body and then carried by the bloodstream to the brain, where it blocks an artery.

Hemorrhagic strokes Strokes caused by blood seeping from a hole in the wall of a blood vessel.

Cerebral hemorrhage Bleeding within the brain that results from a ruptured aneurysm or a head injury.

Subarachnoid hemorrhage Bleeding from a blood vessel on the surface of the brain into the space between the brain and the skull.

RISK FACTORS FOR CARDIOVASCULAR DISEASE

The answer to the problem of cardiovascular disease is prevention. Over the years, researchers have identified risk factors that can increase your risk for developing heart disease. Some risk factors cannot be changed (age, family history, gender), but some can be changed (high cholesterol, cigarette smoking, hypertension, physical inactivity). Factors that cannot be changed are referred to as *unmodifiable* risk factors, whereas factors that can be changed are referred to as *modifiable* risk factors. *Contributing* risk factors are associated with an increased risk of cardiovascular disease, but their significance has not yet been scientifically measured. These factors include diabetes, obesity, and individual response to stress.

Explore 5.3

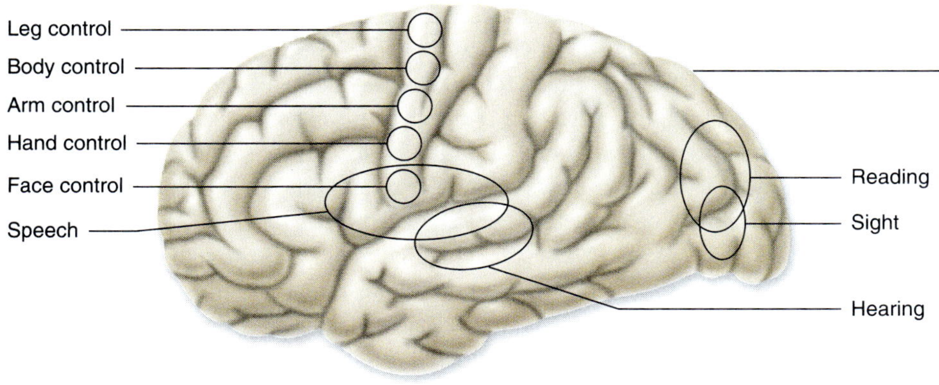

FIGURE 5.6

How Stroke Affects a Person.

SOURCE: American Heart Association. (1996). *Heart and stroke facts.* Dallas, TX: American Heart Association.

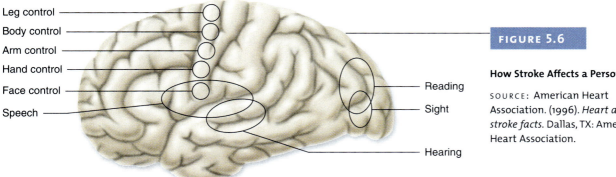

Unmodifiable Risk Factors

7. The three unmodifiable risk factors for CVD are age, family, and gender.

Age The risk of cardiovascular disease increases as we get older (Corti, Guralink, & Bicato, 1996). The majority of people who die of a heart attack are 65 or older. Although you can't change your age, you can change your physical activity, diet, and smoking habits.

Family History There appears to be a hereditary tendency toward heart disease and atherosclerosis. If you have close relatives who have had a heart attack or a stroke before 50 years of age, you are at increased risk for having a heart attack or stroke. Another significant factor is race—African-Americans are two times as likely to have high blood pressure as whites, which increases the risk of cardiovascular disease. Again, despite your genetics, you can choose lifestyle changes to decrease your risk for cardiovascular disease.

Gender Men are more likely than women to develop cardiovascular disease, especially before the age of 40. However, after menopause, women's risk of heart disease increases. Current theory speculates that male hormones (androgens) increase risk, whereas female hormones (estrogens) protect against atherosclerosis.

Modifiable Risk Factors

8. The four CVD risk factors that can be changed are hypertension, cholesterol level, cigarette smoking, and physical inactivity.

physical activity and health connection

Engage
www.pahconnection.com
5.2

Hypertension The relationship between high blood pressure and CVD is a complex one (Lembo et al., 1998). High blood pressure increases the heart's workload, causing the heart to weaken over time. Combine high blood pressure with obesity, smoking, high blood cholesterol, or diabetes and the risk of heart attack or stroke increases several times. Lembo et al. (1998) indicate that reducing high blood pressure alone does not entirely remove the risk of developing coronary heart disease. Hagberg (1997) suggests that the preventive benefit of exercise is probably underestimated, and that "physical activity and physical fitness also appear to diminish the rate of development of hypertension" (p. 117).

There is a direct relationship between sodium intake and hypertension (He et al., 1999). The more sodium you consume, the higher your blood pressure; this tendency is particularly true for people who are overweight. Obesity causes changes in the sympathetic nervous system and other metabolic pathways that result in enhanced sodium reabsorption and sodium retention in the kidneys. While everyone may want to limit their sodium intake, reducing sodium intake may be more beneficial for overweight persons (He et al., 1999.)

Cholesterol Waxy substance that circulates naturally in the bloodstream; when levels are too high, it deposits in the walls of blood vessels.

Lipoproteins Lipid (fatty, insoluble substance in blood) surrounded by a protein; the protein makes it soluble in blood.

Low-density lipoproteins Carriers of harmful cholesterol in the blood; "bad" cholesterol.

High-density lipoproteins (HDL) Carriers of cholesterol that transport cholesterol to the liver, where it can be removed from the bloodstream; "good" cholesterol.

High Blood Cholesterol **Cholesterol** is a fatty, wax-like substance that combines with protein and other lipids called **lipoproteins** and is carried in the blood plasma. There are two types of lipoproteins that carry cholesterol in the blood. **Low-density lipoproteins (LDL),** or so-called bad cholesterol, transport cholesterol from the bloodstream into cells and promote atherosclerosis by transporting cholesterol into the arterial wall. **High-density lipoproteins (HDL),** or *good* cholesterol, remove cholesterol from the cells and carry it to the liver for removal, thus protecting against atherosclerosis. Our HDL helps prevent cholesterol build-up in blood vessels, while low LDL levels increase heart disease risk. Low-density lipoproteins and other risk factors may contribute synergistically to the incidence of CVD (Chien et al., 1999).

One way LDL cholesterol levels become too high in blood is through eating too much of two nutrients: saturated fat (found mostly in animal products) and cholesterol (found only in animal products). Saturated fat raises LDL levels more than anything else in the diet. Cholesterol levels are determined through a chemical analysis of a blood sample. The National Cholesterol Education program has developed a cholesterol classification (Table 5.3).

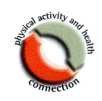

Cigarette smoking Cigarette smoking contributes to heart disease in several ways (Figure 5.7). First, it speeds up the development of atherosclerosis by potentially damaging the arterial walls and allowing cholesterol to deposit. Smoking also decreases the HDL, or good cholesterol, and may contribute to blood clot formation, which can cause a heart attack if the clot becomes lodged in an artherosclerotic artery.

Activities & Assessments 5.1, 5.2

Physical Inactivity Lack of physical activity is a major risk factor for heart disease. Numerous studies have been published during the past 50 years that show people who exercise regularly have better cardiovascular health (Haskell, 1997). Although research results vary from study to study, it is important to note that all studies consistently showed that being physically active does not increase an individual's risk of coronary heart disease. The primary and secondary prevention benefits of physical activity are numerous (Table 5.4). See Chapter 6 for more details about physical activity and cardiovascular health.

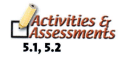

physical activity and health connection

TABLE 5.3 Cholesterol Levels

CHOLESTEROL LEVELS FOR PEOPLE OVER 20 WHO DO NOT HAVE HEART DISEASE*	
Desirable blood cholesterol	• Total blood cholesterol is less than 200 mg/dL • LDL is lower than 130 mg/dL
Borderline high cholesterol	• Total blood cholesterol level is between 200 and 239 mg/dl, OR • LDL is 130 to 159 mg/dL
High blood cholesterol	• Total blood cholesterol level is greater than 240 mg/dL, OR • LDL is 160 mg/dL or higher • LDL above 100 is too high for a patient with heart disease • HDL level less than 35 mg/dL is considered low and increases risk of heart disease

* Cholesterol levels are measured in milligrams per deciliter (mg/dL).

SOURCE: J. Henkel. (1999, Jan–Feb). Keeping cholesterol under control. *FDA Consumer*, 23–27.

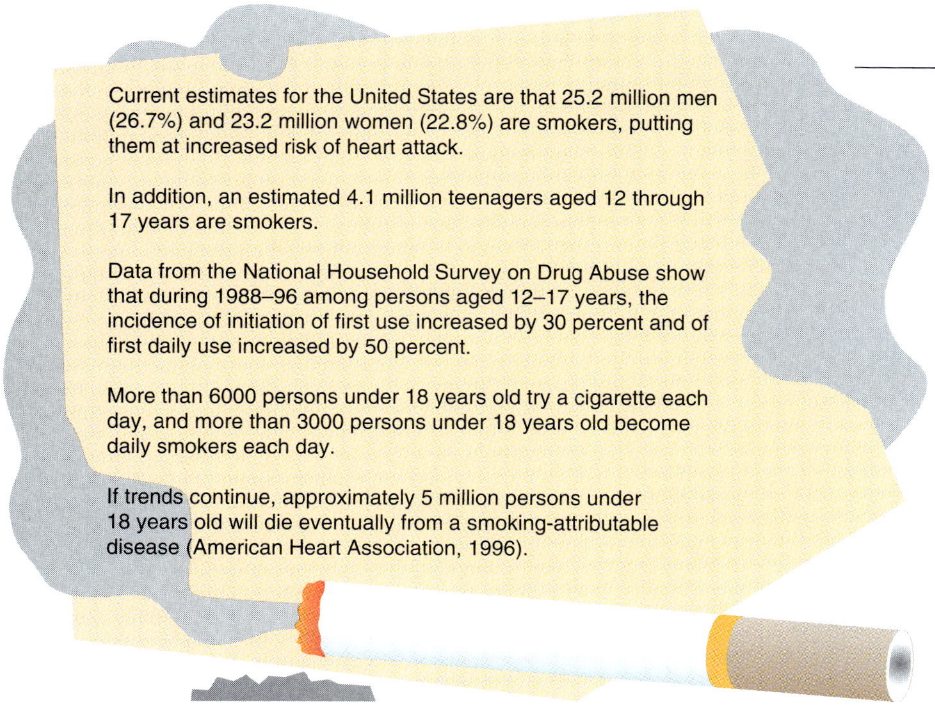
Current estimates for the United States are that 25.2 million men (26.7%) and 23.2 million women (22.8%) are smokers, putting them at increased risk of heart attack.
In addition, an estimated 4.1 million teenagers aged 12 through 17 years are smokers.
Data from the National Household Survey on Drug Abuse show that during 1988–96 among persons aged 12–17 years, the incidence of initiation of first use increased by 30 percent and of first daily use increased by 50 percent.
More than 6000 persons under 18 years old try a cigarette each day, and more than 3000 persons under 18 years old become daily smokers each day.
If trends continue, approximately 5 million persons under 18 years old will die eventually from a smoking-attributable disease (American Heart Association, 1996).

FIGURE 5.7

Some Facts about Cigarette Smoking

9. Diabetes mellitus, obesity, and stress are three contributing risk factors for CVD.

Contributing Risk Factors

Diabetes Mellitus Diabetes mellitus is a disorder of the endocrine system that interferes with the body's production of insulin. Insulin is needed for the body to metabolize glucose (sugar). Diabetes affects cholesterol and triglyceride levels, which explains why a large number of people with diabetes die from some cardiovascular disease. A good diet, physical activity, weight control—and sometimes a prescription medication—can assist in keeping diabetes in control. See Chapter 4 for further information on diabetes.

Obesity Overweight and obesity are increasing globally, with a 25 percent increase noted just over the past three decades (Must et al., 1999). Obesity is a risk factor for heart disease, even if there are no other risk factors present, because carrying excess weight places a strain on the heart.

TABLE 5.4 Biological Mechanisms by Which Exercise May Contribute to the Primary and Secondary Prevention of Coronary Heart Disease

Maintain or Increase Myocardial Oxygen Supply
- Delay progression of coronary atherosclerosis (possible)
- Improve lipoprotein profile (increase HDL-C/LDL-C ratio, decrease triglycerides) (probable)
- Improve carbohydrate metabolism (increase insulin sensitivity) (probable)
- Decrease platelet aggregation and increase fibrinolysis (probable)
- Decrease adiposity (usually)
- Increase coronary collateral vascularization (unlikely)
- Increase epicardial artery diameter (possible)
- Increase coronary blood flow (myocardial perfusion) or distribution (possible)

Decrease Myocardial Work and Oxygen Demand
- Decrease heart rate at rest and submaximal exercise (usually)
- Decrease systolic and mean systemic arterial pressure during submaximal exercise (usually) and at rest (usually)
- Decrease cardiac output during submaximal exercise (probable)
- Decrease circulating plasma catecholamine levels (decrease sympathetic tone) at rest (probable) and at submaximal exercise (usually)

Increase Myocardial Function
- Increase stroke volume at rest and in submaximal and maximal exercise (likely)
- Increase ejection fraction at rest and during exercise (likely)
- Increase intrinsic myocardial contractility (possible)
- Increase myocardial function resulting from decreased "afterload" (probable)
- Increase myocardial hypertrophy (probable); but this may not reduce CHD risk

Increase Electrical Stability of Myocardium
- Decrease regional ischemia or at submaximal exercise (possible)
- Decrease catecholamines in myocardium at rest (possible) and at submaximal exercise (probable)
- Increase ventricular fibrillation threshold due to reduction of cyclic AMP (possible)

* Likelihood that effect will occur for an individual participating in endurance-type training—for 16 weeks or longer, at 65 to 80% of functional capacity, for 25 min or longer per session (300 kcal), for 3 or more sessions per week—ranges from unlikely, possible, likely, probable, to usually.

ABBREVIATIONS: HDL-C = high-density lipoprotein cholesterol; LDL-C = low-density lipoprotein cholesterol; CHD = coronary heart disease; AMP = adenosine monophosphate.

SOURCE: W.L. Haskell. (1997). Physical activity, lifestyle, and cardiovascular health. In A.S. Leon (Ed.), *Physical activity and cardiovascular health: A national consensus*. Champaign, IL: Human Kinetics.

Stress Stress is a given in our society today. The ordinary events at home, on the job, and even at leisure can trigger stress responses as we try to maintain ourselves in an increasingly complex set of circumstances. We may not be able to get away from stress, but we can learn to deal with it (see Chapter 13). Research has not yet revealed exactly how stress effects the heart, but there appears to be a relationship between the occurrence of a heart attack, for instance, and the person's stress level, risky behaviors (cigarette smoking, diet), and socioeconomic status. For instance, an individual may develop high blood pressure due to stress, or may respond to stress by overeating or smoking.

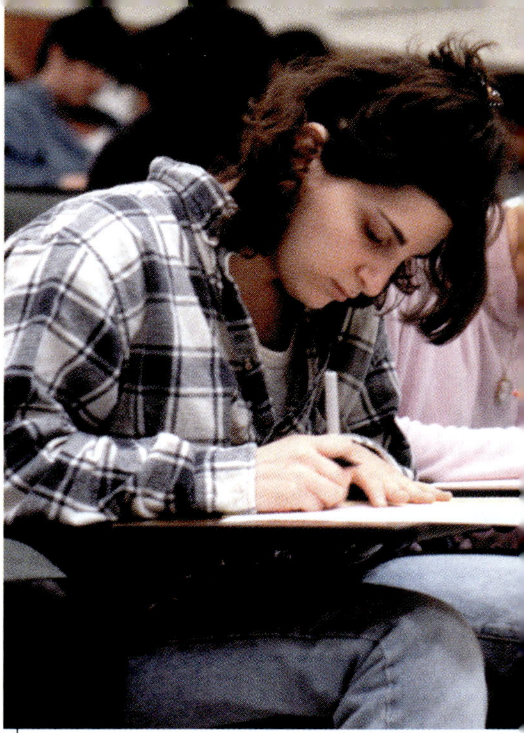

Stress may contribute to heart disease.

DIET AND CARDIOVASCULAR DISEASE

Diet can play a major role in preventing heart disease, especially as it relates to being overweight, obese, or having high blood cholesterol. Of all factors influencing the differences in mortality among populations, nutrition can be considered the most important (Kesteloot, 1999).

10. Diet plays a major role in preventing CVD.

Engage www.pahconnection.com 5.3

Vitamins

Vitamin C has been shown to decrease the prevalence of angina (Simon & Hudes, 1999), and vitamin E increases arterial elasticity, improving the ability of blood to flow through the arteries (Mottram, Shige, & Nestel, 1999).

Fats

Many studies have researched the association between a high intake of saturated fat and the increased incidence of heart disease. However, research suggests that populations with high monounsaturated fat intake (olive oil, for example), such as the Mediterranean cultures, have a lower incidence of CHD. Therefore, experts recommend replacing saturated fat with monounsaturated fat rather than replacing saturated fat with carbohydrates (Perez-Jimenez et al., 1999).

Fruits and Vegetables

The risk of ischemic stroke decreases in both men and women with an increase in fruit and vegetable consumption (Joshipura et al., 1999). No fruit or vegetable in particular has been shown to be more protective than any other. The specific components of fruits and vegetables suggested to be responsible for this beneficial effect include potassium, folate, fiber, and dietary flavonoids (flavonoids are found in abundance in citrus fruit).

TAKING RESPONSIBILITY FOR YOUR HEALTH

Although cardiovascular disease is the leading cause of death in the United States, it can be prevented through not smoking, maintaining a good diet low in cholesterol, maintaining a normal blood pressure, and participating in regular physical activity. Cardiovascular disease is thought of as a lifestyle disease; however, there are some risk factors over which you have no control (age, gender, family history).

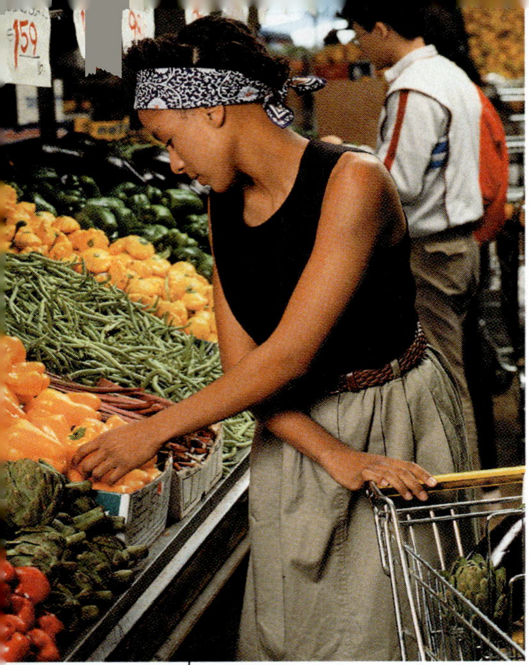

A diet rich in fruits and vegetables may decrease risk for CVD.

PHYSICAL ACTIVITY AND HEALTH CONNECTION

Participation in regular physical activity helps to strengthen the function of all components of your cardiovascular system. This is important not only in terms of cardiovascular efficiency but also in terms of disease protection. Many of the chronic diseases of the cardiovascular system result from disuse. Physical activity stresses the cardiovascular system and makes it more fit. The more fit you are, the easier your cardiovascular system adjusts to the stress of physical exertion. Those who have a fit cardiovascular system are less likely to suffer a heart attack, less likely to die if they have a heart attack, and more likely to recover fully after a heart attack.

Regular exposure to physical activity also benefits the pulmonary system, allowing it to coordinate more efficiently the exchange of oxygen and carbon dioxide with the cardiovascular system. Physical activity also plays an important role in the rehabilitation process for those who have developed cardiovascular disease. Cardiac rehabilitation programs allow individuals to return to a normal lifestyle much more rapidly than in the past.

CONCEPT CONNECTION

1. **The circulatory system consists of the heart, veins, arteries, and capillaries.** The circulatory system is made up of the heart and a network of blood vessels. Arteries carry oxygenated blood from the heart to all the organs and tissues, while veins return blood to the heart after oxygen and nutrients have been exchanged for carbon dioxide and waste products.
2. **There are many forms of cardiovascular diseases (CVD).** Coronary heart disease is the most prevalent form of CVD; it occurs when the coronary arteries become clogged and blood flow is restricted. Heart attack and angina pectoris are most often caused by CHD.
3. ***Angina pectoris* and *heart attack* are not synonymous terms.** Angina is caused by reduced blood flow to the heart; a heart attack results from the complete shutdown of blood supply to the heart.
4. **Hypertension is a major risk factor for coronary heart disease (CHD).** Hypertension, the "silent killer," is a condition where the blood pressure to and from the heart is above the normal range. When the cause of the hypertension is unknown, it is referred to as *primary hypertension. Secondary hypertension* refers to cases in which the cause is known.
5. **Arteriosclerosis and atherosclerosis are key factors in cardiovascular disease.** *Arteriosclerosis* is the hardening of the arteries, which causes the walls of the arteries to thicken and lose their elasticity. *Atherosclerosis* is the most common form of arteriosclerosis and is a slow, progressive disease sometimes beginning in childhood. When the arteries lose their ability to contract and expand, blood flow to the heart is restricted.
6. **Cerebrovascular accident (CVA), or stroke, is a cardiovascular disease that affects the central nervous system.** Stroke is a form of CVD that affects the arteries of the central nervous system. There are two types of stroke: ischemic (caused by clots) and hemorrhagic (caused by blood seeping from a hole in the wall of the blood vessel).
7. **The three unmodifiable risk factors for CVD are age, family, and gender.** Three cardiovascular risk factors that cannot be changed are age, gender, and family history.

8. **The four modifiable CVD risk factors are hypertension, cholesterol level, cigarette smoking, and physical inactivity.** Four cardiovascular risk factors that can be changed include hypertension, cholesterol levels, cigarette smoking, and physical activity (or inactivity).

9. **Diabetes mellitus, obesity, and stress are three contributing risk factors for CVD.** Contributing risk factors such as diabetes, obesity, and stress are associated with an increased risk of cardiovascular disease, but the significance has not yet been scientifically shown.

10. **Diet plays a major role in preventing in CVD.** Diet can play an important role in preventing cardiovascular disease. By eating a nutritious diet that is low in fats, cholesterol, and sodium you can greatly lower your chances of heart disease. Research has also shown that certain vitamins (E and C) and fruits and vegetables may play a protective role against cardiovascular disease.

TERMS

Pericardium, 101
Myocardium, 101
Endocardium, 101
Aorta, 101
Deoxygenated blood, 101
Oxygenated blood, 101
Sinoatrial node, 101
Arteries, 102
Arterioles, 102
Veins, 102
Blood pressure, 102
Blood pressure cuff (sphygmomanometer), 102
Systolic pressure, 102
Diastolic pressure, 103
Venous return, 103
Hemoglobin, 103
Bicarbonate ion HCO_3, 103
Auto-regulation, 103
Pulmonary system, 103
Coronary heart disease, 104
Angina pectoris, 104
Ischemia, 104
Myocardial infarction, 104
Heart attack, 104
Hypertension, 104
Primary hypertension, 105
Secondary hypertension, 105
Arteriosclerosis, 105
Atherosclerosis, 105
Plaque, 106
Stroke, 106
Ischemic strokes, 107
Cerebral thrombosis, 107
Cerebral embolism, 107
Hemorrhagic strokes, 107
Cerebral hemorrhage, 107
Subarachnoid hemorrhage, 107
Cholesterol, 108
Lipoproteins, 108
Low-density lipoproteins (LDL), 108
High-density lipoproteins (HDL), 108

MAKING THE CONNECTION

Richard has learned about the biological mechanisms by which physical activity may contribute to the prevention of coronary heart disease. So, in addition to what he was already doing to prevent cardiovascular disease for the past couple years, he has added a 30-minute walk to his daily routine over the past couple months. Not only does Richard feel better physically as a result of his daily walk, but the internal satisfaction of knowing that he is doing even more to lower his risk of developing coronary heart disease is also very rewarding to him.

CRITICAL THINKING

1. Richard knew that diet, in particular cholesterol, was a factor in lowering his risk for coronary heart disease. Identify three ways in which you can lower your cholesterol.

2. A risk factor of cardiovascular disease is family history. Family history of CVD does not "guarantee" that you will get the disease, nor does it cancel out the importance of a healthy lifestyle (good nutritional balance, regular physical activity, and no smoking). A family history of CVD does predispose you to the disease, so it is important for you to determine your family CVD history. Construct a family tree by listing

your biological parents, siblings, grandparents (maternal and paternal), and aunts and uncles (paternal and maternal). Next to each name, list the CVD disease and the age at which it was discovered. Your family may be helpful with this activity. After completing your tree, you may want to share it with your family and discuss prevention efforts.

3. Melissa is a 21-one year old college student who is very studious. Because her studies are her number one priority (she wants to go to graduate school), Melissa finds it difficult to make time to maintain a healthy lifestyle, despite knowing how important it is. Although Melissa is not a regular smoker, she has a tendency to smoke when under stress (studying for finals), and frequently eats fast food. Melissa was active in high school sports, but she does not seem to find time for sports now that she is in college. As a matter of fact, she has gained about 15 pounds, although she would not be considered overweight. What can you suggest to help Melissa reduce her risk of cardiovascular disease?

REFERENCES

Burt, V.L., Culter, J.A., & Higgins, M. (1995). Trends in the prevalence, awareness, treatment, and control of hypertension in the adult U.S. population. *Hypertension 26:*60–69.

Chien, K.L., et al. (1999). Lipoprotein A level in the population in Taiwan: Relationship to sociodemographic and atherosclerotic risk factors. *Atherosclerosis 143:*(2):267–73.

Corti, M.C., Guralink, J.M., & Bicato, C. (1996). Coronary heart disease risk factors in older persons. *Aging Clinical Experimental Research 9:*75–79.

Hagberg, J.M. (1997). Physical activity, physical fitness, and blood pressure. In Leon, A.S., ed., *Physical Activity and Cardiovascular Health: A National Consensus.* Champaign, IL: Human Kinetics.

Haskell, W.L. (1997). Physical activity, lifestyle, and cardiovascular health. In Leon, A.S., ed., *Physical Activity and Cardiovascular Health: A National Consensus.* Champaign, IL: Human Kinetics.

He, J., Ogdon, L.G., Vupputuri, S., Bazzano, L.A., Loria, C., & Whelton, P.K. (1999). Dietary sodium intake and subsequent risk of CVD in overweight adults. *Journal of the American Medical Association 282*(21):2027–2034.

Joshipura, K.J., et al. (1999). Fruit and vegetable intake in relation to risk of ischemic stroke. *Journal of the American Medical Association 282*(13):1233–39.

Kesteloot, H. (1999). On the determinants of mortality at the population level. *Acta Cardiologica 54*(3):141–49.

Lembo,G., et al.(1998). Systemic hypertension and coronary artery disease: The link. *American Journal of Cardiology 82*(3A): 2H–7H.

Mottram, P., Shige, H., & Nestel, P. (1999). Vitamin E improves arterial compliance in middle-aged men and women. *Atherosclerosis 145*(2):399–404.

Must, A., et al. (1999). The disease burden associated with overweight and obesity. *Journal of the American Medical Association 282*(16):1523–30.

National Heart, Lung, and Blood Institute (1998). *Morbidly and Mortality: 1998 Chartbook on Cardiovascular, Lung, and Blood Diseases.* Bethesda: National Institutes of Health.

National Heart, Lung, and Blood Institute (2000). *NHLBI FY 1999 Fact Book.* Bethesda: National Institutes of Health.

Newschaffer, C.J., Brownson, C.A., & Dusenbury, J. (1998). *Cardiovascular Disease.* In Brownson, R.C., Remington, P.L., & Davis, J.R., eds., *Chronic Disease Epidemiology,* 2nd ed. Washington, DC: American Public Health Association.

Perez-Jimenez, F., et al. (1999). Circulating levels of endothelial function are modulated by dietary monounsaturated fat. *Atherosclerosis 145*: 51–58.

Ross, R. (1993). The pathogenesis of atherosclerosis: A perspective for the 1990s. *Nature 362*:801–810.

Simon, J.A., & Hudes, E.S. (1999). Serum ascorbic acid and cardiovascular disease prevalence in U.S. Adults: The Third National Health and Nutrition Examination Survey. *Annals of Epidemiology 9*(6):358–65.

The Sixth Report of the Joint Committee on Prevention, Detection, Evaluation, and Treatment of High Blood Pressure (1997). *Archives of Internal Medicine 157*:2413–46.

Activities & Assessments

NAME ____________________ SECTION __________ DATE __________

5.1 Check Your Cholesterol and Heart Disease I.Q.

Directions: Are you cholesterol smart? Test your knowledge about high blood cholesterol with the following statements. Mark each true or false. The answers are given on page 116.

	TRUE	FALSE
1. High blood cholesterol is one of the risk factors for heart disease that you can do something about.	☐	☐
2. To lower your blood cholesterol level you must stop eating meat altogether.	☐	☐
3. Any blood cholesterol level below 240 mg/dL is desirable for adults.	☐	☐
4. Fish oil supplements are recommended to lower blood cholesterol.	☐	☐
5. To lower your blood cholesterol level you should eat less saturated fat, total fat, and cholesterol, and lose weight if you are overweight.	☐	☐
6. Saturated fats raise your blood cholesterol level more than anything else in your diet.	☐	☐
7. All vegetable oils help lower blood cholesterol levels.	☐	☐
8. Lowering blood cholesterol levels can help people who have already had a heart attack.	☐	☐
9. All children need to have their blood cholesterol levels checked.	☐	☐
10. Women don't need to worry about high blood cholesterol and heart disease.	☐	☐
11. Reading food labels can help you eat the heart-healthy way.	☐	☐

How cholesterol smart are you?

(continued)

5.1 Check your cholesterol and heart disease I.Q. (cont.)

ANSWERS TO THE CHOLESTEROL AND HEART DISEASE I.Q. QUIZ

1. **True.** High blood cholesterol is one of the risk factors for heart disease that a person can do something about. High blood pressure, cigarette smoking, diabetes, overweight, and physical inactivity are the others.
2. **False.** Although some red meat is high in saturated fat and cholesterol, which can raise your blood cholesterol, you do not need to stop eating it or any other single food. Red meat is an important source of protein, iron, and other vitamins and minerals. You should, however, cut back on the amount of saturated fat and cholesterol that you eat. One way to do this is by choosing lean cuts of meat with the fat trimmed. Another way is to watch your portion sizes and eat no more than 6 ounces of meat a day. Six ounces is about the size of two decks of playing cards.
3. **False.** A total blood cholesterol level of under 200 mg/dL is desirable and usually puts you at a lower risk for heart disease. A blood cholesterol level of 240 mg/dL is high and increases your risk of heart disease. If your cholesterol level is high, your doctor will want to check your level of LDL–cholesterol ("bad" cholesterol). A HIGH level of LDL–cholesterol increases your risk of heart disease, as does a LOW level of HDL–cholesterol ("good" cholesterol). An HDL–cholesterol level below 35 mg/dL is considered a risk factor for heart disease. A total cholesterol level of 200–239 mg/dL is considered borderline-high and usually increases your risk for heart disease. All adults 20 years of age or older should have their blood cholesterol level checked at least once every 5 years.
4. **False.** Fish oils are a source of omega-3 fatty acids, which are a type of polyunsaturated fat. Fish oil supplements generally do not reduce blood cholesterol levels. Also, the effect of the long-term use of fish oil supplements is not known. However, fish is a good food choice because it is low in saturated fat.
5. **True.** Eating less fat, especially saturated fat, and cholesterol can lower your blood cholesterol level. Generally your blood cholesterol level should begin to drop a few weeks after you start on a cholesterol-lowering diet. How much your level drops depends on the amounts of saturated fat and cholesterol you used to eat, how high your blood cholesterol is, how much weight you lose if you are overweight, and how your body responds to the changes you make. Over time, you may reduce your blood cholesterol level by 10–50 mg/dL or even more.
6. **True.** Saturated fats raise your blood cholesterol level more than anything else. So, the best way to reduce your cholesterol level is to cut back on the amount of saturated fats that you eat. These fats are found in largest amounts in animal products such as butter, cheese, whole milk, ice cream, cream, and fatty meats. They are also found in some vegetable oils—coconut, palm, and palm kernel oils.
7. **False.** Most vegetable oils—canola, corn, olive, safflower, soybean, and sunflower oils—contain mostly monounsaturated and polyunsaturated fats, which help lower blood cholesterol when used in place of saturated fats. However, a few vegetable oils—coconut, palm, and palm kernal oils—contain more saturated fat than unsaturated fat. A special kind of fat, called "trans fat," is formed when vegetable oil is hardened to become margarine or shortening, through a process called "hydrogenation." The harder the margarine or shortening, the more likely it is to contain more trans fat. Choose margarine containing liquid vegetable oil as the first ingredient. Just be sure to limit the total amount of any fats or oils, since even those that are unsaturated are rich sources of calories.
8. **True.** People who have had one heart attack are at much higher risk for a second attack. Reducing blood cholesterol levels can greatly slow down (and, in some people, even reverse) the buildup of cholesterol and fat in the wall of the coronary arteries and significantly reduce the chances of a second heart attack. If you have had a heart attack or have coronary heart disease, your LDL level should be around 100 mg/dL which is even lower than the recommended level of less than 130 mg/dL for the general population.
9. **False.** Children from "high-risk" families, in which a parent has high blood cholesterol (240 mg/dL or above) or in which a parent or grandparent has had heart disease at an early age (at 55 years or younger), should have their cholesterol levels tested. If a child from such a family has a cholesterol level that is high, it should be lowered under medical supervision, primarily with diet, to reduce the risk of developing heart disease as an adult. For most children, who are not from high-risk families, the best way to reduce the risk of adult heart disease is to follow a low saturated fat, low cholesterol eating pattern. All children over the age of 2 years and all adults should adopt a heart-healthy eating pattern as a principal way of reducing coronary heart disease.
10. **False.** Blood cholesterol levels in both men and women begin to go up around age 20. Women before menopause have levels that are lower than men of the same age. After menopause, a women's LDL–cholesterol level goes up—and so her risk for heart disease increases. For both men and women, heart disease is the number one cause of death.
11. **True.** Food labels have been changed. Look on the nutrition label for the amount of saturated fat, total fat, cholesterol, and total calories in a serving of the product. Use this information to compare similar products. Also, look for the list of ingredients. Here, the ingredient in the greatest amount is first and the ingredient in the least amount is last. So to choose foods low in saturated fat or total fat, go easy on products that list fats or oil first, or that list many fat and oil ingredients.

SOURCE: National Heart, Lung, and Blood Institute (NHLBI) and National Institutes of Health (NIH) (1995, May). *Cholesterol & heart disease IQ* (NIH Pub. No. 95-3794), [On-line]. Available: http://www.nhlbi.nih.gov/health/public/heart/chol/chol_iq.htm; accessed 1/31/01.

Activities & Assessments

NAME ____________________ SECTION __________ DATE __________

5.2 Check Your Physical Activity and Heart Disease I.Q.

Directions: Test how much you know about how physical activity affects your heart. Mark each statement true or false. See how you did by checking the answer on page 118.

	TRUE	FALSE
1. Regular physical activity can reduce your chances of getting heart disease.	☐	☐
2. Most people get enough physical activity from their normal daily routine.	☐	☐
3. You don't have to train like a marathon runner to become more physically fit.	☐	☐
4. Exercise programs do not require a lot of time to be very effective.	☐	☐
5. People who need to lose some weight are the only ones who will benefit from regular physical activity.	☐	☐
6. All exercises give you the same benefits.	☐	☐
7. The older you are, the less active you need to be.	☐	☐
8. It doesn't take a lot of money or expensive equipment to become physically fit.	☐	☐
9. There are many risks and injuries that can occur with exercise.	☐	☐
10. You should consult a doctor before starting a physical activity program.	☐	☐
11. People who have had a heart attack should not start any physical activity program.	☐	☐
12. To help stay physically active, include a variety of activities.	☐	☐

How well did you do?

(continued)

5.2 Check your physical activity and heart disease I.Q. (cont.)

ANSWERS TO THE PHYSICAL ACTIVITY AND HEART DISEASE I.Q. QUIZ

1. **True.** Heart disease is almost twice as likely to develop in inactive people. Being physically inactive is a risk factor for heart disease along with cigarette smoking, high blood pressure, high blood cholesterol, and being overweight. The more risk factors you have, the greater your chance for heart disease. Regular physical activity (even mild-to-moderate exercise) can reduce this risk.

2. **False.** Most Americans are very busy but not very active. Every American adult should make a habit of getting 30 minutes of low-to-moderate levels of physical activity daily. This includes walking, gardening, and walking up stairs. If you are inactive now, begin by doing a few minutes of activity each day. If you only do some activity every once in a while, try to work something into your routine every day.

3. **True.** Low- to moderate-intensity activities, such as pleasure walking, stair climbing, yardwork, housework, dancing, and home exercises can have both short- and long-term benefits. If you are inactive, the key is to get started. One great way is to take a walk for 10 to 15 minutes during your lunch break, or take your dog for a walk every day. At least 30 minutes of physical activity every day can help to improve your heart health.

4. **True.** It takes only a few minutes a day to become more physically active. If you don't have 30 minutes in your schedule for an exercise break, try to find two 15-minute periods or even three 10-minute periods. These exercise breaks will soon become a habit you can't live without.

5. **False.** People who are physically active experience many positive benefits. Regular physical activity gives you more energy, reduces stress, and helps you to sleep better. It helps to lower high blood pressure and improves blood cholesterol levels. Physical activity helps to tone your muscles, burns off calories to help you lose extra pounds or stay at your desirable weight, and helps control your appetite. It can also increase muscle strength, help your heart and lungs work more efficiently, and let you enjoy your life more fully.

6. **False.** Low-intensity activities—if performed daily—can have some long-term health benefits and can lower your risk of heart disease. Regular, brisk, and sustained exercise for at least 30 minutes, three to four times a week, such as brisk walking, jogging, or swimming, is necessary to improve the efficiency of your heart and lungs and burn off extra calories. These activities are called *aerobic*—meaning the body uses oxygen to produce the energy needed for the activity. Other activities, depending on the type, may give you other benefits such as increased flexibility or muscle strength.

7. **False.** Although we tend to become less active with age, physical activity is still important. In fact, regular physical activity in older persons increases their capacity to do everyday activities. In general, middle-aged and older people benefit from regular physical activity just as young people do. What is important, at any age, is tailoring the activity program to your own fitness level.

8. **True.** Many activities require little or no equipment. For example, brisk walking only requires a comfortable pair of walking shoes. Many communities offer free or inexpensive recreation facilities and physical activity classes. Check your shopping malls, as many of them are open early and late for people who do not wish to walk alone, in the dark, or in bad weather.

9. **False.** The most common risk in exercising is injury to the muscles and joints. Such injuries are usually caused by exercising too hard for too long, particularly if a person has been inactive. To avoid injuries, try to build up your level of activity gradually, listen to your body for warning pains, be aware of possible signs of heart problems (such as pain or pressure in the left or mid-chest area, left neck, shoulder, or arm during or just after exercising, or sudden light-headedness, cold sweat, pallor, or fainting), and be prepared for special weather conditions.

10. **True.** You should ask your doctor before you start (or greatly increase) your physical activity **if** you have a medical condition such as high blood pressure, have pains or pressure in the chest and shoulder, feel dizzy or faint, get breathless after mild exertion, are middle-aged or older and have not been physically active, or plan a vigorous activity program. If none of these apply, start slow and get moving.

11. **False.** Regular physical activity can help reduce your risk of having another heart attack. People who include regular physical activity in their lives after a heart attack improve their chances of survival and can improve how they feel and look. If you have had a heart attack, consult your doctor to be sure you are following a safe and effective exercise program that will help prevent heart pain and further damage from overexertion.

12. **True.** Pick several different activities that you like doing. You will be more likely to stay with it. Plan short-term and long-term goals. Keep a record of your progress, and check it regularly to see the progress you have made. Get your family and friends to join in. They can help keep you going.

SOURCE: National Heart, Lung, and Blood Institute (NHLBI) and National Institutes of Health (NIH) (1996, August). *Physical activity & heart disease IQ* (NIH Pub. No. 96-3795), [On-line]. Available: http://www.nhlbi.nih.gov/health/public/heart/obesity/phy_act.htm; accessed 1/31/01.

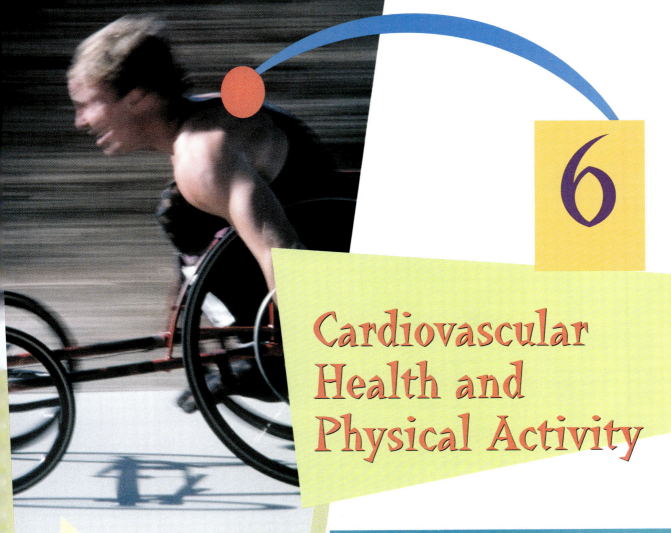

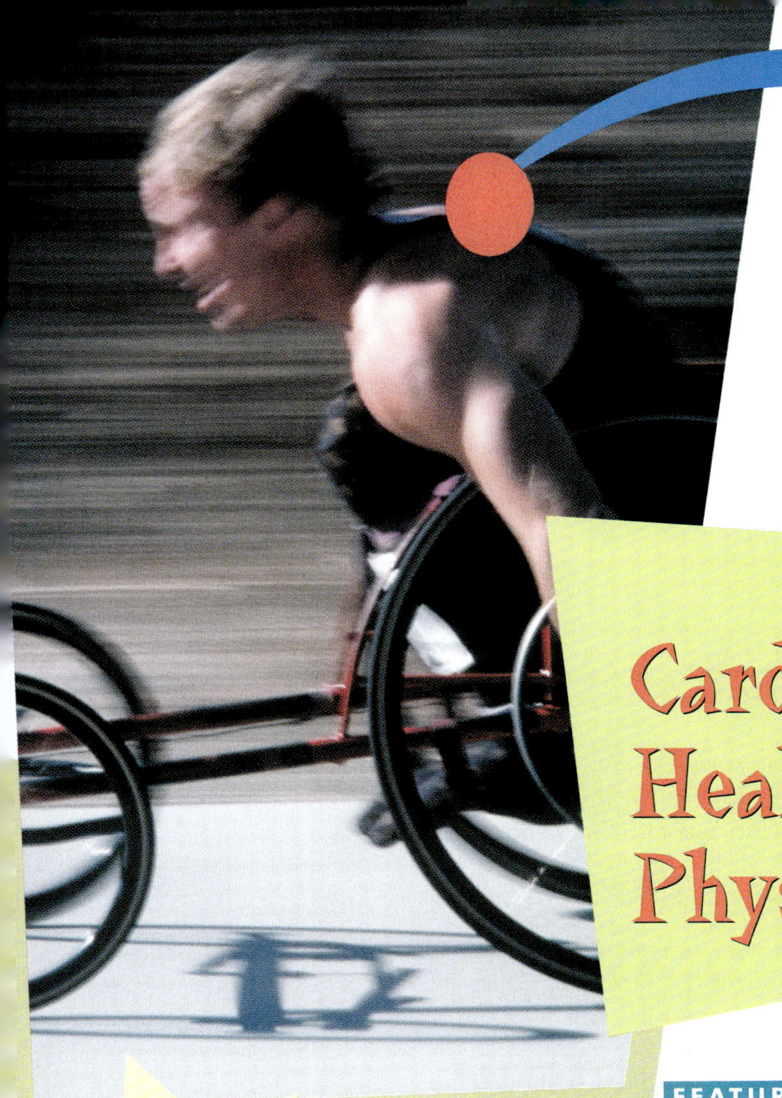

6

Cardiovascular Health and Physical Activity

CONCEPT CONNECTION

1. Physical inactivity is an independent risk factor for cardiovascular disease.
2. The National Institutes of Health say that being physically active helps prevent heart disease.
3. The heart is a specialized muscle made stronger by regular physical activity.
4. Active people are at lower risk for heart disease.
5. Many different activities may be performed to protect your cardiovascular system.

FEATURES

E-Learning Tools: www.pahconnection.com

Engage www.pahconnection.com

- 6.1 Finding your pulse
- 6.2 Determining your target heart rate
- 6.3 Calculating the caloric cost of activities
- 6.4 Assessing your cardiovascular fitness

Experience www.pahconnection.com

- 6.1 Improve your cardiovascular fitness
- 6.2 Evaluate your cardiovascular fitness

Explore www.pahconnection.com

- 6.1 Reserve methods of calculating intensity
- 6.2 Original Rating of Perceived Exertion (RPE) scale
- 6.3 Modified RPE
- 6.4 Using METS to determine intensity
- 6.5 Caloric cost of various activities

Activities & Assessments

- 6.1a Finding your pulse
- 6.1b Target heart rate

WHAT'S THE CONNECTION?

Mike is a former athlete who is concerned about fitness. He knows that physical activity is good for him, but he has only been performing resistance training since his sporting days ended. Mike has decided to incorporate some aerobic exercise into his daily routine, primarily to help maintain optimal body composition but also to help his endurance. Mike had heard that being active also helps his heart, but he is unsure what type of exercise is necessary to provide the benefits he desires.

INTRODUCTION

This chapter explains the role of physical activity in the prevention, management, and rehabilitation of cardiovascular disease. It designed to help you select activities to maximize **cardiovascular fitness** and health.

1. Physical inactivity is an independent risk factor for cardiovascular disease.

Physical Inactivity as an Independent Risk Factor

In the past two decades, several studies have demonstrated that leading a sedentary lifestyle is an **independent risk factor** for the development of cardiovascular disease (Blair, et al., 1989; Paffenbarger Jr., Hyde, Wing, & Hsieh, 1986). The term *independent risk factor* means that if all other potential risks for disease were controlled (or eliminated), living a sedentary lifestyle would, by itself, put you at greater risk for developing cardiovascular disease than if you lived an active lifestyle.

We have known for years the risk of cardiovascular disease associated with cigarette smoking, high cholesterol levels, and hypertension (high blood pressure). If we analyze the percentage of people who have these risks and compare those figures to the percentage of people who live predominantly sedentary lifestyles, we can see that, of all the major cardiovascular disease risk factors, physical inactivity affects the largest percentage of the population (Figure 6.1). If we were to focus on just improving one risk factor, getting more people physically active would have the greatest impact on the health of the population of the United States.

In addition, if we get those people who have other risk factors for cardiovascular disease (CVD) to increase their activity levels, their degree of protection against cardiovascular disease will increase significantly.

2. The National Institutes of Health say that being physically active helps prevent heart disease.

NIH Consensus Statement

The National Institutes of Health (NIH) *Consensus Statement* (1995) was developed by a panel of medical, physical activity, and health experts to report on the status of what is known about the relationship between physical activity and cardiovascular disease. The report concluded that physical inactivity is one of the most important factors that we must deal with if the health of the population is to be improved. The major findings of the NIH *Consensus Statement* are summarized in Table 6.1. These findings support the notion that people need to participate in physical activity on a regular basis to live longer and to live healthier. It also supports the direct relationship between participating in physical activity and cardiovascular health benefits.

Cardiovascular fitness Refers to how well the heart and vascular network can respond to the stress of physical activity. More fit cardiovascular systems can tolerate more physical activity. The ability of the body to utilize oxygen efficiently.

Independent risk factor A disease risk factor that stands alone; by itself, an independent risk factor can cause a disease.

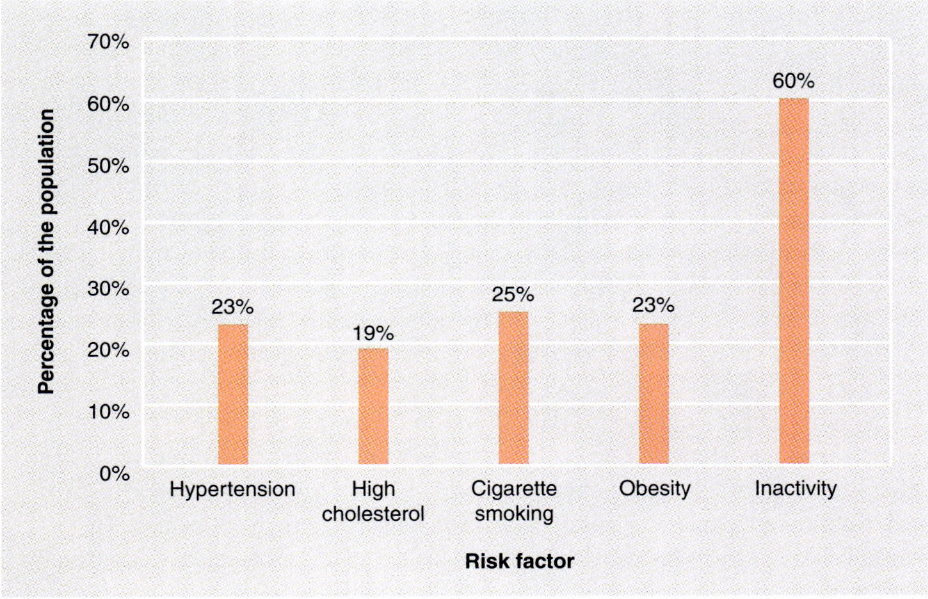

FIGURE 6.1

Disease Distribution and Physical Activity.
Physical inactivity affects the largest segment of our society when compared to the other major causes of disease.

SOURCE: Adapted from S.N. Blair, H.W. Kohl III, R.S. Paffenbarger, D.G. Clark, K.H. Cooper, and L.W. Gibbons. (1989, November 3). Physical fitness and all-cause mortality. *JAMA*, 262(17):2395–2401.

TABLE 6.1 **Major Findings of the NIH Consensus Statement**

- Physical activity protects against the development of CVD and also favorably modifies other CVD risk factors, including high blood pressure, blood lipid levels, insulin resistance, and obesity.
- Physical activity is also important in the treatment of patients with CVD or those who are at increased risk for developing CVD, including patients who have hypertension, stable angina, or peripheral vascular disease, or who have had a prior myocardial infarction or heart failure. Physical activity is an important component of cardiac rehabilitation, and people with CVD can benefit from participation.
- Evidence indicates that physical inactivity and lack of physical fitness are directly associated with increased mortality from CVD. The increase in mortality is not entirely explained by the association with elevated blood pressure, smoking, and blood lipid levels.
- Physical activity increases HDL, normalizes blood pressure, and increases insulin sensitivity. A number of factors that affect thrombotic function—including hematocrit, fibrinogen, platelet function, and fibrinolysis—are related to the risk of CVD. Regular endurance exercise lowers the risk related to these factors.

SOURCE: National Institutes of Health (1995). *NIH Consensus Statement: Physical Activity and Cardiovascular Health,* Vol. 13, No. 3.

CARDIOVASCULAR HEALTH

Physical activity plays an important role in optimizing cardiovascular function. Cardiovascular function responds to physical activity by becoming more efficient, which directly impacts the health of the cardiovascular system.

Cardiac Output, Stroke Volume, and Heart Rate

As stated previously, the heart is a special type of muscle (cardiac muscle). Like the other muscles in your body, the heart responds to the stress of physical activity by

3. The heart is a specialized muscle made stronger by regular physical activity.

Cardiac output The amount of blood ejected from the heart each minute; calculated by multiplying heart rate by stroke volume.

Stroke volume The amount of blood ejected with each contraction of the heart.

Heart rate The frequency at which the heart beats (contracts).

High-density lipoprotein A protective fat-protein substance that helps to remove cholesterol from the blood.

Coronary artery bypass surgery A common surgical technique for people who have had a heart attack. A grafted artery is attached to bypass a blocked coronary artery.

Angioplasty A surgical technique, used to treat CVD, in which a balloon is inserted into an artery to compress formed plaque.

4. Active people are at lower risk for heart disease.

becoming stronger. One of the best measures of your heart's ability to function is its **cardiac output.** Cardiac output refers to the heart's ability to pump out blood every minute. When analyzing cardiac output, the amount of blood squeezed out of the heart with each contraction **(stroke volume)** is important, but so is the rate at which the blood is squeezed out **(heart rate).** With improved fitness, the force with which the heart can contract increases. Another adaptation to regular exercise is the improved ability of the heart to expand and allow more blood to flow into it. This increased contractile force and greater elasticity allows more blood to be squeezed out with each contraction. If you can squeeze more blood out with each contraction (greater stroke volume) the heart doesn't have to beat as often. Therefore, one way to monitor improvement in cardiovascular fitness is to measure your heart rate. The lower your resting heart rate, the higher your stroke volume and the stronger your heart.

With increasing amounts of work, a fit person's heart rate will be lower than an unfit person's heart rate at any workload. The lower heart rate is due to the fit person's heart being stronger (greater stroke volume), so it doesn't have to beat as often. As the workload continues to increase, the unfit person will fatigue before the fit person. The fit person will be able to continue to be active at higher intensities and for a longer time than the unfit person. The unfit person's weaker heart will reach its maximal rate and will not be able to maintain cardiac output. If cardiac output cannot be maintained, the unfit person fatigues. The fit person will be able to be active longer before reaching maximal heart rate because the stroke volume is greater. Therefore, the fit person will be able to postpone fatigue for a longer time.

Controlling our cholesterol and blood lipid levels is one way of reducing the risk for developing cardiovascular disease. It has been shown that participating in regular physical activity can help reduce cholesterol and blood lipid levels. Maintaining a well-balanced diet also helps control both of these factors. Additionally, exercise has been shown to increase your **high-density lipoprotein** levels (HDL-C), which can help prevent the formation of plaque in the arteries by reducing cholesterol levels in the blood. For this reason, HDL-C is sometimes referred to as the "good" cholesterol. For more information on cardiovascular disease, see Chapter 5.

A VO_2 max test can be used to assess cardiovascular fitness.

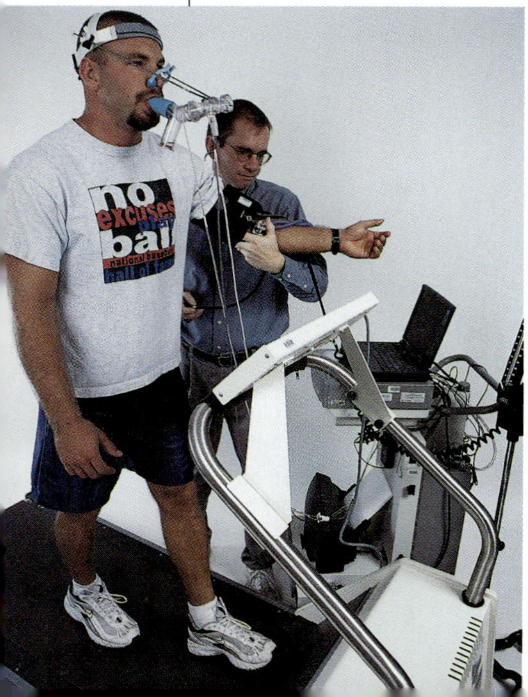

The Role of Physical Activity in Reducing Cardiac Risk

The 1996 *Surgeon General's Report* suggests that physical activity can help to decrease the risk of cardiovascular disease mortality in general, and coronary heart disease mortality in particular. The report also states that participation in regular physical activity prevents or delays the development of high blood pressure, and that exercise reduces blood pressure in people with hypertension (USDHHS, 1996).

Physical activity can play a role in preventing a first heart attack from occurring and reducing the risk of recurrent cardiac events (Haskell, 1995). Physical activity also aids in the recovery of patients following myocardial infarction, **coronary artery bypass surgery,** or cardiac **angioplasty,** through cardiac rehabilitation. Active people are at lower risk of CVD, develop less CVD, develop CVD at a later age, and tend to have less severe forms of CVD compared to those who are inactive (Haskell, 1995).

Physical Activity for Cardiovascular Disease Protection

Only moderate activity is necessary for protection against heart disease. The greatest improvement in protection comes from moving from a sedentary lifestyle to one that is moderately active. We also know that the higher your level of fitness, the more protection you receive from being active.

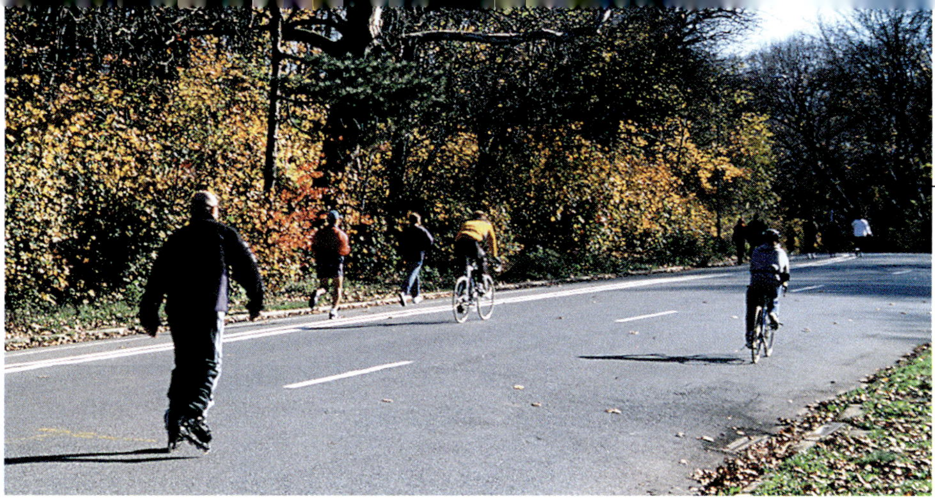

You can select from a variety of activities to improve your cardiovascular system.

Cardiovascular fitness may be defined as the ability of the body to utilize oxygen efficiently. Improvement is measured by assessing changes in VO_2max. Increases in VO_2max may range from 5 to 30 percent when starting a physical activity program. Individuals with low initial levels of fitness will see the greatest percent increase in VO_2max through physical activity. This happens because less fit individuals have more room for improvement.

VO_2max refers to the maximal volume of oxygen you can breathe in and deliver to your muscles. It is the best indicator of your cardiovascular fitness.

Selecting Activities

5. Many different activities may be performed to protect your cardiovascular system.

Recommended forms of activity for improvement of cardiovascular fitness and health are usually focused on the larger muscle masses of the body and include such activities as walking, jogging, hiking, gardening, cycling, and swimming (see Chapter 2). Some believe that the greatest benefit comes from large-muscle dynamic or "aerobic" activity that substantially increases cardiac output with rather small increases in mean arterial blood pressure (Haskell, 1995). These activities not only involve the larger muscles of the body but they are also rhythmical in nature. The cyclical pumping action of the muscles assists blood flow, keeps blood pressure in healthy zones, and allows for the adequate delivery of oxygen. Activities that involve smaller muscle masses (e.g., arm cranking, heavy-resistance weight lifting) may actually restrict blood flow, elevate blood pressure, and retard the delivery of oxygen.

Activities that require the cardiovascular system to perform at a level above its normal resting state for an extended period of time are best for improving cardiovascular function. Such exercises are frequently referred to as being *aerobic* in nature. Examples would include traditional exercises such as walking, jogging, cycling, swimming, roller blading, and cross-country skiing. Other activities that would help you improve your cardiovascular health include house and yard work and physically active recreational pursuits. You can choose any of the activities listed under the activity section at the end of Chapter 2 when exercising to improve cardiovascular fitness. You may wish to engage in several different types of activities to reduce repetitive stress to your bones and joints and to involve a greater number of muscle groups.

See Chapter 2 for the definition of *aerobic*.

The key to using physical activity as a way to prevent CVD is *regularity*. It is important that the heart, lungs, and vascular network are stressed regularly. Remember, it does not take long hours of exhaustive exercise to gain benefit from physical activity in the prevention of coronary disease. You can accumulate 30 minutes of physical activity every day and go a long way toward protecting your heart.

Explore
www.pahconnection.com
6.1

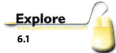

Finding the Right Intensity

As indicated in Chapter 2, the recommended intensity (I) for developing optimal cardiovascular fitness is between 55 and 65 percent, up to 90 percent of your maximum heart rate (determined by subtracting your age from 220) (ACSM, 2000). An alternative

Resting scores of heart rate and VO2 are lower in people who are fit.

VO_2 reserve The difference between maximal oxygen uptake (VO_2max) and resting oxygen consumption.

Heart rate reserve The difference between maximum heart rate and resting heart rate.

way of setting your intensity is to use from 40 and 50 percent up to 85 percent of your **VO_2Reserve** (VO_2R), or **heart rate reserve** (HRR) (ACSM, 2000). All three of these methods may be used to determine your aerobic capacity. Reserve methods utilize a percentage of the difference between your maximal score and your resting score. Reserve methods are preferred over the heart rate maximum method because they include an indirect measure of fitness (the resting score). Exercising at intensities beyond the recommended level shifts you from aerobic exercise into anaerobic exercise. While this may increase your power, aerobic exercise is best for improvements in cardiovascular fitness.

Similar increases in cardiovascular endurance may be achieved by a lower-intensity, longer-duration activity as opposed to higher-intensity, shorter-duration activity. The lower-intensity values—that is, 40–49 percent of VO_2R or HRR, and 55–64 percent of HR_{max}—are most applicable to individuals who are unfit (ACSM, 2000). Higher-intensity, shorter-duration activity is preferred by many people because they can be active for shorter periods of time. The drawback to this type of activity is that you are at greater risk of injury, and it can feel very stressful mentally and physically. Lower-intensity, longer-duration activity will provide the same benefits with a lower risk of injury and less mental and physical stress. The only drawback is that it takes longer to perform.

To reduce the risk of injury and to enhance adherence to your activity program, lower-intensity, shorter-duration activity is typically recommended for beginners. It is also recommended for those with previous injury and those who have no desire for physically challenging activities. However, athletes in training, those of higher fitness levels, and those who enjoy a physical challenge usually perform higher-intensity activities. We also know that the more fit the person, the higher the intensity needs to be to bring about further improvement. For the majority of the healthy adult population, intensities within the range of 70–85 percent HR_{max} or 60–80 percent of HRR are sufficient to achieve improvements in cardiovascular fitness, when combined with an appropriate frequency and duration of training (ACSM, 2000).

Several factors should be considered when determining exercise intensity. These include your level of fitness, any medications you might be taking, your risk for cardiovascular or orthopedic injury, your preference for different types of exercises, and your program objectives (ACSM, 2000). You will learn to modify the intensity of the activity you select to get the best response from your training program.

Monitoring Your Intensity

Heart Rate There are several ways in which you can monitor your cardiovascular response to physical activity. The most common way is by measuring your heart rate response. This will be most accurate when performing exercise of low-to-moderate intensities. During this type of exercise there is a linear relationship between heart rate and oxygen consumption. This means that, as heart rate increases, oxygen consumption increases at the same rate and magnitude. When exercise intensities go beyond the moderate range, heart rate is not a good indicator of cardiovascular response. This is because, as muscles go beyond 60 percent of their force-generating capacity, the muscles spend a longer time compressing the arteries and veins, and blood flow is reduced. Your body tries to compensate for this by having your heart beat more frequently. However, blood flow is still restricted, so heart rate increases at a much faster rate than oxygen delivery. The rise in heart rate is therefore not a good indicator of oxygen consumption at higher intensities of activity.

Engage
www.pahconnection.com
6.1

Activities & Assessments
6.1A, 6.1B

To monitor your exercise response using heart rate, you must first learn how to locate and measure your pulse (Figure 6.2). The next step involves calculating your target heart rate. Your *target heart rate* represents the zone that your heart rate needs to reach in order to receive optimal results from your activity session (Figure 6.3).

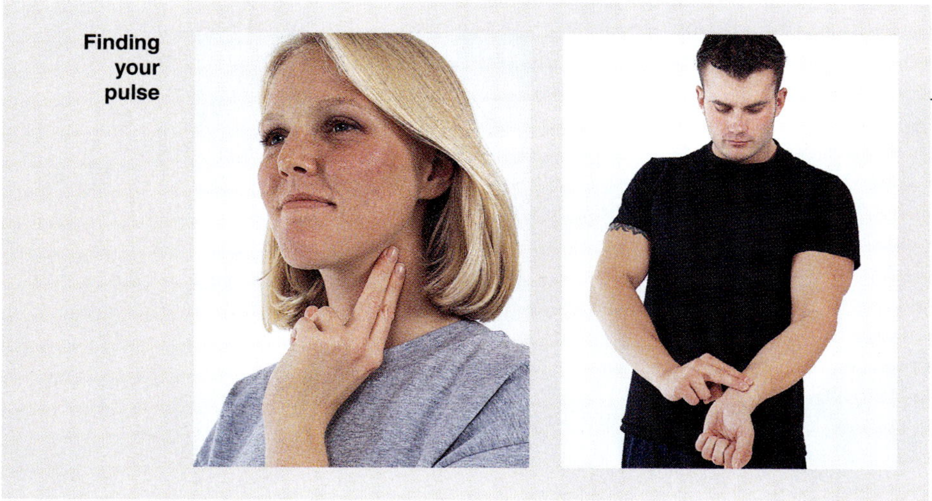
Finding
your
pulse

FIGURE 6.2

How to Find Your Pulse. The (a) carotid artery, and (b) radial artery, are frequently used to monitor heart rate response to physical activity.

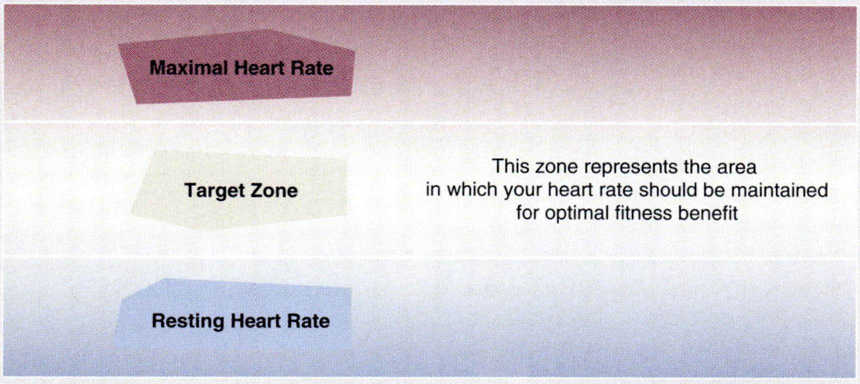
Maximal Heart Rate
Target Zone
This zone represents the area in which your heart rate should be maintained for optimal fitness benefit
Resting Heart Rate

To calculate target heart rate zone:

1. Subtract your age from 220. This gives you your estimated maximum heart rate (MHR).
   Example: 220 − 20 = 200
2. Subtract your resting heart rate from your MHR. This gives you your heart rate reserve (HRR).
   Example: 200 − 65 = 135
3. Multiply your HRR by 50%. This gives you your lower limit factor (LLF).
   Example: 135 × .50 = 67.5 or 68
4. Multiply your HRR by 85%. This gives you your upper limit factor (ULF).
   Example: 135 ×. 85 = 114.75 or 115
5. Add your LLF plus your resting heart rate to get the lower limit of your target zone.
   Example: 68 + 65 = 133
6. Add your ULF plus your resting heart rate to get the upper limit of target zone.
   Example: 115 + 65 = 180
7. You should exercise at a heart rate that falls between 133 and 180 for optimal fitness.

FIGURE 6.3

How to Calculate Your Target Heart Rate. To improve your fitness, try to keep your heart rate in your target zone.

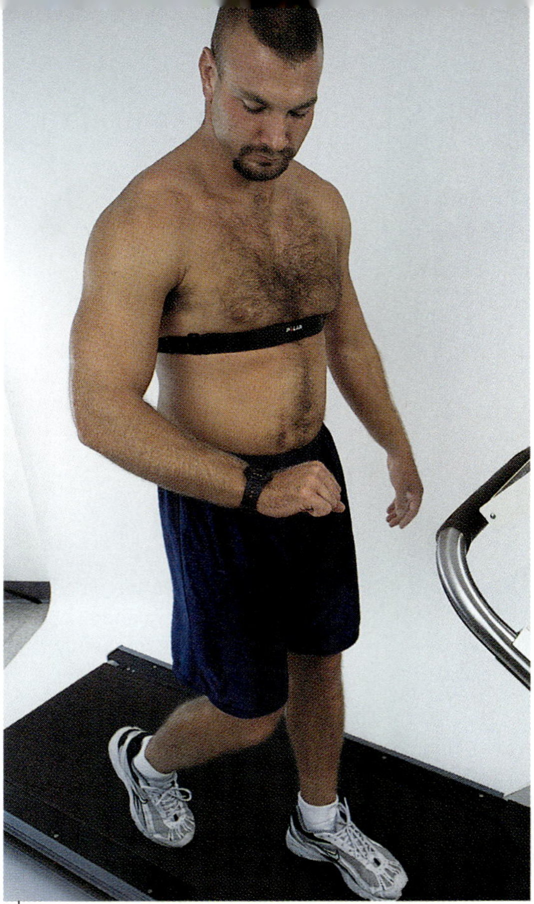

Heart rate can be used to monitor your cardiovascular system's response to physical activity.

The American College of Sports Medicine (2000) reminds us that some people prefer to exercise at the low end of the target heart rate range and focus on long-duration activities to achieve their program goals. This may help adherence in certain populations. We must also remember that different activities bring about different heart rate responses (ACSM, 2000). For example, the target heart rate you might choose while cycling would be different from the target heart rate when swimming. This reinforces the importance of selecting a prescreening test that is similar to the type of activity you plan on performing.

Rating of Perceived Exertion (RPE) You can also monitor your response to exercise by determining your perceived exertion. Swedish scientist Gunnar Borg developed a rating scale, the *rating of perceived exertion (RPE) scale,* that has since gained widespread acceptance and recognition. The original scale was based on a combination of numerical and descriptive associations with feelings of fatigue or exertion (Figure 6.4). To use the RPE scale, you select a number from the chart that corresponds with your perception of overall fatigue or exertion. The descriptors associated with the numbers assist you in selecting the appropriate numbers. There tends to be a relatively good relationship between the number on the RPE scale and exercise heart rate. If you multiply the number from the scale by 10, you will find it relates well with your current exercise heart rate. An RPE rating of 12 to 16 ("somewhat hard" to "hard") is considered to be of moderate intensity and recommended for training to improve cardiovascular fitness (ACSM, 2000).

The original RPE scale has been modified into a zero-based scale that may also be used to monitor exercise response (Figure 6.5). The modified scale was developed to present a baseline measure of zero to represent no exertion. It is used in the same way as the original scale. A rating of 5 to 8 is recommended for improvement of cardiovascular fitness. As with heart rate, RPE scores are specific to the type of activity you perform. Remember that the prescreening test you use to set RPE levels should be consistent with the type of activity you will be performing (ACSM, 2000).

Explore
www.pahconnection.com
6.2, 6.3, 6.4

FIGURE 6.4

The Borg RPE Scale

6	No exertion at all
7	Extremely light
8	
9	Very light
10	
11	Light
12	
13	Somewhat hard
14	
15	Hard (heavy)
16	
17	Very hard
18	Extremely hard
19	
20	Maximal exertion

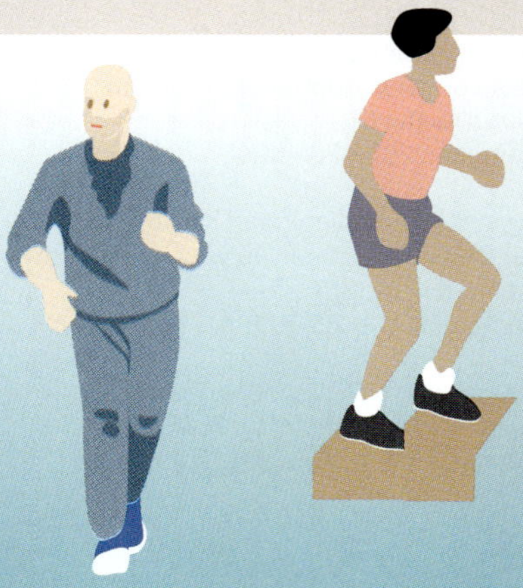

The Borg RPE Scale.
Rating of Perceived Exertion (RPE) can be used to monitor your response to physical activity.

SOURCE: For correct usage of the scale the user must go to the instruction and administration given by Borg, see Borg, G. 1998. *Borg's Perceived Exertion and Pain Scales.* Champaign, IL: Human Kinetics, or to the folder published by Borg on the RPE scale or the CR10 scale, Borg Perception, Furuholmen 1027, 762 91 Rimbo, Sweden.

The Borg CR10 Scale

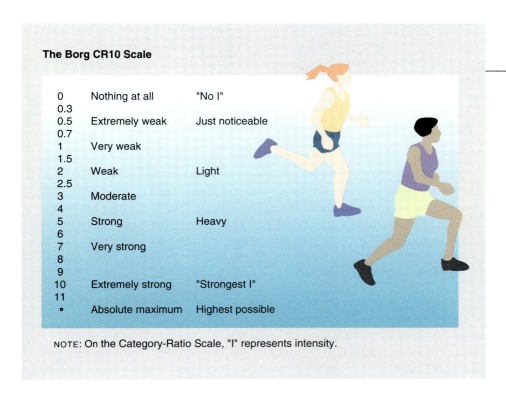

0	Nothing at all	"No I"
0.3		
0.5	Extremely weak	Just noticeable
0.7		
1	Very weak	
1.5		
2	Weak	Light
2.5		
3	Moderate	
4		
5	Strong	Heavy
6		
7	Very strong	
8		
9		
10	Extremely strong	"Strongest I"
11		
•	Absolute maximum	Highest possible

NOTE: On the Category-Ratio Scale, "I" represents intensity.

FIGURE 6.5

The Borg CR10 Scale.
The Borg CR10 scale for RPE is preferred by some people.

SOURCE: For correct usage of the scale the user must go to the instruction and administration given by Borg, see Borg, G. 1998. *Borg's Perceived Exertion and Pain Scales.* Champaign, IL: Human Kinetics, or to the folder published by Borg on the RPE scale or the CR10 scale, Borg Perception, Furuholmen 1027, 762 91 Rimbo, Sweden.

METS You may also use *multiples of your resting metabolism,* or METS, to monitor exercise intensity. One MET is equal to your metabolic rate at rest. Its equivalent in VO_2 is 3.5 mL × kg^{-1} × min^{-1}. Exercising at 10 METS means that your metabolism is working at a rate 10 times its resting level, or at 35 mL × kg^{-1} × min^{-1}. Generally it is recommended that you use MET levels between 50 and 85 percent of your maximal MET capacity for optimal cardiovascular fitness benefit in healthy adult populations (ACSM, 2000). Thus, if a person had a MET capacity of 10 METS, we would suggest that they exercise at an intensity of 5 to 8.5 METS. This represents 5 to 8.5 times your resting metabolic rate.

mL × kg^{-1} × min^{-1} are the units for oxygen consumption. They represent milliliters of oxygen consumed per kilogram of body weight per minute.

Caloric Expenditure Another way of monitoring exercise intensity is through the use of caloric expenditure. All human movement requires the expenditure of energy. In the human body, this energy takes the form of a molecule called **adenosine triphosphate** (ATP). Monitoring caloric expenditure involves estimating the caloric cost of performing physical activity. The unit of heat produced when energy is expended is called a *calorie* (technically it's called a *kilocalorie [kcal]*, but in our metric-phobic society we tend to drop the *kilo* part). The more work we do, the more energy we expend, and the more calories we use. Several charts have been developed for estimating the caloric expenditure of a number of activities.

Caloric expenditure is dependent on body size and sex. Large people expend more energy than small people doing the same activity. Men usually expend more energy than women do when performing the same activity. Additionally, whether your body weight is supported when performing an activity will impact caloric expenditure. For example, running expends more energy per unit of distance traveled than cycling.

Adenosine triphosphate A high-energy phosphate that is the only useable form of energy in the human body.

Generally, it is recommended that we expend approximately 150 to 400 kcal per activity session (ACSM, 2000). This would be equivalent to walking 1.5 to 4 miles. A goal to shoot for is a weekly caloric expenditure between 1000 and 2000 kcal, which has been associated with providing protection against cardiovascular disease. You can

Explore
www.pahconnection.com
6.5

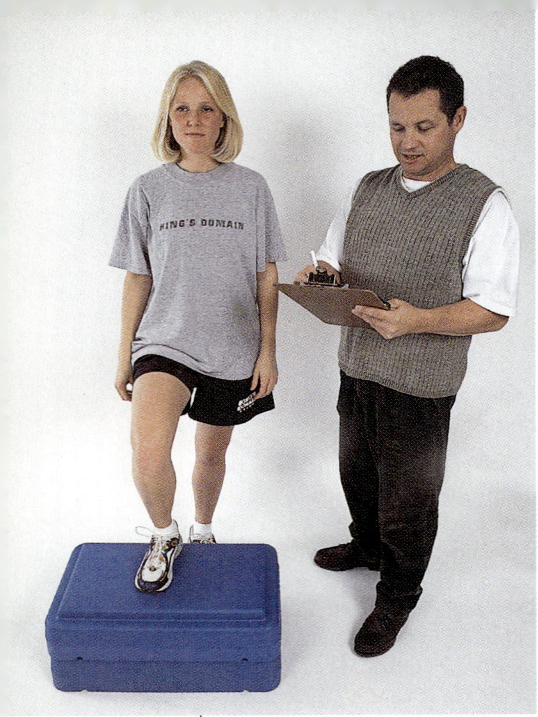

A step test is an easy way to assess your cardiovascular fitness.

Engage
www.pahconnection.com
6.3, 6.4

achieve 2000 kcal by performing activities that expend 400 kcal per session 5 days per week, 500 kcal per session 4 days per week, or any other combination that adds up to 2000 kcal for the week. It is best to spread the 2000 kcal over several days. See the Engage 6.3 and Appendix B on caloric cost of various activities to select the activities that will allow you to achieve this recommendation.

Assessing your Cardiovascular Fitness

To modify your exercise intensity optimally, you must have an accurate understanding of your current fitness level. There are many ways in which you can assess your cardiovascular fitness. Engage 6.4 contains several links to assessments that you may choose to evaluate your fitness status. Remember, if you have not been physically active recently, or if you are not "apparently healthy" (see Chapter 2), check with your physician before performing any of the tests.

Duration of Physical Activity

How long you need to exercise to protect your cardiovascular system will be dependent on the intensity of your activity. The lower the intensity, the longer you need to be active. If you follow the recommendations from the *Surgeon General's Report,* you need to accumulate 30 minutes of moderate-intensity physical activity on most if not all days of the week.

Progression

As pointed out in Chapter 2, it is very important that you progress gradually whenever you start, or make significant changes to, a physical activity program. You must give your body time to adjust to being physically active. If you do not, you run the risk of injury and dissatisfaction with your program.

PHYSICAL ACTIVITY AND HEALTH CONNECTION

This chapter has focused on how physical activity can help to prevent cardiovascular disease. It has been demonstrated that even moderate amounts of physical activity performed regularly will not only lower your risk for developing CVD but also increase the likelihood of surviving a heart attack, should one occur, and assist in the rehabilitation process after a heart attack. The largest jump in protection comes from moving from a category of being predominantly sedentary into one that is moderately active. By accumulating 30 minutes of moderately vigorous physical activity on most if not all days of the week, your risk of suffering a heart attack is diminished significantly.

CONCEPT CONNECTION

1. **Physical inactivity is an independent risk factor for cardiovascular disease.** Physical inactivity, by itself, is a significant risk factor for the development of cardiovascular disease. If all other risk factors for CVD were minimized and you were sedentary, you would still be at increased risk for CVD.

2. **The National Institutes of Health have concluded that being physically active helps to prevent heart disease.** Several government agencies, including the NIH, have issued policy statements supporting the importance of participating in regular physical activity. All of these statements have pointed to the role physical activity plays in helping to prevent heart disease.

3. **The heart is a specialized muscle made stronger by regular physical activity.** The heart is a specialized muscle that responds to the physical stress of being active by becoming stronger and more enduring. By making your heart stronger and more enduring, not only do you improve your ability to be physically active but you also make the cardiovascular system less susceptible to disease.

4. **More active persons appear to be at lower risk for heart disease.** There is a dose-response relationship between physical activity and protection from cardiovascular disease. The more fit a person's cardiovascular system, the greater the degree of protection against disease.

5. **Many different activities may be performed to protect your cardiovascular system.** There is no one perfect activity for improving your cardiovascular system. However, there are many different activities that may be selected to achieve this goal. It is best to vary your activities and incorporate several that use the large muscle masses of the body in a rhythmical pattern for extended periods of time (accumulation of 30 minutes).

TERMS

Cardiovascular fitness, 120
Independent risk factor, 120
Cardiac output, 122
Stroke volume, 122
Heart rate, 122
High-density lipoprotein, 122
Coronary artery bypass surgery, 122
Angioplasty, 122
VO2 reserve, 124
Heart rate reserve, 124
Adenosine triphosphate, 127

MAKING THE CONNECTION

Mike has started a cycling program to supplement his weight workouts. He now knows that the cycling program will provide him with additional protection against cardiovascular disease. Mike has also noticed the added benefit of some fat loss. He thinks this has made his muscles appear bigger.

CRITICAL THINKING

1. In the vignette, Mike added a cycling program to supplement his weight workouts. Why would the addition of aerobic activity help Mike lose fat? How does being physically active reduce Mike's risk for developing CVD?
2. Identify four activities in which you are likely to participate that will enhance your cardiovascular system. Describe how you will incorporate each activity into your daily and weekly routine.
3. Make a list of all the factors that increase your chances of getting CVD. (If you need to, review Chapter 5.) Order the list from the highest to lowest risk. Which risk factors pertain to you? How can you modify or change any of these risk factors?
4. You have been invited to speak at a local high school health class about how physical activity affects heart (cardiovascular) health. In 250 words, explain the impact that physical activity has on heart health.

REFERENCES

American College of Sports Medicine. (2000). *ACSM's Guidelines for Exercise Testing and Prescription,* 6th ed. Philadelphia: Lippincott, Williams & Wilkins.

American College of Sports Medicine. (1998). The recommended quantity and quality of exercise for developing and maintaining cardiorespiratory and muscular fitness, and flexibility in healthy adults. *Medicine and Science in Sports & Exercise 30*(6):975–91.

Blair, S.N., et al. (1989). Physical fitness and all-cause mortality: A prospective study of healthy men and women. *Journal of the American Medical Association 262*(17):2395–2401.

Haskell, W.L. (1995). Physical activity in the prevention and management of coronary heart disease. In Corbin, C., Pangrazi, R., eds., *The President's Council on Physical Fitness and Sports Research Digest,* Series 2, No. 1. Washington, DC: Department of Health and Human Services.

National Institutes of Health (1995). *NIH Consensus Statement: Physical Activity and Cardiovascular Health,* Vol. 13, No. 3. Bethesda, MD: U.S. Department of Health and Human Services.

Paffenbarger Jr., R.S., Hyde, R.T., Wing, A.L., & Hsieh, C. (1986). Physical activity, all-cause mortality, and longevity of college alumni. *New England Journal of Medicine 314*(10):605–613.

U.S. Department of Health and Human Services (1996). *Physical Activity and Health: A Report of the Surgeon General, Executive Summary.* Washington, D.C.

Activities & Assessments

NAME ______ SECTION ______ DATE ______

6.1 Finding Your Pulse and Target Heart Rate

Finding Your Pulse

Directions: You will need a stopwatch, a digital watch, or a watch with a second hand to take your pulse. Your pulse can be located at several places on your body. The two most common locations are the carotid pulse and the radial pulse.

TO FIND YOUR CAROTID PULSE

- Turn your head to one side.
- Feel the point at your neck where the large muscle and tendon stick out when your head is turned.
- Slide the fleshy part of your index, middle, and ring fingers along this tendon until you are on a level equal with your Adam's apple.
- Feel for the pulse. Readjust your fingers if necessary. Don't press too hard because this might alter the pulse.
- Count the number of pulses you feel for 60 sec. This number represents you heart rate in beats per min. If you are rushed for time, you could count the number of pulses you feel in 15 sec and multiply this number by 4. Remember however, that it is more accurate to take a full 60-sec count if possible.

TO FIND YOUR RADIAL PULSE

- Hold your forearm out in front of you with your palm facing you.
- Extend your wrist (move the back of your hand toward the back of your forearm).
- At the top portion of your forearm (nearest the thumb) you should see, or at least be able to feel, a tendon just below the wristbone. This is the radial tendon. Your radial pulse can be found just above your radial tendon near the wrist.
- Slide the fleshy part of your index, middle, and ring fingers along this tendon until you are 1 inch from your wrist.
- Feel for the pulse. Readjust your fingers if necessary. Don't press too hard because this might alter the pulse. Count the number of pulses you feel for 60 sec. This number represents you heart rate in beats per min.

(continued)

6.1 Finding your pulse and target heart rate (cont.)

Finding Your Target Heart Rate

Directions: You can calculate your target heart rate by following the steps outlined below. Your target heart rate represents the recommended heart rate zone in which you should attempt to keep your heart rate when training for cardiovascular fitness.

STEP 1: Select 220 − age = Estimated maximum heart rate (EMHR)
STEP 2: EMHR − resting heart rate (RHR) = heart rate reserve (HRR)

MAKE SURE TO USE THE PROPER INTENSITY FOR YOUR DESIRED OUTCOMES.

- **For those interested in health benefits only,** multiply
  HRR × 40% and HRR × 55%

  Then add your resting heart rate to these figures to arrive at your target training zone

  (HRR × 40%) + RHR = Lower limit of target training zone
  (HRR × 55%) + RHR = Upper limit of target training zone

- **For those interested in optimal health and fitness benefits,** multiply
  HRR × 50% and HRR X 85%

  Then add your resting heart rate to these figures to arrive at your target training zone

  (HRR × 50%) + RHR = Lower limit of target training zone
  (HRR × 85%) + RHR = Upper limit of target training zone

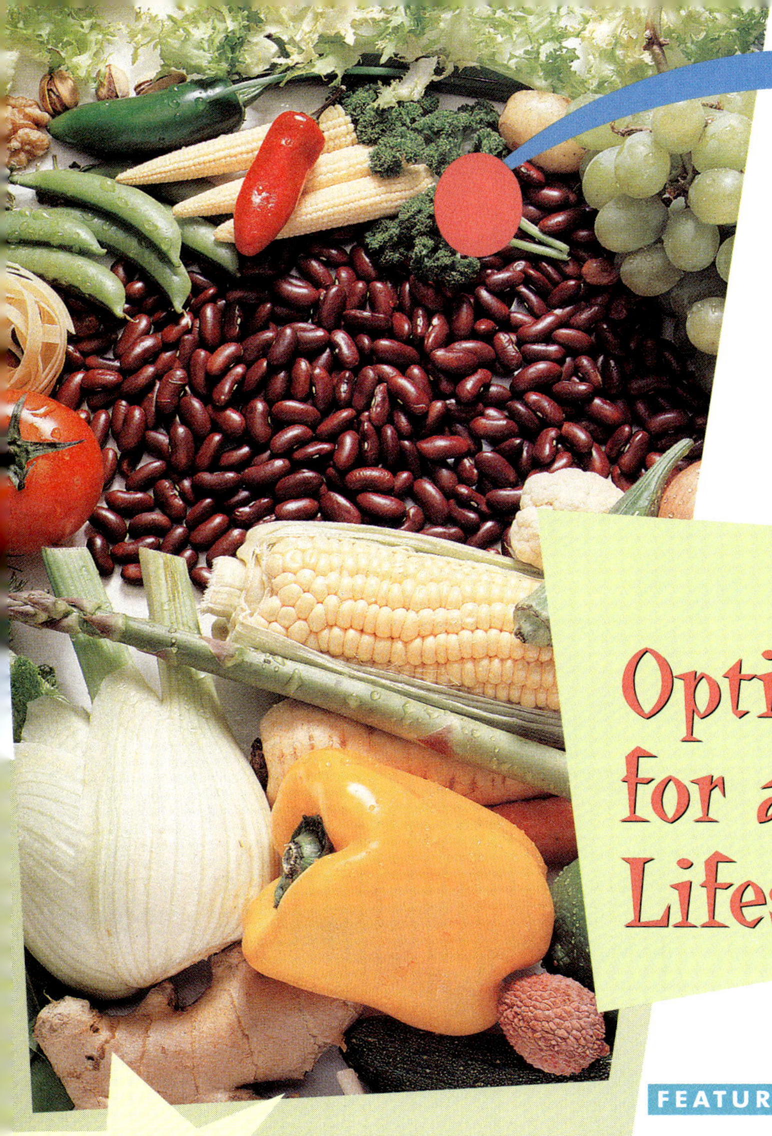

7

Optimal Nutrition for an Active Lifestyle

CONCEPT CONNECTION

1. Nutrition plays a major role in our overall health.
2. Nutrients provide energy, regulate body processes, and nourish tissues.
3. Food can be divided into six classes and each class plays a different role.
4. *Dietary Guidelines for Americans* provides advice about making healthy food choices.
5. The Food Pyramid provides a visual image of the foods Americans need daily.
6. The diet recommended for any healthy individual will support physical activity.
7. You can develop a personal nutrition plan.

FEATURES

E-Learning Tools: www.pahconnection.com

Engage www.pahconnection.com

7.1 Daily iron requirement
7.2 Calculate your recommended level of cholesterol and fat
7.3 The nutrition baseline profile
7.4 The nutritional analysis tool
7.5 Check your eating style
7.6 The healthy eating index

Experience www.pahconnection.com

7.1 American Dietetic Association
7.2 Eat five a day for better health
7.3 USDA food and nutrition information center
7.4 Vegetarian diets

Explore www.pahconnection.com

7.1 American Society for Nutritional Sciences
7.2 Food and nutrition board of the National Academy of Sciences
7.3 The International Food Information Council Foundation
7.4 Center for Food Safety and Applied Nutrition

Activities & Assessments

7.1 Food diary
7.2 My eating habits: Some clues to calories
7.3 Eat for good nutrition
7.4 How does your diet rate for variety?

WHAT'S THE CONNECTION?

Mary is a junior in college and is extremely attentive to her physical health. She began her weekly running program as a freshman and is now in very good physical shape. She runs approximately 20 miles a week and lifts weights twice a week. Mary adheres strictly to the Food Pyramid when selecting foods for her daily diet. In addition, she closely follows the recommended number of servings from each food group, selecting the most nutrient-dense foods from each group. Recently, a number of friends with whom Mary exercises have recommended that she take special vitamin and mineral supplements because she is physically active. Mary is uncertain about whether she needs to supplement her diet. Besides, dietary supplements can be expensive and she is on a tight budget. Mary schedules a meeting with the nutritionist at the university health center. The nutritionist asks Mary to record her food intake for a week so they can analyze Mary's diet.

NUTRITION AND YOUR HEALTH

1. Nutrition plays a major role in our overall health.

"You are what you eat" is a popular phrase, and we are becoming increasingly aware of its implications for health and disease. Nutrition and dietary factors play crucial roles in health promotion and chronic disease prevention. Nutritional and dietary factors contribute substantially to the burden of preventable illness and premature death in the United States. Five major causes of death are associated with dietary factors: coronary heart disease, some types of cancer, stroke, noninsulin-dependent diabetes mellitus, and coronary artery disease (*Healthy People 2010,* 2000) (Figure 7.1). The *Surgeon General's Report* states: "For 2 out of 3 adult Americans who do not smoke or do not drink excessively, one personal choice seems to influence long-term health prospects more than any other: what we eat" (*Surgeon General's Report on Nutrition and Health,* 1988, p.1). During this century, once-prevalent nutrient deficiencies have been replaced by excesses and imbalances of food components in the diet. Today, Americans eat too many calories, with many of these calories coming from foods high in fats and simple sugars, often at the expense of foods high in complex carbohydrates, fiber, and other substances conducive to good health that are found in fruits, vegetables, and grain products (USDA, 2000).

Explore 7.1

"Let food be your medicine and medicine be your food." Hippocrates said this more than two thousand years ago, and it is still meaningful today, as the preventive and therapeutic health values of food relative to the development of chronic diseases are unraveled. In recognition of the role that dietary factors play in causing many major chronic diseases, the U.S. Department of Agriculture (USDA) and the U.S. Department of Health and Human Services (USDHHS) have issued and periodically updated *Dietary Guidelines for Americans* (USDA, 2000). These guidelines encourage Americans to eat diets that emphasize a variety of plant foods, including whole grains, vegetables, and fruits, and to minimize animal foods, especially red meat such as beef, pork, or lamb, in an attempt to lower risk of chronic disease.

In addition to dealing with nutrition's role in chronic disease, the focus of the study and practice of nutrition in the United States also includes addressing nutrient needs for good health throughout the life cycle (Anderson, 1992). The Recommended Dietary Allowances (RDAs), first published in 1943, are undergoing a drastic change related to nutrient needs. The RDAs had been designed to prevent nutritional deficiencies in a gen-

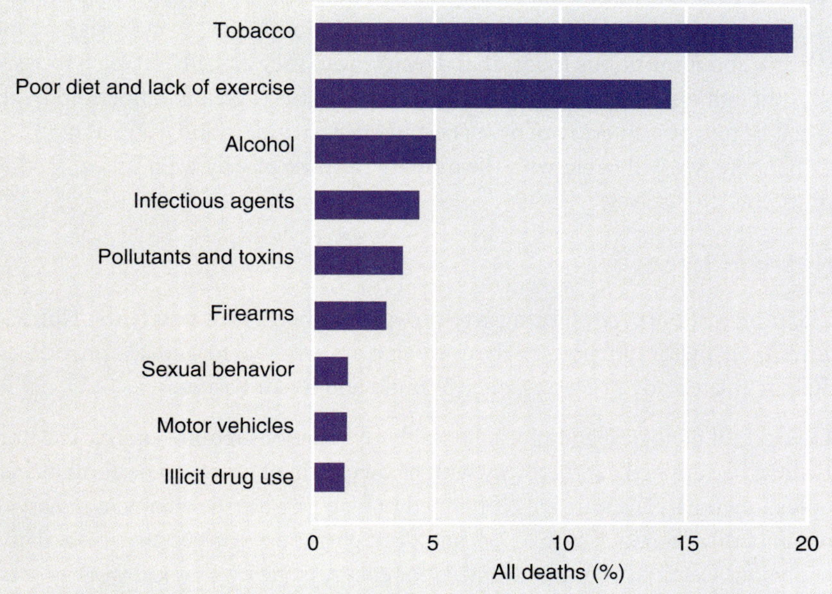

NOTE: The percentages used in the figure are composite approximations derived from published scientific studies that attributed death to these causes.

FIGURE 7.1

Actual Causes of Death in the United States, 1990.

SOURCE: J.M. McGinnis and W.H. Foege. (1993). Actual causes of death in the United States. *JAMA,* 270:2207–2212. (1990 data).

erally healthy population. The new recommendations will incorporate the concept of risk reduction for chronic diseases, not just the prevention of deficiencies. For example, the new RDA for calcium has recently been increased to prevent osteoporosis, an often crippling, disabling, and potentially life-threatening bone disease (see Chapter 10).

Nutrition is also an important component of health and physical activity. People who want to achieve optimal nourishment that will both protect against disease and support maximum physical activity have a twofold task in creating a nutritional plan. First, they must understand the basic biochemical and physiological roles of food, including what nutrients the body needs, in what amounts, and the kinds of foods that supply them. Second, they must study their own behavior and how well their choices meet their body's requirements.

The Council on Food and Nutrition of the American Medical Association (AMA) defines *nutrition* as "the science of food, the nutrients and the substances therein, their action, interaction, and balance in relation to health and disease, and the process by which the organism ingests, digests, absorbs, transports, utilizes, and excretes food substances" (AMA, 1999). This definition stresses the biochemical or physiological functions of the food we eat, but the American Dietetic Association (ADA) notes that nutrition may be interpreted in a broader sense and be affected by our behavior and environment as it relates to these functions (ADA, 1999). So, the second task in creating your nutritional plan includes determining the best ways for you to obtain the nutrients you need in the context of your own lifestyle.

Experience www.pahconnection.com 7.1

Most people know that nutrients in food nourish the body and are essential for promoting health (IFIC, 1989). Nevertheless, most people choose foods for reasons other than their nutrient content. Instead, people's food choices tend to be influenced by a variety of personal factors including: pleasure or preference, emotional comfort, values, attitudes, social pressure, image, habit, ethnic and cultural background, availability, convenience, and cost (Parraga, 1990). In principle, eating well is not difficult. Yet to master that principle and to put it into practice can be challenging because of the powerful influences of personal preferences just noted. Simply put, even though people may know about nutritious foods, that doesn't mean they actually eat such foods all the time. Although our food selection and nutritional status is greatly influenced by these personal factors, it is in every person's best interest to understand optimal nourishment first; therefore, we will begin with the primary purpose of why we must eat food—for the nutrients themselves.

Nutrient Needs

2. Nutrients provide energy, regulate body processes, and nourish tissues.

The principal purpose of eating is to provide our body with **nutrients.** Nutrients perform three major functions in the body that are essential for life: (1) provide energy, (2) help regulate body processes, and (3) build and repair tissues.

Nutrients Elements in foods that are required for energy, growth, and repair of tissues and regulation of body processes.

Digestion Metabolizing of food through a series of complex mechanical and chemical reactions.

Energy All biological and physiological body functions require energy. The human body must be supplied continuously with its own form of energy to perform its many complex functions. The nutrients contained in food provide the energy necessary to maintain bodily functions both at rest and during various forms of physical activity. The most obvious example of our body's need for energy is the mechanical work generated by muscle contraction. Our muscles must be provided with chemical energy from food to accomplish this mechanical work. Your physical functioning related to jogging, swimming, aerobic dancing, and weight lifting is considerably influenced by your capacity to extract energy from food nutrients and deliver it to the skeletal muscles (see Chapter 8).

In addition to the energy required for physical activity, the body requires considerable energy for absorption and assimilation of food nutrients during **digestion,** a series of complex mechanical and chemical reactions. Figure 7.2 depicts the digestive system

FIGURE 7.2

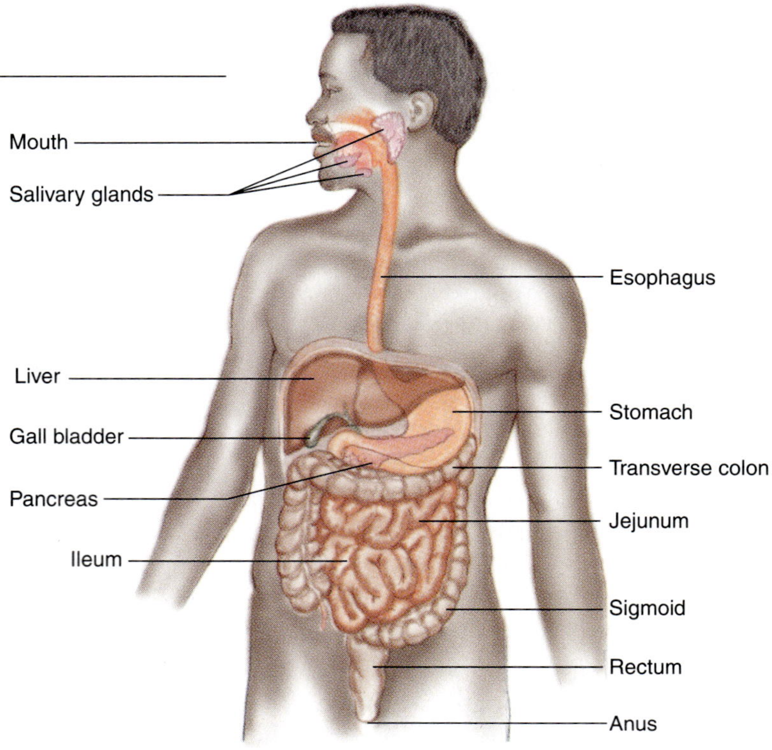

The Human Digestive System. Teeth and glandular secretions in the mouth help break up food, which the esophagus transports to the stomach. The stomach breaks down some of the food molecules and passes the food to the rest of the digestive tube: the duodenum, jejunum, ileum, colon, and rectum. The pancreas secretes enzymes and fluid into the duodenum to help the digestive process. The liver controls release of absorbed nutrients into the body. Undigested material is eliminated from the body at the anus.

and its major organs. The raw fuel for both biological and mechanical energy requirements comes in the form of three **macronutrients:** carbohydrates, fats, and proteins. These energy-yielding nutrients continuously replenish the energy you expend daily from biological and mechanical work.

There are a variety of ways to express the energy value of food. The term used and understood by most people is "calorie." A **calorie** is the amount of heat it takes to raise the temperature of 1 gram of water 1 degree Celsius. Calories are such small units of measurement that nutrition scientists find it easier to express food energy in 1000-calorie units called *kilocalories* (abbreviated kcalories, or kcal). When you see the term *calorie* on a food label, or when you calculate your energy expenditure in calories, you are actually using kilocalories, but since the term *calorie* is commonly used in everyday life we will use it here.

The energy in a particular food depends on how much carbohydrate, protein, and fat the food contains. Carbohydrate and protein yield 4 calories of energy from each gram and fat yields 9 calories per gram (Table 7.1). Once you know the number of grams of each of these substances contained by a certain food, you can derive the number of calories available in that food. Simply multiple the carbohydrate grams times 4, the protein grams times 4, and the fat grams times 9, and add all three together.

Calories are a highly desirable feature of food since they are used to do the body's physiological work or to exercise the muscles. Without calories, we would not survive. A constant flow of energy is so vital to life that other functions are sacrificed to maintain it. The average adult requires about 2000 calories per day to meet energy needs. The

Macronutrients Raw fuel, in the form of protein, carbohydrates, and fats, for biological and mechanical energy requirements.

Calorie Amount of heat it takes to raise the temperature of 1 gram of water 1 degree Celsius.

TABLE 7.1 Classes of Nutrients

NUTRIENT	FUNCTION	MAJOR SOURCES
Proteins (4 kcal/gm)	Form important parts of muscles, bone, blood, enzymes, some hormones, and cell membranes; repair tissue; regulate water and acid-base balance; help in growth; supply energy	Meat, fish, poultry, eggs, milk products, legumes, nuts, soy beans
Carbohydrates (4 kcal/gm)	Supply energy to cells in brain, nervous system, and blood; supply energy to muscles during exercise	Grains (breads and cereals), fruits, vegetables, milk
Fats (9 kcal/gm)	Supply energy; insulate, support, and cushion organs; provide medium for absorption of fat-soluble vitamins	Saturated fats primarily from animal sources, palm and coconut oils, and hydrogenated vegetable fats; unsaturated fats from grains, nuts, seeds, fish, vegetables
Vitamins	Promote (initiate or speed up) specific chemical reactions within cells	Abundant in fruits, vegetables, and grains; also found in meat and dairy products
Minerals	Help regulate body functions; aid in the growth and maintenance of body tissues; act as catalysts for the release of energy	Found in most food groups
Water	Makes up 50–70% of body weight; provides a medium for chemical reactions; transports chemicals; regulates temperature; removes waste products	Fruits, vegetables, and other liquids

physical activity and health connection

Micronutrients Nutrients required in small amounts; includes vitamins and minerals.

Essential nutrients Nutrients the body cannot make for itself; must be obtained from food.

Nonessential nutrients Nutrients made by the body from the foods we eat.

"evil" reputation of calories relates to energy storage in the body and is not deserved. If your body doesn't use all the energy-yielding nutrients to fuel its requirements, it rearranges them into storage compounds, primarily body fat, and puts them away for later use (see Chapter 9). This connection with excess body weight is the way many people think about calories, but it is a distortion of their true value.

Regulate Body Processes The second function of food is to regulate body processes. Although the raw fuel for biological and mechanical work comes from calories in the form of carbohydrates, fats, and proteins (or *macronutrients*), the systematic removal and utilization of energy from these nutrients requires an assortment of additional **micronutrients.** Vitamins, minerals, and water play crucial roles in regulating the body's processes related to activating energy release. The regulating of energy processes and tissue maintenance is referred to as human metabolism. *Human metabolism* is the sum total of all chemical and physical reactions that go on in living cells (Chapter 8). Metabolic processes allow for the release and use of energy from food compounds, the making of new compounds, and the transporting of compounds from place to place. For example, certain vitamins are essential for facilitating the release of the energy found in food and for controlling growth of body tissues. Like vitamins, minerals also play a regulatory role in metabolism and are essential for the synthesis of nutrients.

Maintenance, Repair, and Growth The third function of food is to supply the required nutrients for body tissue maintenance, repair, and growth. Nearly all body cells are constantly being replaced. For example, the red blood cells are useful for about a month and then must be replaced, and the cells that line the intestinal tract live less than a week. Various nutrients must be available to build the new cells for the body tissues: protein is a major material for red blood cells, muscle cells, and various enzymes; certain minerals like calcium and phosphorus make up the cells that form the skeletal system (see Chapter 10).

Essential and Nonessential Nutrients Six classes of nutrients are considered necessary in human nutrition: proteins, fats, carbohydrates, vitamins, minerals, and water (Table 7.1). Some nutritional scientists further distinguish nutrients into **essential nutrients** and **nonessential nutrients.** The term *essential nutrients* describes nutrients the body cannot make for itself and that must be obtained from foods we eat. Table 7.2 lists the specific nutrients currently known to be essential. Essential nutrients are necessary for human life. Inadequate intake of essential nutrients can lead to certain disease states and, eventually, death.

Other nutrients either come from the foods we eat or can be made by the body. For example the body can convert protein or fats into a carbohydrate, if needed. Since it is not crucial that we obtain them from food, we refer to these nutrients as *nonessential nutrients*. This is not to say that nonessential nutrients are unimportant, just that they can be made by the body.

Dietary Reference Intakes

Explore 7.2

So how much of the essential nutrients like Vitamin A or calcium do you really need to eat every day to be healthy? For more than 50 years, the Food and Nutrition Board of the National Academy of Sciences has been reviewing nutrition research and assigning nutrient requirements for healthy people. Until recently, one set of nutrient levels governed: the Recommended Dietary Allowances, or RDAs. First published in 1943, and updated every 5 to 10 years, the RDAs were designed to prevent nutrient deficiencies in large groups of people like the armed forces and children in school lunch programs.

TABLE 7.2 **The Essential Nutrients***

AMINO ACIDS	VITAMINS	MINERALS	FATS	WATER
Isoleucine	Ascorbic acid (vitamin C)	Calcium	Linoleic acid	
Leucine	Biotin	Chlorine	Linoleic acid	
Lysine	Cobalamin (vitamin B_{12})	Chromium		
Methionine	Folic acid	Cobalt		
Phenylalanine	Niacin (vitamin B_3)	Copper		
Threonine	Pantothenic acid Iodine			
Tryptophan	Pyridoxine (vitamin B_6)	Iron		
Valine	Riboflavin (vitamin B_2)	Magnesium		
Arginine†	Thiamine (vitamin B_1)	Manganese		
Histidine†	Vitamin A	Molybdenum		
	Vitamin D	Phosphorous		
	Vitamin E	Potassium		
	Vitamin K	Selenium		
		Sodium		
		Sulfur		
		Zinc		

*Must be obtained from food

†Not essential for adults; needed for growth of children

SOURCE: G. Edlin, E. Golanty, and K. McCormack Brown. (1999). *Health and Wellness,* (6th ed., p. 81). Boston: Jones and Bartlett.

From a statistical standpoint, this means that the RDAs were set to prevent nutritional deficiencies in 97 percent of a population. The RDAs are intentionally set somewhat higher than the body's actual physiological needs. To date, there are RDAs for protein, eleven vitamins, and seven minerals.

Times have changed. In 1993, the Food and Nutrition Board began a major overhaul of the RDAs that continues today. With increased understanding of the relationship between nutrition and chronic disease, the Food and Nutrition Board is redefining nutrient requirements and developing new RDAs based on three overriding principles. The first two principles supporting the current revision include: (1) incorporating the concept of risk reduction for chronic diseases, not just the prevention of nutrient deficiencies; and (2) recommending nutrient intakes that are thought to help people achieve good health by providing multiple reference points for nutrient intake instead of one number for each nutrient. The reference points will be collectively referred to as the **Dietary Reference Intakes** (DRIs). The DRIs serve as an umbrella term that includes the following values.

Dietary Reference Intakes (DRIs) Umbrella term that includes estimated average requirement, recommended dietary allowance, adequate intake, and tolerable upper intake level.

Estimated Average Requirement (EAR) This nutrient intake value, the Estimated Average Requirement (EAR), is estimated to meet the requirement of half the healthy individuals for a specific age-gender group. For example, the iron EAR for women of childbearing age will likely be different than for adult males. The EAR is used to assess nutritional adequacy of intakes of population groups. In addition, EARs are used to calculate RDAs.

Recommended Dietary Allowance (RDA) This value, the Recommended Dietary Allowance (RDA), is a goal for individuals and is based upon the EAR. Unlike earlier RDAs, these are designed to *reduce disease risk,* not just prevent deficiency. It is the daily dietary intake level that is sufficient to meet the requirements of 97 percent of all healthy individuals in a group and is meant for use by individuals. If an EAR cannot be set, no RDA value can be proposed.

Adequate Intake (AI) Adequate Intake (AI) is used when an RDA cannot be determined. In other words, scientific data is not strong enough to come up with a final number, yet there is enough evidence to give a general guideline. Like the RDA, individuals can use this number to set their personal dietary goals.

Tolerable Upper Intake Level (UL) The Tolerable Upper Intake Level (UL) is the highest level of daily nutrient intake that is likely to pose no risks of adverse health effects to almost all individuals in the general population. Anything above the UL might result in toxic reactions. The higher the intake, the higher the risk.

The third principle behind the nutrient revisions is that both essential nutrients and food components—deemed valuable even if not essential nutrients—will be considered. This principle allows the Food and Nutrition Board to consider components such as fiber and carotenoids.

CLASSES OF NUTRIENTS

3. Food can be divided into six classes and each class plays a different role.

As noted earlier, nutritionists divide nutrients into two main groups: macronutrients and micronutrients. Macronutrients, so-called because the body needs more of them, include proteins, carbohydrates, and fats. These are the foods our bodies use for energy and growth. Micronutrients, or nutrients required in only small amounts, include vitamins and minerals. Most foods contain a combination of the two groups. Water is a sixth class of nutrient and provides numerous vital functions in the body. Finally, we will include in this discussion an emerging classification called *functional foods.* Functional foods contain significant levels of biologically active components that impart health benefits beyond the six classes of nutrients.

Proteins

Protein An essential nutrient that the body uses in more ways than any other.

Protein is one of our most essential nutrients. The body uses it in more ways than any other nutrient. Protein was named after the Greek word *proteios,* meaning "of prime importance." The prime importance of protein is reflected by its uses in the body. The body uses proteins for new growth and to build such body proteins as hemoglobin, enzymes, hormones, and antibodies. Proteins constantly help to replace worn-out cells

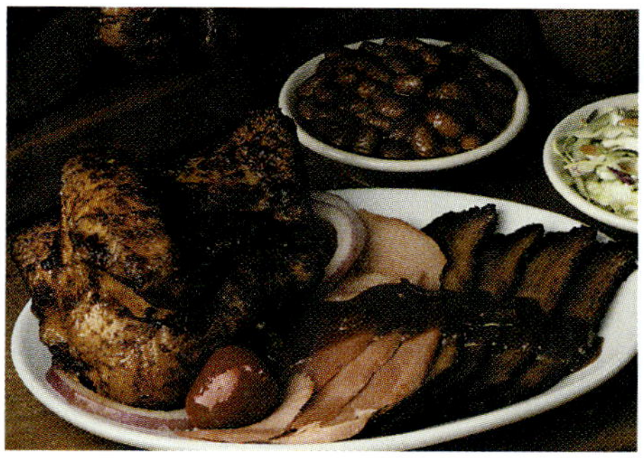
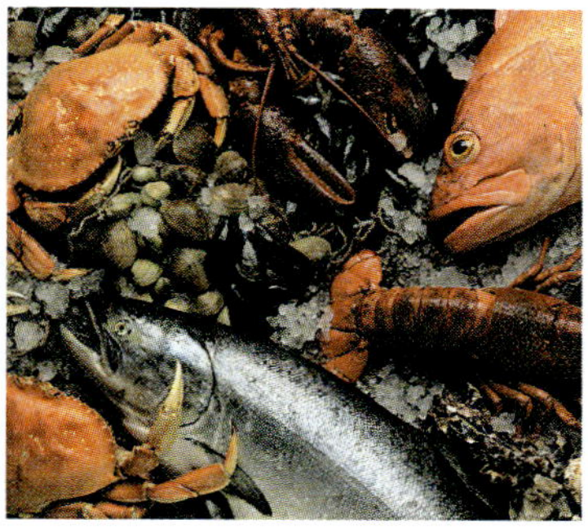
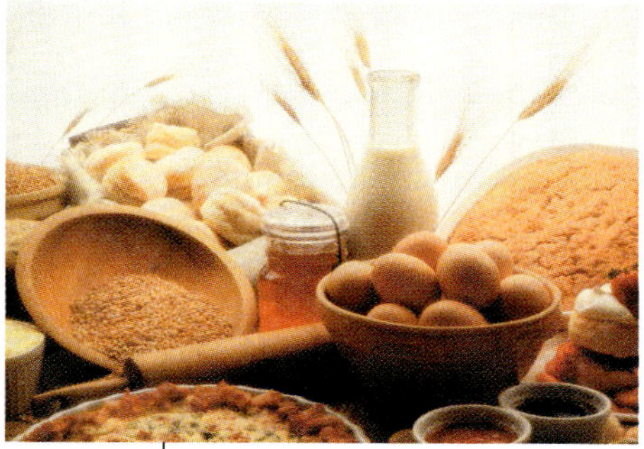

Protein sources consist of fish, meat, poultry, milk, and beans.

in the body. Protein has a number of physiological functions that are essential to optimal physical performance. People think of proteins as body-building nutrients, the material of strong muscles, and rightly so. Protein forms the structural basis for muscle tissue and is a major component of most enzymes in the muscle.

To appreciate the many vital functions of protein, we need to understand its structure. Protein is a complex chemical containing atoms of carbon, hydrogen, oxygen, and nitrogen that are combined in a structure called an **amino acid.** There are twenty different amino acids that are important to human nutrition. Humans can synthesize some amino acids in the body but cannot synthesize others. The nine amino acids that the body cannot make are referred to as **essential amino acids** (Table 7.2). Two of the essential amino acids, *lysine* and *tryptophan,* are poorly represented in most plant proteins. Thus strict vegetarians should make special plans to ensure that their diet contains sufficient amounts of these two amino acids. It should be noted that all twenty amino acids are necessary for protein (synthesis) in the body and must be present simultaneously for optimal maintenance of body growth and function. Protein foods that contain all of the essential amino acids in adequate amount, and in the correct ratio to maintain nitrogen balance and allow for tissue growth and repair, are known as *complete proteins.* Excellent sources of complete protein are eggs, milk, meat, fish, poultry, and soy beans.

Dietary Recommendation for Protein The National Research Council recommends that healthy adults have an RDA of 0.8 grams of protein per kilogram (2.2 lb) of ideal body weight. Ideal weight is used rather than actual weight, because protein is needed for lean body tissues, not for fat tissue. Thus, a 156-lb person needs approximately 56 grams of protein a day. Does the physically active individual or athlete need more protein in the diet? A joint position paper from the American Dietetic Association and the Canada Dietetic Association recommends that all athletes, as well as those who train like athletes, need a little more protein than do sedentary people. They recommend 1.0–1.5 grams of protein per kilogram (0.5–0.8 grams/lb) each day (ADA, 1993). Since many Americans and Canadians consume foods containing plenty of protein, they do not need protein supplements. It is important to realize that additional calories from protein are used for energy or stored as fat; protein is not an efficient source of energy.

Carbohydrates

Carbohydrates are the preferred energy source for most of the body's functions. Carbohydrates are found in all foods, but are especially plentiful in grains, fruits, and vegetables. Carbohydrates are organic compounds that contain carbon, hydrogen, and

Amino acid Complex chemical structure of protein containing atoms of carbon, hydrogen, oxygen, and nitrogen.

Essential amino acids The nine amino acids that the body cannot make.

Carbohydrates Organic compounds that contain carbon, hydrogen, and oxygen.

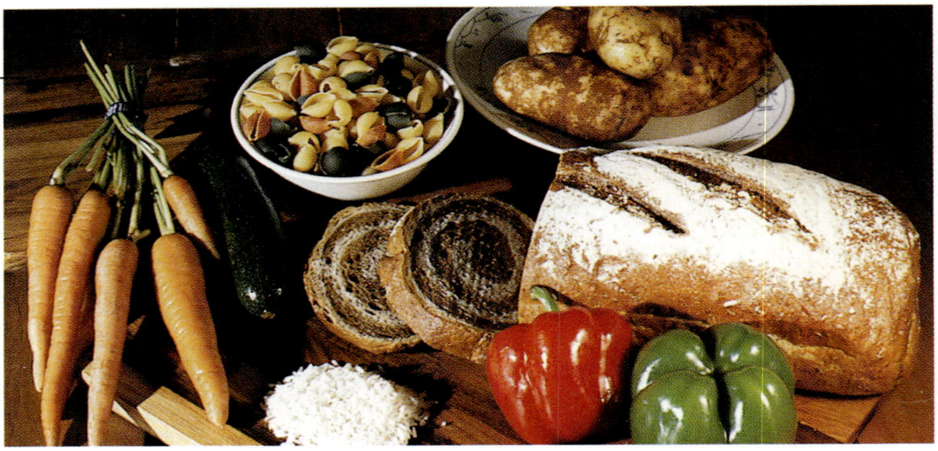

Carbohydrate sources consist of fruit, vegetables, and grains.

Simple carbohydrates Either one-sugar or two-sugar molecules.

Monosaccharide One-sugar molecule.

Disaccharide Two-sugar molecule.

Complex carbohydrates Called polysaccharides, these link three or more sugar molecules.

Starches Storage form of carbohydrates for plants.

Glycogen Storage form of sugar energy for humans and animals.

oxygen. A wide variety exist in nature and in the body. We will divide carbohydrates into two categories: simple and complex.

Simple Carbohydrates **Simple carbohydrates** are divided into one-sugar or two-sugar molecules. A one-sugar molecule is referred to as a **monosaccharide** (saccharide means "sugar" or "sweet"). More than 200 monosaccharides are found in nature, with the most common types being glucose, fructose, and galactose (Figure 7.3). Almost all of the body's cells use glucose as their chief energy source. Fructose is one of the sweetest sugars and is found in fruits and honey. Galactose is produced from milk sugar. Both must be converted to glucose to be used for energy by the cells.

The combination of two monosaccharides yields a **disaccharide,** of which sucrose, maltose, and lactose are formed. All three have glucose as one of their single sugars. Glucose occurs naturally in many fruits and vegetables. The most familiar source of sucrose is table sugar. Table sugar is a concentrated sweetener that is derived by refining the juice from sugar cane. Monosaccharides and disaccharides are known as simple carbohydrates, or simple sugars, because there is only one bond in each that must be broken down by the digestive enzymes before they can be absorbed by the blood.

Complex Carbohydrates **Complex carbohydrates** are known as polysaccharides. The term *polysaccharide* is used when three or more sugar molecules are linked. In fact, from 300 to 26,000 monosaccharides can be linked together to form a complex carbohydrate. The three most common forms of complex carbohydrates are starch, glycogen, and dietary fiber.

physical activity and health connection

Starches are the storage form of carbohydrates for plants. Grains such as wheat, rice, and corn are the richest food sources of starch. Other important sources include the foods from the legume family (peanuts, kidney beans, chickpeas, soybeans) and root vegetables (potatoes, yams).

As starch stores energy for plants, glycogen stores energy for humans and animals. If the blood delivers more glucose than the cells need, the liver and muscles take up a certain amount and build the polysaccharide **glycogen.** Glycogen plays an important role in the body as a readily available source of glucose, especially during physical activity (see Chapter 8). The well-nourished human body can store approximately 400 to 450 grams or 1500 to 2000 calories of energy (Van De Graaff, 1995). Excess glucose beyond what the body is able to use immediately, or deposit as glycogen, is stored as fat.

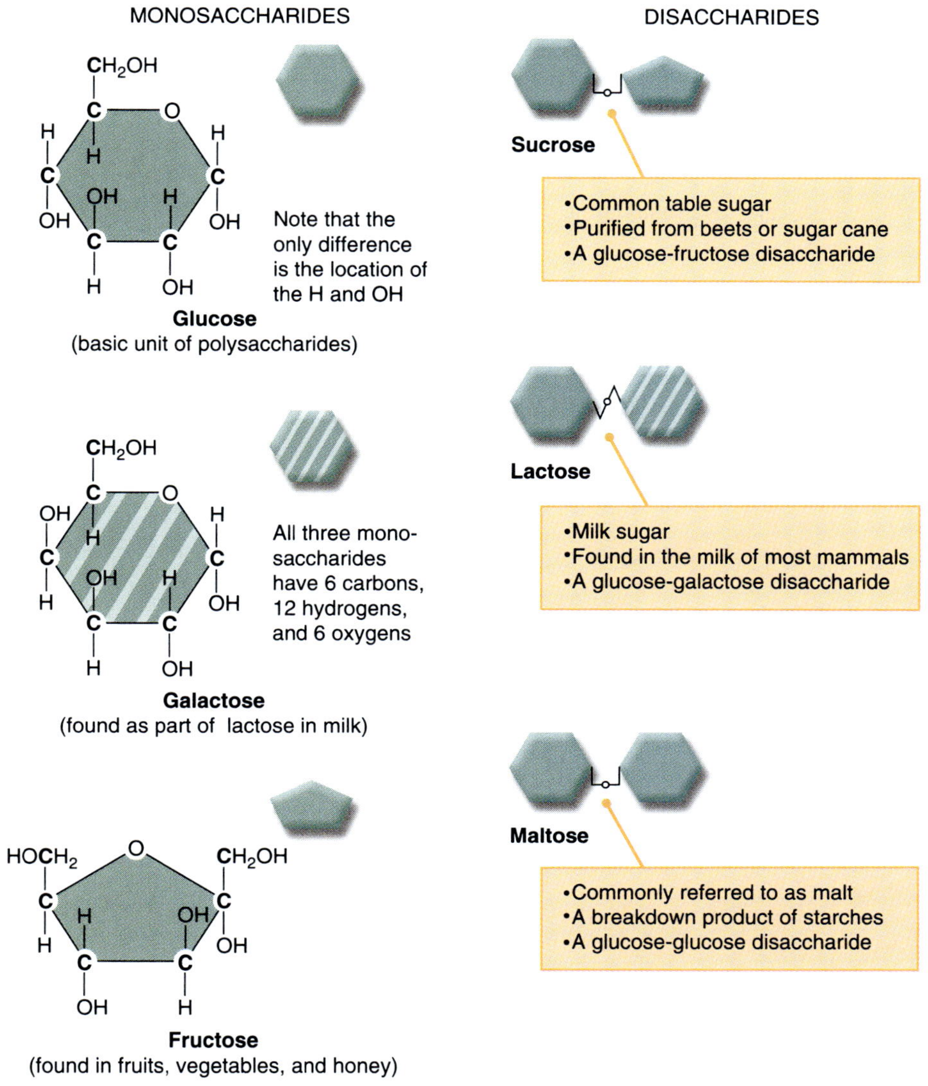
MONOSACCHARIDES
DISACCHARIDES
CH_2OH
Note that the only difference is the location of the H and OH
Glucose
(basic unit of polysaccharides)
All three monosaccharides have 6 carbons, 12 hydrogens, and 6 oxygens
Galactose
(found as part of lactose in milk)
Fructose
(found in fruits, vegetables, and honey)
Sucrose
•Common table sugar
•Purified from beets or sugar cane
•A glucose-fructose disaccharide
Lactose
•Milk sugar
•Found in the milk of most mammals
•A glucose-galactose disaccharide
Maltose
•Commonly referred to as malt
•A breakdown product of starches
•A glucose-glucose disaccharide

FIGURE 7.3

Some Common Sugars. Sucrose and fructose are the most common sugars in our diets.

Dietary fiber is a general term for the diverse carbohydrate polysaccharides of plants that cannot be digested by the human stomach or small intestine. Technically, dietary fiber is not a nutrient, but it has demonstrated benefits for health maintenance and disease prevention. Dietary fiber exists in two basic forms: insoluble and soluble. **Insoluble fibers** are not dissolved in water or metabolized by the intestines; they make the feces bulkier and softer, thus decreasing passage time. They are made up mostly of cellulose, hemicelluloses, and lignins. **Soluble fibers** are dissolved in water and are metabolized in the large intestine; they assists in draining cholesterol from the body. They include pectins, gums, and mucilages.

The ADA recommends 20–35 grams of fiber per day, or 10–13 grams per 1000 calories (ADA Position Paper, 1993). To achieve adequate dietary fiber intake, the ADA recommends you include at least 2–3 servings of whole grains as part of the daily servings of grains, 5 servings of fruits and vegetables daily, and legumes at least twice a week.

Dietary fiber Diverse carbohydrate polysaccharides of plants that cannot be digested by the human stomach or small intestine.

Insoluble fibers Dietary fibers not soluble in water or metabolized by the intestines; makes feces bulkier and softer, promoting decreased passage time.

Soluble fibers Dietary fibers soluble in water, metabolized in the large intestine; assist in removing cholesterol from the body.

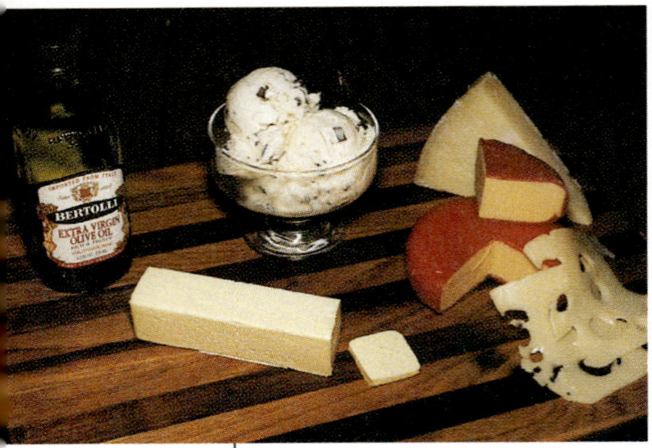

Fats sources include oil, ice cream, cheese, and margarine.

Dietary Recommendation of Energy-Yielding Carbohydrates Dietary recommendations state that carbohydrates should contribute 55–60 percent of the total daily energy intake. Simple refined sugars should account for 10 percent or less of total calories because they supply relatively few nutrients. The sugars in unrefined foods like fruits and vegetables are preferable because they are accompanied by many other nutrients. For active people, and for those involved in exercise training, the majority of carbohydrate calories should come from the complex variety.

Fats

Fats (also known as lipids) are found in foods and in the body. Fats can be categorized into three main groups: triglycerides, cholesterol, and phospholipids. .

Triglycerides When people talk about body fat, or fat in their food, they are usually referring to triglycerides. **Triglycerides** provide many important functions in the body. These fatty acids constitute the body's largest energy store, provide insulation, transport fat-soluble vitamins, and contribute to satiety (satisfaction). More than 95 percent of our body fat is in the form of triglycerides. The chemical name helps explain itself. A triglyceride molecule consists of three fatty acid atoms attached to a glycerol molecule. Fatty acids are chains of carbon, oxygen, and hydrogen atoms (Figure 7.4). Fatty acids chains may differ from one another in two ways: chain length and saturation. The chain length affects the way fat is absorbed and its solubility in water (shorter chains are more soluble). Saturation refers to the chemical structure—specifically, to the number of hydrogens the fatty acid chain is holding. The basic structures of fatty acid molecules are *saturated* and *unsaturated.*

Fats Members of a family of compounds called lipids.

Triglycerides Fatty acids that provide the body's largest energy store, act as insulation, transport fat-soluble vitamins, and contribute to satiety.

FIGURE 7.4

Chemical Structure of Saturated and Unsaturated Fats. Triglyceride consists of a molecule of glycerol with three fatty acids attached. Fatty acids can differ in the lengths of their carbon chains and degree of saturation.

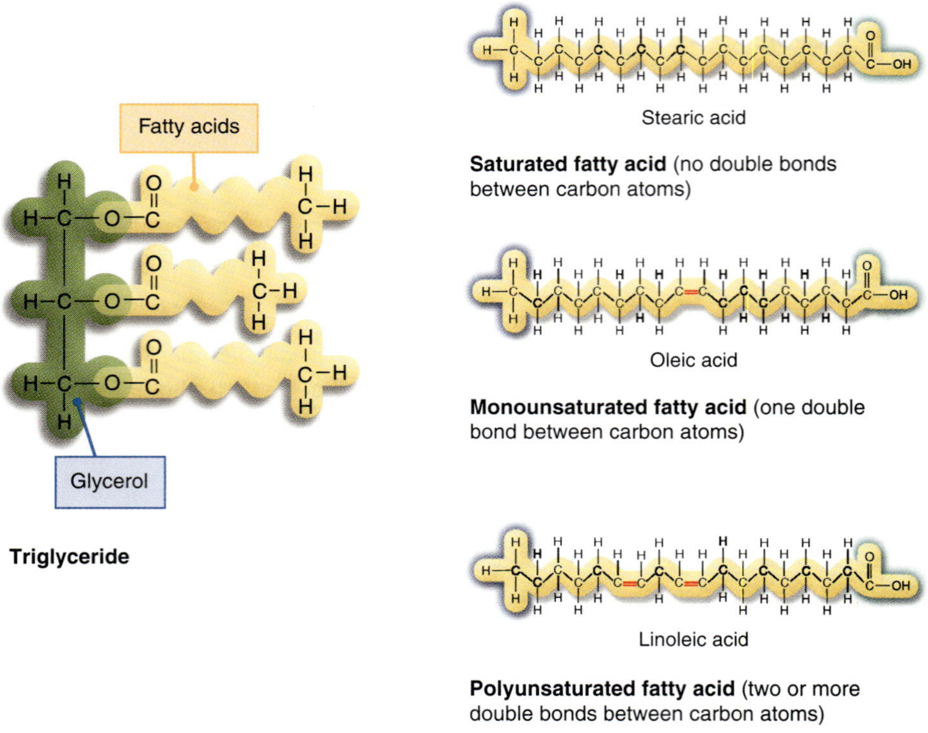

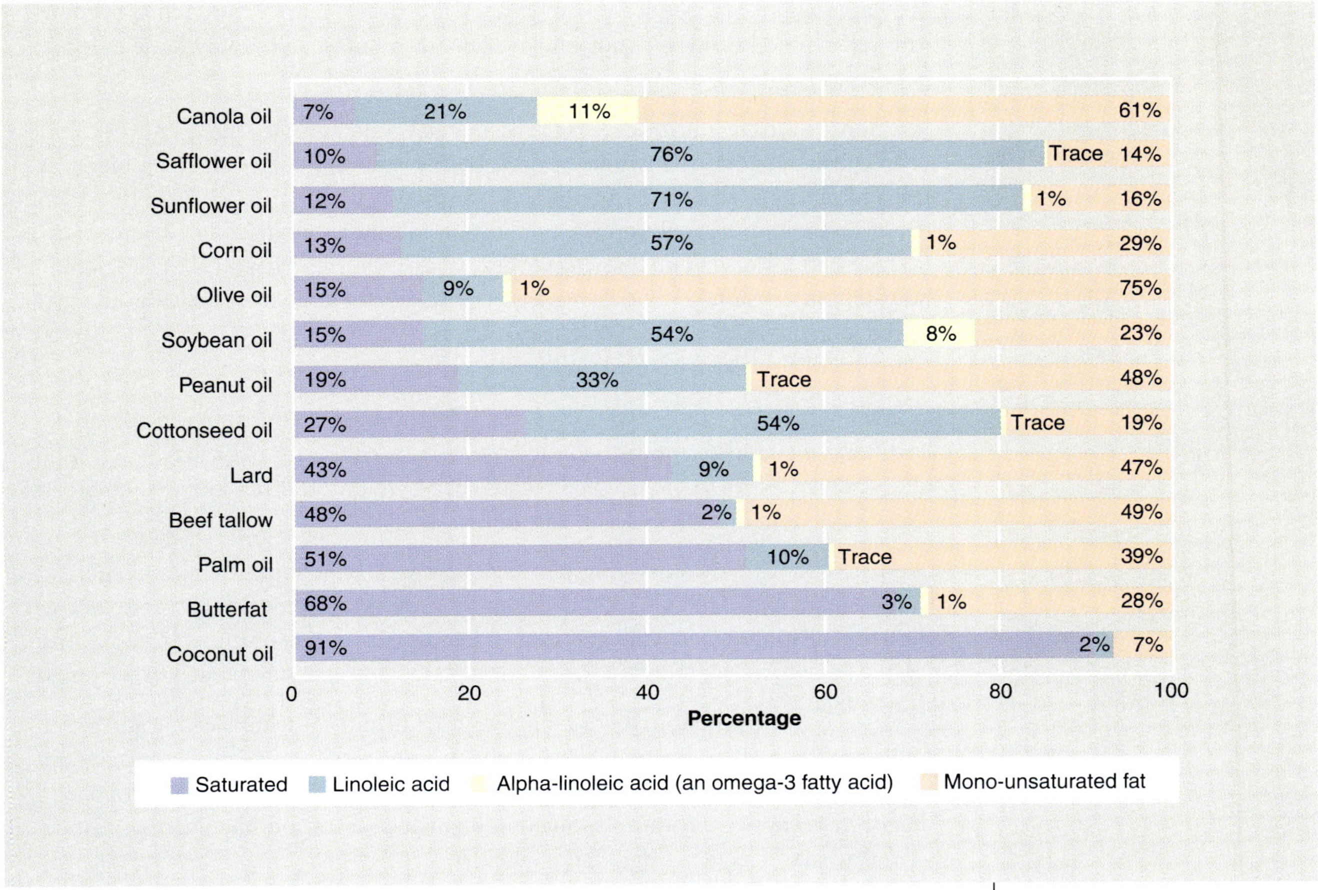

FIGURE 7.5

Comparisons of Dietary Fats.

If every available bond from the carbons is holding a hydrogen atom, the fatty acid is saturated. In some fatty acids chains there is a place where hydrogens are missing; this is the point of unsaturation, and the fatty acid is unsaturated. If there is one point of unsaturation the chain is *monounsaturated* and if there is more than one point of unsaturation the chain is *polyunsaturated*.

Both plants and animals provide ready sources of fat. All dietary fats contain a mixture of saturated and unsaturated fatty acids (Figure 7.5). The type of fatty acid that predominates determines whether the fat is solid or liquid and whether it is characterized as saturated or unsaturated. Coconut and palm kernel oil, for example, contain high levels of saturated fatty acids and are relatively hard at room temperature. Oils such as soybean, canola, cottonseed, corn, and other vegetable oils contain higher levels of unsaturated fatty acids and are liquid at room temperature.

Essential Fatty Acids The body can synthesize all the fatty acids it needs from carbohydrate, fat, or protein except for linoleic acid (omega-6) and alpha-linolenic acid (omega-3). Both are unsaturated fatty acids and, because they must be obtained from food, are referred to as **essential fatty acids** (Table 7.2). These fatty acids are essential for the body because they participate in triggering immune responses, forming cell structures, regulating blood pressure, determining blood lipid concentration, and supporting clot formation. Linoleic acid is found in the seeds of plants and in the

Essential fatty acids Support immune responses, form cell structures, regulate blood pressure, affect blood lipid concentration, and promote clot formation; must be obtained from food.

Cholesterol is vital to the body in a variety of ways. Cholesterol forms part of many important hormones and is an essential structural component of cells. However, like the lecithins, cholesterol can be manufactured by the body and therefore is not an essential nutrient. In addition to the cholesterol made by the body from fats, carbohydrates, or proteins, it can be obtained through eating foods of animal origin, such as eggs, red meat, and fish. Eating saturated fats raises your blood cholesterol level more than anything else in your diet. Elevated blood cholesterol levels have been shown to be related to an increased incidence of coronary heart disease (see Chapter 5). The goal is to encourage people to eat less than 300 mg of cholesterol a day. In addition, less than 10 percent of their fat calories should come from saturated fat.

Dietary Recommendations for Fat Dietary fat is essential for the body because it provides us with a source of essential fatty acids and a means to transport fat-soluble vitamins. Although no specific RDA has been established for the total amount of fat, the National Research Council recommends a minimum daily amount of 3–6 grams, or 1–2 percent of your total calories from linoleic acid. Any diet that contains vegetable oils, seeds, nuts, and whole-grain foods provides enough linoleic acid to meet the body's needs.

The linkage between poor diet and disease was documented earlier in this chapter. A major contributor to many diet-related diseases is the overconsumption of fat, especially saturated fat. Health experts recommend that our total fat consumption be limited to 30 percent or less of total caloric intake. Of this intake, at least 70 percent should be in the form of unsaturated fats. The majority of fat consumption should be monounsaturated (10–15%) and polyunsaturated fat (10%). Saturated fat intake should be limited to less than 10 percent of total caloric intake. Saturated fat is not required for human health and no lower limit has been identified (Dietary Guidelines, 2000).

Vitamins

Vitamins are essential organic substances needed by the body to perform highly specific metabolic processes in the cells. They are indispensable nutrients because they can't be synthesized by the body and must be obtained from food. Additionally, for a substance to be classified as a vitamin its absence from the diet over a period of time must lead to deficiency symptoms. For example, Vitamin A deficiency over an extended period of time can cause blindness, and a lack of niacin can cause mental illness.

Vitamins contribute no energy to the body; instead they assist the enzymes that release energy from carbohydrate, fat, and protein. Thirteen different vitamins have been isolated, analyzed, and synthesized, and their recommended dietary intakes established (Table 7.3). They are needed in small amounts in the diet for normal function, growth, and maintenance of the body. In fact, the body requires only about 350 grams of vitamins from the nearly 1900 pounds of food consumed by the average adult during the year. Vitamins fall into two classes, **fat-soluble** and **water-soluble.** The solubility of a vitamin refers to how it is absorbed and transported, whether it can be stored, and how easily it is lost from the body.

The four **fat-soluble vitamins** (A, D, E, K) are absorbed into the body with fats. These vitamins travel with dietary fats through the bloodstream to reach the cells. They are not readily excreted by the body. Once absorbed, excessive amounts of fat-soluble vitamins are stored in the liver and fat cells until the body needs them. The ability to store fat-soluble vitamins makes daily ingestion of the fat-soluble vitamins unnecessary.

Cholesterol Lipids that form many important hormones and are essential structural components of cells.

Vitamins Essential organic substances needed by the body to perform highly specific metabolic processes in the cells.

Fat-soluble vitamins Vitamins A, D, E, K; must travel with dietary fats in the bloodstream to reach the cells.

Water-soluble Vitamins that can be transported throughout the body by a watery medium.

Nine vitamins are classified as water-soluble because they are transported throughout the watery medium of the body. **Water-soluble vitamins** are more readily excreted than fat-soluble vitamins and are not stored in tissues. Excess water-soluble vitamins are excreted through the urine.

TABLE 7-3 **Water-Soluble and Fat-Soluble Vitamins**

WATER-SOLUBLE VITAMINS	WHY NEEDED?	PRIMARY SOURCES	DEFICIENCY RESULTS IN
Ascorbic acid (vitamin C)	Tooth and bone formation; production of connective tissue; promotion of wound healing; may enhance immunity	Citrus fruits, tomatoes, peppers, cabbage, potatoes, melons	Scurvy (degeneration of bones, teeth, and gums)
Biotin	Involved in fat and amino acid synthesis and breakdown	Yeast, liver, milk, most vegetables, bananas, grapefruit	Skin problems; fatigue; muscle pains; nausea
Cobalamin (vitamin B_{12})	Involved in single carbon atom transfers; essential for DNA synthesis	Muscle meats, eggs, milk, and dairy products (not in vegetables)	Pernicious anemia; nervous system malfunctions
Folacin (folic acid)	Essential for synthesis of DNA and other molecules	Green leafy vegetables, organ meats, whole-wheat products	Anemia; diarrhea and other gastrointestinal problems
Niacin	Involved in energy production and synthesis of cell molecules	Grains, meats, legumes	Pellagra (skin, gastrointestinal, and mental disorders)
Pantothenic acid	Involved in energy production and synthesis and breakdown of many biological molecules	Yeast, meats, and fish, nearly all vegetables and fruits	Vomiting; abdominal cramps; malaise; insomnia
Pyridoxine (vitamin B_6)	Essential fat synthesis, breakdown of amino acids, manufacture of unsaturated fats from saturated fats	Meats, whole grains, most vegetables	Weakness; irritability; trouble sleeping and walking; skin problems
Riboflavin (vitamin B_2)	Involved in energy production; important for health of the eyes	Milk and dairy foods, meats, eggs, vegetables, grains	Eye and skin problems
Thiamine (vitamin B_1)	Essential for breakdown of food molecules and production of energy	Meats, legumes, grains, some vegetables	Beri-beri (nerve damage, weakness, heart failure)
FAT-SOLUBLE VITAMINS	**WHY NEEDED?**	**PRIMARY SOURCES**	**DEFICIENCY RESULTS IN**
Vitamin A (retinol)	Essential for maintenance of eyes and skin; influences bone and tooth formation	Liver, kidney, yellow and green leafy vegetables, apricots	Deficiency: night blindness; eye damage; skin dryness. Excess: loss of appetite; skin problems; swelling of ankles and feet
Vitamin D (calciferal)	Regulates calcium metabolism; important for growth of bones and teeth	Cod-liver oil, dairy products, eggs	Deficiency: rickets (bone deformities) in children; bone destruction in adults. Excess: thirst; nausea; weight loss; kidney damage
Vitamin E (tocopherol)	Prevents damage to cells from oxidation; prevents red blood cell destruction	Wheat germ, vegetable oils, vegetables, egg yolk, nuts	Deficiency: anemia; possibly nerve cell destruction
Vitamin K (phylloquinone)	Helps with blood clotting	Liver, vegetable oils, green leafy vegetables, tomatoes	Deficiency: severe bleeding

SOURCE: G. Edlin, E. Golanty, and K. McCormack Brown. (2000). *Essentials for Health and Wellness,* (2nd ed., p. 76). Boston: Jones and Bartlett.

Minerals

Minerals are inorganic substances that are vital to many body functions. Minerals help build strong bones and teeth, aid in accurate muscle function, help nervous systems transmit messages, help balance the amount of water in the body, and work closely with vitamins to perform our body's chemical and hormonal activities. Like vitamins, minerals do not provide any energy for the body. In the body, minerals are classified as **major minerals** if their requirement exceeds 100 milligrams per day and **trace minerals** if their requirement is less than 100 milligrams per day. Table 7.4 lists the minerals, their major functions, and their food sources.

Minerals can be found in most food items that we eat daily. For example, if you were to consume dark-green leafy vegetables, grain products, and meat and dairy products every day, you would get plenty of the minerals listed in Table 7.4.

Minerals Inorganic substances vital to many body functions.

Major minerals Mineral requirements that exceed 100 mg per day.

Trace minerals Mineral requirements of less than 100 mg per day.

TABLE 7.4 Essential Minerals

MINERAL	WHY NEEDED?	PRIMARY SOURCES	DEFICIENCY RESULTS IN
Calcium	Bone and tooth formation; blood clotting; nerve transmission	Milk, cheese, dark green vegetables, dried legumes	Stunted growth; rickets, osteoporosis; convulsions
Chlorine	Formation of gastric juice; acid-base balance	Common salt	Muscle cramps; mental apathy; reduced appetite
Chromium	Glucose and energy metabolism	Fats, vegetable oils, meats	Impaired ability to metabolize glucose
Cobalt	Constituent of vitamin B_{12}	Organ and muscle meats	Not reported in humans
Copper	Constituent of enzymes of iron metabolism	Meats, drinking water	Anemia (rare)
Iodine	Constituent of thyroid hormones	Marine fish and shellfish, dairy products, many vegetables	Goiter (enlarged thyroid)
Iron	Constituent of hemoglobin and enzymes of energy metabolism	Eggs, lean meals, legumes, whole grains, green leafy vegetables	Iron-deficiency anemia (weakness, reduced resistance to infection)
Magnesium	Activates enzymes; involved in protein synthesis	Whole grains, green leafy vegetables	Growth failure; behavioral disturbances; weakness, spasms
Manganese	Constituent of enzymes involved in fat synthesis	Widely distributed in foods	In animals: disturbances of nervous system, reproductive abnormalities
Molybdenum	Constituent of some enzymes	Legumes, cereals, organ meats	Not reported in humans
Phosphorus	Bone and tooth formation; acid-base balance	Milk, cheese, meat, poultry, grains	Weakness, demineralization of bone
Potassium	Acid-base balance; body water balance; nerve function	Meats, milk, many fruits	Muscular weakness; paralysis
Selenium	Functions in close association with vitamin E	Seafood, meat, grains	Anemia (rare)
Sodium	Acid-base balance; body water balance; nerve function	Common salt	Muscle cramps; mental apathy; reduced appetite
Sulfur	Constituent of active tissue compounds, cartilage, and tendon	Sulfur amino acids (methionine and cysteine) in dietary proteins	Related to intake and deficiency of sulfur amino acids
Zinc	Constituent of enzymes involved in digestion	Widely distributed in foods	Growth failure

SOURCE: G. Edlin, E. Golanty, and K. McCormack Brown. (2000). *Essentials for Health and Wellness,* (2nd ed., p. 76). Boston: Jones and Bartlett.

In general, the human body maintains a proper balance of many minerals through a number of precise control mechanisms, but deficiencies and excesses of any mineral may disturb this balance. Some minerals interact and compete with each other, and consuming excesses of some minerals can affect the absorption of others; this is referred to as a mineral-mineral interaction. For example, iron and magnesium absorption will be hindered if too much calcium is taken in.

Another interaction that is important is the vitamin-mineral interaction. This refers to the importance of certain vitamins and minerals being available at the same time. Iron absorption is improved when it is consumed with vitamin C, and the presence of vitamin D improves the absorption of calcium. Because of mineral-mineral and vitamin-mineral interactions, people should avoid taking individual supplements for minerals unless they have a specific condition that warrants it.

Dietary Recommendations for Vitamins and Minerals A well-balanced diet will satisfy all the vitamin and mineral requirements of most individuals, including those who are physically active. Select a wide variety of foods from all food groups. *For those receiving the RDA of vitamins and minerals, there is no research evidence that supplementation enhances exercise performance.* It is important to remember that excess vitamin and mineral intake does not improve health or exercise performance but it can be toxic. For example, excessive amounts of vitamin A can lead to weakness, headache, nausea, pain in the joints, and liver damage. Too much vitamin D may lead to vomiting, diarrhea, loss of weight, loss of muscle tone, and soft-tissue damage. Vitamin and mineral excesses generally occur as a result of supplementation.

physical activity and health connection

Special Needs for Iron and Calcium Two minerals of special interest, especially for adolescents, adults over 50, and physically active individuals, are iron and calcium. Women need more of both nutrients than men. In all cases, individuals need to be particularly aware of obtaining good sources of nutrients in their diet.

Engage www.pahconnection.com 7.1

The mineral *iron* has many diverse biological functions, but none more important than its role in the transport of oxygen in blood. Iron forms a major part of the hemogloblin in red blood cells. Red blood cells play a major role in aerobic capacity. Nearly 75 percent of the body's iron is found in hemogloblin. If neither diet nor body stores supply the iron needed, hemogloblin concentration levels eventually fall, leading to iron depletion and anemia. **Anemia** is a deficiency in red blood cells and is generally recognized to be the most common single nutritional deficiency, not just in developing countries but around the world.

Several factors are responsible for iron deficiency, including inadequate dietary iron, absorption disturbances, illness, and exercise. Treatment of iron deficiency includes prudent use of the Food Guide Pyramid (see later Figure 7.8) and possibly iron supplements. High-iron foods come from the meat, poultry, fish, dry beans, eggs, and nuts group from the Food Guide Pyramid and from fortified foods like breakfast cereals. Women between the ages of 18 and 50 require 15 milligrams per day. Women over 50 and men over the age of 24 need 10 milligrams of iron daily. The higher RDA for young and middle-aged women is chiefly to counteract menstrual blood loss.

The body contains more *calcium* than any other mineral. Calcium's primary role in the body is that of forming and maintaining bones. Osteoporosis, a major health concern for women, is related to calcium deficiency (see Chapter 10). Calcium is also important for muscle contraction, nerve transmission, and cellular metabolism. Muscles cannot relax after contraction if blood calcium levels fall below a crucial point. Daily calcium intake allows good muscle contractions and relaxations during physical activity.

Anemia Deficiency in red blood cells.

The milk, yogurt, and cheese group of the Food Guide Pyramid and calcium-fortified foods (orange juice, breakfast cereals) provide the best sources of calcium. Adults need between 1000 and 1500 milligrams of calcium daily (Chapter 10, Table 10.1). Surveys indicate that Americans consume only half of this requirement. If you are having difficulty maintaining a well-balanced diet, consider supplementing your diet with calcium.

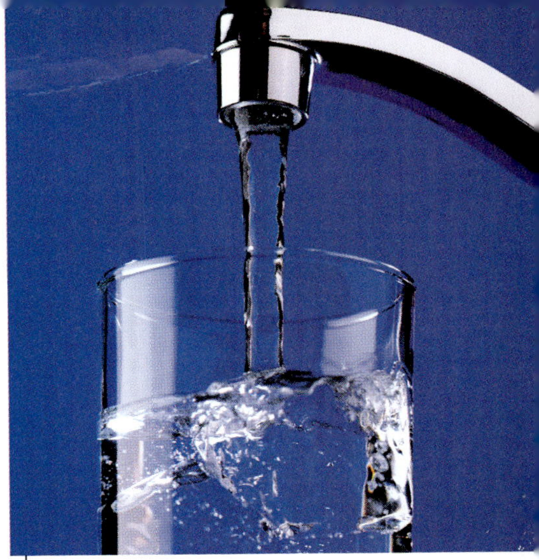

Drink six to eight glasses of water a day.

Water

Water makes up about 60 percent of the body weight and is involved in virtually every body process. Water could be considered the most essential nutrient. Our bodies can survive deficiency of all the other nutrients for a few weeks or more, but can survive only a few days without water. Water serves as the body's transport solvent, distributing nutrients throughout the body and conducting waste products to be excreted through the water in urine and feces. Water serves as the body's reactive medium, participating in every chemical reaction in the body. Water plays a major role in regulating the maintenance of body temperature because it is able to absorb a significant amount of body heat with only a small change in its temperature. Because water is vital to these and other functions, it is essential to maintain a healthy level in the body.

physical activity and health connection

Proper fluid replacement is important for both health and physical activity. The sedentary body loses about 2–3 liters of water each day through urination, perspiration, breathing, and defecation. To replace this water, the RDA recommendation is that, under normal dietary and environmental conditions, the average adult who expends 2000 calories a day should consume 2–3 liters, or about 6–8 glasses, of water each day. In addition to the water people drink, nearly all foods provide water. Fruits and vegetables are generally high in water content, whereas many meats and fatty foods are low.

Water is a crucial nutrient for those engaged in physical activity, especially if the activity is strenuous and performed in extreme environmental temperatures and humidity. To find out how much water you need to replenish from losses occurring during exercise, weigh yourself before and after exercise; the difference is all water. One pound equals approximately 2 glasses of water. Plain cool water is the best choice for drinking because it leaves the digestive system rapidly, is quickly absorbed by tissues, and cools the body.

Functional Foods

We now know that the minimum diet for human growth, energy, and regulating body processes requires six classes of essential nutrients. Within the emerging area of food and nutrition science, however, is the expanding knowledge of the role of other physiologically active components in foods that provide health benefits beyond those supplied by the traditional nutrients. Examples include carotenoids, dietary fiber, flavonoids, and phenols, all of which can be found in fruits and vegetables (Table 7.5). The International Food Information Council defines **functional foods** as those that contain significant levels of biologically active components that provide health benefits beyond basic nutrition (Backgrounder, 1998). The increasing comprehension of the role of physiologically active food components, both from plant *(phytochemicals)* and animals *(zoochemicals)* sources, has notably changed the role of diet in health (IFIC, 1999). Interest in functional foods continues to evolve as food and nutrition science has advanced beyond studying nutritional deficiencies to studying foods for biologically active components that impart health benefits or desirable physiological effects beyond basic nutrition (NAS, 1998). The scientific community is in the early stages of understanding many of the potential benefits from functional foods (IFIC, 1998).

Functional foods Foods that contain significant levels of biologically active components that provide health benefits beyond basic nutrition.

TABLE 7.5 **Examples of Functional Components**

CLASS/COMPONENT	SOURCE*	POTENTIAL BENEFIT
Carotenoids		
Alpha-carotene	Carrots	Neutralizes free radicals that may cause cell damage
Beta-carotene	Various fruits, vegetables	Neutralizes free radicals
Lutein	Green vegetables	Contributes to maintenance of healthy vision
Lycopene	Tomatoes and tomato products (ketchup, sauces)	May reduce risk of prostate cancer
Zeaxanthin	Eggs, citrus, corn	Contributes to maintenance of healthy vision
Collagen hydrolysate		
Collagen hydrolysate	Gelatin	May improve some symptoms associated with osteoarthritis
Dietary fiber		
Insoluble fiber	Wheat bran	May reduce risk of breast and/or colon cancer
Beta glucan**	Oats	Reduces risk of cardiovascular disease (CVD)
Soluble fiber**	Psyllium	Reduces risk of CVD
Whole grains**	Cereal grains	Reduces risk of CVD
Fatty acids		
Omega-3 fatty acids— DHA/EPA	Tuna; fish and marine oils	May reduce risk of CVD & improve mental, visual functions
Conjugated linoleic acid (CLA)	Cheese, meat products	May improve body composition, may decrease risk of certain cancers
Flavonoids		
Anthocyanidins	Fruits	Neutralizes free radicals, may reduce risk of cancer
Catechins	Tea	Neutralizes free radicals, may reduce risk of cancer
Flavanones	Citrus	Neutralizes free radicals, may reduce risk of cancer
Flavones	Fruits/vegetables	Neutralizes free radicals, may reduce risk of cancer
Glucosinolates, Indoles, Isothiocyanates		
Sulphoraphane	Cruciferous vegetables (broccoli, kale), horseradish	Neutralizes free radicals, may reduce risk of cancer
Phenols		
Caffeic acid Ferulic acid	Fruits, vegetables, citrus	Antioxidant-like activities, may reduce risk of degenerative diseases; heart disease, eye disease

Now that you have an understanding of the nutrients you need and why you need them, we'll proceed to a number of educational tools developed by both public and private health organizations to help guide you in making healthy food selections.

DIETARY GUIDELINES FOR AMERICANS

4. *Dietary Guidelines for Americans* provides advice about making healthy food choices.

Under the supervision of the U.S. Departments of Agriculture (USDA) and Health and Human Services (USDHHS), *Dietary Guidelines for Americans* provides advice intended to help consumers make dietary choices most likely to promote their well-being while avoiding or postponing the onset of diet-related chronic diseases for healthy people over the age of 2 (USDA, 2000). The *Dietary Guidelines* were first published in 1980; they are reviewed every five years by a committee of nutrition and health experts who recommend changes based on current knowledge of the influence of diet on disease and health. The most recent guidelines were published in 2000.

TABLE 7.5 (continued)

CLASS/COMPONENT	SOURCE*	POTENTIAL BENEFIT
Plant sterols		
Stanol ester	Corn, soy, wheat, wood oils	Lowers blood cholesterol levels by inhibiting cholesterol absorption
Prebiotics/probiotics		
Fructo-oligosaccharides (FOS)	Jerusalem artichokes, shallots, onion powder	May improve gastrointestinal health
Lactobacillus	Yogurt, other dairy	May improve gastrointestinal health
Saponins		
Saponins	Soybeans, soy foods, soy protein–containing foods	May lower LDL cholesterol; contains anti-cancer enzymes
Soy protein		
Soy protein**	Soybeans and soy-based foods	25 gm/day may reduce risk of heart disease
Phytoestrogens		
Isoflavones—daidzein, genistein	Soybeans and soy-based foods	May reduce menopause symptoms, such as hot flashes
Lignans	Flax, rye, vegetables	May protect against heart disease and some cancers; lowers LDL cholesterol, total cholesterol and triglycerides
Sulfides/thiols		
Diallyl sulfide	onions, garlic, olives, leeks, scallions	Lowers LDL cholesterol, maintains healthy immune system
Allyl methyl trisulfide, dithiolthiones	Cruciferous vegetables	Lowers LDL cholesterol, maintains healthy immune system
Tannins		
Proanthocyanidins	Cranberries, cranberry products, cocoa, chocolate	May improve urinary tract health; may reduce risk of CVD

*Examples are not an all-inclusive list.
**FDA-approved health claim established for component.
SOURCE: International Food Information Council (IFIC). (1999, December). Backgrounder—functional foods [On-line]. Available: http://ificinfo.health.org.index6.htm; accessed 1/30/01. Reprinted from the International Food Information Council Foundation (1999).

The guidelines are presented as three basic messages identified with the ABCs: **A**im for fitness, **B**uild a healthy base, and **C**hoose sensibly—for good health (Figure 7.6). The ABCs for good health are intended to assist you in organizing the guidelines in a memorable and meaningful way. Within each of these three messages are groupings of ten guidelines that mark your way to good health (Figure 7.7).

Aim For Fitness

Aiming for fitness involves two guidelines: (1) aim for a healthy weight, and (2) be physically active each day.

Aim for a Healthy Weight Excess body fat substantially increases the risk of coronary heart disease, stroke, some cancers, diabetes, and hypertension, and is associated with diet (see Chapters 8, 9). For many Americans, the primary culprits of obesity are an over-consumption of calories and physical inactivity. To maintain a healthy weight, a person's intake of calories (calories present in foods) must equal their energy expenditure (calories expended in daily physical activities). This balancing of calories is referred to as the **energy balance equation**; it states that *body weight will remain constant*

Energy balance equation Method for balancing calories to maintain weight.

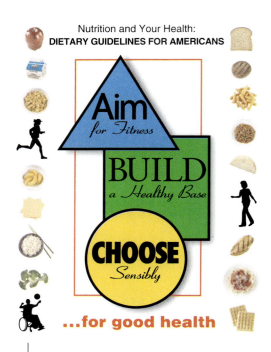

FIGURE 7.6

Dietary Guidelines for Americans.
The USDA's Dietary Guidelines stress the ABC's of health for individuals and families using three basic messages: "Aim for fitness," "Build a healthy base," and "Choose sensibly."

SOURCE: U.S. Department of Agriculture, Agriculture Research Service, Dietary Guidelines Advisory Committee. (2000). *Nutrition and your health: Dietary guidelines for Americans, 2000* (5th ed.). Home and Garden Bulletin No. 232. Washington, D.C.

when caloric intake equals caloric expenditure. If calorie intake exceeds the number of calories expended, the person will gain weight. The achievement of desirable body weight will be discussed in detail in Chapter 9. However, most individuals can follow the USDA's broad calorie-level suggestions:

- 1600 calories is about right for many sedentary women and some older adults
- 2200 calories is about right for most children, teenage girls, active women, and many sedentary men. Women who are pregnant or breastfeeding may need more.
- 2800 calories is about right for teenage boys, many active men, and some very active women.

Table 7.6 shows the number of servings from each food that corresponds to these daily calorie levels and energy intake.

Be Physically Active Each Day The connection between diet and physical activity determines your nutritional health in three important ways. First, physical activity is a significant way to expend energy and therefore can assist in maintaining a healthy weight (see Chapter 9). There is increasing epidemiologic evidence that physical inactivity plays a major role in the rising prevalence of obesity in this country (Weinsier et al., 1998). In fact, physical inactivity may play more of a role in influencing changes in obesity than do dietary intake patterns (Samaras et al., 1999).

TABLE 7.6 **Sample Food Patterns for a Day at Three Calorie Levels**

1600 CALORIES is about right for many sedentary women and some older adults.

2200 CALORIES is about right for most children, teenage girls, active women, and many sedentary men. Women who are pregnant or breastfeeding may need somewhat more.

2800 CALORIES is about right for teenage boys, many active men, and some very active women.

	ABOUT 1600	ABOUT 2200	ABOUT 2800
Bread group servings	6	9	11
Fruit group servings	2	3	4
Vegetable group servings	3	4	5
Meat group servings	5 oz	6 oz	7 oz
Milk group servings	2–3*	2–3*	2–3*
Total fat (grams)*	53	73	93
Total added sugars (teaspoons)†	6	12	18

* Women who are pregnant or breastfeeding, teenagers, and young adults to age 24 need 3 servings.

† Values for total fat and added sugars include fat and added sugars that are in food choices from the five major food groups as well as fat and added sugars from foods in the Fats, Oils, and Sweets group.

SOURCE: A. Shaw, L. Fulton, C. Davis, and M. Hogbin. (1998). *Using the Food Guide Pyramid: A resource for nutrition educators.* U.S. Department of Agriculture, Food, Nutrition, and Consumer Services, Center for Nutrition Policy and Promotion. Available: http://www.usda.gov:80/cnpp/using.htm; accessed 1/30/01.

Second, increasing the calories you use through physical activity permits higher intake of calories, with corresponding essential nutrients, without gaining weight. In this way, physical activity makes it easier for you to get the recommended amounts of nutrients you need. Third, the health benefits of physical activity significantly reduce the risk of developing many chronic diseases that are associated with dietary factors—coronary heart disease, hypertension, colon cancer, type 2 diabetes mellitus, and osteoporosis. Incidences of morbidity and mortality are lower among persons who are physically active than among those who are physically inactive across each of these chronic disease conditions.

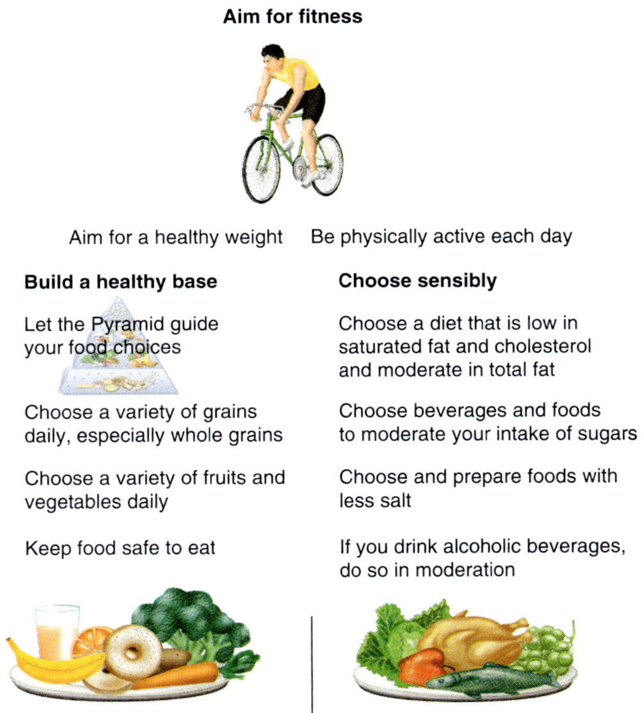

Aim for fitness
Aim for a healthy weight
Be physically active each day
Build a healthy base
Let the Pyramid guide your food choices
Choose a variety of grains daily, especially whole grains
Choose a variety of fruits and vegetables daily
Keep food safe to eat
Choose sensibly
Choose a diet that is low in saturated fat and cholesterol and moderate in total fat
Choose beverages and foods to moderate your intake of sugars
Choose and prepare foods with less salt
If you drink alcoholic beverages, do so in moderation

FIGURE 7.7

Dietary Guidelines for Americans.
The Dietary Guidelines point the way to good health.

SOURCE: U.S. Department of Agriculture, Agriculture Research Service, Dietary Guidelines Advisory Committee. (2000). *Nutrition and your health: Dietary guidelines for Americans, 2000* (5th ed.). Home and Garden Bulletin No. 232. Washington, D.C.

Build a Healthy Base

Building a healthy base involves four guidelines: Let the Pyramid guide your food choices; choose a variety of grains daily, especially whole grains; choose a variety of fruits and vegetables daily; and keep food safe to eat.

Let the Pyramid Guide Your Food Choices An important assumption of this guideline is nutritional adequacy. Different foods contain different nutrients, and no single food can supply all the nutrients you need. The USDA developed the Food Guide Pyramid (Figure 7.8) in 1992 to illustrate its current food guidelines, which includes five major food groups (grains, vegetables, fruits, milk products, meat and meat substitutes) and the foods at the tip, which depicts the relatively small amount of fat and sugar needed in a daily diet and does not constitute a food group (USDA, 1996).

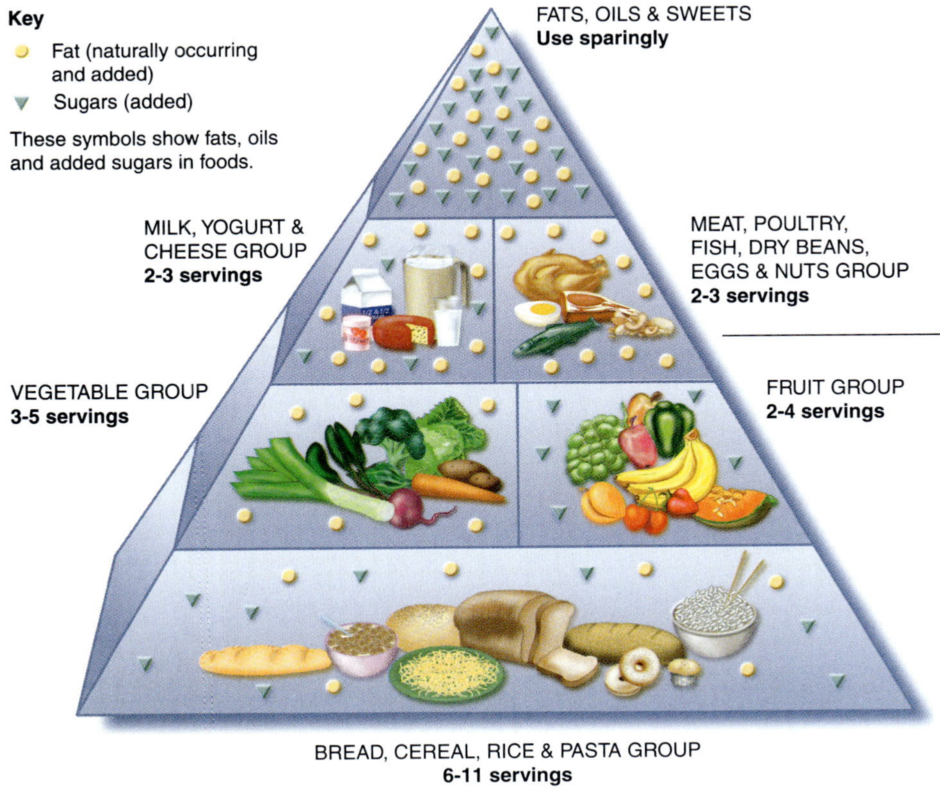

Key
Fat (naturally occurring and added)
Sugars (added)
These symbols show fats, oils and added sugars in foods.
FATS, OILS & SWEETS
Use sparingly
MILK, YOGURT & CHEESE GROUP
2-3 servings
MEAT, POULTRY, FISH, DRY BEANS, EGGS & NUTS GROUP
2-3 servings
VEGETABLE GROUP
3-5 servings
FRUIT GROUP
2-4 servings
BREAD, CEREAL, RICE & PASTA GROUP
6-11 servings

FIGURE 7.8

The Food Guide Pyramid.
The USDA's Food Guide Pyramid is a research-based guidance system that helps consumers put the Dietary Guidelines into action. The pyramid shows how many servings to eat from each food group every day.

SOURCE: U.S. Department of Agriculture/U.S. Department of Health and Human Services.

5. The Food Pyramid provides a visual image of the foods Americans need daily.

The Food Guide Pyramid is flexible and full of food choices. It offers simple, practical advice to help you make choices. More specifically, the Pyramid encourages the basic principles of a healthful diet—variety, balance, and moderation:

- *Variety.* A varied diet includes many different foods from each of the Pyramid's five major food groups. It is generally agreed that people should not eat the same foods day after day, because no single food or foods supplies all the nutrients you need (Table 7.7).

TABLE 7.7 Variety from the Food Groups

BREAD, CEREAL, RICE, PASTA

Whole-grain	Enriched	Grain products with more fat and sugar
Brown rice	Bagels	Biscuit
Buckwheat groats	Cornmeal	Cake (unfrosted)
Bulgar	Crackers	Cookies
Corn tortillas	English muffins	Cornbread
Graham crackers	Farina	Croissant
Granola	Flour tortillas	Danish
Oatmeal	French bread	Doughnut
Popcorn	Grits	Muffin
Pumpernickel bread	Hamburger and hot dog rolls	Pie crust
Ready-to-eat cereals	Italian bread	Tortilla chips
Rye bread and crackers	Macaroni	
Whole-wheat bread, rolls, crackers	Noodles	
Whole-wheat pasta	Pancakes and waffles	
Whole-wheat cereals	Pretzels	
	Ready-to-eat cereals	
	Rice	
	Spaghetti	
	White bread and rolls	

FRUITS

Citrus, Melons, Berries		Other fruits		
Blueberries	Lemon	Apple	Guava	Pineapple
Cantaloupe	Orange	Apricot	Grapes	Plantain
Citrus juices	Raspberries	Asian pear	Mango	Plum
Cranberries	Strawberries	Banana	Nectarine	Prickly pear
Grapefruit	Tangerine	Cherries	Papaya	Prunes
Honeydew melon	Watermelon	Dates	Passion fruit	Raisins
Kiwi	Ugli fruit	Figs	Peach	Rhubarb
		Fruit juices	Pear	Star fruit

VEGETABLES

Dark-green leafy	Deep yellow	Starchy	Dry beans and peas (legumes)
Beet greens	Carrots	Breadfruit	Black beans
Broccoli	Pumpkin	Corn	Black-eyed peas
Chard	Sweet potato	Green peas	Chickpeas (garbanzos)
Chicory	Winter squash	Hominy	Kidney beans
Collard greens		Lima beans	Lentils
Dandelion greens		Potato	Lima beans (mature)
Endive		Rutabaga	Mung beans
Escarole		Taro	Navy beans
Kale			Pinto beans
Mustard greens			Split peas
Romaine lettuce			
Spinach			
Turnip greens			
Watercress			

■ *Balance.* To obtain your needed daily calories and nutrients, a balanced approach that incorporates appropriate amounts of foods from all five groups should be utilized. Balance what you eat over several days and don't worry about just one meal or one day. Your age, sex, and physical activity level make a difference in the number of servings required from each group to maintain a well-balanced diet.

TABLE 7-7 (continued)

VEGETABLES (continued)			
Other vegetables			
Artichoke	Cauliflower	Lettuce	Summer squash
Asparagus	Celery	Mushrooms	Chinese cabbage
Bean and alfalfa sprouts	Cucumber	Okra	Tomato
Beets	Eggplant	Onions (mature and green)	Turnip
Brussels sprouts	Green beans	Radishes	Vegetable juices
Cabbage	Green pepper	Snow peas	Zucchini

MEAT, POULTRY, FISH, AND ALTERNATES		
Meat, Poultry and Fish		**Alternates**
Beef	Pork	Eggs
Chicken	Shellfish	Dry beans and peas (legumes)
Fish	Turkey	Nuts and seeds
Ham	Veal	Peanut butter
Lamb	Luncheon meats, sausage	Tofu
Organ meats		
MILK, YOGURT, AND CHEESE		
Lowfat milk products	**Other milk products with more fat or sugar**	
Buttermilk	Cheddar cheese	Ice milk
Lowfat cottage cheese	Chocolate milk	Process cheeses and spreads
Lowfat milk (1%, 2% fat)	Flavored yogurt	Puddings made with milk
Lowfat or nonfat plain yogurt	Frozen yogurt	Swiss cheese
Skim milk	Fruit yogurt	Whole milk
	Ice cream	
FATS, SWEETS, AND ALCOHOLIC BEVERAGES		
Fats		
Bacon, salt port	Lard	Salad dressing
Butter	Margarine	Shortening
Cream (dairy, nondairy)	Mayonnaise	Sour cream
Cream cheese	Mayonnaise-type salad dressing	Vegetable oil
Sweets		**Alcoholic beverages**
Candy	Maple syrup	Beer
Corn syrup	Marmalade	Liquor
Frosting (icing)	Molasses	Wine
Fruit drinks	Table syrup	
Gelatin desserts	Popsicles and ices	
Honey	Sherbets	
Jam	Soft drinks and colas	
Jelly	Sugar (white and brown)	

SOURCE: A. Shaw, L. Fulton, C. Davis, and M. Hogbin. (1998). *Using the Food Guide Pyramid: A resource for nutrition educators.* U.S. Department of Agriculture, Food, Nutrition, and Consumer Services, Center for Nutrition Policy and Promotion. Available: http://www.usda.gov:80/cnpp/using.htm; accessed 1/30/01.

- *Moderation.* Wise selection of foods and beverages helps you control the amount of calories consumed and the total amount of fat, saturated fat, cholesterol, salt, sugars, and (if consumed) alcohol. Moderation allows you more flexibility to enjoy the variety of foods available to you. You do not have to avoid any food completely; you must only exercise sound judgment as to how much you eat and how often you eat any food. For example, you may enjoy eating pizza. However, if you eat too much pizza, or eat it every day, you may be accumulating too many fat calories in your diet.

Understanding the *Food Guide* Pyramid provides you with an instant and useful visual image of healthy food choices and their quantities. The five food groups in the Food Guide Pyramid depict the variety of foods that make up a healthy diet and the number of servings that should come from each of the food groups. The bread, cereal, rice, and pasta group (6–11 servings) represents the base of the Pyramid, which constitutes the desired preponderance of the daily calories. The next level consists of the vegetable group (3–5 servings) and the fruit group (2–4 servings). These three food groups are derived from grains and plants and should make up approximately 65 percent of your daily servings. The last two food groups, the milk, yogurt and cheese group (2–3 servings) and the meat, poultry, fish, dry beans, eggs, and nuts group (2–3 servings) should make up the remainder of your diet. The majority of the foods from these last two groups come from animal sources. Fats, oils, and sweets (added sugars) appear at the tip of the Pyramid, and are not classified as a group, to indicate that they should be used sparingly because they contain few or no nutrients but still add calories.

The recommended numbers of servings for each food group are expressed as ranges on the Pyramid because nutrient and energy needs vary by age (younger people require more calories than older people), and physical activity (active people need more calories than sedentary people). It is important to choose a variety of foods within a food group to ensure an appropriate assortment of nutrients. Even though the foods are grouped primarily by the nutrients they provide, foods within each group vary regarding nutrient content. For example, some fruits and vegetables are good sources of vitamin A or B, while others are good sources of vitamin C or iron.

Choose a Variety of Grains Daily, Especially Whole Grains The grain group composes the base, the widest part, of the Food Guide Pyramid because it serves as the foundation of a healthy diet (USDA, 1996). These foods are derived mainly from plant sources and should make up the majority of our caloric intake. Most Americans of all ages eat fewer than the recommended number of servings of these foods (*Healthy People 2010,* 2000).

Most grain products (breads, cereals, rice, and pasta) are notable for contributing complex carbohydrates, protein, iron, riboflavin, thiamin, niacin, and magnesium to our diets. The Food Guide Pyramid also encourages greater use of whole-grain products—grains that include the entire seed of the plant. For example whole-wheat bread and brown rice are preferred over refined and milled grains (white bread, white rice) which have been stripped of many of their nutrients. Other whole-grain products include oats, barley, millet, rye, quinoa, and bulgar (Table 7.7).

Experience
www.pahconnection.com
7.2

Choose a Variety of Fruits and Vegetables Daily The second level from the bottom of the Food Guide Pyramid focuses attention on the distinct advantages of another broad category of plant foods, the vegetables and fruits. The vegetable group is notable for its contributions of vitamin A, vitamin C, potassium, magnesium, fiber, and folate, coupled with its lack of fat, saturated fat, and cholesterol. The Food Guide Pyramid encourages consumption of a variety of vegetables, with special focus on dark-green, leafy vegetables. These vegetables include broccoli, brussel sprouts, bean sprouts, cabbage, cucumbers, carrots, spinach, mustard, collard greens, lettuce, and potatoes. Dry beans are included in the meat and nuts group of the Food Guide Pyramid, but they can count toward servings of vegetables instead of meat alternatives since they contribute many nutrients similar to the vegetable group. Eat at least three servings of vegetables each day. The fruit group is notable for its contributions of vitamin A, vitamin C, potassium, fiber, and its lack of fat, saturated fat, cholesterol, and sodium. Fruits include apples, bananas, oranges, strawberries, apricots, cantaloupe, pears, and peaches. Fruit is particularly under-consumed by Americans. Fruits and vegetables can be handy snacks because they require little preparation and are easy to carry. Eat at least two servings of fruit each day.

Keep Food Safe to Eat *Safe* means that the food you eat poses little risk of food-borne illnesses. Food-borne illness is a major preventable public health problem in the United States, and it may be increasing. Nearly 20 percent of food-borne outbreaks that are reported occurred at home (Bean et al., 1996). As a consumer, you can do much to protect yourself from food-borne illnesses by following seven simple actions when preparing, serving, and storing food. These protections are shown in Table 7.8. Each of these simple actions have long been used by the USDA to teach food safety.

Explore www.pahconnection.com **7.3**

Choose Sensibly

Choosing sensibly includes four guidelines: choose a diet that is low in saturated fat and cholesterol and moderate in total fat; choose beverages and foods that limit your intake of sugars; choose and prepare foods with less salt; and, if you drink alcoholic beverages, do so in moderation.

Choose a diet that is low in saturated fat and cholesterol and moderate in total fat. This guideline emphasizes restriction of dietary intake of saturated fats in particular, because saturated fats are the most important dietary factor influencing LDL cholesterol levels and risk of coronary heart disease. Saturated fats are found in meats, whole-milk dairy products, and bakery products that include coconut or palm oil among their ingredients. The average intake of total daily calories from saturated fat

Engage www.pahconnection.com **7.2**

TABLE 7.8 Keep Food Safe to Eat

ADVICE FOR TODAY

Build a healthy base by keeping food safe to eat:

- *Clean.* Wash hands and surfaces often.
- *Separate.* Separate raw, cooked, and ready-to-eat foods while shopping, preparing, or storing.
- *Cook.* Cook foods to a safe temperature.
- *Chill.* Refrigerate perishable foods promptly.
- *Check and follow the label.*
- *Serve safely.* Keep hot foods hot and cold foods cold.
- *When in doubt, throw it out.*

SOURCE: U.S. Department of Agriculture, Agriculture Research Service, Dietary Guidelines Advisory Committee. (2000). *Nutrition and your health: Dietary guidelines for Americans, 2000* (5th ed.) Home and Garden Bulletin No. 232. Washington, DC.

should be less than 10 percent. Monounsaturated fats and polyunsaturated fats are preferred over saturated fats; both kinds of unsaturated fats help keep blood cholesterol low and assist in regulating the balance of saturated fats and cholesterol in your cells.

Dietary cholesterol also affects LDL cholesterol levels and risk of coronary heart disease. Dietary cholesterol should be limited to less than 300 milligrams per day. Dietary cholesterol comes primarily from animal sources, including egg yolks, whole-milk products, meat, poultry, and fish.

It is important to moderate total fat intake because fat contains more than twice as many calories as protein and carbohydrates and thus tends to contribute to obesity. In addition to reducing the risk of chronic diseases, a diet low in total fat makes it easier to consume the variety of foods, such as fruits and vegetables, needed to provide essential nutrients without exceeding caloric needs.

Fats that are represented in the apex of the Food Guide Pyramid should be used sparingly. The fats in this miscellaneous group come from foods like mayonnaise, butter, margarine, snack foods, and desserts that are high in calories but provide few nutrients. It is important to limit your fat options in order to have room for the recommended servings from the five groups in the Food Guide Pyramid. In general, foods that come from animals—the milk and meat groups—are naturally higher in fat than foods that come from plants. Within the milk and meat groups, low-fat options like skim or low-fat milk, poultry, fish, and lean meat are preferred. Visible fat should be trimmed from meats and skin should be removed from poultry. Food preparation methods should minimize or avoid the use of fats; boiling, broiling, or roasting are preferred over frying.

Choose beverages and foods that limit your intake of sugars. Foods that are high in added sugars— table sugar, corn syrup, corn sweetener, sucrose, fructose, maltose, honey—are low in nutrients and can promote tooth decay. These foods include cake, pie, cookies, doughnuts, candy, jelly, ice cream, and soft drinks. Added sugars are included in the apex of the Pyramid and should be used sparingly. It is recommended that simple-sugar consumption be limited to less than 10 percent of total daily calories.

Choose and prepare foods with less salt. Because a high-sodium intake is associated with hypertension, the USDA recommends that the daily sodium intake be limited to 2400 milligrams, or 1 teaspoon, of table salt. A high-sodium diet may also promote calcium excretion. Lowered calcium in the body reduces the ability to control blood pressure and increases the likelihood of osteoporosis. Sodium is found primarily in processed foods and canned foods. To lower your sodium intake, eat fresh fruits and vegetables, which are generally low in sodium. Use spices and herbs to season food instead of table salt.

If you drink alcoholic beverages, do so in moderation. While it is true that moderate amounts of alcohol lower risk of coronary heart disease, the risk of several forms of cancer is increased. Personal decisions about alcohol consumption are complex. If adults elect to drink alcohol, they should consume it in moderate amounts, defined as no more than two drinks a day for men and one drink a day for women. One drink is defined as 12 ounces of regular beer, 5 ounces of wine, or 1.5 ounces of distilled spirits, each of which contains 0.5 ounces of alcohol. It is important to remember that damaging effects occur when alcohol contributes a substantial portion of the energy in a person's diet (see Chapter 14).

Alcoholic beverages contain a substantial number of calories. The body derives energy from alcohol at the rate of 7 calories per gram. The calories from alcohol need to be counted as part of the daily caloric intake. When taken in excess of our body's energy need, alcohol calories are stored as body fat. In addition, alcohol is not a nutrient because it cannot be used in the body to promote growth, repair, or maintenance of tissue.

Food Labeling

Experience
www.pahconnection.com
7.3

You know, as a health-conscious consumer, how important it is to choose foods that offer high nutritional value. But how can you be sure you are making the wisest selections of foods as you roll your grocery cart down the supermarket aisles? Considering that the average supermarket stocks over 40,000 different products and that many food manufacturers use health advertising claims to get you to purchase their products, you have to make many decisions in a short shopping trip.

Fortunately for you, the U.S. government requires that all manufactured foods must be labeled with the product name, name and address of the manufacturer, amount of product in package, ingredients listed in descending order by weight, and the **nutrition facts label.** An ingredients label that contains "wheat flour, malted barley flour, and salt" informs you that wheat flour is proportionally the largest ingredient and that the second largest is barley flour. The nutrition facts label (Figure 7.9) is a simple, graphical nutrition tool that can serve as a key to planning a healthful diet. The label provides comprehensive information on the nutritional composition of food products that facilitates comparison of food products and assists in the selection of foods for a diet that will meet the Dietary Guidelines for Americans.

Nutrition facts label Mandated food labeling designed to help consumers make appropriate choices.

Most of the information needed to adhere to the Food Guide Pyramid is provided on the nutrition facts label. The following fourteen nutrients must be listed: total calories, calories from fat, total fat, saturated fat, cholesterol, sodium, total carbohydrate, dietary fiber, sugars, protein, vitamin A, vitamin C, calcium, and iron. The fourteen mandatory nutrients were selected because they are most relevant to our national health problems. Recently, the FDA proposed amending its regulations on nutrition labeling to require that the amount of trans fatty acids in a food be added to the nutrition facts label. This proposal includes a new nutrient content claim defining "*trans* fat free" and requires that the

FIGURE 7.9

The Nutrition Facts Panel.

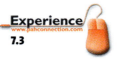

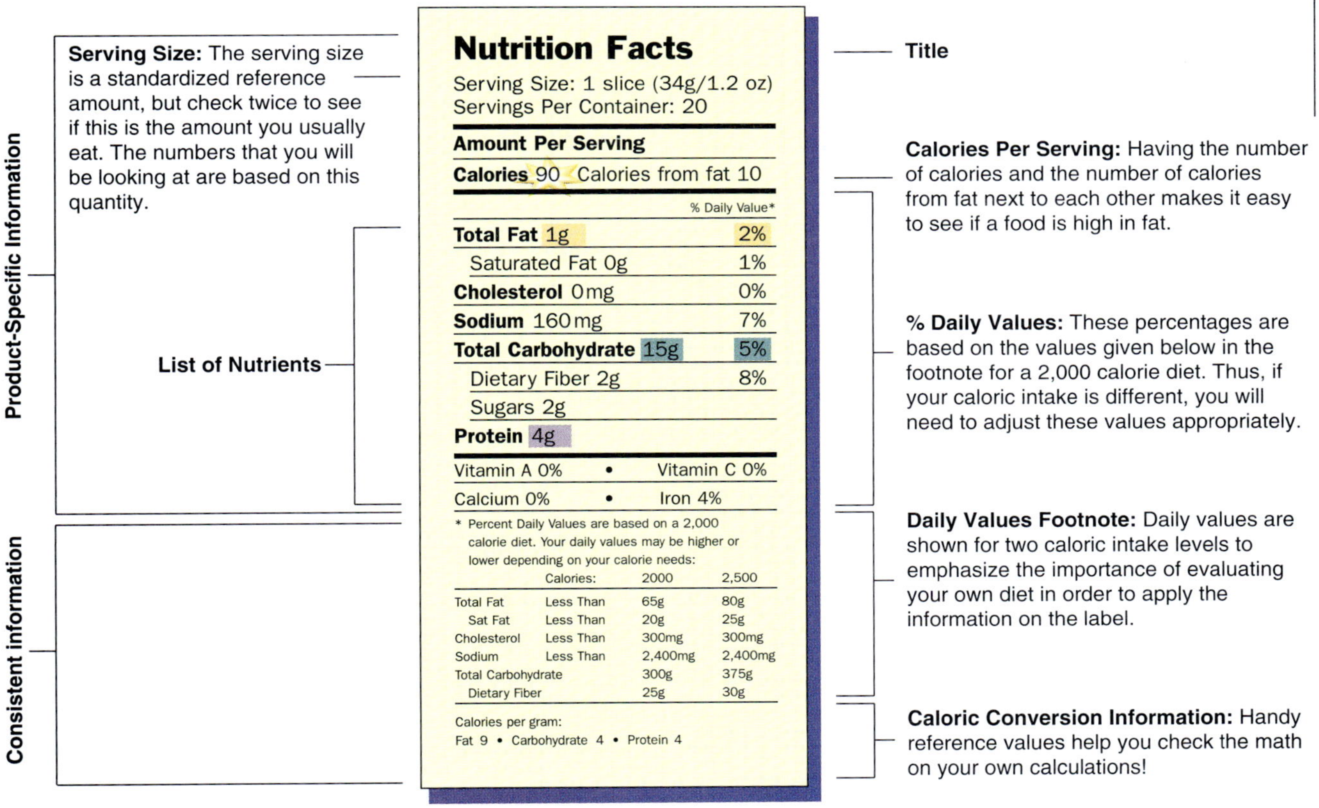

Serving Size: The serving size is a standardized reference amount, but check twice to see if this is the amount you usually eat. The numbers that you will be looking at are based on this quantity.
List of Nutrients
Product-Specific Information
Consistent information
Nutrition Facts
Serving Size: 1 slice (34g/1.2 oz)
Servings Per Container: 20
Amount Per Serving
Calories 90 Calories from fat 10
% Daily Value*
Total Fat 1g 2%
Saturated Fat 0g 1%
Cholesterol 0mg 0%
Sodium 160mg 7%
Total Carbohydrate 15g 5%
Dietary Fiber 2g 8%
Sugars 2g
Protein 4g
Vitamin A 0% • Vitamin C 0%
Calcium 0% • Iron 4%
* Percent Daily Values are based on a 2,000 calorie diet. Your daily values may be higher or lower depending on your calorie needs:
Calories: 2000 2,500
Total Fat Less Than 65g 80g
Sat Fat Less Than 20g 25g
Cholesterol Less Than 300mg 300mg
Sodium Less Than 2,400mg 2,400mg
Total Carbohydrate 300g 375g
Dietary Fiber 25g 30g
Calories per gram:
Fat 9 • Carbohydrate 4 • Protein 4
Title
Calories Per Serving: Having the number of calories and the number of calories from fat next to each other makes it easy to see if a food is high in fat.
% Daily Values: These percentages are based on the values given below in the footnote for a 2,000 calorie diet. Thus, if your caloric intake is different, you will need to adjust these values appropriately.
Daily Values Footnote: Daily values are shown for two caloric intake levels to emphasize the importance of evaluating your own diet in order to apply the information on the label.
Caloric Conversion Information: Handy reference values help you check the math on your own calculations!

amount of *trans* fat per serving be added to the amount of saturated fat per serving so the per-serving value would be based on the total of the two. This limits health claims made on low-saturated-fat items that may also contain *trans* fats (Fact Sheet, *HHS News*, November, 12, 1999). If optional nutrients are listed by the manufacturer in order to make a health claim—for example, naming other essential vitamins and minerals, or whether the food is fortified or enriched with any of them—nutrition figures for these optional nutrients become mandatory as well. The types of descriptive words used to make health-related claims have specific meanings that are clearly defined by regulation (Table 7.9)

Another important way the nutrition facts label helps you meet the Dietary Guidelines is that % daily value is given for each nutrient. The *% daily value* is a measure of the contribution of one serving of the food product to the recommended daily intake of the nutrient,based on a daily intake of 2000 calories. This % daily value information permits comparison of food products without the need for calculations. Also, by scanning the % daily value column, you can see how a product's protein, carbohydrate, fiber, fat, and sodium fits within your total diet. Simple math calculations can help you keep track of how much of each of the various nutrients you have obtained for the day. All of this information can help you balance your food choices and develop improved eating habits.

Serving Sizes Knowing how much food is considered a serving is an important element of any nutrition plan. However, the serving size listed on the nutrition facts label may not be the same as the serving size for the food group in the Food Guide Pyramid. Why do they differ? The serving sizes on the food label and the food guide serve different purposes. The serving size declared on the food label is to allow you to compare

TABLE 7.9 What Words on Product Labels Mean

Calorie-free	Fewer than 5 calories per serving
Light (lite)	1/3 less calories or no more than 1/2 the fat of the higher-calorie, higher-fat version; or no more than 1/2 the sodium of the lighter-sodium version
Fat-free	Less than 0.5 g of fat per serving
Low-fat	3 g of fat (or less) per serving
Reduced/less fat	At least 25% less fat per serving than the higher-fat version
Lean	Less than 10 g of fat, 4 g of saturated fat, and 95 mg of cholesterol per serving
Extra-lean	Less than 5 g of fat, 2 g of saturated fat, and 95 mg of cholesterol per serving
Low in saturated fat	1 g saturated fat (or less) per serving and not more than 15% of calories from saturated fatty acids
Cholesterol-free	Less than 2 mg of cholesterol and 2 gm (or less) of saturated fat per serving
Low-cholesterol	20 mg of cholesterol (or less) and 2 g of saturated fat (or less) per serving
Reduced cholesterol	At least 25% less cholesterol than the lighter-cholesterol version and 2 g (or less) of saturated fat per serving
Sodium-free (no sodium)	Less than 5 mg of sodium per serving and no sodium chloride (NaCl) in ingredients
Very low sodium	35 mg of sodium (or less) per serving
Low sodium	140 mg of sodium (or less) per serving
Reduced/less sodium	At least 25% less sodium per serving that the higher-sodium version
Sugar-free	Less than 0.5 g of sugar per serving
High-fiber	5 g of fiber (or more) per serving
Good source of fiber	2.5 to 4.9 g of fiber per serving

SOURCE: G. Edlin, E. Golanty, and K. McCormack Brown. (2000). *Essentials for Health and Wellness*, (2nd ed., p. 67). Boston: Jones and Bartlett.

serving amounts from similar product categories. The serving sizes must be expressed in consumer-friendly household units, like ounces, cups, or gram weights. This means that all brands of tunafish, for example, must use the same serving size (2 oz) on their labels. The serving sizes in the food guide are specified for each food group, using simple, easy-to-remember household units that allow people to *estimate visually* the amount of food they are eating (Table 7.10). In most cases the serving sizes are similar on food labels and in the food guide. It is important to remember that the "serving size" is a unit of measure and may not be the *portion* an individual actually eats.

If you are not accustomed to judging the amount, or portion, of food you eat, you will find it helpful to weigh and measure foods for a brief time, using a food scale or measuring spoons or cups. This will help you become familiar with visually estimating a recommended serving size. Using the same size and type of bowl, plate, or glass will assist even further in learning to eyeball approximate serving sizes.

TABLE 7.10 **The Pyramid Guide to Daily Food Choices/What Counts as a Serving**

FOOD GROUP	SUGGESTED DAILY SERVINGS	WHAT COUNTS AS A SERVING
Bread, Cereal, Rice, Pasta Whole-grain/enriched	6 to 11 servings from entire group (include several servings of whole-grain products daily)	1 slice of bread 1/2 hamburger bun or english muffin a small roll, biscuit, or muffin 5–6 small or 3–4 large crackers 1/2 cup cooked cereal, rice, or pasta 1 ounce ready-to-eat cereal
Fruits Citrus, melon, berries Other fruits	2 to 4 servings from entire group	a whole fruit such as a medium apple, banana, or orange a grapefruit half a melon wedge 3/4 cup juice 1/2 cup berries 1/2 cup chopped, cooked, or canned fruit 1/4 cup dried fruit
Vegetables Dark-green leafy Deep-yellow Dry beans and peas (legumes) Starchy Other vegetables	3 to 5 servings (include all types regularly; use dark-green leafy vegetables and dry beans and peas several times a week)	1/2 cup cooked vegetables 1/2 cup chopped raw vegetables 1 cup leafy raw vegetables, such as lettuce or spinach 3/4 cup vegetable juice
Meats, Poultry, Fish, Dry Beans and Peas, Eggs, and Nuts	2–3 servings from entire group	Amounts should total 5–7 oz cooked lean meat, poultry without skin, or fish per day. Count 1 egg, 1/2 cup cooked beans, or 2 tablespoons peanut butter as 1 oz of meat.
Milk, Yogurt, Cheese	2 servings (3 servings for women who are pregnant or breastfeeding, teen-agers, and young adults to age 24)	1 cup milk 8 oz yogurt 1.5 oz natural cheese 2 oz process cheese
Fats, Sweets, and Alcoholic Beverages Use fats and sweets sparingly. If you drink alcoholic beverages. do so in moderation.		

NOTE: The guide to daily food choices described here was developed for Americans who regularly eat foods from all the major food groups listed. Some people, such as vegetarians and others, may not eat one or more of these types of foods. These people may wish to contact a dietitian or nutritionist for help in planning food choices.

SOURCE: A. Shaw, L. Fulton, C. Davis, and M. Hogbin. (1998). *Using the Food Guide Pyramid: A resource for nutrition educators.* U.S. Department of Agriculture, Food, Nutrition, and Consumer Services, Center for Nutrition Policy and Promotion. Available: http://www.usda.gov:80/cnpp/using.htm; accessed 1/30/01.

Nutrient Calorie Benefit Ratio

Nutrient calorie benefit ratio Amount of nutrient per energy unit, or the ratio of nutrients to calories.

How can a person get all the essential nutrients without having to eat too many calories? As mentioned before, the nutrient content of foods varies considerably, the differences between food groups being more distinct than the differences between foods in the same group. Therefore the answer lies in selecting the foods within each group that deliver the most nutrients at the lowest calorie cost, foods high in **nutrient-calorie benefit ratio** (NCBR) or nutrient density. *Nutrient-calorie benefit ratio* is defined as the amount of nutrient per energy unit or the ratio of nutrients to calories. In essence, a food with high NCBR possesses a significant amount of a specific nutrient or nutrients per serving compared to its caloric content. We refer to these as "quality" calories. For example eggs have a high nutrient density because they provide an excellent source of protein and a wide range of vitamins and minerals in proportion to their calorie count. Choosing foods that have a high NCBR is important for individuals on low-calorie diets and individuals involved in physical activity.

DIETARY SUPPLEMENTS

physical activity and health connection

With proper food selection and preparation, the need to consume vitamin or mineral supplements is both physiologically and economically wasteful. Most studies show that the intake of protein and major vitamins and minerals is above recommended dietary intake levels in people who are physically active. Physically active people tend to expend more energy and require more calories, to supply their bodies with higher quantities of protein, vitamins, and minerals. The American Dietetic Association has stated that heavy physical activity may increase the need for some vitamins and minerals, but this need is easily met by consuming a balanced diet in accordance with the higher caloric requirement (ADA, 1993).

Can you get too much of the necessary vitamins and minerals? The answer is no, if you eat a balanced diet. However, you can get too much of the needed vitamins and minerals if you incorrectly take supplements. If you wish to take vitamin and mineral supplements, read labels carefully. It is possible to have just as many adverse effects from too many vitamins and minerals as from too few.

Vegetarian Diets

Experience www.pahconnection.com 7.4

Vegan A strict vegetarian who eats no animal products.

Ovovegetarian A vegetarian who includes eggs in the diet.

Lactovegetarian A vegetarian who includes milk in the diet.

Ovolactovegetarian A vegetarian who eats both eggs and milk products.

Semivegetarian A vegetarian who may eat fish and poultry, but not eat red meat.

The shift toward vegetarianism implied by the Food Guide Pyramid is probably becoming increasingly obvious to you. The importance of a plant-based approach to eating is evident by the broad-based area designated on the Food Guide Pyramid for grains, fruits, and vegetables. Vegetarian diets depend largely or entirely on plant products and restrict intake of animal products. There are a variety of ways to be a vegetarian, ranging from being a strict vegetarian, eating no animal products of any kind, to being one who eats certain types of animal products.

Strict vegetarians are known as **vegans** because they eat no animal products. Most nutrients are obtained from breads, cereals, vegetables, fruits, legumes, seeds, and nuts. Less strict vegetarian diets include some foods derived from animals. **Ovovegetarians** include eggs (ovo) in their diet, and **lactovegetarians** include foods in the milk (lacto) group such as yogurt and cheese. An **ovolactovegetarian** eats both eggs and milk products. Finally, **semivegetarians** may eat fish and poultry, but do not eat red meat such as beef and pork.

The American Dietetic Association, in a position paper devoted to vegetarian diets, noted that such diets are healthful and nutritionally adequate, but deficiencies may occur

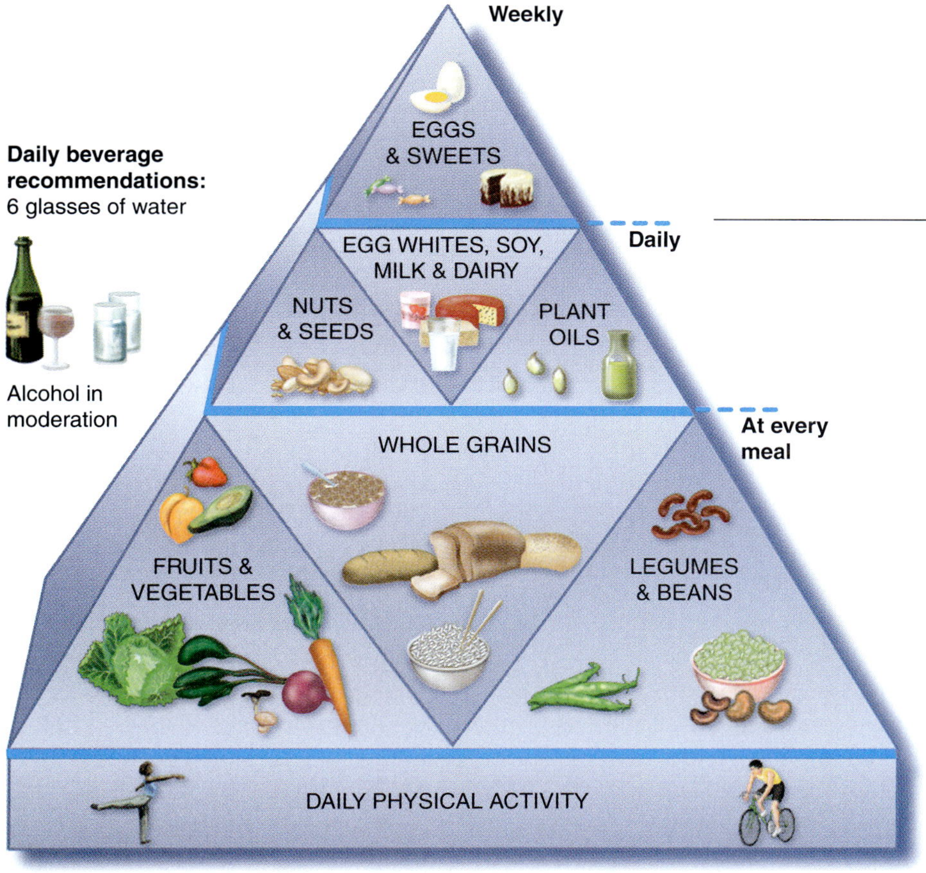

FIGURE 7.10

The Vegetarian Food Guide Pyramid.
With careful planning, a diet that lacks animal products can be nutritionally complete.

SOURCE: Copyright © 2000 Oldways Preservation and Exchange Trust.

if the diet is not planned appropriately. If foods are not selected carefully, the vegetarian may suffer nutritional deficiencies involving calories, vitamins, minerals, and protein. Vegetarians can modify their consumption of foods according to a modified food pyramid (Figure 7.10). The vegetarian pyramid presents a helpful plan for people wishing to avoid meats. The recommended number of servings of grains, vegetables, fruits, and milk products is identical to the recommended amounts on the Food Guide Pyramid. The major difference is the exclusion of meat in favor of legumes, nuts, seeds, and eggs.

NUTRITION AND PHYSICAL ACTIVITY

Good nutrition plays an important role in maximizing your capacity to maintain elevated levels of physical activity. In fact, most researchers feel that proper nutrition ranks right behind proper training principles and heredity in influencing exercise performance (Costill, 1988). This factor, however, may contribute to the widespread belief among those engaging in exercise that additional protein, vitamins, and minerals, sometimes in the form of energy bars or drinks, are necessary for optimal exercise performance. You will discover that the same diet principles that enhance health are advocated for exercise enthusiasts, along with a few commonsense guidelines for managing energy intake and fluid replacement. The following information will help you meet your nutrient needs when you participate in regular physical activity and is presented to dispel some exercise/food–related myths.

6. The diet recommended for any healthy individual will support physical activity.

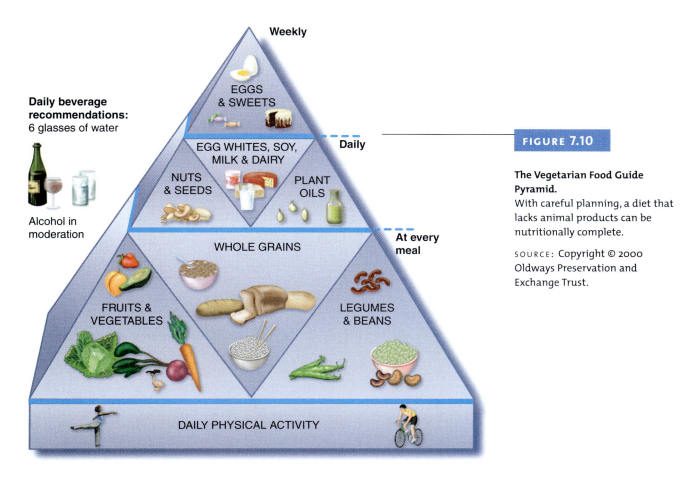

physical activity and health connection

The ideal distribution of protein, carbohydrate, and fat for physically active individuals is comparable to the recommendations provided by the *Dietary Guidelines for Americans* and presented in the Food Guide Pyramid (Figure 7.8). The main difference is in the quantity of calories consumed to produce the extra energy required by increased physical activity (see Chapter 8). As the amount of physical activity increases, so does the amount of energy required to maintain our energy reserves. Individuals who are highly active can expend high levels of daily energy, usually in a short period of time.

Similar to a healthy diet, a high-carbohydrate diet is probably the most important nutritional concern for regular exercisers. Carbohydrates are one of the main sources of energy for working muscles. Additionally, body carbohydrate stores (glycogen) are extremely important for maximizing the muscle glycogen stores that provide greater energy reserve for both aerobic and anaerobic activities. Therefore, heightened glycogen stores are important for increasing endurance and delay of fatigue. Because glycogen synthesis is directly related to dietary carbohydrate intake, it is recommended that 60 to 65 percent of the exerciser's total energy intake should come from carbohydrates.

Many exercisers, especially weight lifters and bodybuilders, feel that extra protein is needed to build muscle mass. Indeed, regular exercisers may require approximately 1.5 grams per kilogram of body weight compared to Recommended Dietary Allowance of 0.8 grams per kilogram of body weight (Paul, 1987). This increased requirement is minor. More important to remember is that the body's protein need is driven more by body-tissue maintenance, repair, and growth (see protein section) than energy needs. During exercise there is relatively little protein loss through energy metabolism. In fact, the limiting factor in the use of protein for tissue growth and repair is energy intake, not protein intake (Butterfield et al., 1992). This means that you must first meet your energy requirements with an adequate intake of carbohydrates and then determine your protein requirements via the biologically driven protein-grams-per-kilogram ratio method. This has been referred to as the *protein-sparing* effect of protein.

Following the serving recommendations of the Food Guide Pyramid for diary products and meat or meat substitutes will provide the necessary daily RDA protein requirements. Americans already eat more protein than they need and do not require protein supplements. Excess protein is used as energy and can be stored as body fat. Furthermore, too much protein can increase calcium loss (contributing to osteoporosis) and put an added burden on the kidneys and liver, which are required to filter out the nitrogen byproduct (ketones) of the protein.

Probably the second most important dietary principle for regular exercisers is to consume the right amount of fluids before, during, and after exercise. Losing as little as 2 to 3 percent of body weight by dehydration can adversely affect exercise performance. Moreover, if exercisers are not careful about avoiding dehydration, they run the risk of heat exhaustion and even heat stroke. Water and fluids are essential to maintaining good hydration and body temperature.

Increased muscular activity from exercise leads to an increase in heat production in the body. The body's chief way to lose heat is evaporation from the skin. To keep the body cool, sweat losses can exceed a liter in a 1-hour period under normal conditions, and be even higher in extremely hot and humid conditions. Any lost body weight during exercise should be replaced with equal amounts of fluids immediately following the exercise. If exercise is longer than an hour or in extremely warm and humid conditions, or if body weight drops more than 3 percent, regular intervals of fluid replacements during exercise is imperative. Cool water (refrigerator cold) is the best choice. The addition of electrolytes (through "sport" drinks like All Sport, Gatorade, and Powerade) is generally not justified. Sweat is about 99 percent water and only 1 percent electrolytes and other substances.

As you learned earlier, vitamins and minerals play an important role in the metabolism of carbohydrates, protein, and fats. Physical activity slightly increases the need for some vitamins and minerals (iron, calcium, ascorbic acid, to name a few) because of the increased metabolism. However, these demands for vitamins and minerals can be easily met through the increased calories consumed from carbohydrate-rich foods. Remember, people who exercise are at an advantage because they need to eat more than sedentary people to account for their increased caloric expenditure, thereby providing their bodies with more vitamins and minerals. Vitamin and mineral supplements are generally not needed if you follow the Food Guide Pyramid.

YOUR PERSONAL NUTRITIONAL PLAN

7. You can develop a personal nutrition plan.

Now that you understand what nutrients the body needs, in what amounts, and the kinds of foods that supply them, you can put together a plan that meets your needs. In this section we provide you with specific strategies to help in developing your personal diet plan. But first it is important to reiterate a key statement in the *Dietary Guidelines for Americans* (2000): "Eating is one of life's greatest pleasures." In an attempt to enable people to feel confident about their food and activity choices, the International Food Information Council (IFIC) (1996) developed six support messages that emphasized the pleasures of eating. These include:

- *It's all about you.* Make healthy choices that fit your lifestyle so you can do the things you want to do.
- *Be realistic.* Make small changes over time in what you eat and the level of activity you do. After all, small steps work better than giant leaps.
- *Be adventurous.* Expand your tastes to enjoy a variety of new foods.
- *Be flexible.* Go ahead and balance what you eat and the physical activity you do over several days. No need to worry about just one meal or one day.
- *Be sensible.* Enjoy all foods, just don't overdo it.
- *Be active.* Walk the dog—don't just watch the dog walk.

These simple messages provide effective nutrition communication, which emphasizes behavior change without overwhelming you with nutritional information.

Strategies To Improve Your Diet

Engage www.pahconnection.com 7.3, 7.4, 7.5

Activities & Assessments 7.1, 7.2

Nutritional Profile First, you need to determine your daily calorie and nutrient intake recommendations based on the RDIs. Then you will know how many calories and nutrients you should be targeting each day based on your individual needs and goals. To complete this activity, go to Engage 7.3, Nutritional Profile, and fill in your name, age, gender, weight, height, frame size, and activity level.

Diet Analysis Record Record your food intake for three consecutive days using the form provided in Activities and Assessments 7.1. Record what you ate, how much you ate, when you ate, and your reasons for eating. Next, analyze your food intake by going to the Nutritional Analysis Tool on the PAH website.

Check Your Present Eating Style Why we eat and how we eat—our eating style—can significantly influence our food choices. To complete this self-assessment activity,

Activities & Assessments
7.3, 7.4

Engage
www.pahconnection.com
7.6

go to the PAH website. The Food Guide Pyramid translates recommendations from *Dietary Guidelines for Americans* into types and amounts of foods people can eat to achieve a healthful diet. The Healthy Eating Index (HEI) analyzes dietary intake relative to servings of the five major food groups in the Food Guide Pyramid. The HEI is based on ten components: grain consumption, vegetable consumption, fruit consumption, milk consumption, meat consumption, total fat intake, saturated fat intake, cholesterol intake, sodium intake, and food variety. Each component of the index has a minimum score of zero and a maximum score of 10. The maximum overall score is 100. To calculate your HEI, go to the Healthy Eating Index web activity (Engage 7.6).

PHYSICAL ACTIVITY AND HEALTH CONNECTION

Sound nutritional advice for good health is also sound nutritional advice for physical activity. Although proper exercise and sound nutrition habits may confer health benefits separately, a reduction in risk factors can be maximized when both are part of a healthy lifestyle. A healthy diet may prevent disease in a variety of ways, but the health benefits multiply when healthful nutrition and proper exercise are combined. For example (see Chapter 9), dieting and aerobic exercise may combat obesity independently, but together sound eating practices and participation in a physical activity program are more effective.

Proper nutritional practices may complement physical activity as a means to enhance health status. Nutrition forms the foundation for physical activity; it provides both the fuel for mechanical work and the elements for extracting and using the potential energy contained within the fuel. Food also provides the essential elements for the synthesis of new tissue and the repair of existing cells. A nutrient-dense diet provides the minerals for strong bones and muscles. Adequate consumption of water helps keep you hydrated when you are active in warm climates. Expending energy through physical activity helps maintain healthy body composition. As you increase your level of physical activity, you will find that you are much more successful if you are also following sound nutritional practices.

CONCEPT CONNECTION

1. **Nutrition plays a major role in overall health.** Five major causes of death are associated with dietary factors: coronary heart disease, some types of cancer, stroke, noninsulin-dependent diabetes mellitus, and coronary artery disease
2. **Nutrients perform three functions in the body.** Nutrients play three major functions in the body that are essential for life: (1) they provide energy, (2) they build and repair tissues, and (3) they help regulate body processes.
3. **Food can be divided into seven classes and each class plays a different role.** Proteins, carbohydrates, fats—the raw fuel for both biological and mechanical energy requirements comes in the form of these three macronutrients. Vitamins, minerals, and water play crucial roles in regulating the body's processes related to activating energy release. Functional foods contain significant levels of biologically active components that provide health benefits beyond basic nutrition.

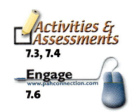

4. ***Dietary Guidelines for Americans* provides advice about making healthy food choices.** Eat a variety of foods; balance the food you eat with physical activity; maintain or improve your weight; choose a diet with plenty of grain products, vegetables, and fruits; choose a diet low in fat, saturated fat, and cholesterol; choose a diet moderate in sugars; choose a diet moderate in salt and sodium; and, if you drink alcoholic beverages, do so in moderation.

5. **The Food Guide Pyramid provides a visual image of the foods Americans should eat daily.** The Food Pyramid specifies daily food choices from five major food groups and takes into account both nutrient adequacy and excesses. The Pyramid is designed to be practical and useful to consumers by providing a visual image of the variety of foods that Americans should eat daily; it suggests ranges in the numbers of servings from each group so that everyone can meet their needs from one basic menu. The specific nutrient levels targeted in the Pyramid are protein, vitamins, minerals, and dietary fiber, without excessive amounts of calories, fat, saturated fat, cholesterol, sodium, added sugars, and alcohol. The Pyramid is based on ideas highlighted by the *Dietary Guidelines* and by consensus reports of authoritative health organizations. The Food Guide Pyramid is flexible and full of food choices. It offers simple, practical advice to help you make choices that are consistent with the seven dietary guidelines for Americans. The Pyramid encourages the basic principles of a healthful diet: variety, balance, and moderation.

6. **The diet recommended for the person who participates in physical exercise differs little in composition from the diet advised for any healthy individual.** The most important dietary concerns for regular exercisers are meeting their increased caloric requirements with complex carbohydrates and drinking enough fluids before, during, and after exercise to ensure proper hydration.

7. **You can develop a personal nutrition plan.** Completing a nutritional profile, checking your present eating habits, and analyzing your diet will help you develop your personal nutrition plan.

TERMS

Nutrients, 136
Digestion, 136
Macronutrients, 137
Calorie, 137
Micronutrients, 138
Essential nutrients, 138
Nonessential nutrients, 138
Dietary Reference Intakes (DRIs), 139
Protein, 141
Amino acid, 141
Essential amino acids, 141
Carbohydrates, 141
Simple carbohydrates, 142
Monosaccharide, 142
Disaccharide, 142
Complex carbohydrates, 142
Starches, 142
Glycogen, 142
Dietary fiber, 143
Insoluble fibers, 143
Soluble fibers, 143
Fat, 144
Triglycerides, 144
Essential fatty acids, 145
Trans fats, 146
Phospholipids, 146
Cholesterol, 147
Vitamins, 147
Fat-soluble vitamins, 147
Water-soluble, 147
Minerals, 149
Major minerals, 149
Trace minerals, 149
Anemia, 150
Functional foods, 151
Energy balance equation, 153
Nutrition facts label, 161
Nutrient-calorie benefit ratio, 164
Vegan, 164
Ovovegetarian, 164
Ovolactovegetarian, 164
Semivegetarian, 164

MAKING THE CONNECTION

Meeting with the nutritionist at the university health center, Mary learns that she is meeting all of her daily nutrient requirements for vitamins and minerals, including iron and calcium. Mary is relieved to discover that, by following the Food Guide Pyramid and its basic principles of variety, balance, and moderation, she is obtaining all the needed nutrient requirements to maintain her physically active lifestyle.

CRITICAL THINKING

1. Like Mary, we sometimes rely on dietary supplements. What supplements are you currently taking, or have you taken? For each supplement, list natural foods that you could have eaten that would have provide you the same nutritional value as the supplement.

2. Identify three barriers you face in trying to follow the *Dietary Guidelines for Americans*. For each barrier, identify a strategy and timeline to overcome each barrier.

3. You are one of twelve students at your university who are asked to assist the dietetics staff in developing healthy, nutritious, and appealing meals for college students. Using your nutrition knowledge, develop a well-balanced menu for breakfast, lunch, and dinner.

4. Go to a local health food store (these are often found in a shopping mall). Walk through the store, looking at the products and their health claims. Find two products, identify the claims made, and note any scientific research that support the claim. Would you, based on the information provided, use this product? Why or why not?

REFERENCES

ADA Reports. (1993). Position of the American Dietetic Association and the Canadian Dietetic Association: Nutrition for physical fitness and athletic performance for adults. *Journal of the American Dietetic Association* 93:691–96.

American Medical Association. (1999). Nutritional basics: Nutrition information that will make a difference in your health. Online: http://www.ama-assn.org/insight/gen_hlth/nutrinfo/nutrinfo.htm

International Food Information Council Foundation. (1998). Backgrounder: Functional Foods. In: *Food Insight Media Guide*. Washington, DC..

Bean, N.H., Goulding, J.S., Lao, C., & Angulo, F.J. (1996). Surveillance for foodborne disease outbreaks, United States, 1988–1992. *Morbidity and Mortality Weekly Report* 45:1–66.

Butterfield, G., Cady, D., & Moynihan, S. (1992). Effect of increasing protein intake on nitrogen balance in recreational weight lifters. *Medicine in Science and Sports Exercise* 24(S71):S14–S22.

Costill, D.L. (1988). Carbohydrates for exercise: Dietary demands for optimal performance. *International Journal of Sports Medicine* 9:1–18.

Deckelbaum, R.J., et al. (1999). Summary of a scientific conference on preventive nutrition: Pediatrics to geriatrics. *Circulation 100*:450–56.

National Academy of Sciences, Institute of Medicine. (1998). *Dietary Reference Intakes: Thiamin, Riboflavin, Niacin, Vitamin B_6, Folate, Vitamin B_{12}, Pantothenic Acid, Biotin, and Choline.* Washington, DC: National Academy Press.

Obesity Education Initiative, National Heart, Lung, and Blood Institute. (1998). *Clinical Guidelines on the Identification, Evaluation, and Treatment of Overweight and Obesity in Adults.* Bethesda, MD: National Institutes of Health. Online: http://www.nhlbi.nih.gov/nhlbi/cardio/obes/prof/guidins/ob_home.htm.

Paul, G.L. (1987). Dietary protein requirements for physically active individuals. *Sports Medicine* 8:154–76.

Samaras, K, Kelley, P., Chiano, M., Spectro, T., & Campbell, L. (1999). Genetic and environmental factors on total-body and central abdominal fat: The effect of physical activity in female twins. *Annals of Internal Medicine 130*: 873–82.

Schmidt, D.B., Morrow, M.M., & White, C. (1997). Communicating the benefits of functional foods. *Chemtech 20*: 40–44.

The Surgeon General's Report on Nutrition and Health. (1988). Washington, DC: U.S. Department of Health and Human Services. DHHS (PHS) Publication No. 88-50210.

U.S. Department of Agriculture, Agriculture Research Service, Dietary Guidelines Advisory Committee. (2000). *Nutrition and Your Health: Dietary Guidelines for Americans, 2000,* 5th ed. Home and Garden Bulletin No. 232. Washington, DC.

U.S. Department of Agriculture, Food, Nutrition, and Consumer Services, Center for Nutrition Policy and Research. (1996). Using the food guide pyramid: A resource for nutrition educators. Washington, DC.

United States Department of Health and Human Services (2000). *Healthy People 2010* , Conference Edition, 2 vols. Washington, DC.

Van DeGraaff, K.M. & Fox, S.I. (1995). *Concepts of Human Anatomy and Physiology.* Dubuque, IA: Wm. C. Brown.

Weinsier, R.L., Hunter, G.R. Heini, A.F., Goran, M.I. Sell, S.M. (1998). The etiology of obesity: Relative contribution of metabolic factors, diet, and physical activity. *American Journal of Medicine 105*:145–50.

Activities & Assessments

NAME ______________________ SECTION ____________ DATE ____________

7.1 Food Diary

Data Collection: For 2 days, keep a list of everything you eat. Choose days that are representative of your usual food-consumption patterns. Record the quantity of each food item, the time of day it was consumed, whether consumption was part of meal or a snack, whether you ate because of hunger or for other reasons, your feelings at the time you ate, and the social circumstances surrounding eating (alone, with friends, with family).

FOOD	QUANTITY	TIME OF DAY	MEAL OR SNACK	OTHER? HUNGRY?	FEELINGS?	SOCIAL?
Cereal	bowlful	6:30 am	meal	hungry	sleepy	alone
Banana	one	6:30 am	meal	hungry	sleepy	alone
Milk, skim	cup	6:30 am	meal	hungry	sleepy	alone

DATA ANALYSIS

Analyze the nutrient content of a representative meal from your food diary:

1. Choose a representative meal.
2. Log on to the Nutritional Analysis Calculator at the University of Illinois and submit your meal for a nutrition analysis. You can find the link to the calculator on the Health and Wellness website.
3. Print out the analysis.
4. Write a one-page paper in which you compare your food intake (the number of servings in each category) with the guidelines offered by the Food Guide Pyramid (see page 155).

SOURCE: G. Edlin, E. Golanty, and K. McCormack Brown. (1999). *Health and Wellness* (6th ed., p. 543). Boston: Jones and Bartlett.

Activities & Assessments

NAME ____________ SECTION ____________ DATE ____________

7.2 My Eating Habits: Some Clues to Calories

Calories come from food—all kinds of food. Do you get enough? More than you need? Think about your eating patterns and why you eat what you eat. Check all the answers that describe your eating patterns.

What Do I usually Eat?

____ A varied and balanced diet.

____ A diet with only moderate amounts of fats and sugars.

____ Deep-fat-fried and breaded foods.

____ "Extras," such as salad dressings, potato toppings, spreads, sauces, and gravies.

____ Sweets and rich desserts, such as candies, cakes, and pies.

____ Snack foods high in fat and sodium, such as chips and other "munchies."

____ Soft drinks.

When Do I Usually Eat?

____ At mealtime.

____ While studying.

____ While preparing meals or clearing the table.

____ When spending time with friends.

____ While watching TV or participating in other activities.

____ Anytime.

Where Do I Usually Eat?

____ At home at the kitchen or dining room table.

____ In the school cafeteria.

____ In fast-food places.

____ In front of the TV or while studying.

____ Wherever I happen to be when I'm hungry.

Why Do I Usually Eat?

____ It's time to eat.

____ I'm hungry.

____ Foods look tempting.

____ Everyone else is eating.

____ Food will get thrown away if I don't eat it.

____ I'm bored or frustrated.

Changes I Want to Make

1. ____________________

2. ____________________

3. ____________________

SOURCE: U.S. Department of Agriculture. (1992). *Dietary guidelines and your health: Health educator's guide to nutrition and fitness.* Washington, DC: U.S. Government Printing Office.

Activities & Assessments

NAME ____________ SECTION ____________ DATE ____________

7.3 Eat for Good Nutrition

Are you "in action"? Are you ready to stay in shape—for a lifetime? From these statements, check seven guidelines for smart eating that can help you stay healthy.

____ Use salt and sodium only in moderation.

____ Choose a diet low in fat, saturated fat, and cholesterol.

____ Avoid snacking.

____ Eat an apple a day for good health.

____ Use sugars only in moderation.

____ Avoid desserts.

____ Maintain a healthy weight.

____ Avoid alcoholic beverages.

____ Eat green vegetables every day.

____ Avoid candy, chips, and soft drinks.

____ Choose a diet with plenty of vegetables, fruits, and grain products.

____ Eat a variety of foods.

____ Avoid fast foods.

I want to follow the dietary guidelines so I stay healthy.
Here's how I'll eat smart:

____

____

____

____

Signed ____

Date ____

SOURCE: U.S. Department of Agriculture. (1992). *Dietary guidelines and your health: Health educator's guide to nutrition and fitness.* Washington, DC: U.S. Government Printing Office.

Activities & Assessments

NAME ____________________ SECTION __________ DATE __________

7.4 How Does Your Diet Rate for Variety?

A varied diet is a healthful diet. How would you describe the variety in your food choices?

	SELDOM OR NEVER	1 OR 2 TIMES A WEEK	3 TO 4 TIMES A WEEK	ALMOST DAILY
How often do you eat:				
1. At least six servings of bread, cereals, rice, crackers, pasta, or other foods made from grains (a serving is one slice of bread or a half cup cereal or rice) per day?	☐	☐	☐	☐
2. Foods made from whole gains?	☐	☐	☐	☐
3. Three different kinds of vegetables per day?	☐	☐	☐	☐
4. Cooked dry beans or peas?	☐	☐	☐	☐
5. A dark-green vegetable, such as spinach or broccoli?	☐	☐	☐	☐
6. Two kinds of fruit or fruit juice per day?	☐	☐	☐	☐
7. Three servings of milk, yogurt, or cheese per day?	☐	☐	☐	☐
8. Two servings of lean meat, poultry, or fish, or eggs, dry beans, or nuts per day?	☐	☐	☐	☐
Count the number of check marks in each column. TOTAL	____	____	____	____

To eat a varied diet, I will

____

____

____

____

SOURCE: G. Edlin, E. Golanty, and K. McCormack Brown. (1999). *Health and Wellness* (6th ed., p. 544). Boston: Jones and Bartlett.

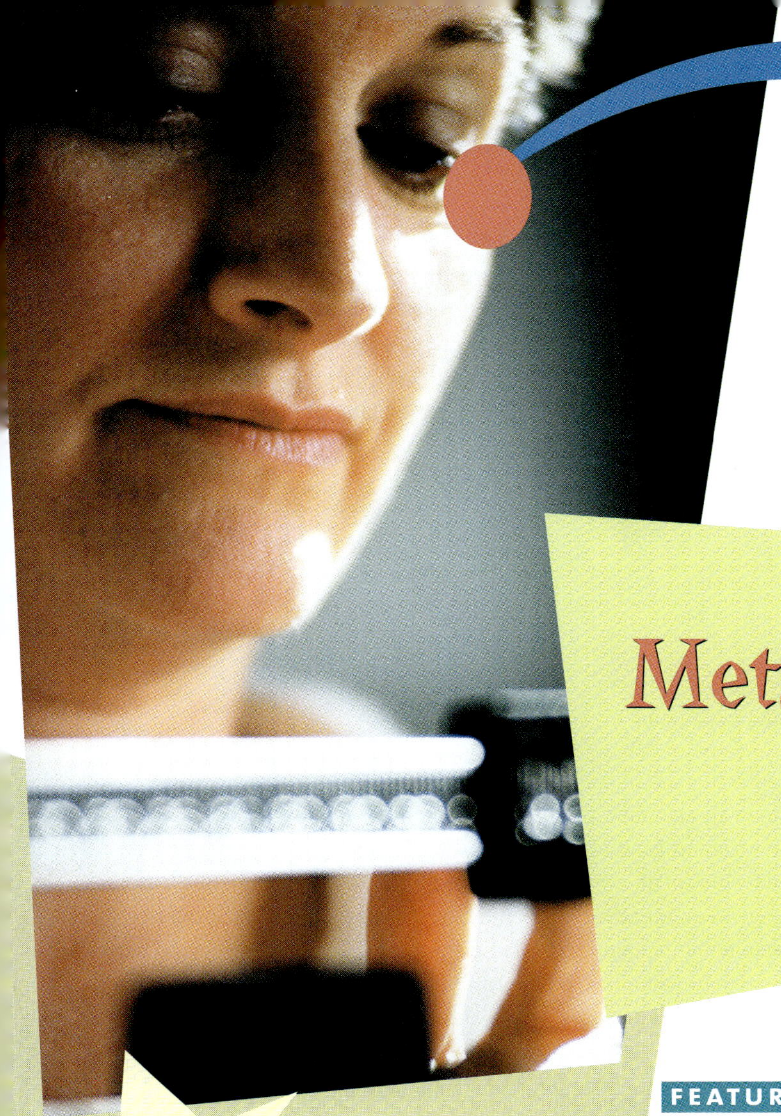

8

Metabolic Health

CONCEPT CONNECTION

1. Metabolism is the transfer, storage, and utilization of energy in the human body.
2. Your metabolism at rest is called the *resting metabolic rate,* or RMR.
3. Physical activity has a profound effect on your metabolism.
4. Metabolic disorders may lead to obesity, eating disorders, and other conditions that can negatively impact your health.
5. We are in the midst of an obesity epidemic in the United States.

FEATURES

E-Learning Tools: www.pahconnection.com

Engage www.pahconnection.com

8.1 How much energy do I expend daily?
8.2 How much energy do I consume daily?
8.3 Eating disorder checklist

Experience www.pahconnection.com

8.1 Energy values (calories) for foods
8.2 Metabolic energy expenditure levels

Explore www.pahconnection.com

8.1 Caloric values of various foods
8.2 Eating disorders
8.3 Shape up America!

Activities & Assessments

8.1a Estimating your Resting Metabolic Rate (RMR)
8.1b Changing your Resting Metabolic Rate

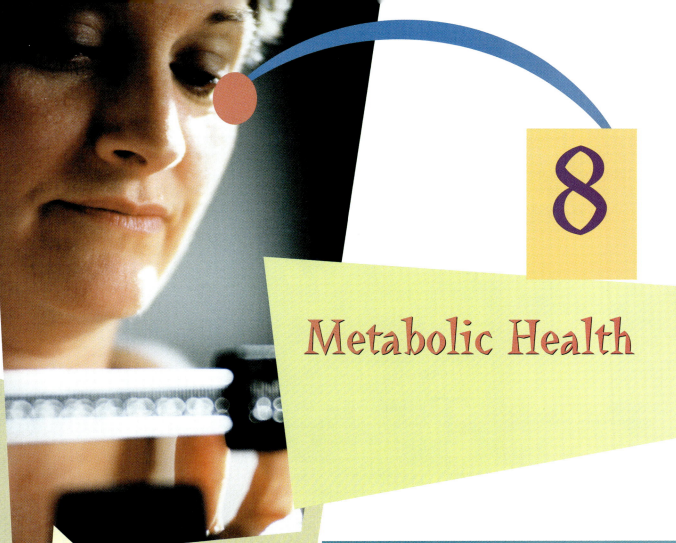

WHAT'S THE CONNECTION?

Fred noticed that some people could eat just about anything and never put on weight, while some who became overfat didn't appear to eat any more than their slim friends. Fred knew the answer had something to do with how energy is used and stored in the body, but he wasn't sure what factors make people use and store energy differently. As part of a class project, Fred decided to research the process by which energy is utilized in the human body. He thought this might help him to understand why some people store excess fat and others don't.

1. Metabolism is the transfer, storage, and utilization of energy in the human body.

Metabolism Process whereby the body takes in energy, converts it to a useable form, stores what is needed, and eliminates what is not.

First Law of Thermodynamics Energy can neither be created nor destroyed.

INTRODUCTION

This chapter will establish the link between your metabolism and your health. In order to function, all living beings must take in energy, transfer it into a useable form, store what is needed, and eliminate what is not. This process is referred to as **metabolism.** There are many factors that influence your metabolism, including genetics, gender, body size, eating habits, and physical activity. Physical activity has a profound effect on energy intake, storage, and utilization (metabolism). This chapter also touches on several metabolic disorders and explains how they may affect your metabolic health.

ENERGY BALANCE, TRANSFER, AND STORAGE

Our ability to balance, transfer, and store energy determines, to a large extent, our fitness, our health, and our body composition. The intensity of our activities is limited by how rapidly we can transfer energy. Our energy intake and our energy expenditure regulate whether we gain or lose weight. The importance of our metabolic health cannot be overlooked (Kaplan & Dietz, 1999).

FIRST LAW OF THERMODYNAMICS

The **first law of thermodynamics** states that energy can neither be created nor destroyed. The energy used by the human body for movement and to power biological work comes from the food we eat. The three sources of food energy used by humans are carbohydrates, fats, and proteins (Chapter 7). When our body uses energy, we don't destroy it. Rather, we transfer the energy into a useable form (adenosine triphosphate, or ATP), send it to our surrounding environment (heat energy), or store it in our bodies (most commonly as adipose tissue). Your ability to balance the transfer, utilization, and storage of energy determines your metabolic health.

When we consume carbohydrates, fats, or proteins, we must first break them down to **substrates** that can be used by the body. Carbohydrates are reduced to glucose, fats to triglycerides, and proteins to amino acids. Of these three fuel sources, fats supply the most energy per unit of weight. For example, 1 gram of either carbohydrate or protein will contain approximately 4 kilocalories (kcal) of energy. For each gram of fat we consume, we receive 9 kcal of energy. Therefore, more energy is available in foods higher in fat than in foods higher in either protein or carbohydrate.

Heat is one of the byproducts when food is broken down and used for energy. The heat production can actually be measured, and this **thermic effect** of breaking down food, transferring it, using it to power biological work, storing excess amounts in the body, and exchanging energy with our environment determines your metabolic rate. Sweating during physical activity releases the body's heat produced during the transfer of energy.

Your metabolic rate is composed of three factors: (1) the thermic effect of feeding [TEF], (2) your resting metabolic rate [RMR], and (3) the thermic effect of physical activity [TEA] (Wilmore, 1994). Of these three, the greatest contributor to daily energy expenditure is your resting metabolic rate (Figure 8.1).

The Thermic Effect of Feeding

The process of digesting food requires energy. The warming sensation that we feel after eating is due to the release of heat produced through the digestive process. This warming sensation also explains why we feel a bit drowsy after eating. Warmth relaxes the body. Roughly 10 percent of your daily energy expenditure is due to the thermic effect of feeding (Wilmore, 1994).

Resting Metabolic Rate and Basal Metabolism

Two terms are commonly used to describe your metabolic rate. The first term, **resting metabolic rate (RMR)**, reflects your energy expenditure in a normal rested state. The second term, **basal metabolic rate (BMR)**, represents your energy expenditure under

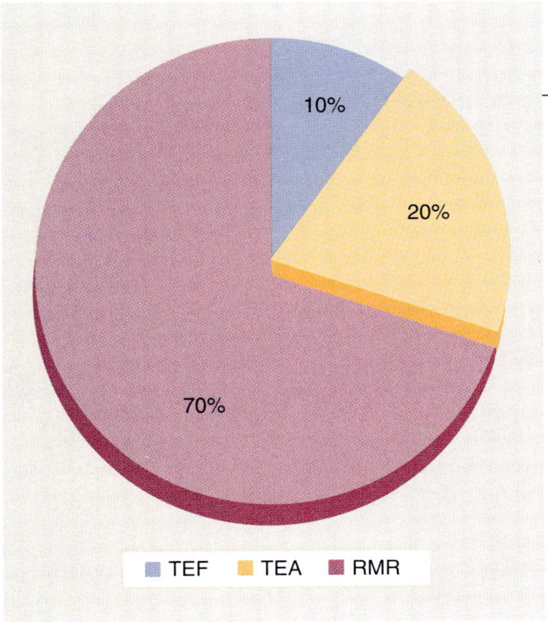

FIGURE 8.1

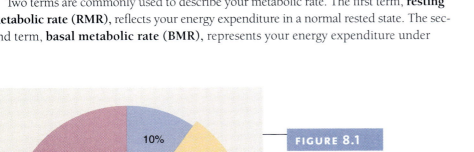

Components of Energy Expenditure.
Three major factors contribute to our daily energy expenditure: the thermic effect of feeding (TEF), the thermic effect of physical activity (TEA), and your resting metabolic rate (RMR).

SOURCE: Data from J.H. Wilmore. (May 1994). Exercise, obesity, and weight control. In C. Corbin, R. Pangrazi (Eds.), *The President's Council on Physical Fitness and Sports Research Digest*, Series 1, No. 6.

Substrates Sources of energy that can be used by our bodies.

Thermic effect A warming effect; occurs when physically active, digesting food, or increasing energy expenditure in any other way.

Resting metabolic rate Your rate of energy use at rest.

Basal metabolic rate Basic energy requirement necessary to sustain life.

Explore
8.1

2. Your metabolism at rest is called the resting metabolic rate, or RMR.

carefully controlled conditions, in which a person spends the night in a clinical facility, fasts for 12 hours, has no activity preceding measurement, and minimizes emotional excitement. Your BMR reflects the basic energy requirements of the body necessary to sustain life. Measurement of BMR is difficult and must be performed in a strictly controlled environment.

Most research on metabolism focuses on the resting metabolic rate. Your RMR accounts for 60 to 75 percent of the total energy you expend each day (Wilmore, 1994). It reflects the normal energy requirement of your body while it is in a state of rest. The RMR is usually low per unit of time when compared to energy expenditure while we are active, but because we spend a greater proportion of our time in a rested state our RMR contributes significantly to total daily energy expenditure.

Activities & Assessments 8.1A, 8.1B

physical activity and health connection

Several factors influence the RMR. Large people tend to have higher metabolic rates because they have more mass that requires energy. People with a great concentration of lean muscle mass also have higher metabolic rates because muscle is more active tissue than fat and it expends more energy, even in a resting state. We also know that RMR remains elevated for a period of time following physical activity. Men tend to have higher metabolic rates than women and young people have higher metabolic rates than seniors. Your genetics will also influence your metabolic rate. The rate at which cellular processes occur in your body is determined by a combination of genetic and environmental factors. Your genetics provide the blueprint for all cellular processes and set up the necessary conditions for these processes to occur. Your environment supplies the necessary triggers for genetic expression to occur. For example, if you have the genetics to be tall, cellular processes will cause growth to occur at a rate greater than in a person with the genetics to be short. However, if we don't provide the proper environmental stimuli (good nutrition, physical activity, lack of disease), the growth may be stunted.

Engage www.pahconnection.com 8.1

Your natural resting metabolic rate will be influenced by your genetics. However, your RMR may be altered by environmental factors to which you are exposed. Being physically active will raise your RMR. The advantage of having a higher metabolic rate is that more of the energy you consume will be used to sustain the body and less will end up stored as adipose tissue.

3. Physical activity has a profound effect on your metabolism.

The Thermic Effect of Activity

The thermic effect of activity (TEA), the energy expended above your RMR, represents the energy necessary to accomplish a given task or activity and includes anything from a small turn of the head while seated to an all-out physical workout. Your TEA accounts for the remainder (15–30%) of your daily energy expenditure (Wilmore, 1994). You may also experience a carryover effect from physical activity on your metabolic rate. Some evidence suggests that physical activity causes a higher metabolic rate that remains elevated for a period of time after the activity has been completed.

Diet and Metabolic Rate

The body will adjust each of these three components of total energy expenditure when there are major increases or decreases in the energy intake. With very low calorie diets, your RMR, TEF, and TEA decrease. Your body attempts to conserve its energy stores to balance the lowered energy consumption associated with dieting. Resting metabolic rate may decrease by 20 to 30 percent or more within weeks after someone begins a very low calorie diet (Wilmore, 1994). With overeating, RMR and TEF increase to prevent the unnecessary storage of a large number of calories, although the adjustment may not be large enough to prevent an increase in body fat. It is speculated that these adaptations are under the control of the **sympathetic nervous system** (controls involuntary bodily functions) and play a major role in controlling weight around a given **set point** (concept that your body prefers to maintain a certain body weight) (Wilmore, 1994).

Sympathetic nervous system Part of the autonomic nervous system; helps prepare the body for physical activity.

Set point Level of resting metabolism that your body naturally prefers. Some research suggests that our metabolic rate will return to its set point even if we try to change our metabolism through modifying our diet.

Energy Balance

To maintain a healthy metabolic profile, you must balance your energy intake with your energy expenditure. If you expend more than you consume, you decrease energy stores in your body. If you consume more than you expend, you increase energy stores in your body.

The typical human consumes an average of 2500 kcal per day, or nearly 1 million kcal per year. We also know that the average adult gains 1.5 pounds of fat each year. This gain represents an imbalance between energy intake and expenditure of only 5250 kcal per year, or less than 15 kcal per day (Wilmore, 1994). It has been proposed that body weight is regulated within a narrow range similar to the way in which body temperature is regulated. When people go to extremes of food consumption by eating too much or going on a starvation diet, they usually return to their original weight when allowed to go back to their normal eating patterns (Wilmore, 1994).

Engage
www.pahconnection.com
8.2

ATP, or adenosine triphosphate, is a high-energy compound that is used by the body to perform work. When ATP is broken down by enzymes, energy is released. This energy allows us to move.

Energy Transfer

Energy transfer in the human body involves the breakdown of carbohydrates, fats, and proteins for the eventual formation of ATP. The breakdown of ATP causes the release of energy that powers all biologic work. Our metabolic systems function to ensure that we have an adequate amount of ATP available when the body needs it.

Our approach to eating helps to determine our metabolic health.

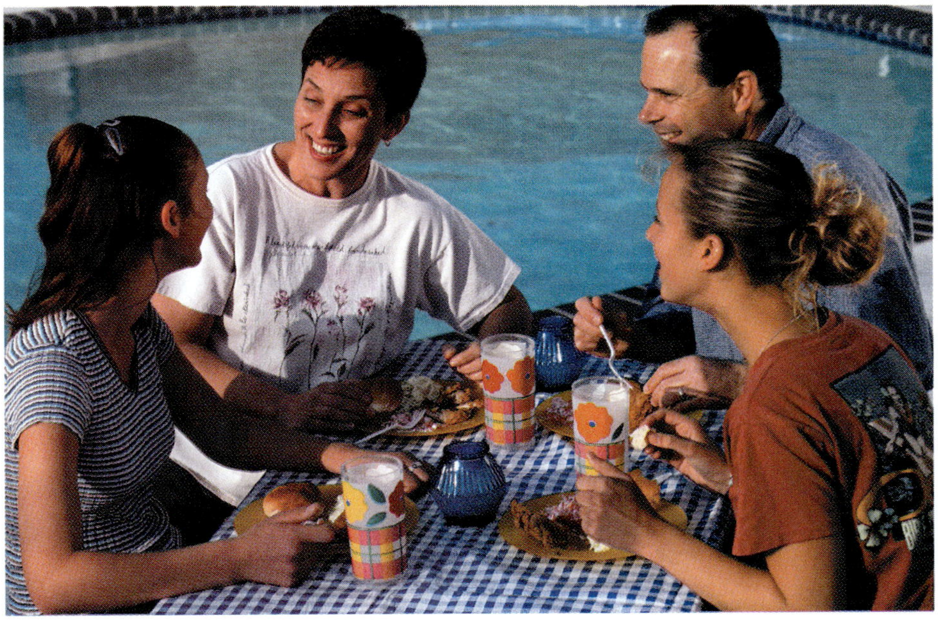

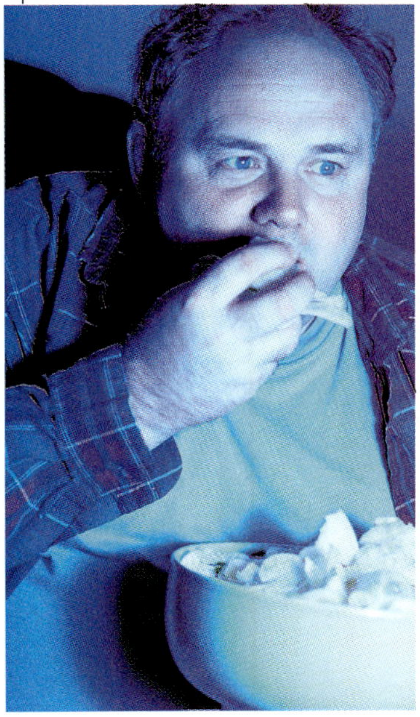

When we initially require energy for movement, we draw upon stores of ATP in the muscle (intramuscular ATP). We only have limited amounts of intramuscular ATP, so we must quickly replenish these stores by breaking down **creatine phosphate,** glucose, triglyceride, and amino acids. Small amounts of creatine phosphate in our muscles require that we rely primarily upon glucose, triglyceride, and amino acids. Carbohydrate is the preferred fuel source because it can be used with or without oxygen present. We rely on carbohydrate when intensity of physical activity is high. However, the amount of carbohydrate we have stored in the body is limited, so we eventually turn to triglyceride to power long-term physical activity.

Most people have almost unlimited energy stored in their body in the form of adipose tissue. Adipose tissue is the stored form of triglyceride. Each pound of adipose tissue contains 3500 kcal of energy. To expend this amount of energy, you would have to run 35 miles! In fact, when we tire during physical activity, it is not because we do not have adequate amounts of energy in our body. It is usually because we have run low on carbohydrates or are experiencing orthopedic stress (pounding on our joints).

To utilize body fat as a fuel source, low-level metabolism of carbohydrate must be occurring. This is because a byproduct of the breakdown of carbohydrates is required to break down fat (triglycerides); thus, we must maintain a baseline level of carbohydrate metabolism if we wish to utilize our stored fat. The statement "Fats burn in a carbohydrate flame" expresses this relationship.

Creatine phosphate Fuel source used in the body to replenish ATP; stored in small amount, it depletes rapidly.

Glycogen Stored form of glucose, a primary carbohydrate used for energy by the human body.

Lactic acid Byproduct of the anaerobic breakdown of carbohydrate; it upsets the acid-base balance in tissues and disrupts muscle function.

Energy Storage

Energy from the food we eat is stored in our bodies in three ways. *Carbohydrates* are usually stored as either glucose (in the muscles and blood) or **glycogen** (in the muscles or liver). *Protein* is stored as lean muscle tissue. *Fat* is stored as adipose tissue. Remember that excess energy from any food source can be converted and stored as adipose tissue. Thus it is important not only to avoid consuming excessive amounts of fat but also to avoid excessive carbohydrates and proteins.

The energy needed to power physical activity is drawn first from the energy stores in muscle, second from energy circulating in the blood, and third from energy stores throughout the body. Because carbohydrate is the only fuel source that can be used without oxygen present, it plays a crucial role in energy utilization. If we eat a low-carbohydrate diet, or exercise to extreme levels, we start to burn muscle tissue as fuel in an attempt to make up for low levels of carbohydrate.

Since carbohydrates are required to metabolize fat, eating a diet that does not contain adequate amounts of carbohydrate prevents us from using fat as a fuel source. We are then forced to break down muscle tissue to meet the energy needs of the body.

ANAEROBIC METABOLISM

Anaerobic metabolism refers to the transfer of energy when there is a limited amount of oxygen available. This occurs when we are first starting to move and also when we are active at high intensity. At these times, the need for energy is greater than the speed at which the blood can deliver oxygen. The only fuel source that can be used anaerobically is carbohydrate. Physical activity of high intensity (sprinting, weight lifting) is referred to as anaerobic exercise. When we use carbohydrate anaerobically, one of the byproducts is an accumulation of **lactic acid.** The hydrogen ions released during the formation of lactic acid upsets the acid-base balance in the body, leading to muscle fatigue. This explains why we can only be active at high intensities for short periods of time. As the intensity of the activity diminishes, adequate amounts of oxygen are delivered and the lactic acid is reconverted to **pyruvic acid**, which can then be used as a fuel source.

Pyruvic acid Byproduct of the breakdown of glucose metabolism. If oxygen is not present, pyruvic acid is converted into lactic acid. If oxygen is present, pyruvic acid is further broken down to provide energy for movement.

AEROBIC METABOLISM

Aerobic metabolism refers to the process whereby energy is transferred in the presence of oxygen. In aerobic metabolism, energy demand does not outpace oxygen delivery. Your heart and circulatory system are able to deliver oxygen in sufficient quantities to meet the body's needs for energy transfer. In this circumstance, you initially use carbohydrate as a fuel source and then shift to fat as the primary source. If the intensity remains relatively low, this type of activity can go on indefinitely. The only limiting factors will be orthopedic stress and low levels of carbohydrate.

PHYSICAL ACTIVITY AND METABOLISM

When we are physically active, our metabolic rate increases to meet the energy demands of the activity. If we are engaged in high-intensity physical activity, our metabolic rate is higher per unit of time. If we engage in lower-intensity, longer-duration activity, our metabolic rate is elevated for a longer period of time. In both cases, our energy expenditure is significantly higher than at rest. Understanding this concept is important to understanding energy balance in the body. From an energy storage–energy reduction standpoint, the total caloric output at the end of the day is the primary determinant of whether you gain or lose body fat. Although higher-intensity activity may result in greater energy expenditure per unit of time, the short duration during which we can maintain high-intensity activity may result in lower total energy expenditure at the end of the day compared to performing lower-intensity activity for longer periods of time. For this reason, and because it is safer for most people, it is usually recommended that people interested in reducing adipose tissue stores participate in low-to-moderate intensity activity for longer periods of time. For those interested in optimal fitness, or for those with time restrictions that do not allow longer activity sessions, higher-intensity activities are an option. Remember that you can break your activity session into multiple segments and still receive the same benefits as if all the activity were performed during one extended session.

Physical activity has an impact on your RMR and the thermic effect of food. However, the contribution of physical activity to total daily energy expenditure is primarily a result of increased energy expenditure during the activity (Melby & Hill, 1999). In other words, while being active may impact your metabolic rate during recovery, and in some cases even during rest, physical activity has its greatest impact on energy expenditure during the time in which you are active. The energy expended in physical activity will vary both with the characteristics of the activity (frequency, intensity, duration) and the individual (body weight, aerobic capacity, skill level) (Melby & Hill, 1999). More activity results in greater energy expenditure.

An active lifestyle helps to maintain a healthy metabolism.

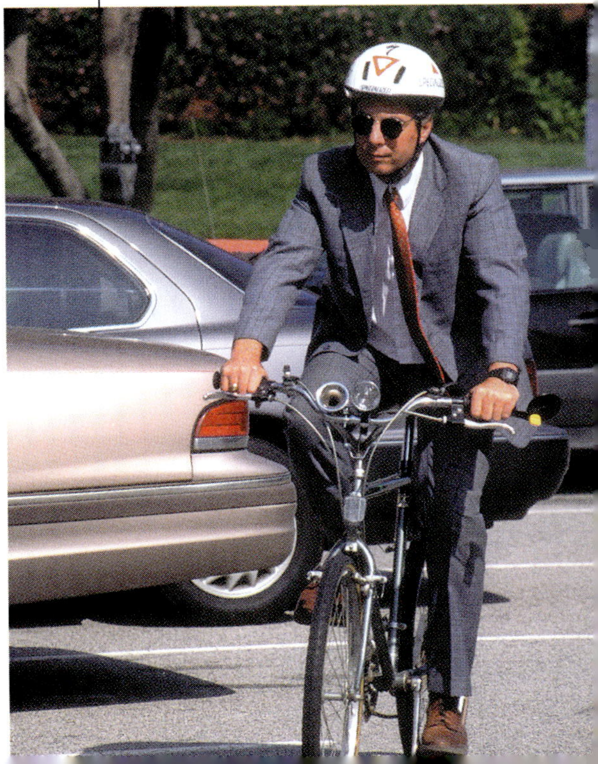

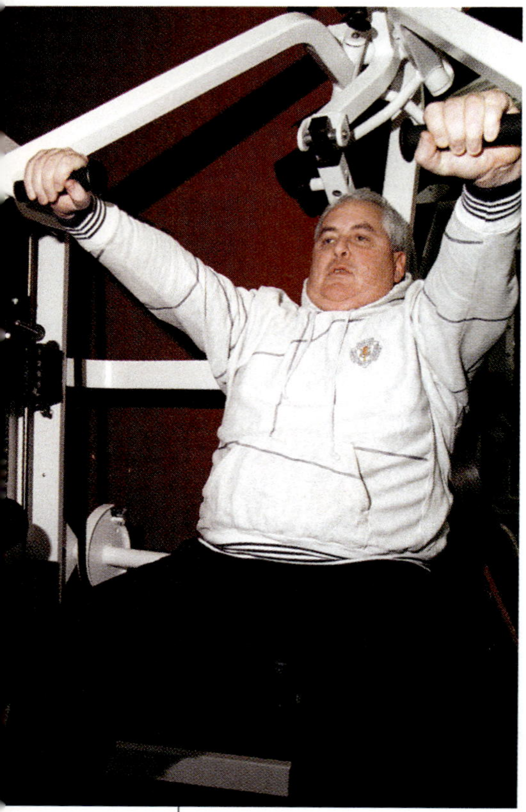

Resistance training is an important component of fat-loss programs.

Energy expenditure does not return to baseline levels immediately following physical activity. How much physical activity contributes to the magnitude and duration of post-activity energy expenditure is controversial and appears to be related to the frequency, intensity, duration, and type of activity performed (Melby & Hill, 1999). Some research suggests that physical activity will raise your resting metabolic rate for an hour or longer after you finish working out, while other research suggests that your metabolic rate returns to normal levels much more rapidly.

The intensity of your physical activity affects the magnitude of the post-activity elevation of metabolic rate more than the duration of the activity. The intensity and duration of the types of activity sessions engaged in by most nonathletes typically results in a return of metabolic rate to baseline values within 5 to 40 minutes following the activity (Melby & Hill, 1999). In individuals capable of performing high-intensity, long-duration activities, the post-activity energy expenditure may be higher and could be a significant contributor to total energy requirements (Melby & Hill, 1999).

Less is known about the effects on post-activity energy expenditure following resistance training, but recent data suggest that high-intensity weight lifting may elevate energy expenditure above baseline values for several hours. However, novice weight lifters may not be capable of training at the intensities required to bring about a prolonged elevation of post-activity energy expenditure (Melby & Hill, 1999). For those individuals who experience increases in muscle mass as a result of resistance training, increases in resting metabolic rate usually result. Because muscle tissue is metabolically more active than adipose tissue, if you increase the percentage of muscle mass in your body, you increase your metabolic rate. Therefore, resistance training should be incorporated as one component of fat and body composition management programs.

Building Muscle Mass

The ability to gain lean body mass is dependent on four major factors, including (1) proper nutrition, (2) overload resistance training, (3) genetic predisposition, and (4) secretion of the **hormones** associated with tissue growth. A variety of other factors, including body mass, gender, and motivation, will also have an impact on how much muscle you can gain.

Hormones Substances secreted by the glands of the endocrine system that regulate cellular function.

In some people, it is possible to observe body mass increases of approximately 20 percent during the first year of regular heavy resistance training (Butterfield, Kleiner, Lemon, & Stone, 1995). These initial gains usually occur at a faster rate and to a greater magnitude than subsequent gains. The reduction in the degree of further benefit occurs because, once you have started a resistance training program, you have less room for improvement. In other words, you tend to approach your genetic potential. After a few years of systematic training, gains may be only 1 to 3 percent per year (Butterfield et al., 1995).

Impact of Physical Activity on TEF and RMR

Changes in chronic physical activity may influence the other components of energy expenditure, specifically the TEF and RMR. It is likely that the effect of physical activity on TEF is fairly small, with the benefits on weight control of being active resulting more from the increased energy expenditure during the activity, rather than from its impact on TEF (Melby & Hill, 1999).

There is some uncertainty as to whether changes in physical activity alter RMR independently of changes in fat-free mass (Melby & Hill, 1999). Some data suggest that RMR may be chronically elevated in individuals who engage in daily, high-intensity, prolonged physical activity. It is unclear whether the increase in RMR is caused by the residual effects of acute activity or by an actual long-term change in metabolism. It has been speculated that the amount of activity performed by nonathletes for the purpose of weight control is typically of much lower intensity and duration than would be needed to increase RMR permanently (Melby & Hill, 1999).

INACTIVITY AND METABOLISM

In direct opposition to the relationship of physical activity and metabolism, we see that being inactive lowers the metabolic rate and increases the likelihood of storing excess adipose tissue. Inactivity results in a lower lean-mass percentage of body composition. Muscle responds to physical activity by becoming stronger and **hypertrophying.** Muscle also responds to inactivity by becoming weaker and **atrophying.** As your percentage of muscle tissue decreases, your metabolic rate also decreases.

We also know that as your activity level declines a greater percentage of your day is spent in an inactive state. Since physical activity itself has a thermic effect, this component of daily energy expenditure is also decreased. The end result is that your total caloric expenditure is lower when you are inactive than when you are active. Based on the relationship of total caloric expenditure and total caloric consumption, we can see that, if we lower caloric expenditure by being inactive, we must either decrease caloric consumption by eating less or see an increase in adipose tissue storage (increased percentage of body fat). As we increase our percentage of body fat, our metabolism is decreased further, a vicious circle that leads to obesity.

physical activity and health connection

Hypertrophy Increase in cell size. Adipose tissue (fat cells) hypertrophies when there is too much food; muscle cells hypertrophy when stressed through resistance training.

Atrophy Decrease in cell size. Adipose tissue atrophies when activity increases; muscle cells atrophy when activity decreases.

4. Metabolic disorders may lead to obesity, eating disorders, and other conditions that can negatively impact your health.

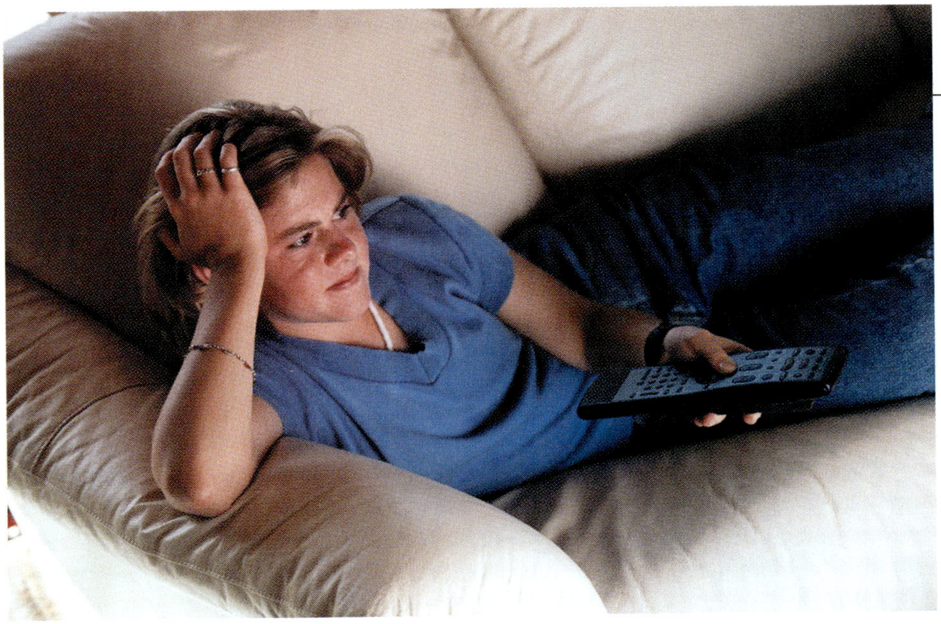

Inactivity may result in many metabolic disorders.

METABOLIC ABNORMALITIES

A healthy metabolic rate is necessary for good health. If your metabolic rate wanders from its natural state, your health may suffer. A metabolic rate that is either too high or too low can bring on several conditions that may be detrimental to your health.

Body Composition

Overweight Having a body weight above levels recommended for a certain height.

Underweight Having a body weight below levels recommended for a certain height.

Overfat Having body fat levels above recommended levels for good health.

Underfat Having body fat levels below what is recommended for good health.

Body composition refers to the components that make up the human body. (For more information on body composition management, see Chapter 9.) Generally speaking, these components are divided into a two-component model (fat and fat-free mass) or a four-component model (fat, mineral, muscle, and water). Body composition is more important than body weight when determining the health of an individual. Weight only informs someone of how much they weigh, it does not inform them of the composition (how much is fat, bone, and muscle) of the weight.

To understand the importance of knowing your body composition, you need to understand the concepts of **overweight** and **underweight** versus **overfat** and **underfat.** Traditionally, people have compared their weight to a height-weight chart. These charts were originally developed by life insurance companies to establish premiums. They categorize people as being underweight, overweight, or of acceptable weight. The concern with these charts is that a person's weight does not always accurately represent the composition of that weight. Individuals who are very muscular, have dense bones, or are in optimal physical condition may be labeled as being overweight and therefore unhealthy. On the other hand, someone who has poor muscular development, porous bones, and is not in optimal physical condition might be categorized as being of acceptable weight and considered to be healthy. In terms of metabolic health, being overfat or underfat is a health problem, while being overweight or underweight may not be a problem, depending on the composition of the weight.

Body fat is normally categorized as either essential or nonessential. *Essential fat* is the fat necessary for normal physiologic functioning. Body fat plays an important role in thermal insulation, vitamin transfer and storage, nervous system function, reproductive function, hormone synthesis, cell structure, and energy storage and utilization (Chapter 7). Having too little essential fat in your body can lead to physiological dysfunction.

Excess energy stored in your body in the form of adipose tissue is not necessary for normal physiological function. This additional storage fat is referred to as *nonessential fat*. Too much non-essential fat leads to overfatness and obesity.

Determining how much body fat we should have is open to debate. Several standards, ranging from traditional normative data to criterion-referenced standards, have been proposed. Normative data are based on comparing your body fat score to data gathered on a representative population. In others words, a researcher might collect body composition data on a large group of adults. Your body composition score would then be compared to this data set. The potential problem with using normative data is that it only tells you how you compared to the data set. Normative data provides little information about your health status. You may find out that your score is equal to the average score of the data set; however, you don't know if the average score of the data set is overfat, underfat, or falls into a healthy fatness zone.

Due to the limitations of normative data in body composition analysis, experts who study this area of health and fitness have begun relying more on criterion-referenced standards. *Criterion-referenced standards* are standards that have been developed through an analysis of **epidemiological studies**, expert opinion, and normative data. The experts have determined levels of body fatness that are related to health and disease and not so closely associated with averages. Criterion-referenced standards define healthy zones of body fatness and zones where one would be considered at increased risk for disease. These standards also help to demonstrate that it is just as dangerous to be underfat as it is to be overfat (Table 8.1).

Epidemiological studies Studies of diseases, their causes and their spread.

Regional Fat Distribution and Disease

Body fat is stored in various locations throughout the human body. The majority is stored directly under the skin *(subcutaneously)*. This layer of fat provides for cushioning, makes a body feel soft, and provides thermal insulation. We also store fat around our internal organs *(viscerally)*. Several factors determine where we store our fat and how much fat we store, including genetics, activity levels, food consumption, and hormones.

Android and Gynoid Patterns Men and women tend to store fat in different locations. Men typically store extra fat around the abdominal region. Women tend to store additional fat in the hips, thighs, and buttocks. The male pattern of fat storage is referred to as the *android* (derived from a Greek word meaning "male") pattern. The female pattern of body fat storage is termed the *gynoid* pattern. You will also hear these patterns referred to as the apple-shaped pattern (male) and pear-shaped pattern (female). These patterns are determined by secretion of the hormones responsible for the development of secondary sexual characteristics. In fact, as men and women age and hormone secretion levels diminish, their body fat storage patterns start to resemble each other more closely.

Recent research has indicated that the android pattern is associated with a higher risk for the development of cardiovascular disease. This is thought to be related to the fact that the android pattern represents visceral fat storage around the internal organs, whereas, the gynoid pattern is more peripheral and away from internal organs.

Metabolic Abnormalities and Disease

There are several factors that can lead to metabolic abnormality and disease. These include genetic predisposition, lifestyle patterns (eating and activity patterns), and environment (access to nutritious foods). Genetic factors may *predispose* us, or put us at higher risk, for the development of metabolic abnormalities. If we have the genetic predisposition for metabolic disease, it does not mean that we are doomed to develop the disease. It does mean that we must be extremely vigilant and avoid exposing ourselves to environmental factors that could trigger the disease. For instance, if we come from a long line of obese individuals, we are not necessarily doomed to be obese. However, for people with the genetic predisposition for obesity, it can be more difficult to maintain

TABLE 8.1 Criterion-Referenced Standards for Healthy Fat Zones

	ESSENTIAL FAT*	HEALTHY FAT ZONE	OVERFAT
Men	3%	3–25%	>25%
Women	12%	12–30%	>30%

* If your body fat percentage drops below this level, you are considered underfat and are putting yourself at increased health risk.

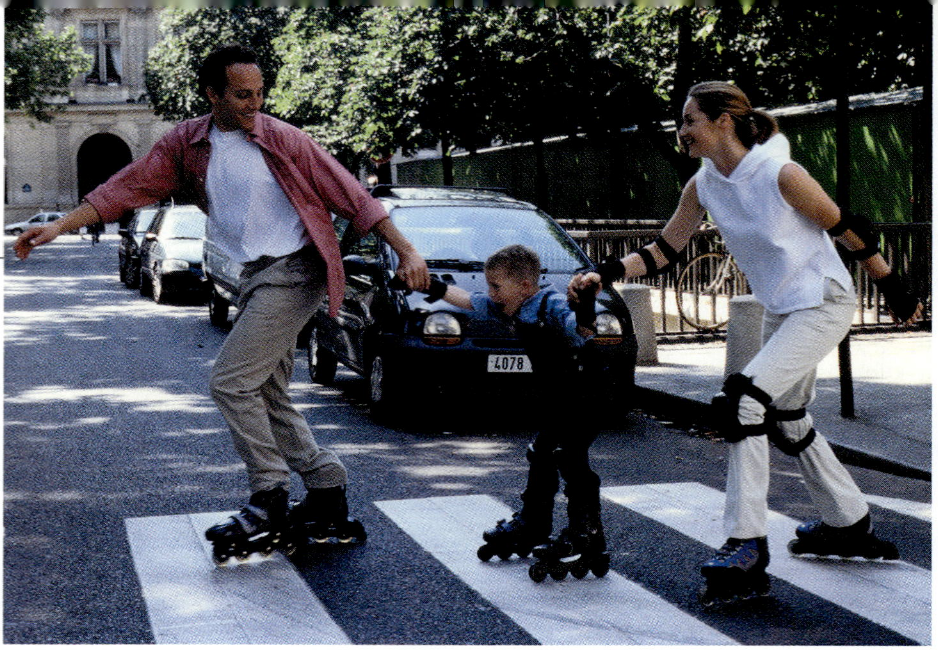

A modest amount of physical activity provides a lot of protection against degenerative diseases.

a healthy body composition. These individuals must be more careful to eat moderately and nutritiously while making regular physical activity an important part of their lives. If people with a genetic predisposition for obesity carefully watch how much and what they eat and maintain an active lifestyle, they limit their risk for the development of this metabolic disorder.

We must also realize that if most of our relatives are large people the chances of our becoming very thin are not good. Many people put themselves through much anxiety, and even choose unwise weight loss and diet techniques, in an attempt to change their body type. This may be nothing short of impossible and thus potentially very harmful. We must think of weight (body fat) in much the same way we think of height. If all of our relatives are short, the odds are against our being tall.

Some common forms of metabolic disorder and disease include hyperinsulinemia, elevated levels of cholesterol and blood lipids, increased blood pressure, and obesity (Chapter 5). *Hyperinsulinemia* is a condition in which there is an excessive amount of insulin in the blood. This can result in low blood sugar levels and possibly lead to insulin shock. Elevated levels of blood cholesterol and blood lipids are dangerous because they may increase the likelihood of plaque forming within the arteries, potentially leading to a heart attack or stroke. Obesity (severe overfatness), is related to all of the metabolic disorders just mentioned. Being obese places you at a greater risk for numerous diseases.

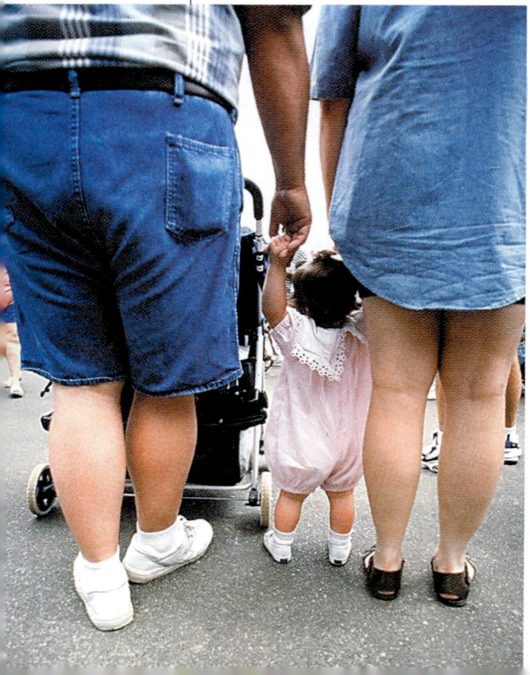

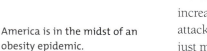

America is in the midst of an obesity epidemic.

Obesity

Obesity is associated with 5 of the 10 leading causes of death and disability in the United States: heart disease, some forms of cancer, type 2 diabetes, stroke, and high blood pressure (Shape Up America, 2000). The laws of thermodynamics dictate that an energy surplus is the cause of all obesity; if we take in more energy from eating than we expend through physical activity, then we will store energy (Melby & Hill, 1999). An energy surplus occurs when food consumption increases, energy expenditure decreases, or both. The best research available suggests that a low level of physical activity is a major factor contributing to the high prevalence of obesity in the United States. A sedentary lifestyle resulting in fewer kcal expended than consumed leads to the excess kcal being stored in the body as adipose tissue or fat. It must be understood that physical activity contributes to weight loss only if it creates a negative energy balance. A negative energy balance will not occur if we start eating more to

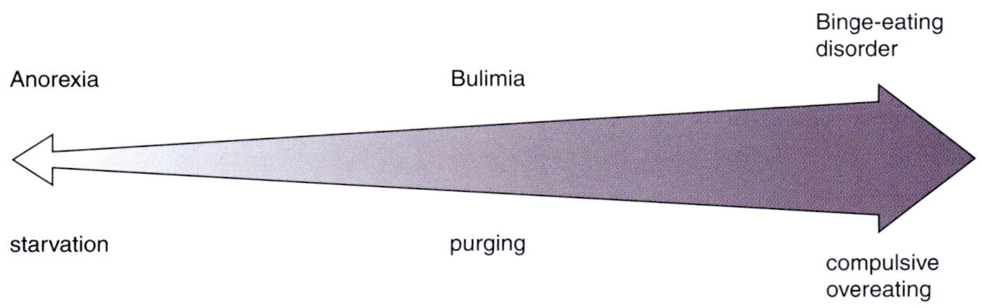

FIGURE 8.2

The Eating Disorder Continuum. Anorexia and bulimia are part of a continuum of disordered eating that also includes binge eating.

meet the energy demands brought on by physical activity and/or if physical activity levels decline (Melby & Hill, 1999). Chapter 9 presents the challenge of achieving and maintaining a healthy body composition in more detail.

Engage www.pahconnection.com 8.3

Explore www.pahconnection.com 8.2

Eating Disorders

In our society, metabolic health disorders are not only associated with excessive consumption of food but also with the underconsumption of food (Figure 8.2). Certain segments of our society are under constant pressure to be thin. This pressure may come from society, from families and peers, or it may be self-imposed. Individuals may practice nutritional behaviors that are unhealthy in an attempt to achieve thinness. Two eating disorders are associated with the drive to be thin. The first, **anorexia nervosa,** is a condition that occurs when an individual develops a severe misconception of their body image and perceives that they are too fat even if their body fat levels are dangerously low. Anorexic individuals starve themselves in an attempt to reduce their weight. This leads to malnutrition and the person's health will suffer correspondingly. Anorexia nervosa may be fatal.

Bulimia nervosa is another condition related to metabolic health. Bulimic individuals binge-eat and then force themselves to vomit, so the energy in the food will not be absorbed. Bulimia is an attempt to lose weight while continuing to eat more than the body requires. In addition to the likelihood of being malnourished, a bulimic individual may also sustain throat and mouth injury due to the vomiting of stomach acids, and eye injury from ruptured blood vessels.

Anorexia and bulimia are conditions that require professional counseling and treatment. If someone you know practices these behaviors, they should be referred to qualified practitioners for treatment. For more information on anorexia and bulimia, see Chapter 9 and the PAH website.

5. We are in the midst of an obesity epidemic in the United States.

AN OBESITY EPIDEMIC

The citizens of the United States are the fattest population on earth. Over the last 20 years, Americans have gotten progressively fatter (Figure 8.3). Current figures indicate that approximately 60 percent of the adult population is overfat, and one-third are obese. Perhaps even more alarming are the statistics that indicate that over one-quarter of adolescents are overfat. If these trends continue, we will see increasing health care costs, higher insurance rates, and a greater percentage

Anorexia nervosa Eating disorder in which individuals incorrectly believe they are overfat; resultant excessive dieting leads to health problems.

Bulimia nervosa Eating disorder in which individuals binge-eat and then force themselves to vomit.

FIGURE 8.3

Rise in Overweight in the United States.
The incidence of overweight has increased over the last three decades.

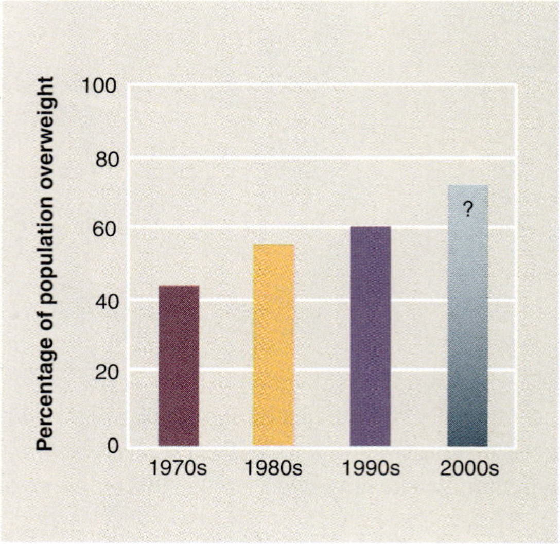

of our population dying from obesity-related diseases. Some people are quick to blame genetics for this increased rate of obesity. However, the increased rate of obesity has far outdistanced the rate at which genetics can change.

C. EVERETT KOOP'S *SHAPE UP AMERICA*

Americans are dying as an indirect result of having access to and eating too much food. The American public spends billions of dollars each year overeating, and then spends billions more attempting to lose the resultant excess weight (Wilmore, 1994). In an attempt to heighten awareness of the obesity epidemic gripping the United States, C. Everett Koop, former surgeon general of the United States, started a program called *Shape Up America*. The three primary objectives of *Shape Up America* are:

1. Promote a new understanding by Americans of the health importance of achieving and maintaining a healthy weight and increasing physical activity;
2. Inform Americans of the logical, proven ways to achieve a healthy body weight;
3. Increase cooperation among national and community organizations committed to advancing healthy weight and increased physical activity as major public health priorities.

Explore 8.3

The purpose of *Shape Up America* is to educate the public on the importance of the achievement and maintenance of a healthy body weight through the adoption of increased physical activity and healthy eating. The stated ultimate goal of *Shape Up America* is to stimulate behavior change by focusing on redefining weight management through encouraging increased physical activity and healthy eating for all Americans. *Shape Up America* promotes small lifestyle changes that provide immediate health dividends such as lower blood cholesterol levels, increased independence, greater productivity, and reduced demands for health care services.

PHYSICAL ACTIVITY AND HEALTH CONNECTION

Your metabolism is directly connected to your health. If your metabolic system is functioning properly, your body will be able to transfer, store, and utilize energy efficiently. However, if you have a metabolic disorder, you may develop several conditions that can lead to life-threatening situations. Physical activity is an important component of metabolic health. To prevent metabolic disorders such as obesity, you must make sure that your energy expenditure balances your energy consumption. Physical activity plays a major role in increasing your metabolic rate and total energy expenditure. Being active makes it easier to ensure that your energy expenditure keeps pace with your energy consumption.

CONCEPT CONNECTION

The transfer, storage, and utilization of energy in the human body is referred to as *metabolism*. Our bodies need energy to function. Proper metabolic function is important for good metabolic health.

1. **Your metabolism at rest is referred to as your resting metabolic rate, or RMR.** In all living bodies, there is a baseline rate of cellular activity required to keep the body functioning. All cellular activity requires the exchange of energy. The rate of energy exchange when the body is in a relaxed state is your resting metabolic rate.
2. **Physical activity has a profound effect on your metabolism.** Any increase in cellular function increases your metabolism. Physical activity increases your rate of cellular function while active and results in an elevated metabolic rate during the recovery period following physical activity. Performing physical activity that builds muscle mass will even impact your resting metabolic rate. Muscle is more active tissue than fat, even at rest. By increasing your muscle mass, you increase the percentage of metabolically active tissue in your body.
3. **Metabolic disorders may result in obesity, eating disorders, and several other conditions that can have a negative impact on your health.** Your body typically does an amazing task in balancing energy expenditure against energy consumption. However, in certain individuals, factors including lifestyle, genetics, and societal pressures may lead to the development of metabolic disorders. Metabolic disorders such as obesity, anorexia, and bulimia can have severe consequences. It is important to identify symptoms of metabolic disorders and seek treatment as soon as possible.
4. **We are in the midst of an obesity epidemic in the United States.** Figures indicate that close to two-thirds of the adult population is overfat and approximately one-third may be clinically obese. This alarming information demonstrates the need for action to reduce the negative consequences associated with obesity. Obesity is related to several serious medical conditions and results in increasing health care costs for all Americans. The best recommendation for reducing the incidence of obesity is to encourage physical activity and good nutritional habits.

TERMS

Metabolism, 176
First Law of Thermodynamics, 176
Substrates, 177
Thermic effect, 177
Resting metabolic rate, 177
Basal metabolic rate, 177
Sympathetic nervous system, 179
Set point, 179
Creatine phosphate, 180
Glycogen, 180
Lactic acid, 180
Pyruvic acid, 181
Hormones, 182
Hypertrophy, 183
Atrophy, 183
Overweight, 184
Underweight, 184
Overfat, 184
Underfat, 184
Epidemiological studies, 185
Anorexia nervosa, 187
Bulimia nervosa, 187

MAKING THE CONNECTION

Fred now understands why people develop different body builds. He plans to use the information he has learned about energy transfer, storage, and utilization to his advantage. Fred has decided to begin a program designed to lower his body fat and increase his muscle mass through healthy eating and increased physical activity. He thinks he will be able to stick with his new program because his goals are realistic and based on what he has learned about energy metabolism and health.

CRITICAL THINKING

1. Like Fred, we can find information a powerful tool in understanding ourselves. Identify 3 factors that affect metabolism. For each, describe how this factor may or may not affect your metabolism.
2. There are many different body builds. Looking at your parents, siblings, and friends, what are some possible explanations for the different body build each has.

REFERENCES

Butterfield, G., Kleiner, S., Lemon, P., & Stone, M. (1995). Roundtable: Methods of weight gain in athletes. *Sports Science Exchange, 6*(3). Gatorade Sports Science Institute.

Kaplan, J.P., & Dietz, W.H. (1999). Caloric imbalance and public health policy. *Journal of the American Medical Association 282*(16):1579–81.

Melby, C.L., Hill, J.O. (1999). Exercise, macronutrient balance, and body weight regulation. *Sports Science Exchange 12*(1). Gatorade Sports Science Institute.

Shape Up America. (2000). http://www.shapeup.org/

Wilmore, J.H. (May 1994). Exercise, obesity, and weight control. In Corbin, C., Pangrazi, R., eds., *The President's Council on Physical Fitness and Sports Research Digest,* Series 1, No. 6.

Activities & Assessments

NAME ____________ SECTION ____________ DATE ____________

8.1 Estimating and Changing Your Resting Metabolic Rate

Estimating Your Resting Metabolic Rate

Directions A simple calculation can provide a rough estimate of your resting metabolic rate (RMR). However, remember that your RMR can vary greatly from this estimate due to your fitness level, sex, size, body composition, pregnancy status, age, whether you have eaten recently, environmental temperature, drugs and medications, hormone secretion status, and health status.

TO CALCULATE RMR

1. Measure your body weight (BW) in kilograms. ____________
2. Measure your height (HT) in centimeters. ____________
3. Record your age in years. ____________
4. Insert those items into the appropriate equation below and perform the calculation. The result is your RMR in kcal.

Men RMR = 66.473 + 13.751 (BW) + 5.0033 (HT) − 6.755 (age)

Women RMR = 655.0955 + 9.463 (BW) + 1.8496 (HT) − 4.6756 (age)

This calculation is valid for adults 20–40 years of age.

SOURCE: J.A. Harris and F.G. Benedict. (1919). *A biometric study of basal metabolism in man* (Pub. No. 279). Washington, DC: Carnegie Institute

(continued)

8.1 Estimating and Changing Your Resting Metabolic Rate (cont.)

Changing Your Resting Metabolic Rate

Directions The most effective way to increase your resting metabolic rate (RMR) is through resistance training. By performing strength training exercises, you add muscle mass to your body. Muscle tissue is more active tissue than adipose tissue, so your metabolic rate will increase. In addition, larger people tend to have higher RMRs than smaller people.

TO SEE HOW A 10 LB ADDITION OF MUSCLE MASS WILL IMPACT YOUR RMR

1. Measure your body weight (BW) in kilograms (kg). __________
2. Add 4.5 kg to that number (BW+). __________
3. Measure your height (HT) in centimeters. __________
4. Record your age in years. __________
5. Insert those items into the appropriate equation below and perform the calculation.

The result is your new RMR. In fact, adding 10 lb of muscle will potentially bring about an even higher RMR.

Men RMR = 66.473 + 13.751 (BW+) = 5.0033 (HT) − 6.755 (age)

Women RMR = 655.0955 + 9.463 (BW+) + 1.8496 (HT) − 4.6756 (age)

SOURCE: This calculation is a modification of J.A. Harris and F.G. Benedict. (1919). *A biometric study of basal metabolism in man* (Pub. No. 279). Washington, DC: Carnegie Institute

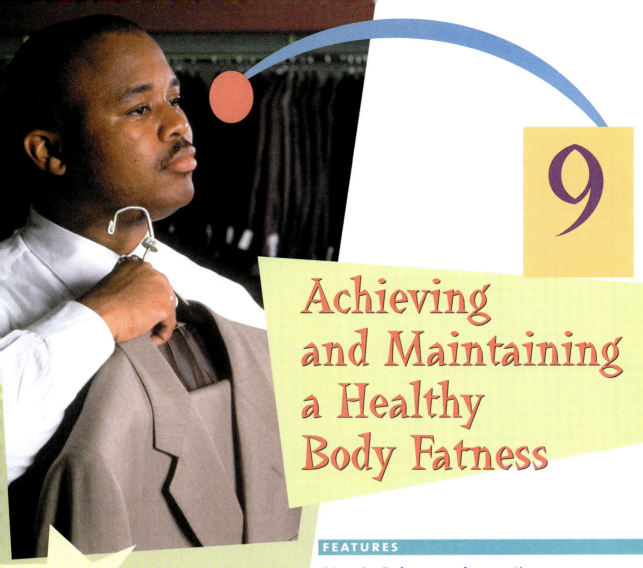

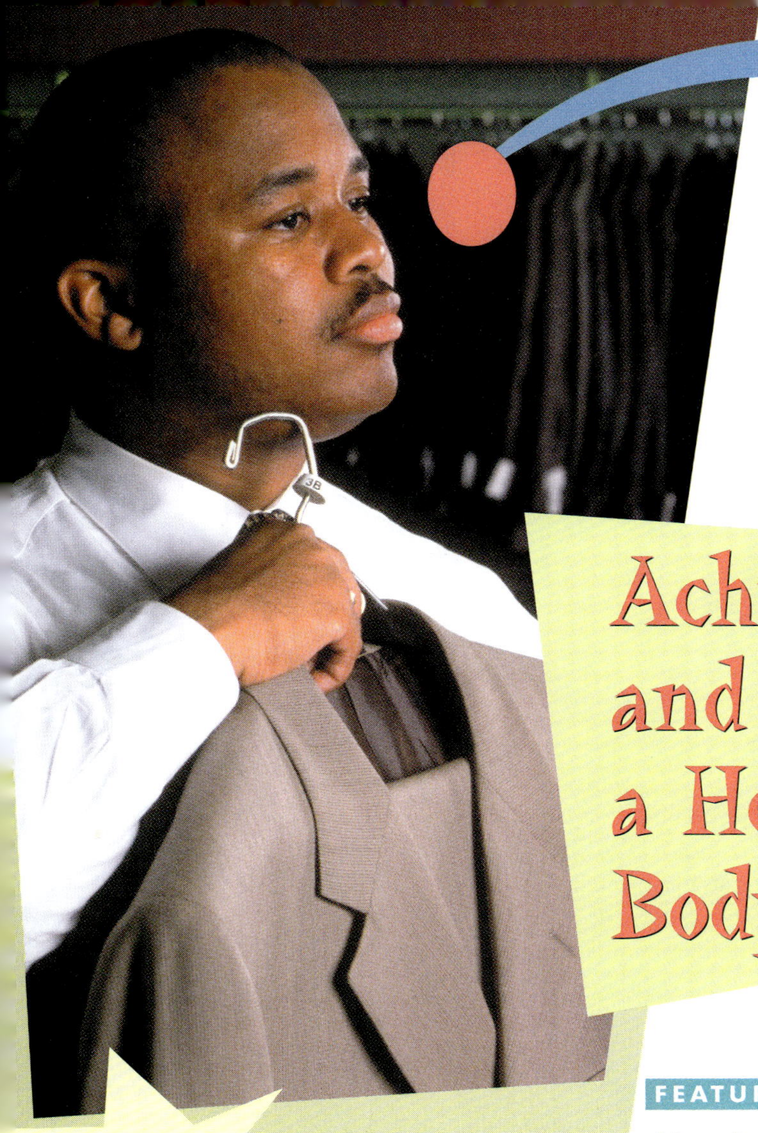

9 Achieving and Maintaining a Healthy Body Fatness

CONCEPT CONNECTION

1. An acceptable or optimal weight is one that leaves us free from disease, is realistic, and is attained and maintained through physical activity and a healthy diet.
2. Excess body fat is associated with a number of morbid conditions.
3. Your body requires some body fat for healthy functioning.
4. Obesity is influenced by our genetics (nature) and our environment (nurture).
5. Health risk related to obesity can be determined in a number of ways.
6. Regular physical activity and a healthy nutritious diet are the most important components to fat loss and control.
7. Behavioral modification strategies should be included in a personal fat loss program.
8. A negative sign of dissatisfaction with body weight is the development of eating disorders.

FEATURES

E-Learning Tools: www.pahconnection.com

Engage www.pahconnection.com

9.1 Determining your Body Mass Index (BMI)
9.2 Weight wellness profile
9.3 Determining your readiness to lose fat
9.4 7-day food record
9.5 Average daily caloric and nutrient intake
9.6 Daily energy expenditure
9.7 Eating style questionnaire
9.8 Testing your body image perception

Experience www.pahconnection.com

9.1 Underwater weighing
9.2 Bioelectrical impedance analysis

Explore www.pahconnection.com

9.1 The National Heart, Lung, and Blood Institute (NHLBI) Obesity Education Initiative (OEI)
9.2 Shape up America!
9.3 Weight loss and obesity on the Internet
9.4 National Association of Anorexia Nervosa and Associated Disorders

Activities & Assessments

9.1 Estimating healthy body fatness
9.2 Assessing your body image

WHAT'S THE CONNECTION?

Melinda is a freshman in college; she is 5'6" tall and weighs about 130 pounds. Previously, when Melinda was happy, she looked in the mirror and thought "Hey, I am not that bad!" However, if Melinda was in a bad mood, she would think "I am so fat!" and get mad at herself. Recently, things are not going well in Melinda's life and, when she looks in the mirror, she often sees herself as fat. It seems to her that the weight is piling on and she cannot stop it. To Melinda, every part of her body looks bigger—her legs, her arms, her face—and she hates it. Melinda thinks "I just want to be thin. I never really noticed how fat I was until yesterday when I looked in the mirror." Melinda is not sure what to do. "I don't eat that much. Really I eat only a little, and I'm not sure why I even eat that." Melinda is thinking about stopping eating altogether so she can lose all this weight.

INTRODUCTION

1. An acceptable or optimal weight is one that leaves us free from disease, is realistic, and is attained and maintained through physical activity and a healthy diet.

Most of us do not ask ourselves "What is my ideal body fatness?" But many of us ask "What is my ideal body weight?" We all believe that there is an ideal weight for our body based on our height, structure, and sex. But what criteria do we use to define our ideal weight? Do we base our weight on reducing the burden of a number of preventable physical morbidities or illnesses? Do we base our weight on what our culture considers attractive and sexually desirable—even if it unrealistic? Do we base our weight on what best contributes to enhancing our athletic performance?

Health professionals use the term **healthy weight** to describe a weight that protects you from developing a number of serious chronic diseases (Figure 9.1). Healthy weight is based on the principle that your body composition needs to include an optimal amount of body fat—not too little and not too much. The *Dietary Guidelines for Americans* goal "Aim for a healthy weight" encourages evaluating your body weight in three ways—each with the objective of reducing illness from being overfat. The first recommended technique is using a "weight-corrected-for height" measure that is related to your body mass and structure, termed your **body mass index (BMI).** As you will learn later, BMI is easy to calculate and a good estimator of body fat in assessing health risk for the average adult. A second method focuses on regional fat distribution and encourages you to measure your waist circumference. Waist circumference addresses "abdom-

Healthy Weight Describes a weight that protects you from disease and supports wellness; based on the principle that your body composition avoid fatness.

Body Mass Index (BMI) An estimate of body fatness that uses a "weight-corrected-for height" calculation related to body mass and structure.

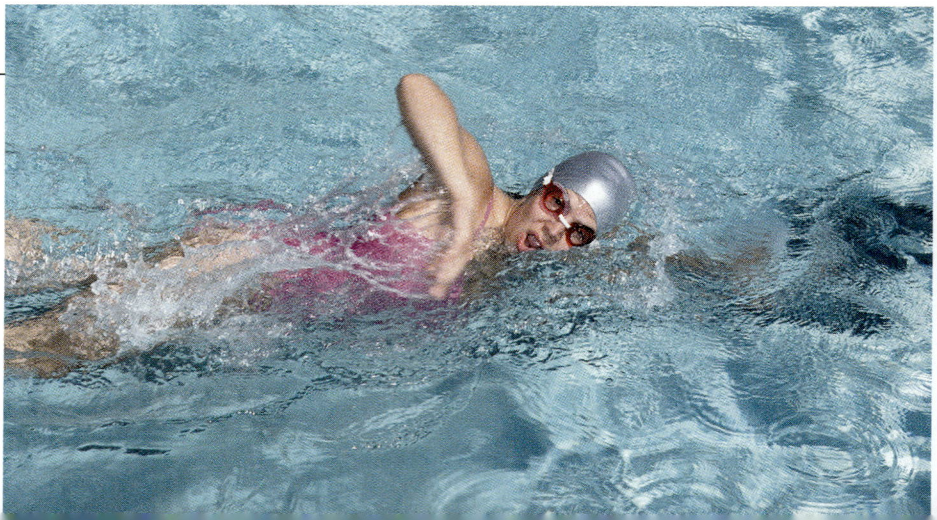

Ideal body composition may vary across different types of physical activity.

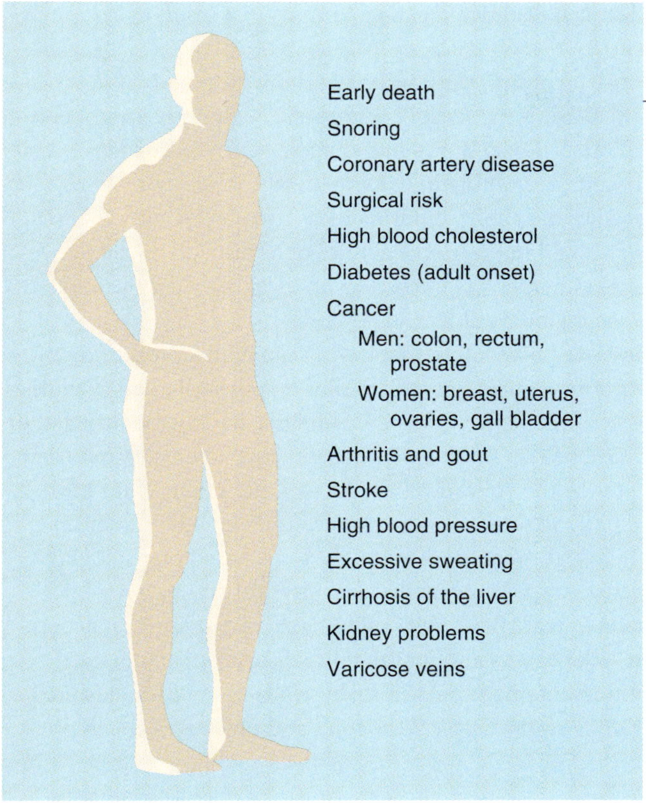

Early death
Snoring
Coronary artery disease
Surgical risk
High blood cholesterol
Diabetes (adult onset)
Cancer
Men: colon, rectum, prostate
Women: breast, uterus, ovaries, gall bladder
Arthritis and gout
Stroke
High blood pressure
Excessive sweating
Cirrhosis of the liver
Kidney problems
Varicose veins

FIGURE 9.1

Health Problems Arising from Obesity.
Overweight people have a greater likelihood of developing certain health problems than do people of normal weight.

inal obesity," which increases the risk for developing a number of serious chronic diseases. Finally, you are encouraged to evaluate other risk factors related to body fat composition. The greater the number of risk factors, the more you are likely to benefit your health by losing fat.

Another group of people may believe a body composition where extra body weight is in the form of muscle may be an advantage for a chosen recreational or athletic activity in which they participate. For example, increased strength may allow them to perform at higher levels in football, basketball, or weight lifting, to name a few (Chapter 11). Therefore, these individuals may attempt to increase their amount of lean-tissue body mass in the hope of elevating their level of enjoyment from performing such activities. They too are altering their body composition. A number of techniques (skinfold, underwater weighing) are available in fitness centers and exercise physiology laboratories to measure your body composition.

Finally, an increasing number of Americans attempt to achieve an unrealistic weight and shape based on the fashion industry's "ideal" body. This "ideal" standard is one of extreme thinness for females and exaggerated muscularity for males. These so-called ideals have been created by the fashion and advertising industries to sell products. For people who try to live up to this standard of "perfection," the defining characteristic for ideal weight and size is *perceived body image*. People should not attempt to base their weight or shape on our society's glamour approach.

Tools to assess the "ideal" body generally use silhouettes or models' pictures to measure the difference between the current "I look like this" and the desired "I'd like to look like this." Researchers have shown that, the wider the gap between these two body satisfaction measures (especially in women), the greater the risk of psychological and physiological problems. We will discuss how this "dissatisfaction gap" caused by a wholesale

The "ideal" body promoted by the fashion industry may influence distorted images in individuals, particularly women.

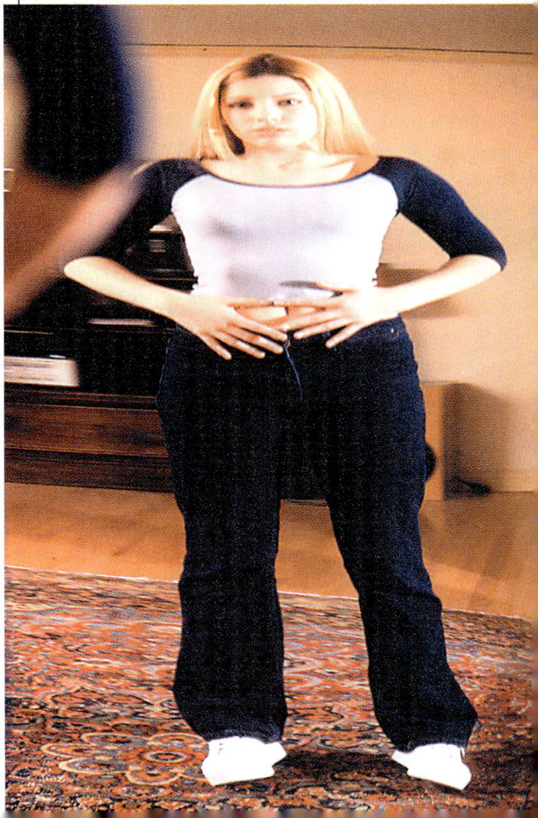

pursuit of aesthetic "ideals" leads to disordered eating patterns that result in extremely serious conditions.

We can begin to see that instead of the question "What is my ideal body weight?" a preferable focus should be on "What is my ideal body fatness?" Our body weight consists of fat, muscle, bone, and other tissue. But in this chapter our main concern is with the proportion of body fat, because accumulating too much fat (obesity) or having too little fat (malnutrition) can lead to metabolic abnormalities (Chapter 8) and other disease conditions. However, we should not neglect the roles of healthy diet (Chapter 7), bone (Chapter 10), and muscle (Chapter 11) in shaping an ideal body composition, because each contributes to weight and health.

Returning to our focus on fatness, we know that having too high a proportion of body weight as fat may contribute to increased risk of illness (physical and psychological) as well as to limitations on athletic performance. Similarly, having too little fat, or being too thin, can also increase risk of illness (physical and psychological) and limit athletic performance. How you define your ideal weight—or, preferably, your ideal body composition related to body fatness—is critical, because it greatly influences how you decide to manage it. Weight management ought to be based on achieving and maintaining the weight that supports a high level of physical and psychological health at each stage of a person's life (Dalton 1997). This ideal of pursuing an **acceptable** and/or **optimal weight**—defined as a weight that leaves us free from disease, is realistic, and is attained and maintained through a physically active lifestyle and healthy diet—is consistent with *Healthy People 2010* goals and objectives (*Healthy People 2010*, 2000).

This chapter looks at obesity in terms of health risk, causes of obesity, evaluating your body composition (with a special emphasis on the amount of body fat relative to your weight), and the attainment and maintenance of healthy body fatness. The principles and recommendations provided in this chapter apply to the overfat individual who wants to shed excess body fat so as to decrease his risk of disease, as well as to the person with a healthy level of body fatness who wants to maintain the level for her optimal psychological and physical function.

AMERICA'S NUMBER 1 HEALTH CONCERN

2. Excess body fat is associated with a number of morbid conditions.

Being overweight or obese is the most common chronic health concern in America. More than half (55%) of the U.S. adult population is overweight. Within this overweight population, more than 40 percent, or nearly 1 in every 4 Americans, is classified as obese (Flegal et al., 1998). Moreover, the condition of obesity is worsening in the United States. Since 1980, the number of U.S. adults who are obese has risen more than 50 percent, from 14.5 to 22.5 percent. Presently, 1 in 5 adult males and 1 in 4 adult females are now obese (Table 9.1).

Overweight and **obesity** significantly increase a person's risk for developing a number of diseases, including seriously morbid conditions like high blood pressure, dyslipidemia (high levels of fat in the blood), diabetes mellitus, and osteoarthritis (Figure 9.1). These morbid conditions usually lead to serious illness and premature death. Many overweight and obese people do not know they are at greater risk for serious illness and are cutting their lives short. In fact, obesity is the second leading cause of death in the United States, killing an estimated 300,000 Americans annually (Allison et al., 1999).

Acceptable or optimal weight A weight that supports health, is realistic, and promotes a physically active life.

Overweight Excess amount of body weight, including both fat and fat-free mass, in relationship to a standard or "ideal" weight for height.

Obesity Condition of excess body fat relative to body composition; increases risk for developing certain diseases.

TABLE 9.1 Combined Prevalence of Overweight and Obesity (BMI ±25.0 kg/m²) among Adults Age 20 to 80+ Years,by Gender, Race/Ethnicity, and Age: United States, 1960–1994.

GENDER, RACE/ETHNICITY, AGE 20 YEARS AND OLDER, AGE ADJUSTED	NHES I 1960–62 (AGE 20–74)	NHANES I 1971–74 (AGE 20–74)	NHANES II 1976–80 (AGE 20–74)	NHANES 1982–84 (AGE 20–74)	NHANES III 1988–94 (AGE ≥20)
Both Sexes	43.3	46.1	46.0		54.9
Men	48.2	52.9	51.4		59.4
Women	38.7	39.7	40.8		50.7
White men	48.8	53.7	52.3		61.0
White women	36.1	37.6	38.4		49.2
Black men	43.1	48.9	49.0		56.5
Black women	57.0	57.6	61.0		65.8
White, non-Hispanic men			52.0		60.6
White, non-Hispanic women			37.6		47.4
Black, non-Hispanic men			48.9		56.7
Black, non-Hispanic women			60.6		66.0
Mexican-American men				59.7	63.9
Mexican-American women				60.1	65.9
Age and gender-specific categories:					
Men					
20–29	39.9	38.6	37.0		43.1
30–39	49.6	58.1	52.6		58.1
40–49	53.6	63.6	60.3		65.5
50–59	54.1	58.4	60.8		73.0
60–69	52.9	55.6	57.4		70.3
70–79	36.0	52.7*	53.3*		63.1
80+	N/A**	N/A**	N/A**		50.6
Women					
20–29	17.0	23.2	25.0		33.1
30–39	32.8	35.0	36.8		47.0
40–49	42.3	44.6	44.4		52.7
50–59	55.0	52.2	52.8		64.4
60–69	63.1	56.2	56.5		64.0
70–79	57.4	55.9*	58.2*		57.9
80+	N/A**	N/A**	N/A**		50.1

* Prevalence for age 70 to 74 years
** Not available

SOURCE: National Heart, Lung, and Blood Institute (NHLBI). (1998). *Obesity education initiative expert panel clinical guidelines on the identification, evaluation, and treatment of overweight and obesity in adults.* (NIH Pub. No. 98-4083). Washington, DC: NHLBI.

3. Your body requires some body fat for healthy functioning.

Essential body fat Fat that is required for normal healthy functioning.

Storage fat Body fat, above essential levels, that accumulates in adipose tissue.

physical activity and health connection

FIGURE 9.2

Body Fatness of a Typical Man and Woman.

SOURCE: Data compiled from Nutrition for physical fitness and athletic performance for adults—Position of ADA and the Canadian Dietetic Association. (1993). *Journal of the American Dietetic Association* 93:691–697.

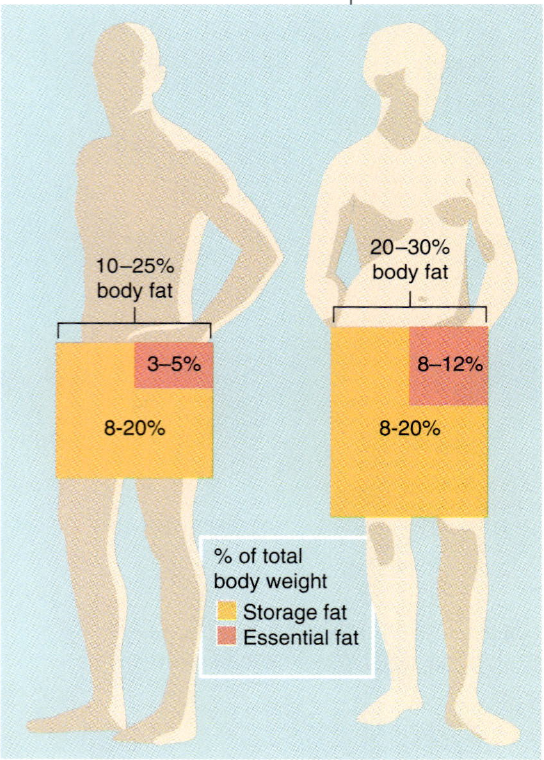

Health and Body Fat

How much fat is too fat? The composition of fat can range between 2 and 70 percent of body weight. Determining cutoff points for acceptable body percentages requires first considering **essential body fat** and **storage fat** allowances. *Essential body fat* is required for normal healthy functioning. Fat is necessary for transporting vitamins and regulation of various body processes (Chapter 7). In addition, females require additional fat for "sex-specific" functions associated with reproduction. Essential fat is stored in a number of major organs and in tissue, including the heart, lungs, liver, bone, muscle, liver, and central nervous system. Authorities agree that essential fat should compose 3 to 5 percent of the total body weight for men and 8 to 12 percent of total body weight for women (Going & Davis, 1998).

Storage fat is body fat above essential fat levels that accumulates in adipose tissue (fat cells). Some storage fat is advised for both males and females. Storage fat is needed for protection of organs and insulation of the body (Chapter 7). This type of fat is an excellent source of energy, providing 3500 calories in every pound of adipose tissue. Storage fat accumulates when energy intake (calories consumed) exceeds energy expenditure. Desirable storage levels are estimated to be between 8 and 20 percent of total body weight.

Summing the contributions of essential fat and storage fat supplies us with desirable ranges for body fat percentages: for men, between 10 and 25 percent; for women, 20 to 30 percent. An ideal body fat percentage is one that meets your body's fundamental energy needs but does not create health risks. Health problems have been found to develop most often when body fat percentage exceeds 25 percent in males and 30 percent in females (Figure 9.2). *Obesity* is the term used to define this excessive accumulation of body fat that places your health at risk. Morbid or malignant obesity is used to define a condition when body fat percentage exceeds 50 percent. The major health risks of obesity, as well as the conditions associated with obesity, become worse with increasing overfatness. Fortunately, even minor fat reduction at all levels of obesity reduces risk and improves the conditions associated with obesity.

Storage Fat and Energy Balance

The laws of thermodynamics (Chapter 8) govern the energy processes in the human body. The basic mechanism for obesity is an imbalance in the energy equation (Figure 9.3). If people consume less energy in calories from food than they expend in metabolic processes, then they are in negative energy balance and will lose weight. If people consume a higher caloric intake from food than they expend in metabolic processes, they are in positive energy balance and will gain weight. It is only when the amount of energy consumed as food exceeds the daily energy requirements that excess energy in the form of calories is stored as fat in the adipose cells.

We have revisited the energy balance equation and the factors that influence a positive energy balance or weight gain: diet, metabolic factors, and physical activity. As you learned in Chapter 8, each factor interacts with the other to influence the energy balance equation. Furthermore, both genetics (nature) and environment (nurture) influence each factor.

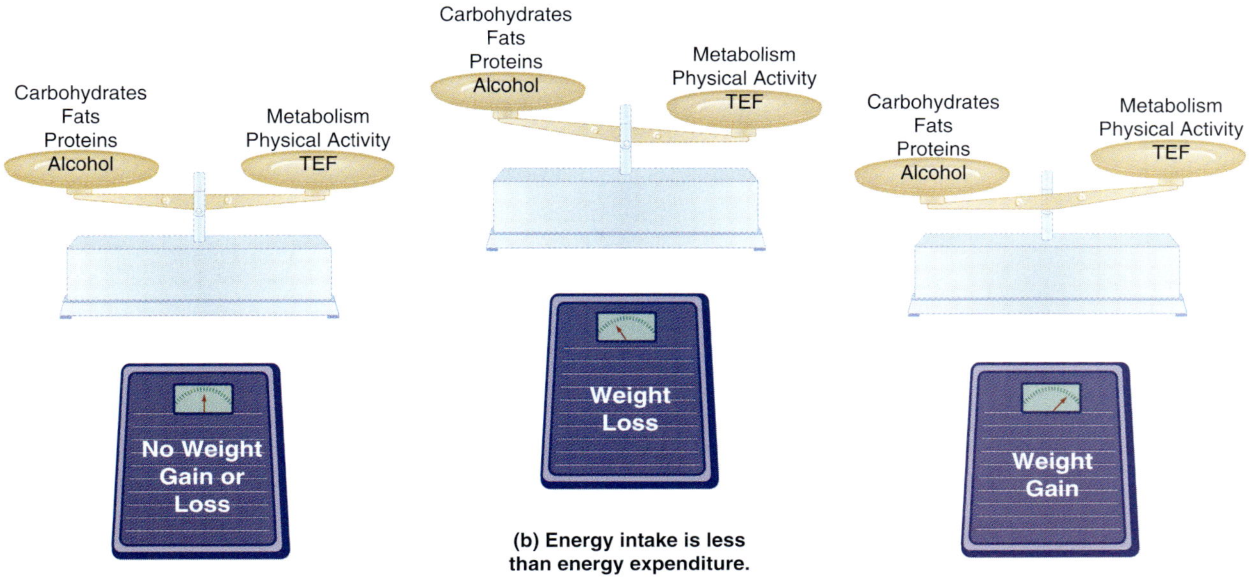

(a) Energy is in balance.

(b) Energy intake is less than energy expenditure.

(c) Energy intake exceeds energy expenditure.

FIGURE 9.3

Energy Balance Equation. (a) When energy expenditure equals energy intake, the body maintains its weight. (b) When energy expenditure is greater than energy intake, the body loses weight. (c) When energy expenditure is less than energy intake, the body gains weight.

CAUSES OF OBESITY

What is becoming increasingly difficult for researchers to explain is why this imbalance in the energy balance equation occurs. Until recently, the major causes of obesity were thought to be behavioral in nature—that is, due to excessive caloric intake and deficient energy expenditure (people eating too much and exercising too little). This idea led many health professionals and, thus, the public to believe that excess weight reflects a lack of willpower on the part of the obese. However, recent research provides evidence that physiological, biochemical, and genetic factors also affect obesity. We will now look at the various factors that may contribute to a positive energy balance related to fat in the body.

4. Obesity is influenced by our genetics (nature) and our environment (nurture).

Genetic, Physiological, and Biochemical Factors

The research related to genetic, physiological, and biochemical factors that contribute to fat accumulation demonstrates that obesity is not a simple problem of willpower, as was sometimes charged in the past, but a complex disorder of appetite regulation and energy metabolism. This research aids in helping us recognize that our body fatness is not totally under our voluntary control.

Recent research documents that body fat is controlled genetically. Bouchard (1994) estimates that genetics accounts for 25 to 40 percent of the factors regulating body weight. Genetic factors, including influences on fat metabolism and the regulation of certain hormones, may affect appetite and contribute to obesity. Inherited attributes include the way fat is distributed, metabolic rates, and changes in energy response to overeating.

Although genetic discoveries related to obesity, made possible by recent technological advances, are particularly promising for a better understanding of obesity, they still signal only a tendency for obesity or a predisposition for becoming obese. Our genes may permit us to become obese, but our environment determines if we actually do become obese. In other words, while recognizing that genetic differences may predispose an individual toward obesity, we must understand that these differences can be overcome by environmental factors such as being physically active and eating right. Remember that the prevalence of obesity has dramatically increased over the past three decades and our genes have not changed appreciably within that time. Most cases of obesity occur now in people with normal physiology who live in a sociocultural environment characterized by mechanization, sedentary lifestyles, and ready access to abundant food. Concurrent with the increase in obesity, the proportion of overweight adults who report using exercise and diet to lose weight has declined (*Healthy People Review,* 1998–99).

Interest in physiological factors related to obesity focus on the concept of the set point theory. The set point theory proposes that a regulatory system exists in the human body that is designed to maintain body weight at some fixed level. Similar to other regulated physiological variables in the body (blood glucose, body temperature) that are maintained within certain limits, the body seeks to protect against pressures to be too heavy or too thin. The level of the body's fat stores is thought to be governed by a mechanism in the brain called the **adipostat.** The adipostat establishes a set point for a fixed amount of body fat just as a thermostat regulates heat according to a preset temperature. The brain maintains this set point by regulating the expenditure or storage of energy until fat stores meet the level determined by the adipostat. A set point above the ideal healthy weight presents a difficult struggle for the obese individual. Unknown to the person who has been diligently dieting, the brain is busily undermining the efforts by working to restore weight to the set point. The adipostat may do this by activating the sensation for hunger, so that more calories are consumed, or by slowing the metabolism.

physical activity and health connection

Adipostat Brain mechanism that establishes a set point for a fixed amount of body fat.

Recently, the belief regarding where the set point originates has changed. Instead of a genetic determination, set point is now believed to be under control of more external factors like lifestyle and thus lends itself to be altered (Bennett, 1995). The external factor that can lower the set point more than any other is regular physical activity. The concept of a set point is theoretical, but it is appealing to researchers because it may aid in a search for factors that regulate body weight.

Our eating patterns are regulated by feeding and satiety centers located in the hypothalamus and pituitary glands of the brain that respond to signals indicating high fat stores and hunger (Figure 9.4). Substances critical to this process include glucose (sugar),

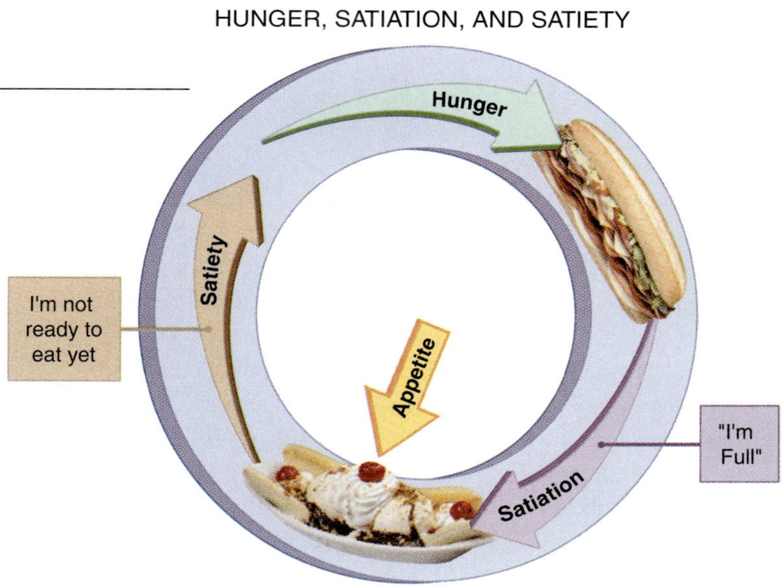

FIGURE 9.4

Hunger, Satiation, and Satiety. Hunger, satiation, and satiety are internal cues that influence eating behavior.

insulin, and leptin. Leptin has many functions that are of great interest in the study of obesity. This hormone is released by fat cells. Rising levels appear to signal the hypothalamus to suppress appetite and falling levels to stimulate appetite. Leptin is made in fat cells by a gene called the *ob* gene.

The findings just presented seem to indicate that weight and fat distribution are strongly influenced by genetic and biological factors. However, the increase in the prevalence of obesity in the past couple of decades cannot be explained by changes in our genetics and biology. Many environmental and lifestyle influences have contributed to our obesity epidemic. In other words, our genetics and biology permit us to become obese, but our environment enables us to become obese.

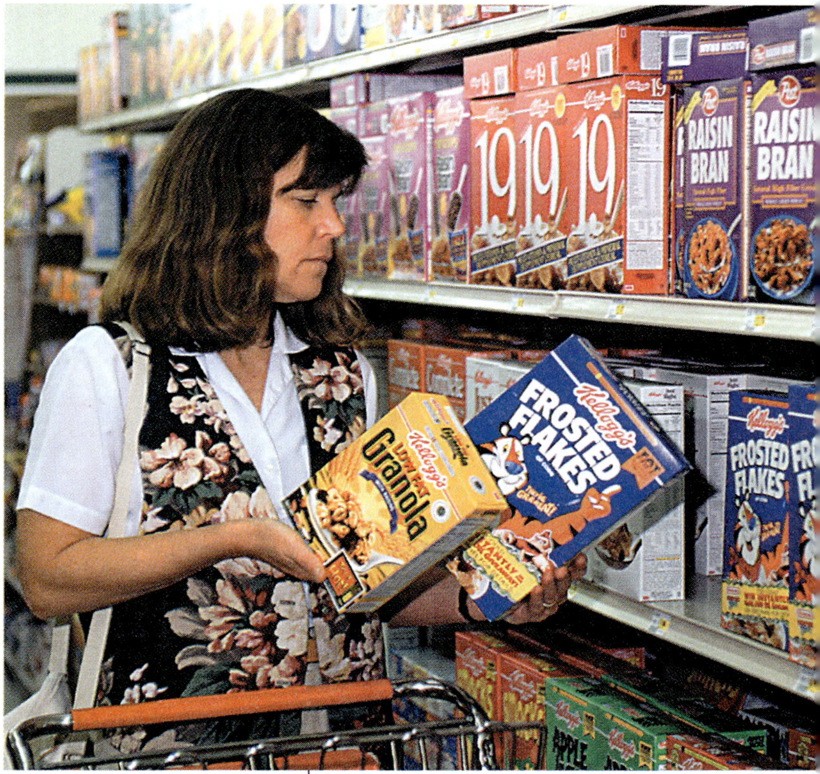

Reading food labels to compare calorie content is important to understanding your overall caloric intake.

Dietary Factors

The Centers for Science in the Public Interest (CSPI) have reported that Americans are eating between 100 and 300 calories more per day than we were in the 1970s (Liebman, 1996). Foods that are high in fat and calories and low in nutrients are common in our daily diets (Chapter 7). Food manufacturers know how taste, smell, and texture increase the human appetite and engineer food accordingly (Sclafani, 1996). Increased availability of convenience foods, changes in food preparation, and eating out more often are additional factors that contribute to obesity among Americans (Harnack, 2000). These factors support a 15 percent increase in per capita per day availability of food energy since 1970. This upward shift in energy intake is consistent with trends of obesity in America. Decreasing calorie intake to match our drastically reduced energy expenditure from our sedentary lifestyles is a difficult challenge.

physical activity and health connection

Physical Inactivity

Despite a number of public health campaigns that have encouraged people to become more physically active in the past decade, the majority of people lead sedentary lives. Systematic survey trend data collected over the last two decades regularly indicate that about 60 percent of U.S. adults report not engaging in regular physical activity and about 25 percent report not participating in physical activity at all (USDHHS, 1996). In addition, it was reported that only 8 percent of adults aged 18 to 65 exercise regularly. Thus, the available evidence suggests that reduced physical activity related to energy expenditure is a potentially important contributor to obesity.

Everyone who has a sedentary lifestyle is at risk for obesity. A sedentary lifestyle and obesity play against each other in a no-win game; that is, lack of physical activity contributes to fat gain and fat gain makes it more difficult to be physically active. The tendency in America is toward an unhealthy weight gain with age. As you age, bone and muscle mass tend to decrease. A sedentary lifestyle accelerates the problem of bone and muscle loss. All physical activity involves muscular movement that requires the expenditure of calories and contributes to lean-tissue maintenance. In other words, body fatness is not only responsible for general weight gain in sedentary individuals but also for making up more of the lean weight they may have once had.

To summarize, the increased prevalence of obesity in America has been largely attributed to an increased consumption of energy-dense food, which is both flavorful and pleasurable, and a decreased level of caloric expenditure due to a sedentary lifestyle (PiSunyar, 1994). In other words, a major reason for obesity in America is that Americans are increasingly having trouble controlling their appetite and being physically active. This overeating and lack of physical activity leads to an unbalancing of the energy equation. Both inherited and lifestyle factors contribute to appetite and physical inactivity (Weinsier et al., 1998). However, the tendency for obesity and its extent (whether inherited or due to lifestyle) can be significantly influenced by physical activity and diet.

MEASURING OBESITY AND HEALTH RISK

Engage www.panconnection.com 9.1

5. Health risk related to obesity can be determined in a number of ways.

Recognized since 1985 as a chronic disease, obesity is the second leading cause of preventable death in the United States, exceeded only by cigarette smoking. Overweight and obesity affects more than half of all U.S. adults and the prevalence is increasing (Must et al., 1999). Currently, several measures are used to determine a person's obesity status and potential health risk. A complete evaluation includes assessments of height and weight, fat distribution and composition, and the presence or absence of other health problems and risk factors. Each appraisal provides unique information that can be used to improve health status. For everyone, the higher the cumulative risk status, the greater the risk to health. The obesity health risk gradient ranges from minimal, to low, to moderate, to high, to very high, to extremely high.

Weight-Corrected-For-Height Measure

An increase in death from all causes is associated with higher body weight (Lew & Garfinkel, 1979). In studies on large groups of people, the body mass index (BMI) is the approved measure of excess weight to estimate relative risk of disease because BMI relates highly with both morbidity (disease) and mortality (death). BMI is a "weight-corrected-for-height measure" and is based on the concept that most overweight people are also obese (IOM, 1995). BMI is a direct calculation based on the concept that a person's weight should be proportional to height and is not gender specific.

Activities & Assessments 9.1

Explore www.panconnection.com 9.1

BMI is calculated manually by dividing body weight in kilograms (W) by height measured in meters squared (H^2):

$$BMI = W/H^2$$

or by using the chart shown in Figure 9.5. Height should be measured without shoes and weight obtained wearing only undergarments.

The National Heart, Lung, and Blood Institute (NHLBI) identifies overweight as a BMI of 25–29.9 kg/m^2, obesity as a BMI of 30 kg/m^2, and extreme obesity as a BMI of 40 or greater (NHLBI, 1998) (Table 9.2). This classification system relates BMI to the risk of disease.

Figure 9.6 documents the increased risk for serious disease conditions in women and men. The higher one's BMI, the greater the health risk. The lowest morbidity and mortality rates for both sexes occur in persons with a BMI of 22–25 kg/m^2. An exceptionally low BMI can also be indicative of a health concern, such as an eating disorder.

If an individual's BMI is less than 19, it may be wise for the person to be screened by a physician.

The advantages of using BMI to measure risk from being overweight is that it is simple, quick, inexpensive, and provides a good estimate of body fat for most adults. Because of these benefits, it is the method used for measuring obesity in large populations—but it does have important limitations. First, BMI should not be the sole measure used in estimating overweight and obesity related to one's health risk. Other important independent assessments, such as regional fat distribution and obesity related disease contribute to predicting health risk. Second, BMI should not be used with heavily muscled athletes, pregnant or lactating women, children, or inactive seniors. People who are muscular or pregnant may classify as "overweight" when they are actually healthy and fit. On the other hand, sedentary seniors may be classified in a "healthy weight" category according to their BMI even though they may have lost valuable muscle mass from being inactive. To determine whether an individual is obese from simply being overweight because of increased muscle mass, or being underweight because of a lack of muscle tissue, requires specific techniques for quantifying fat mass and fat-free mass. These techniques will be described following elaboration of regional fat distribution and other risk factors related to obesity.

FIGURE 9.5

Body Mass Index (BMI). BMI measures weight in relation to height.

SOURCE: Report of the Dietary Guidelines Advisory Committee on the Dietary Guidelines for Americans. (2000).

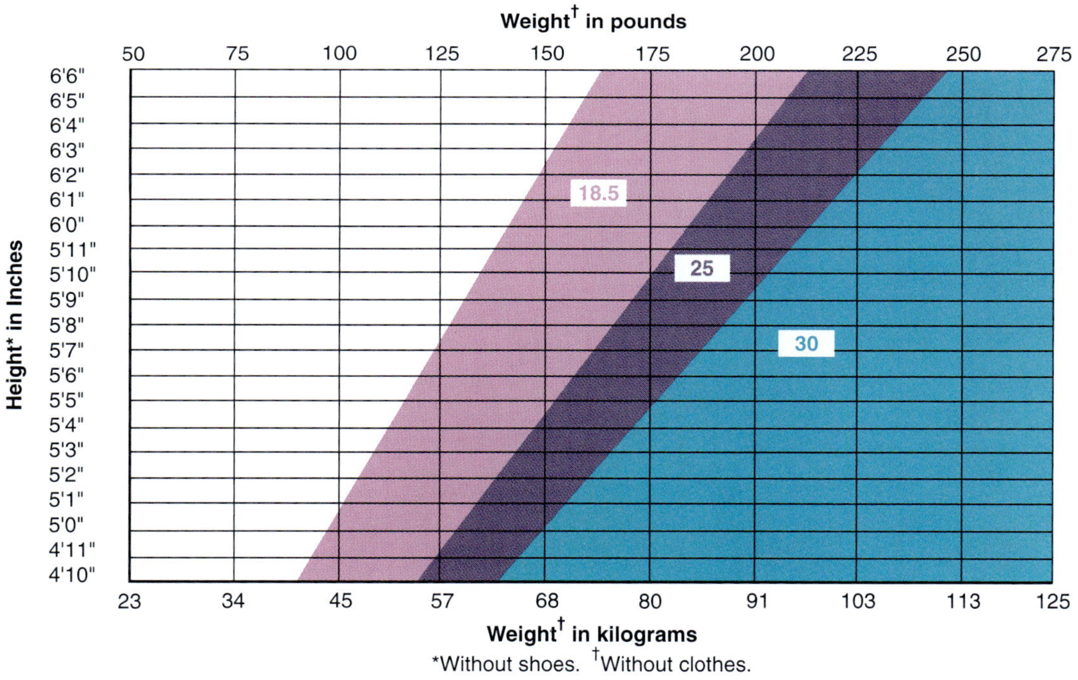

Directions: Find your weight on the bottom of the graph. Go straight up from that point until you come to the line that matches your height. Then look to find your weight group.

- **Healthy weight** BMI from 18.5 up to 25 indicates a healthy weight.
- **Overweight** BMI from 25 up to 30 indicates overweight.
- **Obese** BMI 30 or higher indicates obesity.

TABLE 9.2 **Classification of Overweight and Obesity by BMI, Waist Circumference, and Associated Disease Risk***

	BMI (KG/M²)	OBESITY CLASS	DISEASE RISK* (RELATIVE TO NORMAL WEIGHT AND WAIST CIRCUMFERENCE) MEN ≤40 IN (≤102 CM) WOMEN ≤35 IN (≤88 CM)	>40 IN (>102 CM) >35 IN (>88 CM)
Both sexes	43.3	46.1	46.0	54.9
Men	48.2	52.9	51.4	59.4
Women	38.7	39.7	40.8	50.7
White men	48.8	53.7	52.3	61.0
Underweight	< 18.5		—	—
Normal†	18.5 –24.9		—	—
Overweight	25.0–29.9		Increased	High
Obesity	30.0–34.9	I	High	Very high
	35.0–39.9	II	Very high	Very high
Extreme obesity	≥ 40	III	Extremely high	Extremely high

* Disease risk for type 2 diabetes mellitus, hypertension, and CVD.

Increased waist circumference can also be a marker for increased risk even in persons of normal weight.

SOURCE: National Heart, Lung, and Blood Institute (NHLBI). (1998). *Obesity education initiative expert panel clinical guidelines on the identification, evaluation, and treatment of overweight and obesity in adults.* (NIH Pub. No. 98-4083, p. 17). Washington, DC: NHLBI.

FIGURE 9.6

BMI and Mortality.
People with a very low or high BMI have a higher relative mortality rate.

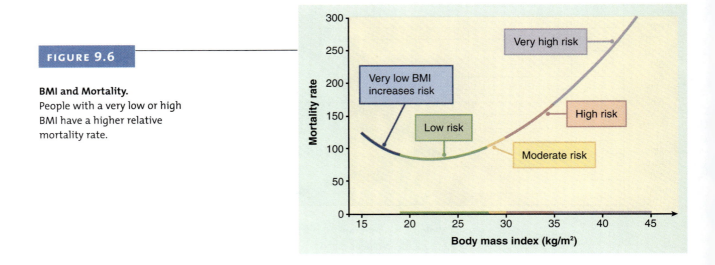

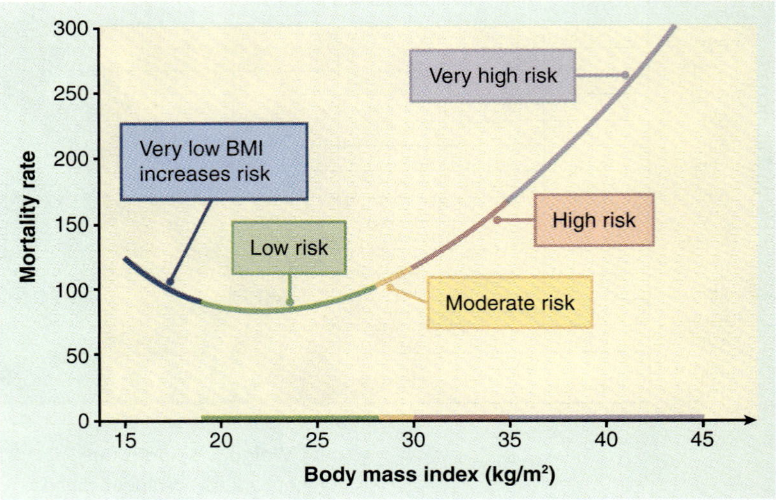

Regional Distribution of Fat

Activities & Assessments 9.1

Where we store fat greatly affects obesity-related health risks (Chapter 8). Fat located in the abdominal area is related to greater risk of heart disease, high blood pressure, and type 2 diabetes than fat located in any other region. Waist circumference provides the most practical means of assessing abdominal fat. To assess waist circumference, locate the upper hip and place a measuring tape in a horizontal plane around the waist. The measurement should be made with the abdominal muscles relaxed (not pulled in). Men who have waist circumferences greater than 40 inches and women who have waist circumferences greater than 35 inches are at higher risk.

Although waist circumference and BMI are interrelated, the waist circumference contributes to the risk factors additionally and independently. Table 9.2 integrates both BMI and waist circumference in overweight and obesity classification, along with an index of disease risk. In mild-to-moderate obesity BMI classifications (25.0–29.9 and 30.0–34.9), the inclusion of waist circumference increases disease risk. In fact, it has been shown that increases or decreases in waist circumference measures, even in the absence of BMI changes, are important predictors of cardiovascular risk factors (Lemieux et al., 1996).

Presence of Other Risk Factors or Health Problems

The preferred course of action is to *prevent obesity from occurring* rather than treating it after the fact. Research has shown that as Americans age we gain a disproportionate amount of weight and fat. However, just because the average value of body fat increases with age, this should not dictate that people expect to get fatter as they go through life. Events that predispose a person to becoming obese include the following: being physically inactive, binge eating, seeing a recent gain of 10 pounds or more, having a family history of obesity, recently quitting smoking, recently giving birth, and nearing menopause (Table 9.3). Lower levels of excess weight can also constitute a health risk, particularly in the presence of obesity-associated diseases (co-morbidities) like diabetes, high blood pressure, and heart disease (Table 9.4). The higher the number of risk factors, the greater the risk.

TABLE 9.3 Other Risk Factors for Chronic Disease

The more of these risk factors you have, the more you are likely to benefit from weight loss if you are overweight or obese.

Do you have a personal or family history of heart disease?

Are you a male older than 45 years or a postmenopausal female?

Do you smoke cigarettes?

Do you have a sedentary lifestyle?

Has your doctor told you that you have
- high blood pressure?
- abnormal blood lipids (high LDL cholesterol, low HDL cholesterol, high triglycerides)?
- diabetes?

SOURCE: U.S. Department of Agriculture, Agriculture Research Service, Dietary Guidelines Advisory Committee (2000). *Nutrition and your health: Dietary guidelines for Americans, 2000* (5th ed.) Home and Garden Bulletin No. 232. Washington, D.C.

TABLE 9.4 Classification of BMI, with Health Risk and Co-morbidities

BMI	HEALTH RISK	WITH CO-MORBIDITIES**
<25	Minimal	Low
25 – <27	Low	Moderate
27 – <30	Moderate	High
30 – <35	High	Very high
35 – <40	Very high	Extremely high
>40	Extremely high	Extremely high

** Hypertension, cardiovascular disease, dyslipidemia, Type 2 diabetes, sleep apnea, osteoarthritis, infertility, other conditions

SOURCE: National Heart, Lung, and Blood Institute (NHLBI). (1998). *Obesity education initiative expert panel clinical guidelines on the identification, evaluation, and treatment of overweight and obesity in adults.* (NIH Pub. No. 98-4083, p. 17). Washington, DC: NHLBI.

Activities & Assessments 9.1

Engage www.pahconnection.com 9.1

Experience www.pahconnection.com 9.1

Skinfold technique Measure of subcutaneous fat at various body sites using special calipers.

Underwater weighing Technique to measure body fat percentage that requires weighing a person underwater as well as on land.

The skinfold technique requires special calipers and an experienced tester.

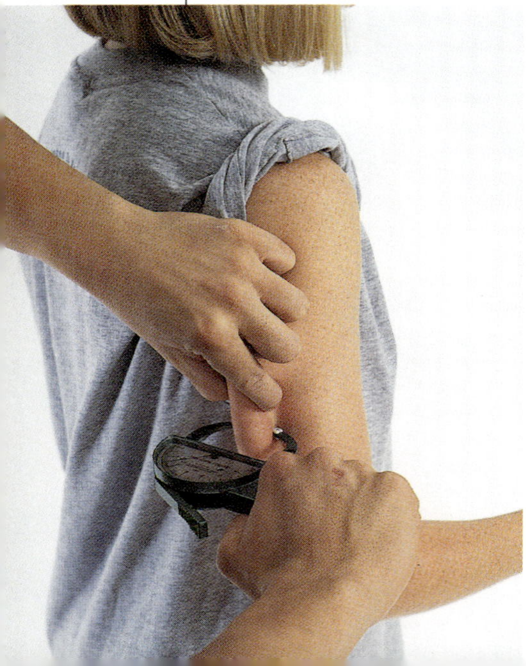

ASSESSING BODY FATNESS

The preceding facts on body mass index, waist circumference, and obesity-associated diseases provides an important understanding on how scientists estimate the risks related to the condition of obesity. Their research supplies valuable information for making inferences related to health status based on risk factor calculation. The measures used in these studies are uncomplicated and easy to implement, so they have been readily accepted. There are a wide variety of methods that use more specific measures to determine body fat. The majority are based on seeing the body as two separate components: fat weight and fat-free weight. Body fat percentage is obtained by dividing body fat mass and fat-free mass (Lukaski, 1987).

Skinfold Testing

Because approximately 50 percent of body fat is stored under the skin (subcutaneous fat), measuring skinfold thickness at various body sites allows an estimate of total body fat. The **skinfold technique** requires special calipers and an experienced tester. The tester lifts a fold of skin and fat between the thumb and forefinger, pulls it away from the underlying muscle, and then measures the fold (Photo 9.4). The five most common measured sites are the triceps (back of upper arm), subscapular (upper back), suprailiac (just above the hip bone), abdomen (either side of the umbilicus), and the frontal thigh. The values obtained are inserted into an appropriate formula to calculate the body-fat percentage.

Underwater Weighing

The most widely used laboratory procedure for measuring body fatness is **underwater weighing** (Photo 9.5). This technique is considered a more precise assessment of body fatness than skinfolds but requires special equipment and highly trained personnel. The procedure for this technique requires weighing a person underwater as well as on land. Since lean tissue is more dense than fat tissue, a person with more muscle and bone will weigh more in water. From this density measurement, the percent of body fat can be calculated.

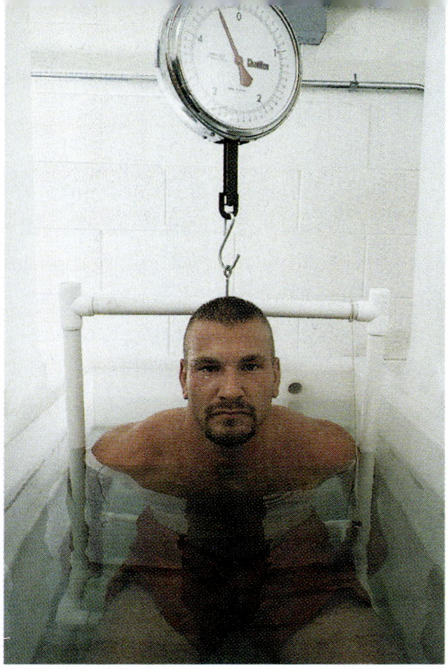

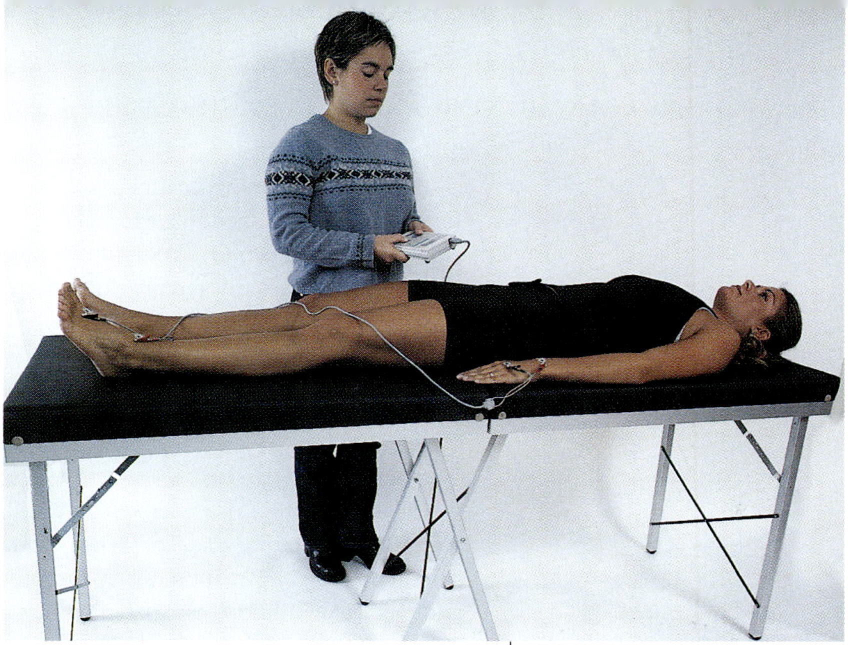

(Left) Body fat is measured using the underwater weighing method. (Right) Bioelectrical impedence is another method used to measure body fat.

Bioelectrical Impedance

Since body fat contains less water and fewer electrolytes than lean body mass, it exhibits a greater resistance (impedance) to the flow of an electrical current. In **bioelectrical impedance,** a harmless, low-level, single-frequency electric current is passed through a person's body by electrodes placed on the wrist and an ankle (Photo 9.6). The amount of resistance, and the body size, are used to calculate body fat percentage. The greater the resistance to the flow, the greater the percentage of body fat.

You may want to check with your university fitness center or exercise science program to see if they offer either the skinfold, underwater weighing, or bioelectrical impedance body-fat analyses as one of their services.

Experience
www.pahconnection.com
9.2

LIFESTYLE AND WEIGHT MAINTENANCE

Primary prevention lies in avoiding becoming overweight or obese in the first place. Voluntary weight maintenance efforts should focus on behaviors related to a healthy diet and regular physical activity. The American Dietetic Association position (1994) on successful weight maintenance for adults is that it requires a lifelong commitment to healthful lifestyle behaviors emphasizing eating practices and regular physical activity that are sustainable and enjoyable. The goal of maintaining a healthy weight through these preventive efforts is desirable for good physical and psychological health and to avoid the effects of creeping obesity or the negative consequences of repeated weight gains and losses.

6. Regular physical activity and a healthy nutritious diet are the most important components to fat loss and control.

Explore
www.pahconnection.com
9.2

In contrast to weight maintenance, the primary purpose of obesity treatment is to reduce the risk associated with increased morbidity (illness) and mortality (death) by decreasing body fatness (NHLBI, 1998). To meet these fat loss goals, strategies must be employed that allow for the reduction in body fatness in an incremental manner (small changes over time) that are maintainable. The term *weight loss* does not discriminate between lean body tissue (bone, muscle, water) and fat mass. For example, inappropriate dieting (low-calorie or low-nutrient-to-calorie ratio diets) and lack of or improper exercising (under or overtraining) can decrease the weight of the body's lean healthy tissue. These behaviors may lead to an increase in overall body fat percentage, thus increasing your risk of disease and decreasing your overall appearance of health.

Bioelectrical impedance
Technique to measure body fat percentage that passes a harmless, low-level, single-frequency electrical current through the body using electrodes placed on the wrist and ankle.

Rather than defining treatment solely in terms of general weight loss, a more fitting focus would be on shedding excess body fatness that increases your overall weight. Any plan to shed excess body fat should include strategies for maintaining or enhancing the level of lean body tissues to provide a more healthy weight. This approach requires a thorough understanding of body fatness and health. This pattern of thinking is consistent with recent efforts that minimize the emphasis on body weight loss and focus on healthy living (Robinson, 1997 and NIH, 1992).

Preliminary Self-Assessments

An assessment of risk related to overweight and obesity is an important first step in the process of setting goals for weight management or weight loss. This assessment should include information related to body fatness and the impact of lifestyle habits and medical conditions associated with obesity.

Engage www.pahconnection.com 9.2

Activities & Assessments 9.1

Body Mass Index (BMI) As discussed earlier, body mass index (BMI) is a popular tool currently used by health professionals to screen adults for their health risks and degree of obesity. It is based upon a relationship between weight and height, excluding frame size and muscle mass. The BMI is not a valid assessment of health risk during childhood, pregnancy, or lactation. It must also be interpreted carefully for heavily muscled athletes and sedentary elderly adults. To review determining your BMI, complete Engage 9.2 or Activities and Assessments 9.1A, "Determining Your Body Mass Index." Then compare your BMI to Table 9.4 to determine your health risk status.

Waist Circumference It is not only important to look at your healthy weight range based on your BMI measure but also to take into account where you carry that weight. Regional patterns of fat deposit are controlled genetically and differ between, and among, men and women (Figure 9.7). Determine your **waist circumference** by placing a measuring tape snugly around your waist. Your health risk increases with a waist measurement of over 40 inches if you are a man and over 35 inches if you are a women. Additionally, if your BMI measurement was above 25, you could be at even a greater health risk for obesity-related diseases (Table 9.2).

Waist circumference Estimate of regional fat distribution at the abdomen.

Weight Wellness Profile Your physical activity levels, eating habits, smoking behavior, and medical history provide further information related to your health risk. To determine your weight wellness profile, complete Engage 9.3.

FIGURE 9.7

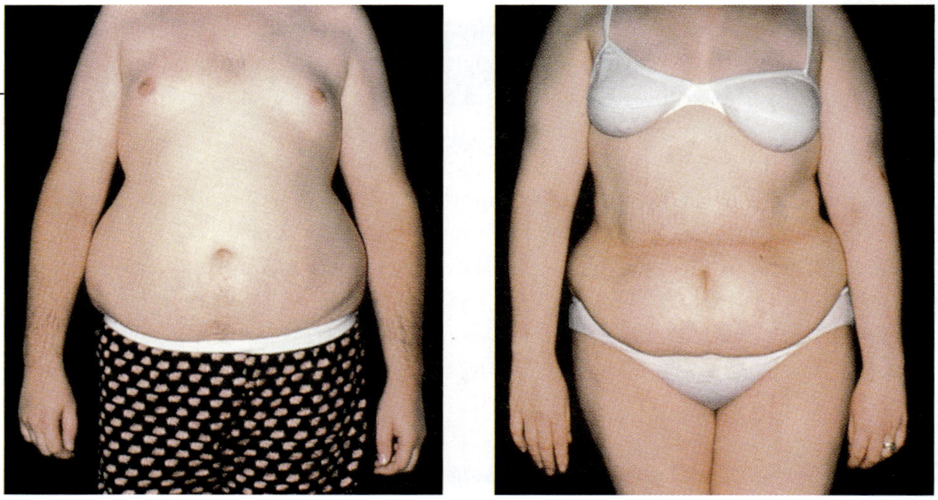

Regional Fat Distribution.
Fat located in the abdominal area is related to greater risk of heart disease, high blood pressure, and type 2 diabetes than fat located in any other region.

Setting Realistic Goals

Engage
www.pahconnection.com
9.3, 9.4

Based on your self-assessments, you may want to maintain your weight at its current level or reduce it to a level that diminishes your health risk. If you are already somewhat lean and at low risk, then the following recommendations may help reinforce what you are already doing. If you have determined that you may be at risk, you need to set realistic goals and then take action toward achieving them.

The American Health Foundation's expert panel on healthy weight has proposed a BMI of 25 as a generous upper limit to protect against development of chronic diseases (AHF, 1996). If your BMI exceeds the target of 25, a BMI that is two units below your current BMI (equivalent to approximately 5 to 10% of your initial body weight) is recommended. Even though a lower BMI might be more desirable to you at this time, the health advantages of setting an obtainable and maintainable goal outweigh the risk of setting unrealistic goals that increase the likelihood of your regaining weight. Furthermore, it is recommended that, when you reach your new BMI goal, you attempt to maintain it for more than 6 months before further attempts to lower your BMI.

Determining Your Readiness The next step, after you have documented your BMI and set a reasonable goal, is to assess your readiness to achieve this goal. *Readiness* is your level of motivation related to losing body fat and includes whether your commitment to losing fat can be sustained across each of the steps required to meet and maintain your goal. Deciding if the time to begin your fat loss program is right requires considering several components, including your reason, how responsible you are, the dieting process, the types of food to eat, the type of exercise, your self-image, and your attitude and commitment. To help you determine if you are truly prepared to begin a fat-loss program, complete Engage 9. 4, "Determining Your Readiness to Lose Fat." For each item, click on the statement that best describes your feelings related to your level of readiness to begin a fat-reduction program. If you are not ready, you should not begin a fat-loss program right now, and you can reassess your level of readiness in a few weeks. If you feel that you are ready to begin a fat-loss program right now, you can begin the preparation stage (determining your energy intake and expenditure) for the behavioral strategies (diet and exercise modification) that follow.

Regular walking is a good way to burn calories.

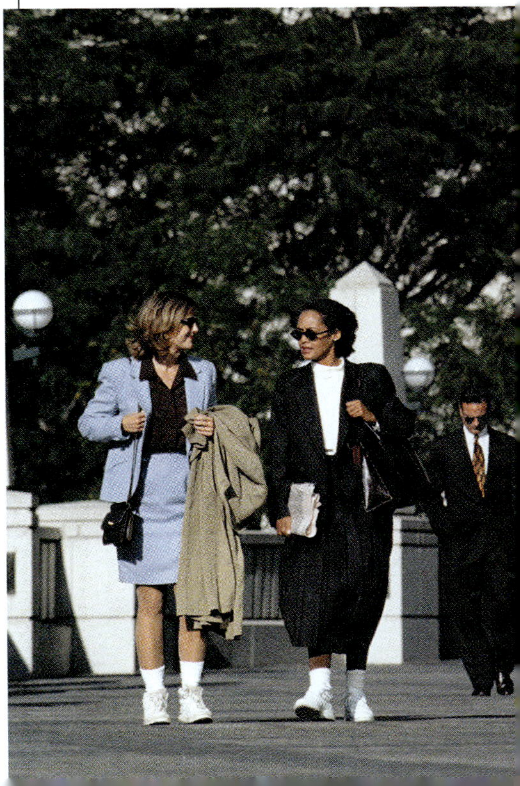

Lifestyle and Fat Loss

The lifestyle approach to fat loss and control focuses on developing a lifelong commitment to a lifestyle that achieves and maintains a stable level of body fat relative to your physical and psychological health. Without a doubt, the amount of physical activity and your dietary habits are the most important components of any healthy lifestyle fat-loss and maintenance program. These two behaviors are crucial in determining your initial fat loss as well as your long-term success. The following steps give you a lifestyle approach to fat loss and control that is both achievable and maintainable.

Determining Your Energy Balance Equation An objective assessment of your average daily energy intake and energy expenditure provides the basis for *unbalancing* the energy equation in order to achieve fat loss. To determine your average daily calorie intake, keep a careful 7-day food intake record using Engage 9.5 "7-Day Food Record." If you are like most people, you eat differently on weekdays than on weekends. When it comes to healthy eating, it's what you take in over a number of days that counts, not just one day. Withhold judgement regarding the analysis of your diet until you have completed the 7-day record. By avoiding early analysis, you can learn much about your individuality related to your food habits, which is an important aspect of the fat loss

Engage www.pahconnection.com **9.5, 9.6, 9.7**

process. In addition, your food intake record will provide a more accurate picture of your average daily caloric and nutrient intake. To determine your average daily calorie and nutrient intake, complete Engage 9.6 .

Next you must determine your average daily calorie expenditure. To determine your average daily calorie expenditure, keep a careful 7-day physical activity record. Use Engage 9.7, "Daily Energy Expenditure," to determine your average daily expenditure.

Unbalancing the Energy Equation The recommended *maximum* value of fat loss in a week is 2 pounds. Since there are 3500 calories in a pound of fat, you would need a deficit of 7000 calories for the week, or 1000 calories for the day, to lose 2 pounds. Generally, you do not want to shed more than 1 pound of body fat per week (3500 weekly calorie deficit or 500 daily-calorie deficit) in order to maximize fat loss and minimize lean tissue loss. Increasing the weekly energy deficit above 3500 calories could cause a significant loss of muscle tissue and be counterproductive to your body composition goal (Kleiner, 1998). As discussed earlier, although either the lowering of caloric intake (dietary modification) or increasing energy expenditure (physical activity) can be effective independently in obtaining the recommended 3500 weekly calorie deficit, a combination of the two produces the best results. As you will discover in the next sections, the advantages of one technique counterbalance the disadvantages of the other. For example, caloric restriction produces a rapid reduction of resting metabolic rate, substantially decreasing energy expenditure, whereas exercise increases resting metabolic rate, thereby negating the dietary effects. Hence, a comprehensive fat-loss program involving both a dietary and physical activity schedule is highly recommended by major health-related organizations like the American College of Sports Medicine, The National Heart, Lung, and Blood Institute, The American Heart Association, and the American Dietetic Association.

PHYSICAL ACTIVITY AND FAT LOSS

physical activity and health connection

Without a doubt, physical activity is one of the most important components of any fat-loss program. In addition, accumulated evidence has shown that physical activity is the best predictor for maintaining weight loss (Pate et al., 1996). Therefore, describing the benefits of physical activity related to fat loss and maintenance will provide you with added incentives to become, or stay, physically active.

Physical Activity Burns Calories

The immediate function of physical activity in a fat-loss program is simply to increase the level of energy expenditure—helping to unbalance the caloric equation so that there is a greater amount of energy output. Physical activity is the most important way to increase the calories you burn. The calorie-expending effects of physical activity are cumulative and substantial. This means that even mild-to-moderate increases in physical activity can be beneficial. For example, 40 to 60 minutes of walking expends approximately 350 calories. Performing this activity five times a week would contribute to 1750 calories expended or shedding half a pound of fat. Increasing the intensity or duration of physical activity (or participating in a formal exercise program) can further increase the number of calories burned.

Physical Activity Ameliorates Obesity-Associated Diseases

Physical activity benefits your health even if you don't lose weight. Physical activity has positive effects on blood pressure, blood fat levels, and insulin insensitivity (type 2 diabetes), independent of those produced by weight loss alone.

Physical Activity Compensates for RMR Decline

A well- documented change that occurs during dietary restriction of calories is a considerable reduction in resting metabolic rate (RMR) (Chapter 8). This decline can reach up to 40 percent of RMR after a brief time, significantly reducing overall calorie expenditure by the body. Physical activity increases the metabolic rate both during activity and afterward.

Physical Activity Minimizes Loss of Lean Body Mass

Muscle is metabolically active—it requires calories. The more muscle you have, the more calories you need to sustain it, and the more calories you can eat and still lose weight. The use of physical activity in a weight loss program provides protection against a loss of lean tissue routinely seen with diet-only weight loss programs. Aerobic and weight-resistance activities contribute to the conservation of lean tissue in different ways. Aerobic physical activities utilize the oxygen energy system that requires the mobilization and metabolism of the body's fat storage (Chapter 8). Weight-resistance activities (weight training) burn calories as well. In addition, weight-resistance activities helps stimulate muscular development (Chapter 11), preventing significant losses of lean body tissue that generally occur during calorie-restricting diets.

Physical Activity Suppresses Appetite

To some degree, regular physical activity appears to contribute to the normal functioning of the brain's feeding control mechanisms. A sensitive balance between energy expenditure and food intake is apparently not maintained very well in physically inactive people. This lack of precision in regulating food intake may account for some of the increasing obesity observed in America (Weinsier et al., 1998). Individuals who are regularly physical active are better able to match daily energy intake with daily expenditure.

Physical Activity Can Lower Set Point

The set point theory proposes that a regulatory system exists in the human body that maintains body weight at some fixed level. Instead of a simply genetic determination, set point is now believed to be under control of environmental factors. The environmental factor that can lower set point more than any other is regular, sustained physical activity (Bennet, 1995). A lower set point can make maintaining a lower percentage of body fat much easier.

Physical Activity Improves Psychological Well-Being

A weight problem or poor body image may contribute to lower self-esteem, guilt, depression, anxiety, and distress. Physical activity can enhance self-esteem and reduce depression, anxiety, and stress through both physiological and psychological mechanisms (Chapter 13). Increased psychological well-being can enhance compliance with a weigh loss program as well as helping the individual to cope with societal pressure.

As you can see, physical activity plays an integral role in a healthy weigh loss program. Another key component is healthy eating.

Physical activity of any kind is generally considered the most important component in a fat-loss program.

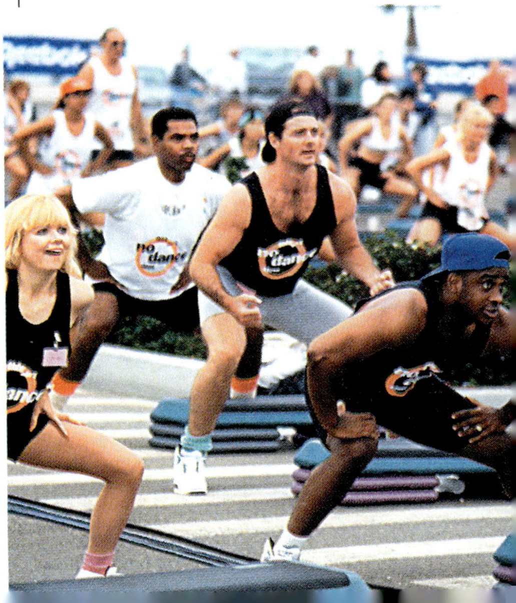

HEALTHY EATING FOR FAT LOSS

The foundation for any healthy eating plan for fat loss should be built from the *Dietary Guidelines for Americans* and the Food Guide Pyramid (Chapter 7). To incorporate their guidelines into a fat-loss program, particular attention must be given to serving size and to choosing mainly from food groups that appear in the lower half of the Food Pyramid.

Food Intake Modification

Using your estimated daily caloric intake, develop a daily caloric plan that reduces your calories by 250 each day. (Avoid daily caloric restriction plans of 1200 calories or less.) As for the diet itself, the cornerstone of any meal plan should be the Food Guide Pyramid, which builds upon and complements the *Dietary Guidelines* (Chapter 7). The Food Guide Pyramid recommends a variety of foods, with a notable emphasis on grains, fruits, and vegetables. Moreover, the Food Guide Pyramid helps you establish a tolerable, enjoyable, and stable eating pattern that is consistent with a healthy lifestyle approach to fat loss. Finally, the *Dietary Guidelines* advocate the moderation of fat, sugar, and alcohol consumption, all of which are all-important in weight loss.

While not designed to be calorie-specific management tools, both the Food Guide Pyramid and the *Dietary Guidelines* are relevant and valuable tools for healthy menu planning related to body fat loss. You just need to pay special attention to the serving size and select food items from each group that are low in fat.

Explore www.pahconnection.com **9.3**

The key principle is to select foods with a high nutrient-calorie benefit ratio (Chapter 7). This can easily be accomplished by choosing natural and unrefined foods from the base of the Food Guide Pyramid. Avoid refined and processed foods (refined sugar) as much as possible. Since you will be encouraged to participate in a regular physical activity program, it is important to maintain a good macronutrient ratio comprised of 55 to 65 percent of your total calories from carbohydrates (preferably complex carbohydrates), 20 to 25 percent from protein, and 10 to 20 percent from fat (Kleiner, 1998). Dietary fat is not a terrible thing, but when you are limiting your calories, as on a fat-loss program, the calories are better spent on carbohydrates (to fuel your activity) and protein (to maintain your muscle tissue). Research has shown that, during negative energy balance, slightly more protein (1.2 grams per 2.0 pounds of body weight) is required to maintain muscle mass. Finally, sources of complex carbohydrates, such as grain products and vegetables, not only allow you to feel energetic for longer periods of time but also are generally higher in other important nutrients.

Eating Style Modification

Engage www.pahconnection.com **9.8**

Obesity is as much a result of how we eat as it is of what we eat. While what we eat contributes to our fat loss efforts, so do our eating styles. Eating styles can be hard to change. Correcting problem areas will make a big difference in your success with fat loss. Therefore, it is important to evaluate your eating styles. Complete Engage 9.8, "Eating Style Questionnaire," to learn more about your eating style and how it may affect your diet.

Emotional Eating

One of the primary reasons for keeping a food diary is to have a written record of your moods and the events occurring just prior to eating. How you feel and what's going on around you before you eat are significant; our emotions strongly influence our eating behavior. By keeping an accurate food diary that includes this information, your eating style will become more visible to you. This may include eating when we are stressed or depressed. Once you become aware of the precursors causing unnecessary eating behaviors, a conscious effort can be made to avoid them.

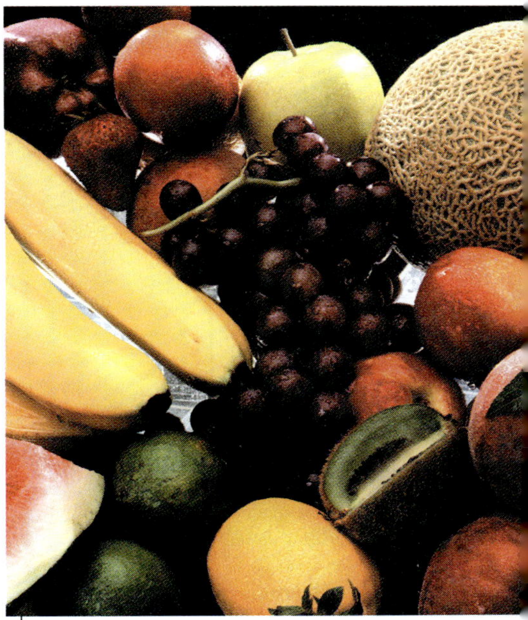

Fruits and vegetables make excellent snacks.

Focus on Body Fat, Not Weight

Do not build everything around "losing weight." Too many people focus their dietary restriction program on weight loss and not fat loss. They get up every day and check their weight on the scale. They are depressed if they did not lose anything and elated if they lost weight. You want to focus on losing body fat. You could lose weight and get fatter if you are dieting incorrectly! What matters is your level of body fatness, not your weight.

Eat Smaller, More Frequent Meals

Do not skip meals or go more than 3 to 4 hours without eating. Skipping a meal often leads to bingeing at the next meal, which initiates an up-and-down energy and nutrient pattern. When meals are more than 6 hours apart, plan strategic healthy snacks. You can obtain many nutrients, and energy, by choosing your snacks wisely and eating them in moderation. Include fresh fruits and vegetables and avoid cookies, candies, ice cream, and potato chips.

Eat Slowly

You will probably overeat if you eat too quickly. It takes about 20 to 30 minutes for your stomach to signal the brain that you are full. Put your eating utensil down between bites and chew your food thoroughly.

BEHAVIORAL MODIFICATION REVISITED

Personal fat-loss treatment strategies should include behavioral modification, which assists in choosing healthier diets and increasing activity levels (Chapter 3). Fat loss strategies that include lower calorie diets and increased physical activity are based on achieving a negative energy balance of 3500 calories per week, or 500 calories per day (NIH, 1992, and ADA, 1995). This can be accomplished in three ways:

7. Behavioral modification strategies should be included in a personal fat loss program.

- Reducing daily caloric intake by 500 calories
- Reducing daily caloric intake by 250 calories and increasing daily physical energy expenditure by 250 calories (or a combination of the two that equals a 500-calorie deficit)
- Increasing physical activity expenditure by 500 calories a day

This traditional intervention strategy for fat loss is built on the sound premise that individuals can control their own behaviors related to managing and maintaining a focus on healthful eating and increased activity. However, it is often difficult to motivate people with this sound traditional approach when they read or hear about such quick fixes as "lose 10 pounds in 1 week" or "lose 30 pounds in 1 month." These ads may lead people to abandon basic-fat loss principles.

8. A negative sign of dissatisfaction with body weight is the development of eating disorders.

Engage www.pahconnection.com 9.9

Activities & Assessments 9.2

BODY IMAGE

Body image is the picture we have of our of body, what it looks like to us, and how we think it looks to others. This image can be accurate or inaccurate and is often subject to change. The relationship between body image and weight is complicated. Choosing unrealistic weight loss goals in response to societal ideals can set you up for failure and perpetuate unhealthy choices. To improve body image, as well as self-esteem, it is important to learn to like ourselves and to take care of ourselves through healthy lifestyle choices that do not emphasize weight loss at the expense of psychological and physical health.

The relationship of eating and weight management to emotional and physical well-being is complex. An eating disorder can greatly impact an individual's effort to manage weight; conversely, a person's intense effort to control weight can lead to an eating disorder. People with a history of anorexia nervosa or bulimia nervosa should receive specialized care and avoid addressing weight problems on their own. Find out if whether your feelings about your body image perception are normal using Engage 9.9, or Activities and Assessments 9.2 .

FIGURE 9.8

The Progression of Anorexia.

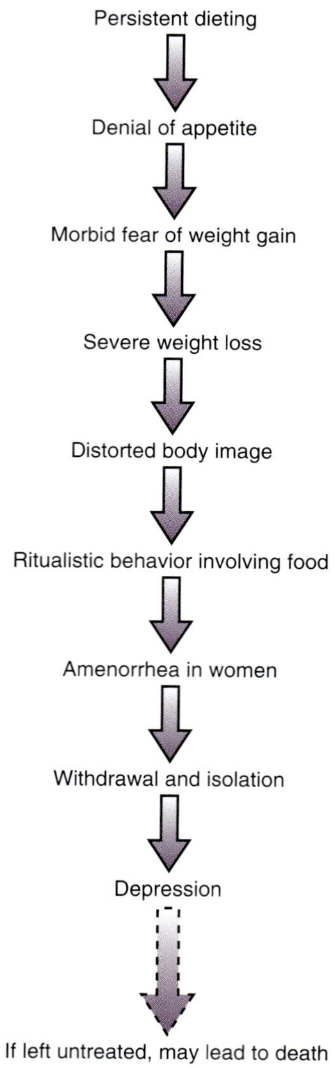

EATING DISORDERS

Concerns with body weight and weight maintenance are not limited to excessive accumulation of body fat. As you read in the introduction, we are assaulted daily by the media with images of the "ideal" body. The "ideal" body is presented as extreme thinness for females and extreme muscularity for males. Many people have become image conscious, and they feel pressured to match the "ideal" portrayed in magazines and on television. This can lead to major discontent with body weight. A recent survey indicated that 15 percent of women and 11 percent of men sampled said they would sacrifice more than 5 years of their life to be at an ideal weight (Psychology Today, 1997). A negative sign of dissatisfaction with body weight is the development of **eating disorders.** *Eating disorders* refers to a wide range of harmful eating behaviors used in the attempt to lose weight or achieve a lean appearance (ACSM, 1997). The eating behaviors range from severe restriction of food intake to binge eating and purging.

Eating disorders patterns are far-reaching and escalating, now affecting more than 7 million women and 1 million men in the United States (ANAD, 2000). Nearly 90 percent of these destructive eating patterns begin before the age of 20, with the majority (77%) lasting anywhere from 1 to 15 years. Anorexia nervosa and bulimia nervosa are the two most severe forms of eating disorders.

Anorexia Nervosa

Anorexia nervosa literally means "loss of appetite." This definition is misleading, in that a person with anorexia nervosa becomes hungry, but repudiates the hunger because of an irrational fear of eating and becoming fat. **Anorexia nervosa** is characterized by a distorted body image, self-starvation, and extreme weight loss (Figure 9.8).

Because of extreme weight loss, females with anorexia nervosa often suffer from a lack of menstrual periods (amenorrhea) due to to little body fat. Furthermore, excessive weight loss increases rates of bone loss (osteoporosis), muscle loss, and dehydration. When body fat is severely limited and muscle tissue is lost, the body turns to its organs in a critical search for energy, and the vicious cycle of wasting away continues. Victims lose the ability to function effectively and put themselves in a life-threatening physical condition. It is estimated that about 4 to 8 percent of people with anorexia nervosa die prematurely.

Eating disorder Refers to a wide range of harmful eating behaviors used in the attempt to lose weight or achieve a lean appearance.

Anorexia nervosa Extreme eating disorder in which individuals literally starve themselves due to an irrational fear of eating and becoming fat.

Bulimia nervosa Extreme eating disorder characterized by uncontrollable cycles of binge eating followed by purging through forced vomiting or abuse of laxatives and diuretics.

Bulimia Nervosa

Bulimia means to "eat like an ox." **Bulimia nervosa** is characterized by uncontrollable cycles of binge eating followed by purging through forced vomiting or the abuse of laxatives and diuretics. During a binge, individuals lose control over their eating and may quickly consume large amounts of food—up to 20,000 calories in a single binge. Bulimic individuals are afraid of being fat and follow the binge with efforts to redress uncontrolled eating by purging the food from their bodies or by fasting (Figure 9.9).

The person suffering from bulimia nervosa is usually in a normal weight range, but may suffer from weight fluctuations of 10 or more pounds over short periods of time due to alternating binges and purging/fasting (Figure 9.9). This binge-purge cycle puts a tremendous strain on the body. In repeated vomiting, the stomach acid can erode tooth enamel and even the esophagus. Additionally, nutrient deficiencies may occur from vomiting and the use of laxatives.

Compulsive Overeating

Compulsive eaters are similar to those with bulimia nervosa in that they may eat large amounts of food in a short period of time and exhibit a lack of control regarding their eating. However, compulsive eaters do not purge, and thus they usually become obese, thereby encountering all the health risks of obesity. They may eat continually throughout the day as a means to cope with stress and other emotionally issues.

Treatment for Disordered Eating

The treatments for disordered eating patterns are complex and most often require professional help. Anorexia nervosa treatment, depending on the duration of the illness, generally begins with medical treatment to address the physical destruction and to restore the body to a sufficient weight. This generally requires hospitalization. Once health is stabilized, the psychological factors underlying the anorexia nervosa need to be addressed through psychotherapy.

Initial treatment for bulimia nervosa or compulsive eating disorders involves the elimination of the eating pattern. Unlike anorexia nervosa, most bulimia nervosa and compulsive eating disorders do not require hospitalization. They do, however, require

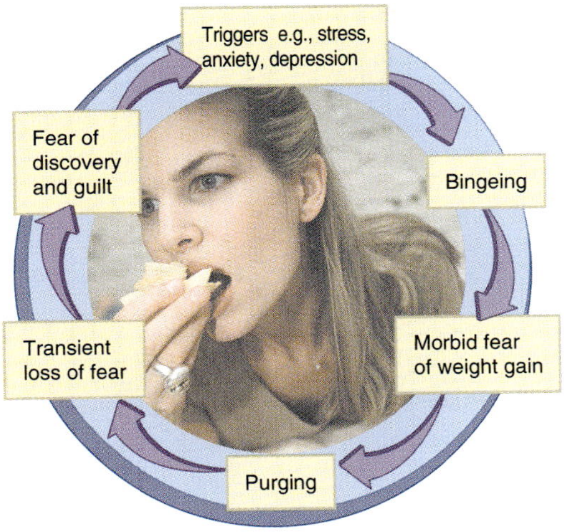

FIGURE 9.9

The Binge–Purge Cycle of Bulimia.

Explore
www.pahconnection.com
9.4

professional assistance to uncover the system of thinking that led to the disordered eating. Changing the thinking pattern is necessary for successful treatment.

Self-help and supports groups are extremely beneficial adjuncts to treatment by professionals. Family, friends, and support groups all play an important role in helping the person with disordered eating to start and maintain a treatment program.

PHYSICAL ACTIVITY AND HEALTH CONNECTION

Body composition management includes a lifelong commitment to a healthy lifestyle. Two elements involved in attaining and maintaining a healthy body composition are eating a nutritious diet and performing physical activity. Adequate nutrition and decreased calorie intake are important goals of diet modification for decreasing body fatness. Sufficient physical activity is equally important because it expends excessive fat storage and enhances lean body mass. Moreover, physical activity offsets the harmful effects of a number of morbid conditions that are attributed to excessive body fat storage. The goals of physical activity related to achieving and maintaining a healthy body composition should be based on activities that are enjoyable and can be performed consistently.

CONCEPT CONNECTION

1. **An acceptable or optimal weight is one that leaves us free from disease, is realistic, and is attained and maintained through physical activity and a healthy diet.** Answering the question "What is my ideal body composition?" should include both physical and psychological considerations. Weight management ought to be based on the weight that supports a high level of physical and psychological health at each stage of a person's life.

2. **Excess body fat is associated with a number of morbid conditions.** Excess body fat is highly associated with morbid conditions including high blood pressure, dyslipidemia (high levels of fat in your blood), diabetes mellitus, and osteoarthritis. These diseases can lead to serious illness and premature death.

3. **Your body requires some body fat for healthy functioning.** Determining cut off points for acceptable body percentages requires first considering essential body fat and storage fat allowances. Essential body fat is required for healthy functioning. Authorities agree that essential fat should compose 3 to 5 percent of the total weight for men and 8 to 12 percent of total body weight for women. Storage fat is body fat above essential fat levels that accumulates in adipose tissue (fat cells). Some storage fat is advised for both males and females. Storage fat is needed for protection of vital organs and insulation of the body. Desirable storage levels are estimated to be between 8 to 20 percent of total body weight.

4. **Obesity is influenced by our genetics (nature) and our environment (nurture).** Research indicates that weight and fat distribution are strongly influenced by genetic and biological factors. However the increase in the prevalence of obesity in the past couple of decades cannot be explained by changes in our genetics and biology. Many environmental and lifestyle influences have contributed to our obesity epidemic. Our genetics and biology permit us to become obese, but our environment enables us to become obese. The increased prevalence of obesity in America has been largely attributed to an increased consumption of energy-dense food, which is both flavorable and pleasurable, and a decreased level of caloric expenditure due to a sedentary lifestyle.

5. **Health risk related to obesity can be determined in a number of ways.** Body mass index, waist circumference, and the precence of obesity-associated diseases provide an important understanding on how research scientists estimate the risks related to the condition of obesity. Their research supplies valuable information for

making inferences related to health status based on risk factor calculation. The measures used in these studies were uncomplicated and easy to implement, hence their popularity in field settings.

6. **A lifestyle approach that includes regular physical activity and a healthy nutritious diet is the most important component of fat loss and control.** The lifestyle approach to fat loss and control focuses on developing a lifelong commitment to a lifestyle that achieves and maintains a stable level of body fat relative to one's physical and psychological health. Voluntary weight maintenance efforts related to lifestyle should to focus on behaviors a healthy diet and regular physical activity.

7. **Behavioral modification should be included in personal fat loss strategies.** Personal fat-loss treatment strategies should include behavioral modification to assist in helping people obtain healthier diets and increased activity levels. Fat-loss strategies that include lower-calorie diets and increased physical activity are based on achieving a negative energy balance of 3500 calories per week, or 500 calories per day.

8. **A negative sign of dissatisfaction with body weight is the development of eating disorders.** Anorexia nervosa and bulimia nervosa are the two most severe forms of eating disorders. If individuals have a history of anorexia nervosa or bulimia nervosa, they should receive specialized care and avoid going it alone.

TERMS

Healthy Weight, 194
Body Mass Index (BMI), 195
Acceptable or optimal weight, 196
Overweight, 196
Obesity, 196
Essential body fat, 198
Storage fat, 198
Adipostat, 200
Skinfold technique, 206
Underwater weighing, 206
Bioelectrical impedance, 207
Waist circumference, 208
Eating disorder, 214
Anorexia nervosa, 214
Bulimia nervosa, 215

MAKING THE CONNECTION

Melinda realizes that what is important related to her health is her ideal body fatness and not necessarily her weight. In recognizing this important difference she decides to have a body composition assessment completed. She schedules an appointment with the university wellness center, choosing the skinfold technique. Furthermore, she decides to make an appointment to discuss her self-image with the university's counseling center.

CRITICAL THINKING

1. From the vignette, how would you assess Melinda's preoccupation with her weight? What factors influence her concerns about her weight? Do you believe she has an unhealthy obsession with her weight?
2. On your campus, identify and briefly describe the resources available for students regarding healthy weight management and eating disorders.
3. We have learned that we should be asking ourselves "What is my ideal body fatness?" not "What is my ideal body weight?" Based on this, what measures can you take to better understand your body weight?
4. Your housemate, Joan, goes on a new fad diet that was recently reported by a respected national morning TV show. Joan reports that this new diet will allow her to lose 10 pounds by Saturday (6 days from now). Explain to Joan why this fad diet will not work, and if she were to lose the 10 pounds in 6 days, what would likely happen.
5. As a residence hall assistant (RA) you have been asked by your floor to talk about obesity and how as college freshmen they can manage their weight sensibly. In your talk discuss healthy weight, overweight and obesity, body mass index, and the importance of good nutrition and physical activity.

REFERENCES

Allison, D.B., Fontaine, K.R., Manson, J.E., Stevens, J., & Van Itallie, T.B. (1999). Annual deaths attributable to obesity in the United States. *Journal of the American Medical Association 282:*1530–38.

American College of Sports Medicine. (1997). The female athlete triad: Position stand. *Medicine and Science in Sports and Exercise 29:*(5):1–10.

American College of Sports Medicine. (1995). *ACSM's Guidelines for Exercise Testing and Prescription,* 5th ed. Baltimore: Williams & Wilkins.

American Health Foundation Roundtable on Healthy Weight. Report of an expert panel discussion. *American Journal of Clinical Nutrition 63:*409s–477s.

Alpert, M.A. & Hashimi, M.W. (1993). Obesity and the heart. *American Journal of Medical Sciences 306*(2):117–23.

Bennett, W.I. (1995). Beyond overeating [editorial]. *New England Journal of Medicine 332:*621.

Centers for Disease Control. (1994). Prevalence of overweight among adolescents—United States, 1988–91. *Morbidity and Mortality Weekly Report 43:*818–21.

Flegal, K.M., Carrol, M.D., Kuczmarski, R.J., & Johnson, C.L. (1998). Overweight and obesity in the United States: Prevalence and trends, 1960–1994. *International Journal of Obesity* 22(1):39–47.

Food and Nutrition Board, Institute of Medicine. (1995). Weighing the options: Criteria for evaluating weight management programs. Committee to develop criteria for evaluating the outcomes of approaches to prevent and treat obesity. Thomas, P.R. (ed.). Washington, DC: National Academy Press.

Going, S., Davis, R. (1998). Body Incomposition. In Roitman, J.L., ed., *ACSM's Resource Manual* (3rd ed.). Baltimore: Williams & Wilkins.

Goldstein, D. J. (1992). Beneficial effects of modest weight loss. *International Journal of Obesity 16:*397–415.

Harnack, L. J. (2000). Temporal trends in energy intake in the United States: An ecologic perspective. *American Journal of Clinical Nutrition 71:*1478–84.

King, A.C., & Tribble, D.L. (1991). The role of exercise in weight regulation in nonathletes. *Sports Medicine 11:*331–49.

Kleiner, S.M. (1998). *Power eating.* Champaign, IL: Human Kinetics.

Kuczmarski, R.J. (1994). Increasing prevalence of overweight among U.S. adults. The national health and nutrition examination survey, 1960–1991. *Journal of the American Medical Association 272:*205–211.

Lemieux, S., Prudhomme, D., Bouchard C, Tremblay, A, & Despres, J. (1996). A single threshold value of waist girth identifies normal-weight and overweight subjects with excess visceral adipose tissue. *American Journal of Clinical Nutrition 64:*685–93.

Liebman, B. (1996). Zoning out on the new diet books. *Center for Science in Public Interest Nutrition Action Newsletter 23:*6–8.

Must, A., et al. (1999). The disease burden associated with overweight and obesity. *Journal of the American Medical Association 282:*1523–29.

National Heart, Lung, and Blood Institute. (1998). Obesity education initiative expert panel clinical guidelines on the identification, evaluation, and treatment of overweight and obesity in adults. NIH Pub. No. 98-4083. Washington, DC.

National Institute of Health, Technology Assessment Panel. (1993). Method of evaluating weight-loss and control. *Annuals of Internal Medicine 19:*764–70.

National Task Force on Prevention and Treatment of Obesity. (1994). Toward prevention of obesity: Research directions. *Obesity Research 2:*571–84.

Pate, R.R., Pratt, M., & Blair, S.N. (1995). Physical activity and health. A recommendation from the Centers for Disease Control and Prevention and the American College of Sports Medicine. *Journal of the American Medical Association 273:*402–407.

PiSunyar, X. (1994). The fattening of America. *Journal of the American Medical Association 272:*283.

Revicki, D.A., & Israel, R.G. (1986). Relationship between body mass index indices and measures of body adiposity. *America Journal of Public Health 76:*992–94.

Robinson, J. (1997). Weight management: Shifting the paradigm. *Journal of Health Education 28*(1):28.

Sclafani, A. (1996). Dietary obesity. In Stunkard, A. J., Wadden, T. A. (eds.), *Obesity Theory and Therapy,* 2nd ed. 126-136. Philadelphia: Lippencott-Raven.

Weinsier, R.L., Hunter, G.R., Heini, A.F., Goran, M.I., Sell, S.M. (1998). The etiology of obesity: Relative contribution of metabolic factors, diet, and physical activity. *American Journal of Medicine 105:*145–50.

Activities & Assessments

NAME ____________________ SECTION __________ DATE __________

9.1 Estimating Healthy Body Fatness

DETERMINING YOUR BODY MASS INDEX (BMI)

Directions

STEP 1: Measure your height in inches (without shoes). ____________

STEP 2: Measure your weight in pounds (without shoes). ____________

STEP 3: Determine your BMI using the chart in Figure 9.5. ____________

STEP 4: Determine your health risk using Figure 9.6. ____________

DETERMINING YOUR WAIST CIRCUMFERENCE (REGIONAL FAT DISTRIBUTION)

Directions

STEP 1: Locate the upper hip and place a measuring tape in a horizontal plane around the waist. The measurement should be made with the abdominal muscles relaxed.

STEP 2: Determine your health risk using Table 9.2. ____________

PERSONAL HEALTH EVALUATION PROFILE

Directions

My current weight puts me at an:

☐ Increased ☐ High ☐ Very high ☐ Extremely high

risk for health problems.

LOWERING YOUR HEALTH RISK

Directions

Select a target BMI that is one to two units below your current BMI.

My current BMI is ________.

My target BMI is ________.

I need to lose ________ pounds to achieve my goal. (This can be read right from the BMI chart).

Activities & Assessments

NAME ______________________ SECTION __________ DATE __________

9.2 Body Image: How do you feel about the appearance of these regions of your body?

	OUITE SATISFIED	SOMEWHAT SATISFIED	SOMEWHAT DISSATISFIED	VERY DISSATISFIED
Hair	☐	☐	☐	☐
Arms	☐	☐	☐	☐
Hands	☐	☐	☐	☐
Feet	☐	☐	☐	☐
Waist	☐	☐	☐	☐
Buttocks	☐	☐	☐	☐
Hips	☐	☐	☐	☐
Legs and ankles	☐	☐	☐	☐
Thighs	☐	☐	☐	☐
Chest or breasts	☐	☐	☐	☐
Posture	☐	☐	☐	☐
General attractiveness	☐	☐	☐	☐

1. Which of your thoughts and actions enhance your body image?

____

____

2. Which of your thoughts and actions are detrimental to your body image?

____

____

3. What societal forces (expectations of friends and parents, advertising, celebrities and professional athletes, etc.) influence your body image most strongly?

____

____

4. What could you do to become more satisfied with your body image?

____

____

SOURCE: G. Edlin, E. Golanty, and K. McCormack Brown. (1999). *Health and Wellness,* (6th ed., p. 546). Boston: Jones and Bartlett.

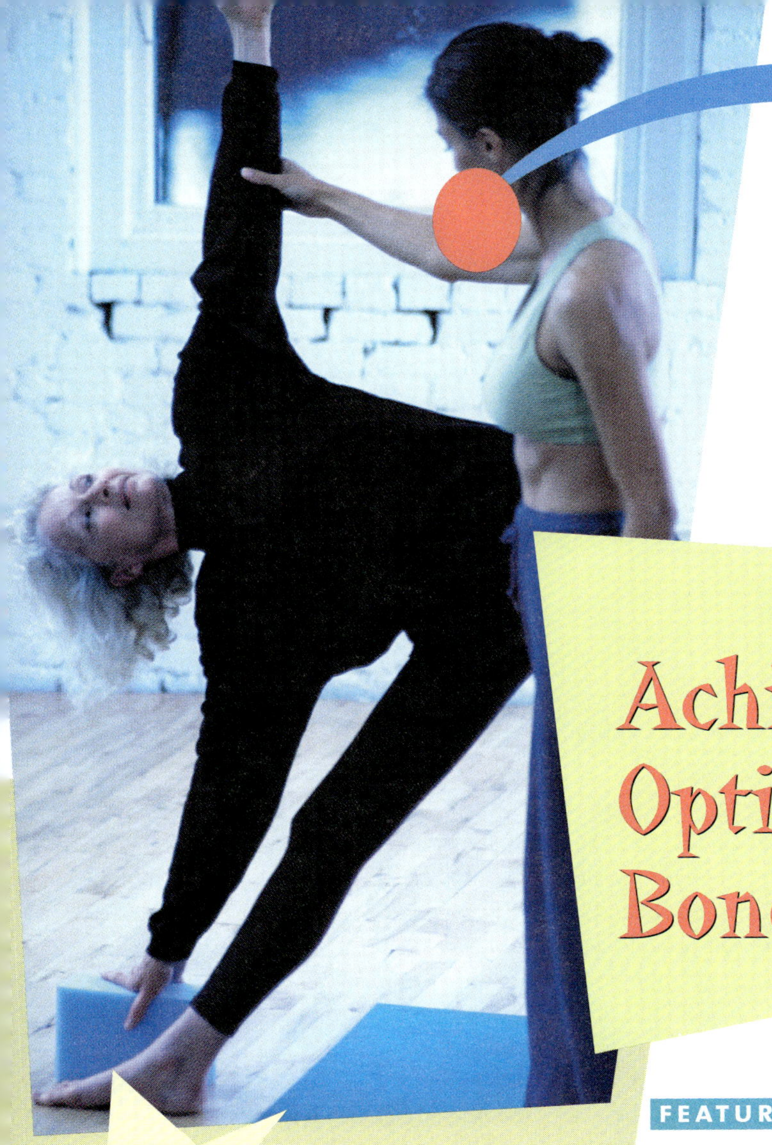

10

Achieving Optimal Bone Health

CONCEPT CONNECTION

1. Bones do more than provide structural support; they protect vital organs and support essential metabolic processes.
2. Three types of cells are involved in bone formation and resorption: osteoblasts, osteocytes, and osteoclasts.
3. To maintain bone mass, bone formation must be at the same rate as bone resorption.
4. Osteoporosis is excessive bone loss that can be prevented.
5. Osteoporosis can be affected by genetic, hormonal, nutritional, and lifestyle factors.

FEATURES

E-Learning Tools: www.pahconnection.com

Engage www.pahconnection.com

10.1 Calcium calculator
10.2 Test your calcium IQ

Experience www.pahconnection.com

10.1 Conditions men get too
10.2 Osteoporosis: progress and promise

Explore www.pahconnection.com

10.1 National Institutes of Health: osteoporosis and related bone diseases national resource center
10.2 National Osteoporosis Foundation

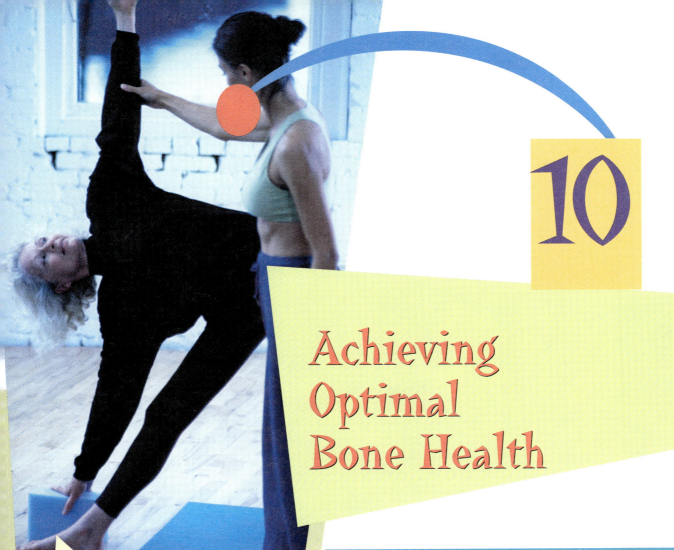

WHAT'S THE CONNECTION?

Julie is a sophomore in college and concerned about women's health issues. One of her biggest worries is developing osteoporosis, a metabolic disease that causes bone loss and subsequent skeletal fragility, so that the bones fracture easily. Julie is aware that osteoporosis can have a crippling effect, especially in older women. She knows the importance to good bone health of calcium and vitamin D, and makes sure that she fulfills her daily requirement of each. However, Julie lives a sedentary lifestyle. Recently, Julie has heard with interest that physical activity can aid her in developing good bone health.

INTRODUCTION

Strength and energy are lasting benefits of a healthy and active lifestyle. In addition to achieving cardiovascular fitness, optimal bone health should be a priority as you develop healthful habits. Genetics can play an important role in developing a healthy skeleton; skeletal disorders, such as osteogenesis imperfecta, are caused by genetic mutations and cannot be "fixed" through nutrition or exercise. In other instances, only surgical intervention can improve the strength of certain bones. However, if you have a healthy skeleton, environmental factors play a key role in the continued building and maintenance of bone health. This chapter reviews the development of the skeleton, the nutritional and physical activity requirements for maintaining a healthy skeleton, and the effects of aging and metabolic changes on bone health.

UNDERSTANDING BONE PHYSIOLOGY

1. Bones do more than provide structural support; they protect vital organs and support essential metabolic processes.

Beyond the structural support provided by the skeleton, some of the bones (ribs, skull) protect our vital internal organs (heart, lungs, brain). Bone also plays a major role in daily metabolic processes: bones produce cells that contribute to the formation of red and white blood cells and platelets, store fat needed for cellular energy production, and both release and absorb calcium to regulate blood levels.

Bone Structure

Bone and cartilage are forms of connective tissue in the human body. **Cartilage** is a semi-rigid connective tissue that provides firm, flexible support. Bone is a more specialized and harder form of connective tissue (Ackermann 1992; Rhoades & Pflanzer, 1996). Healthy bone is light, rigid, of high tensile strength, and not brittle (Ng, Romas, Donnan, & Findlay, 1997). As fetal development begins, the skeleton is made entirely of cartilage. This cartilaginous framework serves as the template for the bone to come later. Mature bone consists of inorganic bone minerals, calcium, and phosphate precipitates that are

Cartilage Semi-rigid tissue that provides support.

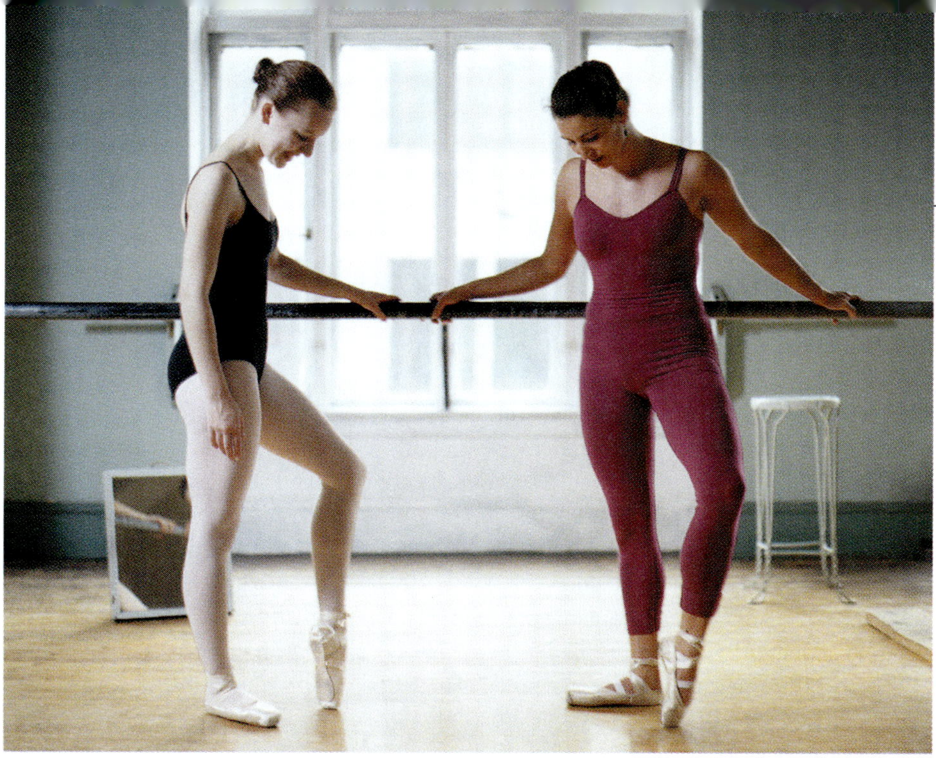

Bones are formed early in life.

incorporated into the organic support material known as *osteoid*. **Collagen** makes up 95 percent of the osteoid substance (Ackermann, 1992; Rhoades & Pfanzler, 1996).

Bone Cells Three types of cells are involved both in bone formation and in **resorption** of mature bone: osteoblasts, osteocytes, and osteoclasts.

Osteoblasts are immature bone cells that deposit new bone around the outside of the bone. When they are surrounded by mineralized bone, they become mature bone cells and are then called **osteocytes. Osteoclasts** digest, or absorb, bony tissue. They remove old bone tissue so that its components can be absorbed into the circulation. This process is known as resorption.

Bone Formation

While the diameter of bones can change throughout our lifetimes, bones grow in length only while the skeleton develops; this growth usually ends in adolescence. Longitudinal bone growth occurs at the ends of long bones at the epiphyseal plate (Ackermann, 1992). The epiphyseal plate is where cartilage synthesis and bone replacement form an area of active growth. Chrondrocytes, or chondroblasts (cells like osteoblasts), synthesize the cartilage. Bone replacement, by osteoblasts, begins in the center of the cartilage and proceeds outward (Rhoades & Pflanzer, 1996). This process of bone formation occurs in layers. As chondrocytes are surrounded and trapped by the cartilage, new chondrocytes replace them on top of the cartilage for continued synthesis of the collagen matrix. The cartilage calcifies, the chondrocytes begin to die off, and the calcified material begins to erode. Osteoblasts move into the area and begin bone replacement. This continuous activity of cartilage synthesis, calcification, erosion, and osteoblast invasion forms the zone of active bone formation (Rhoades & Pflanzer, 1996).

Chondrocyte activity is greatly influenced by hormones. Growth hormone is considered the major stimulus to bone growth and is an important regulator in the growth of young children (Ackermann, 1992; Rhoades & Pflanzer, 1996). Around puberty, the epiphyseal plates of long bones begin to stop responding to hormonal stimulus (Rhoades & Pflanzer, 1996). When adult height is reached, the epiphyseal plate is sealed from the marrow by a thin plate of bone (Ackermann, 1992). Bone formation is now complete, and the process of **bone remodeling** begins.

Collagen The principle substance in connecting fibers and tissues, and in bones.

Resorption The loss of substance (bone, in this case) through physiological or pathological means.

Osteoblasts Bone-forming cells.

Osteocytes A bone cell responsible for the maintenance and turnover of the mineral content of surrounding bone.

Osteoclasts A cell in developing bone concerned especially with the breaking down of unnecessary bone parts.

Remodeling The ongoing dual processes of bone formation and bone resorption after cessation of growth.

2. Three types of cells are involved in bone formation and resorption: osteoblasts, osteocytes, and osteoclasts.

Bone Remodeling

Bones are remodeled throughout our lives to meet the stresses of growth and everyday living. The skeleton provides a reservoir for minerals that are to be reabsorbed into the circulation. Calcium and phosphate are the two chief minerals balanced by the process of remodeling. All cells require calcium and phosphate for proper functioning and well-being. When circulating calcium falls below adequate levels to maintain cells, osteoclasts work to dissolve the minerals from bone to be reabsorbed into the system. Through remodeling, bone structure and density are modified (Boskey, Wright & Blank, 1999). Remodeling is the lifelong renewal process to preserve the mechanical integrity of the skeleton. It is the continuous removal of bone followed by synthesis of new bone matrix and mineralization (Ng et al., 1997). Bone strength, organizational patterns of the minerals, and organic components determine the mass of bone. Maintaining adequate levels of nutrients for the renewal of bone is an important component of good health. Inherited alterations of collagen synthesis and nutritional factors can alter bone density and bone mechanical process (Boskey et al., 1999).

Bone health is one more example of the importance of balance within the body. Bone formation must occur at the same rate as bone resorption to preserve bone mass and shape. It is when this balance is altered—bone formation is not meeting the rate of bone resorption—that pathologic conditions such as osteoporosis ensue (Ng et al., 1997).

3. To maintain bone mass, bone formation must be at the same rate as bone resorption.

Bone remodeling can be triggered by mechanical forces (trauma), and by hormonal responses to changes in calcium and phosphorous levels (Raisz, 1999). Many systemic hormones regulate calcium; however, estrogen is probably the most important hormone in bone maintenance because it produces a decrease in bone formation and remodeling and at the same time increases bone mass (Raisz, 1999).

NUTRITION AND PHYSICAL ACTIVITY FOR BONE HEALTH

To achieve optimal bone health, and to continue to build new bone as you get older, good nutrition and consistent physical activity are necessary.

Nutritional Recommendations

Good nutrition is not only critical for strong bones but also for proper functioning of the heart, muscles, and nerves. Nutrients that are key for bone health are calcium and vitamins D and C.

Calcium Intake Calcium balance is important for achieving peak bone mass and maintaining that bone mass throughout your life. Bone contains 99 percent of the body's calcium (Ng et al., 1997). Calcium is considered essential in the diet regardless of gender or age, and may be particularly beneficial in the diet of children, adolescents, and young adults to ensure maximal bone density at maturity (Finn, 1987). When calcium levels are low, the body compensates by adjusting serum calcium levels at the expense of skeletal calcium (Finn, 1987). Table 10.1 contains the dietary recommendations for calcium established by the National Institutes of Health (NIH).

After the age of 35, women lose calcium at the rate of 25 milligrams per day. After menopause, they lose 50 milligrams per day until, by age 65, there is a cumulative bone loss of 410 grams. This equates to 40 percent of the 1000 grams of total body cal-

TABLE 10.1 Optimal Calcium Requirements

The preferred source of calcium is through calcium-rich foods such as dairy products. Calcium-fortified foods and calcium supplements are other means by which optimal calcium intake can be reached in those who cannot meet their need by ingesting conventional foods.

GROUP	OPTIMAL DAILY INTAKE (IN MG OF CALCIUM)
Infant	
Birth-–6 months	400
6 months–1 year	600
Children	
1–5 years	800
6–10 years	800–1200
Adolescents/Young Adults	
11–24 years	1200–1500
Men	
25–65 years	1000
Over 65 years	1500
Women	
25–50 years	1000
Over 50 years (postmenopausal)	
With estrogen replacement	1500
Without estrogen replacement	1000
Over 65 years	1500
Pregnant and nursing	1200–1500

SOURCE: NIH Consensus Development Panel on Optimal Calcium Intake. (1994). NIH concensus conference on optimal calcium intake. *JAMA* 272:1942–1948.

cium in the young adult (Marcus, 1982). There is, however, a level of toxicity associated with calcium intake. Most people may tolerate up to 2000 milligrams per day without consequence, but this amount is not recommended and appears unnecessary. An increase in calcium intake during the critical time between menarche and late adolescence will aid in achieving optimal bone density, which is thought to reduce the risk of future osteoporosis (Wardlaw, 1993).

Explore www.pahconnection.com 10.1

Calcium Sources The largest source of calcium is milk and dairy products. Many foods contain calcium, but the amounts of calcium and the absorption rates vary. Dairy foods provide approximately 73 percent of the daily calcium needed (Gerrior & Bernie, 1997). Fruits, vegetables, and grains also provide calcium, but at a much lower level. For example, it would take 7.75 cups of spinach to yield the same amount of calcium as 1 cup of milk.

Engage www.pahconnection.com 10.1

It is difficult for most Americans to achieve optimal calcium intake exclusively from fruits, vegetables, and grains. Calcium-fortified foods and/or supplements may be instrumental in providing adequate calcium for individuals who choose not to eat dairy products (NIH Osteoporosis and Related Bone Diseases Resource Center, 1999). The amount you need depends on how much you obtain through food sources. Two commonly available calcium compounds used as supplements are calcium carbonate and

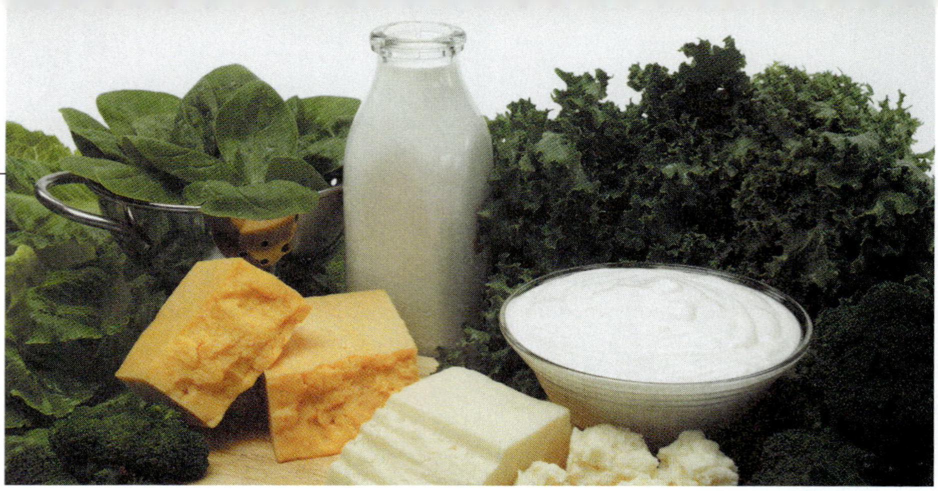

Good nutrition is essential for optimal bone health.

calcium citrate. All calcium supplements are absorbed better when taken in small doses several times during the day, versus one large dose one time a day.

Vitamin D Vitamin D is essential to the absorption of calcium and bone metabolism. Vitamin D can be obtained in two ways: sunlight and diet (NIH Osteoporosis and Related Bone Diseases Resource Center, 1999). It is readily available through 15 minutes of exposure to sunshine daily. Through your diet, the consumption of egg yolks, liver, saltwater fish, and vitamin D–fortified dairy products can provide the recommended daily amounts (between 400 and 800 IU). It is not recommended to take more (unless prescribed by your physician), as massive doses may be harmful.

Vitamin C Vitamin C is essential in collagen formation. When the body lacks vitamin C, premature collagen fibers are secreted into the bone (Weber, 1999). Collagen fibers could be likened to to steel cables within a cement wall—they lend strength to the structure. With weakened collagen, bones are brittle and may easily fracture.

"Bone Robbers" You need not only be aware of nutrients that build strong bones but must also be aware of substances that deplete nutrients from your body, referred to as "bone robbers" (McIlwain & Bruce, 1998). Common bone robbers are sodium, protein, and caffeine. A diet high in sodium and protein may cause increased urinary loss and a negative calcium balance. Coffees and colas containing caffeine may be bone robbers of concern today. A diet with a high caffeine intake also causes loss of bone calcium. Recent studies suggest that excessive caffeine intake may contribute to osteoporosis.

Weight-bearing activity is key for maintaining bone density.

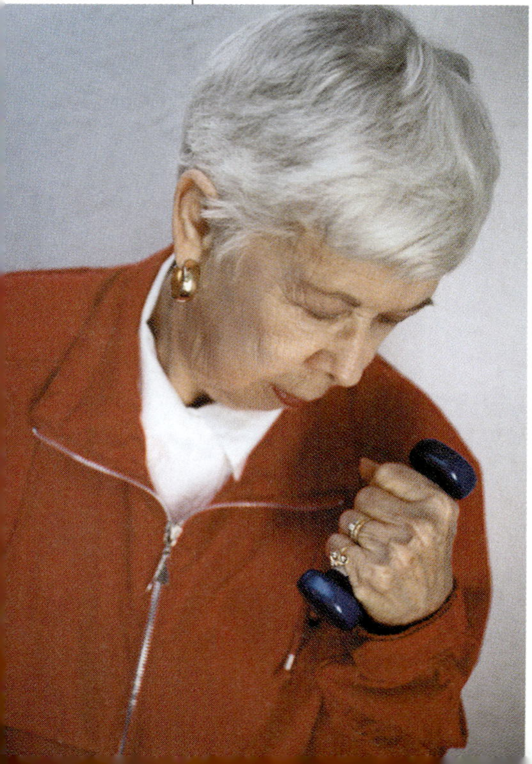

Physical Activity Recommendations

Many studies have investigated the role of physical activity and bone health and reported that physical activity is necessary for bone acquisition and maintenance throughout adulthood (Osteoporosis Prevention, Diagnosis, & Therapy, 2000). The effects of physical activity on bone may result in increased bone enzyme activity, increased breaking strength, or inhibition of bone growth under high-intensity training programs (Foss & Keteyian, 1998). Bone mineral deposition as a result of weight-bearing activity is specific to the site bearing the mechanical load. For example, an Olympic long jumper would be expected to have greater bone mineral density of the femur than a swimmer. Tennis players should present with more forearm bone mass than nonplayers. Physical training also increases the breaking strength of both ligaments and tendons. Not only have ligaments and tendons been shown to strengthen, but attachments to bones (junction strength) have also shown to increase after training (Foss & Keteyian, 1998). This research suggests that through regular weight-bearing exercise our bodies can sustain greater stresses, and we can reduce our risk of injury.

The intensity of training and exercise is dependent on the purpose of the regimen. For osteoporosis, low-impact aerobic exercises and exercises aimed specifically at improving balance, such as tai chi, are useful (Juby, 1999). Postural retraining teaches the proper ways to bend and lift. Immobilization should be avoided because it can result in increased calcium excretion and bone loss. It is recognized that when a body region is paralyzed or immobilized, the bones involved atrophy (Meunier, 1998). Using bone is important for its maintenance. However, moving around may be especially difficult for those with chronic pain and recurrent fractures. Community exercise programs are important for encouraging the elderly to continue to exercise (Juby, 1999).

Using strength training machines, or lifting weights, strengthens bones. While strength training is a slow process, it is an important component of an exercise program. Layne and Nelson (1999) reviewed numerous studies that looked at physical activity and bone health. Resistance training was shown to be positively associated with **bone mineral density (BMD).**

Sharkey, Williams, and Guerin (2000) suggest that the main objective of physical activity is to delay the onset of osteoporosis and prevent fractures. Ideally, physical activity early in life may build greater amounts of bone that will take longer to be resorbed—whereas, physical activity later in life may provide the stimulus to maintain current bone density.

OSTEOPOROSIS

Osteoporosis, literally meaning "porous bones," is a metabolic disease characterized by excessive skeletal fragility, as noted earlier. Bone loss is so common that most people consider it a normal process of aging. However, osteoporosis is a preventable and unnecessary occurrence in most individuals (McIlwain, Bruce, Silverfield, & Burnette, 1988).

The onset of osteoporosis occurs most often in women after menopause. As the U.S. population ages, the incidence of osteoporosis will increase, with a subsequent increase in cost to the healthcare industry. Since osteoporosis is a painful and debilitating disease that lowers a person's quality of life, prevention and early treatment are important issues for all ages. Some changes in bone health are considered permanent; therefore, prevention becomes the primary "cure" for osteoporosis (Figure 10.1).

4. Osteoporosis is excessive bone loss that can be prevented.

Bone mineral density (BMD) Usually expressed as the amount of mineralized tissue in the scanned area, it is a risk factor for fractures.

Osteoporosis Literally means "porous bones"; a metabolic disease resulting in bone loss and bones that fracture easily.

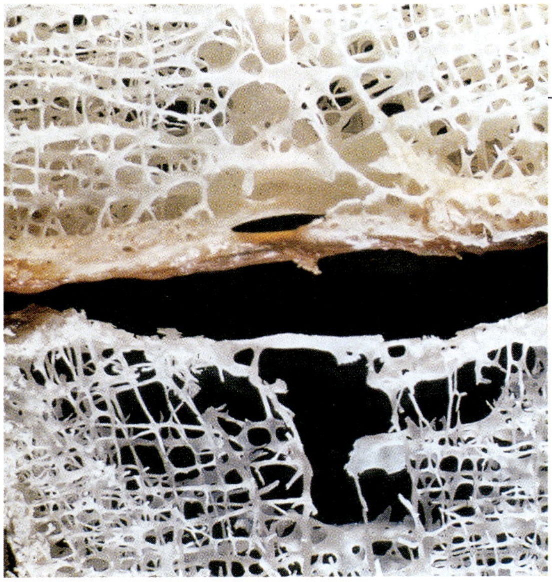

FIGURE 10.1

Osteoporosis. Microscopically, normal bone (top) is much stronger than osteoporotic bone (bottom).

Explore 10.2 www.pahconnection.com

Experience 10.1 www.pahconnection.com

Postmenopausal osteoporotic individuals undergo a high rate of bone turnover. Osteoblastic activity cannot meet the rate of osteoclastic bone resorption. Bones are thin and brittle due to the loss of mineralization. The decreased bone mass puts the individual at an increased risk for fracture, most often fractures of the hip, spine, and wrist (Figure 10.2).

The annual cost of osteoporosis in the United States is estimated to be $14 billion (Woodhead & Moss, 1998). Currently, 10 million Americans are affected, and 18 million more have low bone mass, placing them at risk for osteoporosis (Osteoporosis Prevention, Diagnosis and Therapy, 2000). This cost of osteoporosis is expected to increase over the next decades due to the overall aging of the population. Part of the cost of osteoporosis is related to the morbidity of the disease. Only 50 percent of individuals who suffer a hip fracture are able to return home or live independently after injury, and the estimated cost of hip fractures could reach $240 billion by the year 2040.

Osteoporosis affects both men and women, however 80 percent of those affected are women. While postmenopausal women may exhibit bone loss due to estrogen deficiency, men entering their older years may develop osteoporosis due to testosterone deficiency. Men may be treated with testosterone therapy; however, this treatment puts them at a risk for enlargement of the prostate (Francis, 1999).

Researchers suggest there may be a link between sodium/calcium intake and bone density. There appears to be an increase in bone resorption with elevated sodium. Thus, reducing sodium intake may not only reduce the risk of cardiovascular disease but also osteoporosis (Mizushim, Tsuchida & Yamori, 1999).

Since osteoporosis is often not diagnosed until fractures occur, prevention is considered the most cost-effective approach. Prevention focuses on two main objectives: (1) achieving optimal bone density in the first two to three decades of life, and (2) maintaining bone density and decreasing rate of bone loss in later years. Physical activity and good nutrition are key elements in meeting these preventive strategies.

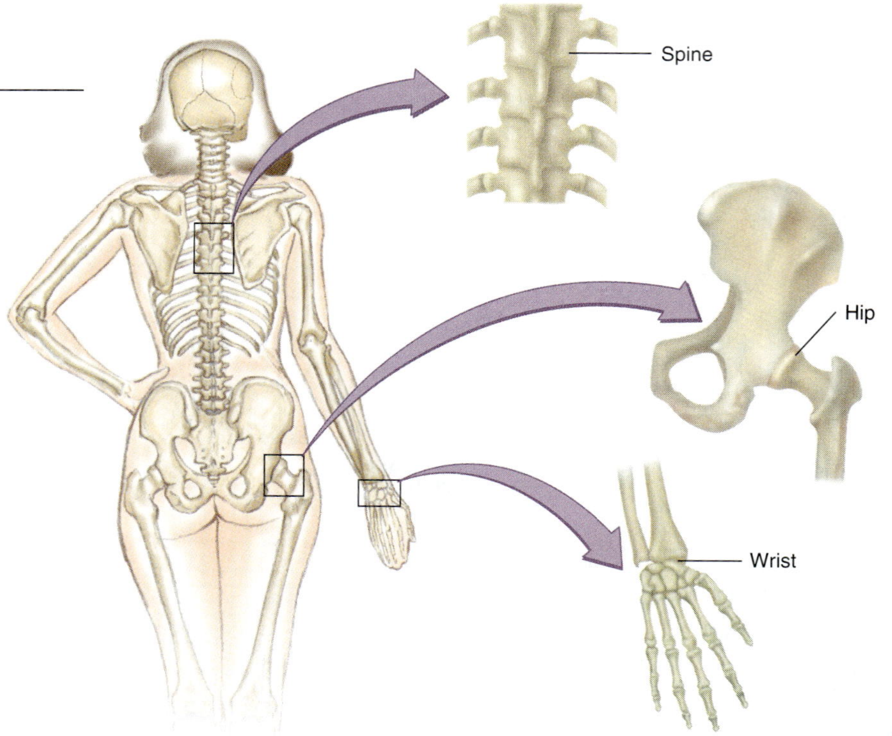

FIGURE 10.2

Postmenopausal Risk for Fracture.
The wrist, spine, and hip are easily fractured in someone with osteoporosis.

Risk Factors

The many risk factors that influence osteoporosis can be grouped into four categories: genetic, hormonal, nutritional, and lifestyle factors.

5. Osteoporosis can be affected by genetic, hormonal, nutritional, and lifestyle factors.

Genetic Factors Race, heredity, and gender influence bone fragility. Typically, white and Asian women are at greater risk for developing osteoporosis and related fractures (Juby, 1999); Hispanic and black women have greater bone mineral density (BMD) and are at less risk for developing osteoporosis (however, they are still at some risk). In addition, women with a family history of osteoporosis are considered to be at increased risk. Daughters of women with spinal fractures generally have lower BMD in the spine. Although most research has focused on the mother's history of osteoporosis, research shows that the father's history is also important (Matkovic, Fontana, Tominac, Goel, & Chesnut, 1990). Furthermore, women with relatives who have a dowager's hump or have incurred low trauma fractures have a positive family history of osteoporosis (Lappe, 1994).

Gender also plays a major role in bone fragility. The prevalence of osteoporosis and related fractures is substantially greater in women than in men. This is a result of lower bone mass and bone density among women. Why? Men have larger skeletons; their bone loss starts later in life and progresses more slowly; and they do not experience menopause.

Hormonal Factors Hormonal status greatly influences bone fragility, and menstrual history is a key component. Risk of bone fragility also increases for women after menopause because bone loss accelerates with reduction in estrogen production (Woodhead & Moss, 1998). Hormonal changes of menopause cause the loss of about 11 percent of bone during the first 5 years after menopause and an additional 5 percent during the next 20 years (Nordin, Need, Chatteron, Horowitz, & Morris, 1990). Men with hypogonadism are at special risk for bone loss.

Hypogonadism is a failure of the testes to function normally. It is treated with replacement testosterone therapy.

Amenorrhea is a condition associated with BMD that may result from excessive exercise or eating disorders. Achieving high bone mineral density is critical during adolescence, but amenorrhea lowers estrogen levels, which can cause a loss of bone mass and increase the risk of osteoporosis later in life. Amenorrhea in young women is of concern because achieving peak bone mass in the second and third decades seems to be an important indicator for lifetime fracture risk (Wardlaw, 1993.) While physical activity may affect estrogen hormone levels and indirectly affect bone density, low body fat is more likely the culprit.

Estrogen and other sex hormones have been reported to stimulate osteoblastic activity weakly (Wardlaw, 1993). Estrogens are female sex hormones that are responsible for the development and maintenance of a woman's secondary sex characteristics (development of breasts, for example), and following menstruation, estrogens stimulate the rebuilding of the uterine lining. Ovaries are the primary source of estrogen. Estrogens are probably the most important hormone controlling bone mass loss. Estrogens inhibit bone resorption by modifying osteoclast function (McCaw, 1999). Estrogen replacement therapy is one treatment used to prevent the onset of osteoporosis; however, its many side effects make it an unpopular treatment for many women.

A condition referred to as *female athlete triad* is chronic overexercising accompanied by disordered eating, amenorrhea, and osteoporosis (Beck & Shoemaker, 2000). Chronic overexercising has been associated with reduced bone mass in premenopausal women. The overexercising and unbalanced diet disrupts the body's hormones enough to impair the influence of estrogens on the skeletal system. Despite the weight-bearing exercise, the lack of estrogen accelerates bone resorption and bone loss.

Amenorrhea Absence of menstrual periods.

Nutritional Factors As noted earlier, a general well-balanced diet is recommended, with special attention to adequate calcium, vitamin C, and vitamin D.

Lifestyle Factors Another risk factor for osteoporosis is physical inactivity. Prolonged inactivity decreases bone mass. Regular exercise has been shown to stimulate bone formation and retard bone mass reduction (Goodman, 1987). Studies also support the principle that weight-bearing exercise can promote and preserve bone strength (Katz & Sherman, 1998).

A multimodal exercise program involving both weight-bearing aerobic exercise and resistance training is part of optimal osteoporosis management (Katz & Sherman, 1998). Brisk walking is an ideal weight-bearing exercise for someone with osteoporosis. The full benefits of walking come from a regular walking schedule, 3 or 4 days per week for at least 15–20 minutes. Kannus (1999) best summarizes physical activity and osteoporosis: "Overall, the evidence strongly suggests that regular physical activity, especially if started early in childhood and adolescence, is the only cheap, safe, readily available, and largely acceptable way of both improving bone strength and reducing the propensity to fall (p. 205)."

Experience www.pahconnection.com 10.2

Engage www.pahconnection.com 10.2

Use of cigarettes, alcohol, and certain medications (for example, long-term use of glucocorticoids in treating arthritis, asthma, lupus and other diseases of the lungs, kidneys, and liver) also affect bone mass negatively. Women who smoke cigarettes experience an earlier menopause, a higher incidence of vertebral compression fractures, a decreased bone mineral density, and a lower urinary estrogen level (Daniell, 1976). Alcohol abuse, a lifestyle factor, has devastating effects on bone mass. On average, alcoholics exhibit low BMD and a subsequent increased risk of fracture (Wardlaw, 1993). First, alcohol is thought to depress bone formation by directly reducing osteoblastic activity. Second, dietary intakes of heavy drinkers are often lacking in essential nutrients. Finally, alcohol intoxication gives rise to social situations that favor accidents and falls (Laiteinen & Valimaki, 1991).

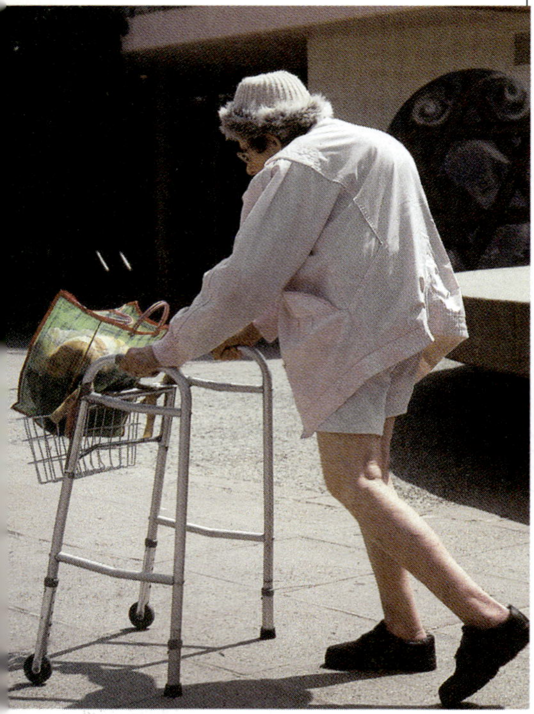

FIGURE 10.3

Spinal Osteoporosis. Osteoporosis is characterized by loss of stature.

Prevention and Detection of Osteoporosis

By the age of 20, most women have built 98 percent of their bone mass (Fishman, 2000). A healthy lifestyle, which includes no smoking, limited alcohol consumption, weight-bearing exercise, and a well-balanced diet, is important in preventing osteoporosis. In the past, osteoporosis was often not diagnosed until a fracture occurred. Today, with a better understanding of osteoporosis, measures can be taken to detect bone density early.

Osteoporosis diagnosis often begins with a thorough physical examination, which includes an oral history, recording of complaints of height loss, a review of overall nutrition and medication intake, and observations of stature, carriage, and spine curvature (Woodhead & Moss, 1998). Spinal osteoporosis is often characterized by loss of stature (Figure 10.3).

Bone Mineral Density (BMD) Tests Bone mineral density tests measure bone density in various body sites, the hip, spine, wrist, finger, kneecap, shinbone, and heel. A bone density test can detect osteoporosis before a fracture occurs, predict your risk of fracturing in the future, and determine your rate of bone loss and/or monitor the effect of treatment. The test is conducted at intervals of 1 year.

The BMD tests vary in the type of bone measured (trabecular, cortical, or both), precision (deviation based on multiple measurements, generally represented on a percentage basis as a coefficient of variation), accuracy (variation in quality of bone measured versus real content of bone), and radiation dose (Black, Cummings, Genant, Nevitt, Palermo, & Browner, 1992) (Table 10.2).

What do your BMD test results mean? A normal bone density is called a "T-score" (Figure 10.4). This means you have the bone density of a normal young adult and have no risk for fractures. The World Health Organization (WHO) (1994) has established the following mineral density diagnostic criteria for women who have experienced no fragility fractures. These criteria provide a basic diagnostic framework:

- Normal bone mineral density is within 1 standard deviation (SD) of the young adult mean.
- **Osteopenia,** or low bone mass, is a bone mineral density between 1 and 2.5 SD of the young adult mean.
- Osteoporosis is defined as a value greater than 2.5 SD below the young adult mean.

Standard deviation is a measure of variation in a distribution.

Osteopenia Low bone mass.

TABLE 10.2 Types of BMD Tests

ACRONYM	NAME	MEASURES
DXA	Dual-energy X-ray absorptiometry	Spine, hip, or total body
SXA	Single-energy X-ray absorptiometry	Wrist or heel
RA	Radiographic absorptiometry	Uses an X-ray of the hand and a small metal wedge to calculate bone
DPA	Dual photon absorptiometry	Spine, hip, or total body
SPA	Single photon absorptiometry	Wrist
QCT	Quantitative computed tomography	Wrist

FIGURE 10.4

Bone Mass Density T-Scores. The lower the T-score, the higher the likelihood of osteoporosis. The photos show bone mass density in women of varying ages.

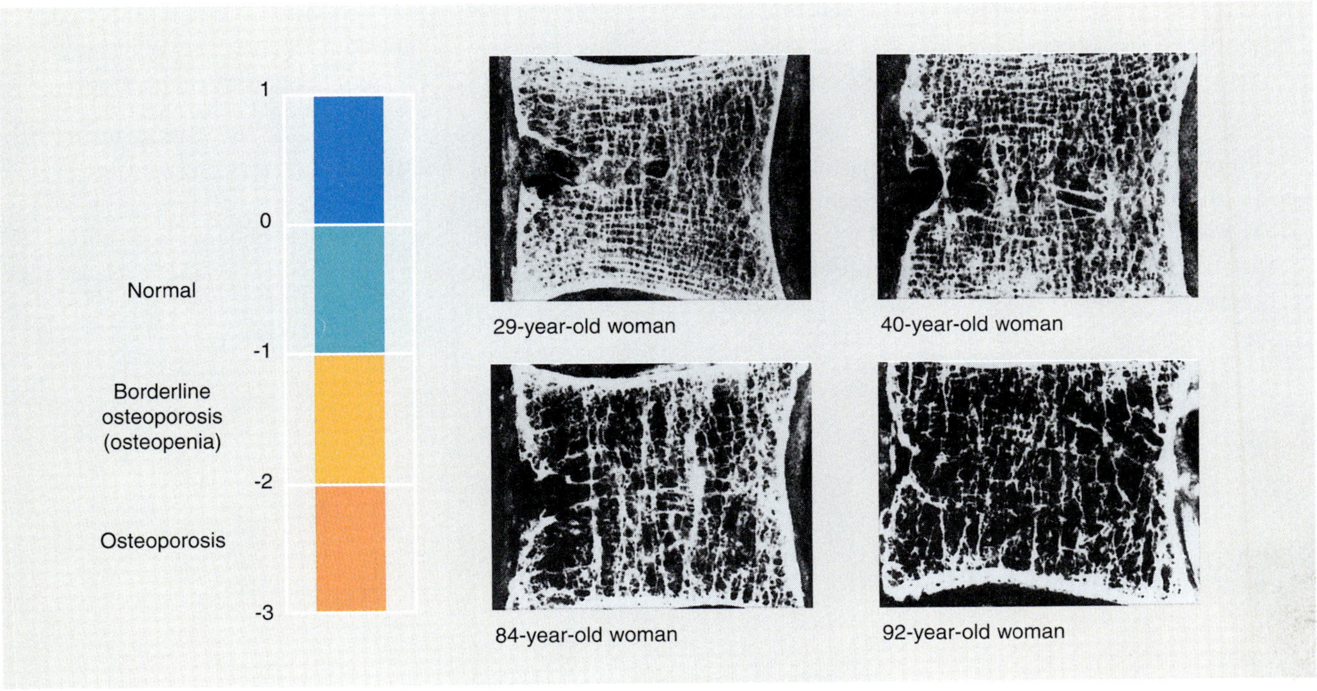

PHYSICAL ACTIVITY AND HEALTH CONNECTION

Maintaining optimal bone health requires a healthy lifestyle that includes a balanced diet and a healthy physical activity program. A diet that pays close attention to calcium intake through dairy and other foods is important. If the diet does not contain enough calcium naturally, calcium supplements may be needed.

Bone is a living tissue that responds to exercise by becoming more dense and stronger. Weight-bearing and resistance exercises increase bone mass and density. Therefore, weight-bearing physical activities (dancing, walking) and resistance activities (weight lifting, swimming) are essential for improving and maintaining optimal bone health.

CONCEPT CONNECTION

1. **Bones do more than provide structural support.** Bones contain cells that help form blood cells, store fat, and release and absorb calcium. Bone formation and remodeling are important factors in understanding the development, treatment, and prevention of osteoporosis.
2. **Three types of cells are involved in bone formation and resorption: osteoblasts, osteocytes, and osteoclasts.** *Osteoblasts* are immature cells that when surrounded by mature bone cells become osteocyctes. *Osteoclasts* absorb bony tissue.
3. **To maintain bone mass, bone formation must occur at the same rate as bone resorption. Bone remodeling is the lifelong renewal process of the skeletal system.** This process allows for bone to be removed and new bone generated. This process of new bone forming at the same rate as resorption is critical, because without this balance osteoporosis can take place.
4. **Osteoporosis is excessive bone loss that can be prevented.** Although considered by many as part of the aging process, osteoporosis can be prevented. Millions of Americans suffer from osteoporosis and the bone fractures that result from osteoporosis. Optimal physical activity and nutrition habits when young are key elements to an osteoporosis prevention program.
5. **Osteoporosis can be affected by genetic, hormonal, nutritional, and lifestyle factors.** Recognizing common osteoporosis risk facts will help in understanding effective prevention strategies and will be useful in decreasing the incidence and prevalence of osteoporosis.

TERMS

Cartilage, 222
Collagen, 223
Resorption, 223
Osteoblasts, 223
Osteocytes, 223
Osteoclasts, 223
Remodeling, 224
Bone mineral density (BMD), 227
Osteoporosis, 227
Amenorrhea, 229
Osteopenia, 231

MAKING THE CONNECTION

Julie now knows that, while her bones may seem to be rigid and unchanging, they are actually more like muscles, capable of strengthening with use or weakening without use. Each time a bone is moved, it bends ever so slightly, just enough to stimulate electrical and biochemical changes that stimulate bone formation. The more force, the greater the bending, the greater the stimulus for new bone formation (up to a point). In addition to maintaining the Recommended Daily Intake (RDI) for calcium, Julie knows that a regular physical activity program keeps the density of bone constant or contributes to increased bone mass. Julie now understands that the threat of osteoporosis doesn't just come from a low calcium intake, but from a sedentary lifestyle.

CRITICAL THINKING

1. Like Julia, many people do not understand that both physical inactivity and low calcium intake are key factors in the development of osteoporosis. You have been asked by a local ninth-grade health teacher to explain to her students the importance of physical activity and nutrition in preventing osteoporosis (a condition that is the last thing on most ninth-graders' minds). In 250 words or less, explain their importance.
2. Review the factors that affect osteoporosis (genetic, hormonal, nutritional, and lifestyle). Review your family history to determine if you are at risk of osteoporosis. Then select two other factors and, based on your current behaviors, decide what behaviors you could change that would assist in preventing osteoporosis. List them.
3. "Physical activity and nutrition are key elements in achieving optimal bone density during the first 20 to 30 years of life and maintaining bone density throughout life." Provide information that supports that statement.

REFERENCES

Ackermann, U. (1992). *Essentials of Human Physiology.* St. Louis: Mosby–Year Book.

Beck, B.R., & Shoemaker, M.R. (2000). Osteoporosis: Understanding key risk factors and therapeutic options. *The Physician and Sportsmedicine* 28(2): 69ff.

Black, D.M., et al. (1992). Axial and appendicular bone density predict fractures in older women. *Journal of Bone Mineral Research* 7(6):633–38.

Boskey, A.L., Wright, T.M., & Blank, R.D. (1999). Collagen and bone strength. *Journal of Bone and Mineral Research 14*(3):330–35.

Daniell, H. (1976). Osteoporosis of the slender smoker. Vertebral compression fractures and loss of metacarpal cortex in relation to postmenopausal cigarette smoking and lack of obesity. *Archives of Internal Medicine 136*(3):298–304.

Finn, S. (1987). Osteoporosis and nutrition. *American Association of Occupational Health Nurses 35*(12):536–37.

Fishman, T.D. (March 2000). Osteoporosis and other metabolic bone diseases. *Podiatry Medicine,* pp. 111–18.

Foss, M., & Keteyian, S.J. (1998). *Fox's Physiological Basis for Exercise and Sport.* New York: McGraw-Hill.

Francis, R.M. (1999). The effects of testosterone on osteoporosis in men. *Clinical Endocrinology 50*(4): 411–14.

Gerrior, S., & Bernie, L. (1997). Nutrient content of the U.S. food supply: 1909–1994. Home Economics Research Report No. 53. Washington, DC: U.S. Department of Agriculture.

Goodman, C. (1987). Osteoporosis and physical activity. *American Association of Occupational Health Nurses 35*(12):539–42.

Juby, A. (1999). Managing elderly people's osteoporosis. *Canadian Family Physician 45*:1526–36.

Kannus, P. (1999). Preventing osteoporosis, falls, and fractures among elderly people. *British Medical Journal 318*:205-206.

Katz, W.A., & Sherman, C. (1998). Osteoporosis: The role of exercise in optimal management. *The Physician and Sportsmedicine, 26*(2):33–42.

Laiteinen, K., & Valimaki, M. (1991). Alcohol and bone. *Calcified Tissue International 49*(suppl):S70–S73.

Lappe, J. (1994). Bone fragility: Assessment of risk and strategies for prevention. *Journal of Obstetric, Gynecologic, and Neonatal Nursing* 23(3):260–68.

Layne, J.E., & Nelson, M.E. (1999). The effects of progressive resistance training on bone density: A review. *Medicine and Science in Sports and Exercise 31*(1):25–30.

Marcus, R. (1982). The relationship between dietary calcium to the maintenance of skeletal integrity in man: An interface of endocrinology and nutrition. *Metabolism: Clinical and Experimental 31*(1):93–102.

Matkovic, V., Fontana, D., Tominac, C., Goel, P., & Chestnut, C.H. (1990). Factors that influence peak bone mass formation: A study of calcium balance and the inheritance of bone mass in adolescent females. *American Journal of Clinical Nutrition* 52(5):878–84.

McCaw, S.T. (1999). Aging, osteoarthritis, and osteoprosisis: A teaching packet. Normal, IL: Illinois State University.

McIlwain, H.H., Bruce, D.F., Silverfield, J.C., & Burnette, M.C. (1988). *Osteoporosis: Prevention, Management, Treatment.* Toronto: Wiley.

McIlwain, H.H., & Bruce, D.F. (1998). *The Osteoporosis Cure.* New York:Avon.

Meunier, P.J. (1998). *Osteoporosis: Diagnosis and Management.* London: Martin Dunitz.

Mizushim, S., Tsuchida, K., & Yamori, Y. (1999). Preventive nutritional factors in epidemiology: Interaction between sodium and calcium. *Clinical and Experimental Pharmacology and Physiology 26*(7):573–75.

National Institutes of Health Osteoporosis and Related Bone Diseases National Resource Center (1999). *Calcium and vitamin D: Important at every age.* Washington, DC.

Ng, K.W., Romas, E., Donnan, L., & Findlay, D.M. (1997). Bone biology. *Bailliere's Clinical Endocrinology and Metabolism 11*(1):1–22.

Nordin, C., Need, A., Chatterton, B., Horowitz, & Morris, H. (1990). The relative contributions of age and years since menopause to postmenopausal bone loss. *Journal of Clinical Endocrinology 70*(1):83–88.

Osteoporosis Prevention, Diagnosis, and Therapy (2000). NIH Consensus Statement, March 27-29; [Online] http://odp.od.gov/consensus/cons/111/111/_statement .htm

Raisz, L.G. (1999). Physiology and pathophysiology of bone remodeling. *Clinical Chemistry 45*(8):1353–58.

Rhoades, R., & Pflanzer, R. (1996). *Human Physiology.* Philadelphia: W.B. Sanders.

Sharkey, N.A., Williams, N.J., & Guerin, J.B. (2000). The role of exercise in the prevention and treatment of osteoporosis and osteoarthritis. *Nursing Clinics of North America 35*(1):209–221.

Wardlaw, G.M. (1993). Putting osteoporosis in perspective. *Journal of the American Dietetic Association 93*(9): 1000–1006.

Weber, P. (1999). The role of vitamins in the prevention of osteoporosis: A brief report. *International Journal for Vitamin and Nutrition Research 69*(3):194–97.

Woodhead, G.A., & Moss, M.M. (1998). Osteoporosis: Diagnosis and prevention. *The Nurse Practitioner 23*(11):18–35.

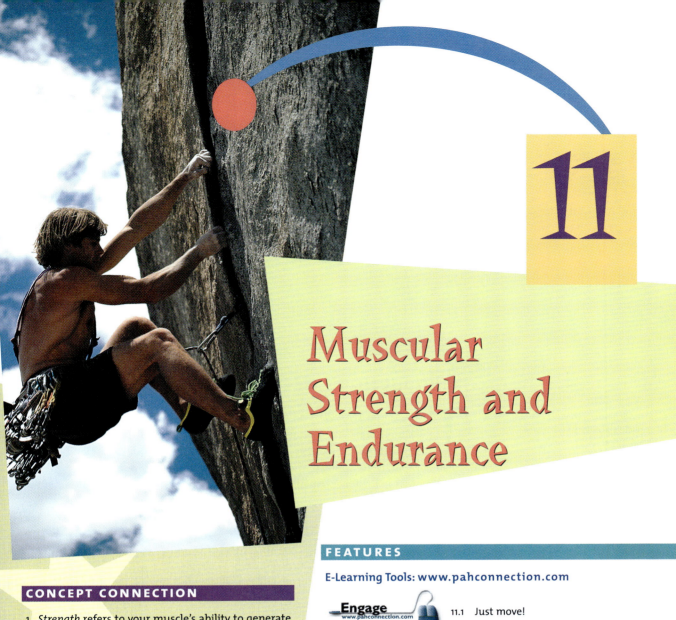

11

Muscular Strength and Endurance

CONCEPT CONNECTION

1. *Strength* refers to your muscle's ability to generate maximal force.
2. Significant health benefits are associated with resistance training.
3. Muscles that are stressed by resistance training get stronger and increase in size (hypertrophy), while muscles that are neglected get weaker and shrink in size (atrophy).
4. You can develop muscular strength and endurance through a variety of resistance training programs.
5. Individuals of any age can benefit from resistance training.

FEATURES

E-Learning Tools: www.pahconnection.com

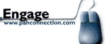

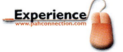

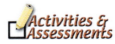

Engage www.pahconnection.com

11.1 Just move!
11.2 Strength and power assessment

Experience www.pahconnection.com

11.1 Resistance training
11.2 Resistance training for older individuals
11.3 Resistance training for youth

Explore www.pahconnection.com

11.1 General information
11.2 Fitness online
11.3 National Strength and Conditioning Association
11.4 American College of Sports Medicine (ACSM)
11.5 Sample exercises

Activities & Assessments

11.1 Finding your one-rep max for the bench press
11.2 Muscular endurance assessment for abdominal fitness

WHAT'S THE CONNECTION?

Beth wants to improve her muscular strength to lessen the possibility of developing osteoporosis as she ages. She's interested in including resistance training in her activity program. Beth has toyed with weights at the health club on occasion, but has never really been serious about performing resistance training with goals and outcomes in mind. She decides to search the Internet for information on how to get the most out of a resistance training program. Beth knows she has to be careful to screen suggestions from the Internet, but hopes she can get the information she needs.

INTRODUCTION

1. *Strength* refers to your muscle's ability to generate maximal force.

This chapter will focus on the importance of good muscular strength and endurance and their relationship to good health. It will provide information on how to assess your muscular strength and endurance and how to formulate a program to optimize the development of these important concepts.

Muscles provide the force that allows our bodies to move. As muscles contract they pull on the bones to which they are connected. The many complex physical movements of which the human body is capable are the result of this simple action. **Muscular strength** refers to your muscle's ability to generate maximal force. The stronger a muscle, the more force it can generate. **Muscular endurance** refers to a muscle's ability to sustain a given force over an extended period of time or to repeat a muscle action for several repetitions.

2. Significant health benefits are associated with resistance training.

Muscle fitness is important in many ways. Fit muscles allow us to perform the tasks of daily living with less stress; help to protect our joints from injury; aid in sport and activity performance; assist in developing and maintaining strong bones, thereby reducing the risk for osteoporosis (Chapter 10); and have a positive effect on our metabolism (Brill et al., 2000; Stone et al., 2000).

Building muscles that are strong and have good endurance can improve your health. In addition to increasing bone mineral density, regular resistance training lowers your percentage of body fat, increases your lean body mass (LBM), decreases your insulin response to changing levels of glucose, lowers your baseline insulin levels, and increases your insulin sensitivity (Pollock & Vincent, 1996). The last three factors are related to your body's ability to use sugars as fuel and aid in the prevention of diabetes. Resistance training maintains or improves your HDL levels, maintains or decreases your LDL levels, regulates your diastolic blood pressure at rest, increases your VO_2max **(circuit weight training)**, improves your endurance, improves your physiologic function, and increases your basal metabolism (Mayo & Kravitz, 1999; Pollock & Vincent, 1996). All of these factors help to insure a healthy cardiovascular system and guard against cardiovascular disease.

Muscular strength Force-generating ability of a muscle.

Muscular endurance Ability of a muscle to repeat or sustain an action.

Circuit weight training Method of training that involves moving from station to station, performing different exercises at each station.

Seniors who perform regular resistance training have discovered that it helps to improve their ability to resist falls, improves their balance, and helps to prevent (or rehabilitate) low-back pain (Pollock and Vincent, 1996). These improvements are vital in maintaining independent living.

MUSCULAR ANATOMY AND PHYSIOLOGY

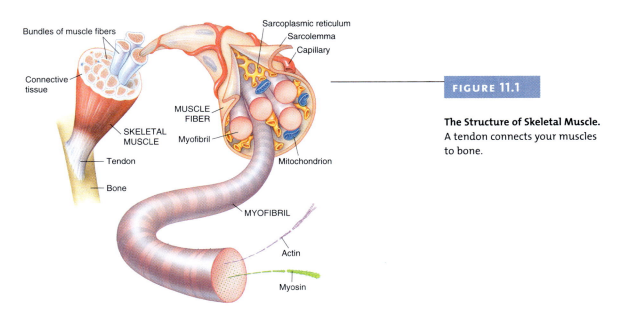

To understand how muscles get stronger and more enduring, we must look at some basic muscular anatomy and physiology. Muscles are composed of water, **protein filaments,** and several key minerals. Tendons are connective tissues that function to connect muscle to bones (Figure 11.1). The membranes that form the tendons both surround, and are a part of, the muscles. When the muscles contract, the tendons exert forces on the bones, causing the bones to moves.

Protein filaments Strands of protein (actin and myosin) that give muscle its structure and functional ability.

Actin Thin protein filament found in muscle; plays an important role in muscle movement.

Sarcomere The functional unit of a muscle. The site where muscle movement takes place.

Myosin Thick protein filament found in muscle; plays an important role in muscle movement.

Sliding Filament Theory

It is the protein filaments, located within the muscles, that cause muscle movement to occur. The filaments responsible for movement are called *actin* and *myosin*. **Actin** filaments are made of thin protein and located within the functional unit of a muscle cell, or **sarcomere. Myosin** filaments are thicker protein strands that must connect with the actin for movement to happen. Oar-like projections (myosin cross bridges) extend from the myosin and connect to active sites on the actin when the muscle is stimulated by an electrical impulse. As the muscle is stimulated, energy is released, and the connected cross bridges swivel and rotate (Figure 11.2). This pulls the actin filaments over the myosin filaments and the muscle shortens. As long as the muscle remains stimulated and energy is released, the muscle will remain in this shortened state. When the stimulus is removed, the cross bridges detach and the filaments slide back over each other until they regain their elongated, resting state. The process of protein filaments moving over the top of each other is referred to as the *sliding filament theory of muscle contraction*.

Muscle Fibers and Motor Units

The protein filaments found within our muscles join together to form muscle fibers. There are two types of muscle fibers: slow-twitch and fast-twitch. Most muscles in our body have a composition that contains both slow- and fast-twitch fibers. The function of the muscle and our genetics determine which one is available in the greater quantity.

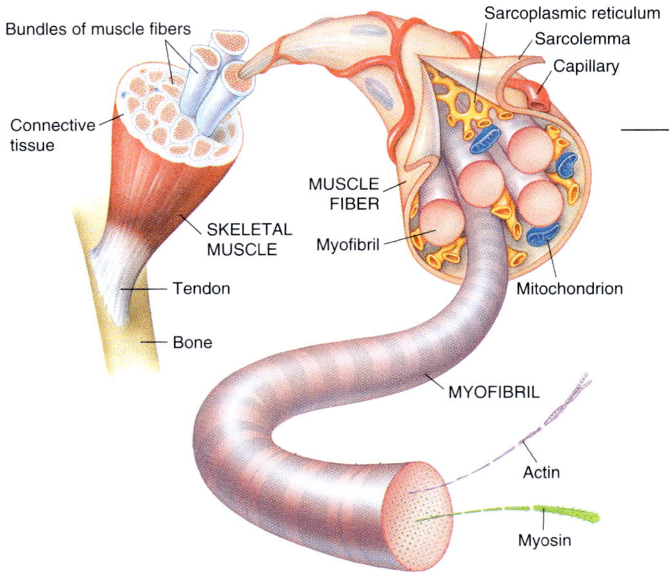

FIGURE 11.1

The Structure of Skeletal Muscle. A tendon connects your muscles to bone.

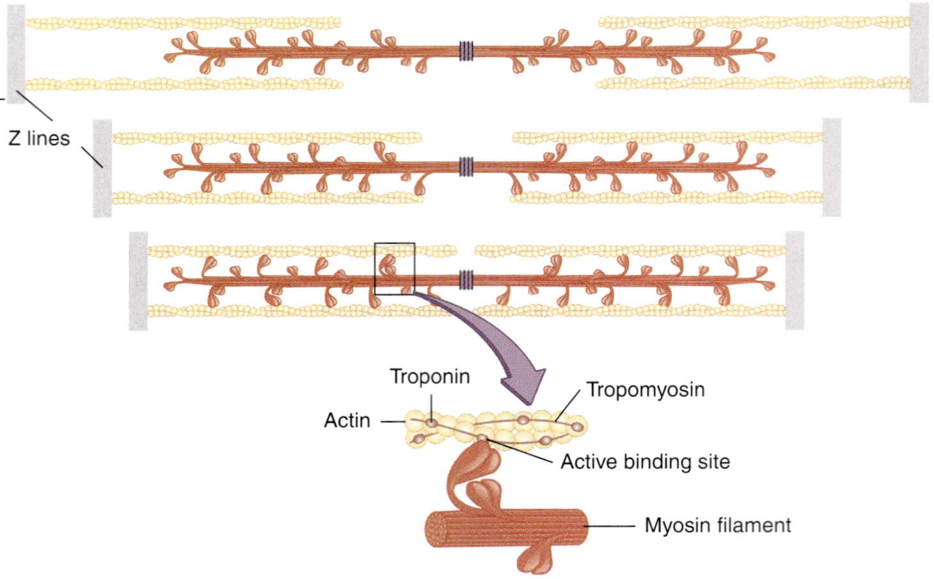

FIGURE 11.2

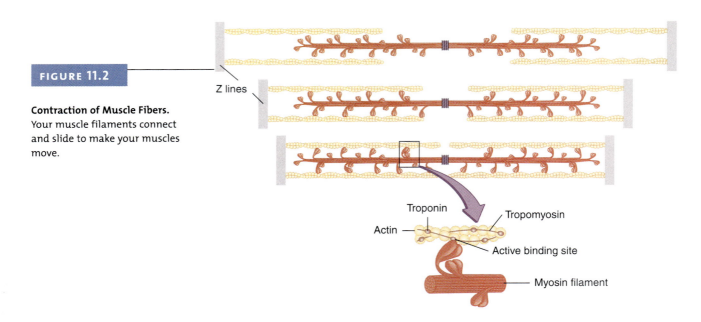

Contraction of Muscle Fibers. Your muscle filaments connect and slide to make your muscles move.

Slow-twitch fibers are endurance fibers. They have a better blood supply than fast-twitch fibers, more mitochondria (sites of energy transfer), and greater aerobic capacity. Muscles that perform aerobic activities and muscular endurance training improve the functional abilities of the slow-twitch fibers. Slow-twitch fibers allow us to perform activities for extended periods of time or to repeat an activity again and again.

Fast-twitch fibers are the power fibers. They allow us to generate a great deal of force in a short period of time. Since their blood supply is not as rich as slow-twitch fibers, fast-twitch fibers fatigue more rapidly. Sprint training and heavy resistance training develop the functional capacity of our fast-twitch fibers.

A motor unit is comprised of a nerve and all of the fibers in a muscle that are *innervated* (connected to the nervous system) by that single nerve. Some motor units contain relatively few muscle fibers. These tend to be slow-twitch motor units. Motor units that contain large numbers of muscle fibers tend to be fast-twitch motor units. The more muscle fibers in a motor unit, the greater the force-generating capacity of that motor unit. One reason fast-twitch motor units are capable of generating a great deal of power is because each motor unit contains many muscle fibers. Fast-twitch motor units also have larger nerves than do slow-twitch motor units. This allows for greater speed of conduction of the nervous impulse that controls the muscle.

Eccentric and Concentric Muscle Action

Static contraction Muscle develops tension but does not move (see also isometric).

Concentric muscle action Muscle movement in which the muscle shortens while under tension.

Eccentric muscle action Muscle movement in which the muscle lengthens while under tension.

A muscle can be in one of four states of motion. The first is the normal relaxed state in which muscle activity is at a minimum. The second is when the muscle develops tension, but does not move. This is referred to as a **static contraction.** The third is when the muscle shortens under tension. This state is called a **concentric muscle action.** For example, when you bend your arm at the elbow to lift an object from a table, your biceps brachii muscle undergoes concentric movement (Figure 11.3).

The fourth state is when the muscle lengthens under tension. This state is called an **eccentric muscle action.** For example, when you are lowering an object back to a table and controlling how fast the object is moving by regulating how slowly you allow your arm to straighten out, your biceps muscle is undergoing eccentric muscle action (Figure 11.4). Eccentric muscle action is more stressful to the muscle than concentric muscle action because the myosin cross bridges are being stretched while they are under tension (Dolezal, Potteiger, Jacobsen, & Benedict, 2000). Many people believe that eccentric muscle activity may be responsible for the soreness you sometimes feel when you do too much resistance training too soon (Dolezal et al., 2000).

Focusing the early stages of a resistance training program on proper form, using light resistance, and emphasizing the concentric portion of a lift can minimize this pain. Once the body has adapted to the stress of regular resistance training, greater emphasis may be placed on eccentric muscle action with less likelihood of pain. It has been demonstrated that eccentric resistance training is important is achieving maximal benefit from a strength training program. Eccentric muscle action adds to the total work of resistance training and the use of typical concentric-eccentric repetitions contributes to enhanced muscle strength and muscle fiber size (Kraemer, 1992).

Agonist Muscle that acts as the prime mover; the muscle most responsible for a movement.

Antagonist Muscle that resists the agonist; helps to maintain joint stability.

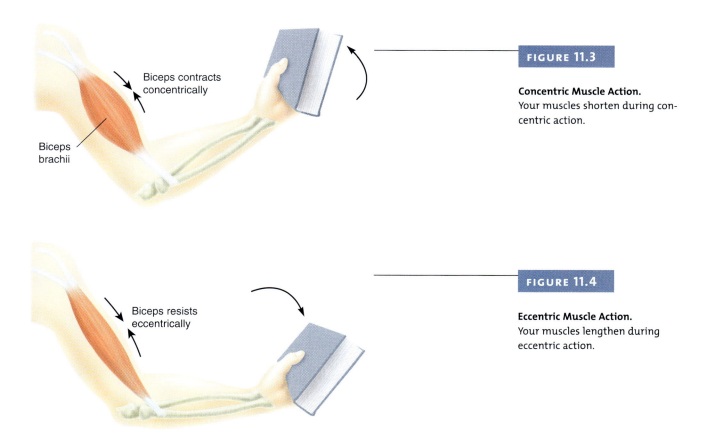

Agonists, Antagonists, Synergists, Neutralizers

Muscles can perform many different functions, depending on the demands placed upon them (Figure 11.5). If a muscle is called upon to be responsible for the primary action of a desired movement, it is called the **agonist,** or prime mover. A muscle that resists the prime mover and helps to maintain joint integrity is called an **antagonist.**

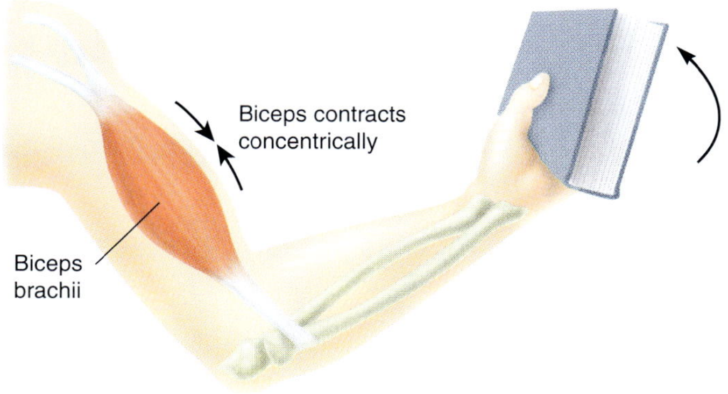

FIGURE 11.3

Concentric Muscle Action. Your muscles shorten during concentric action.

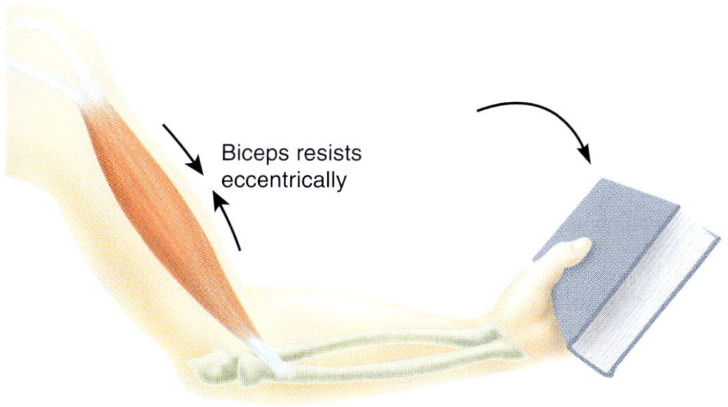

FIGURE 11.4

Eccentric Muscle Action. Your muscles lengthen during eccentric action.

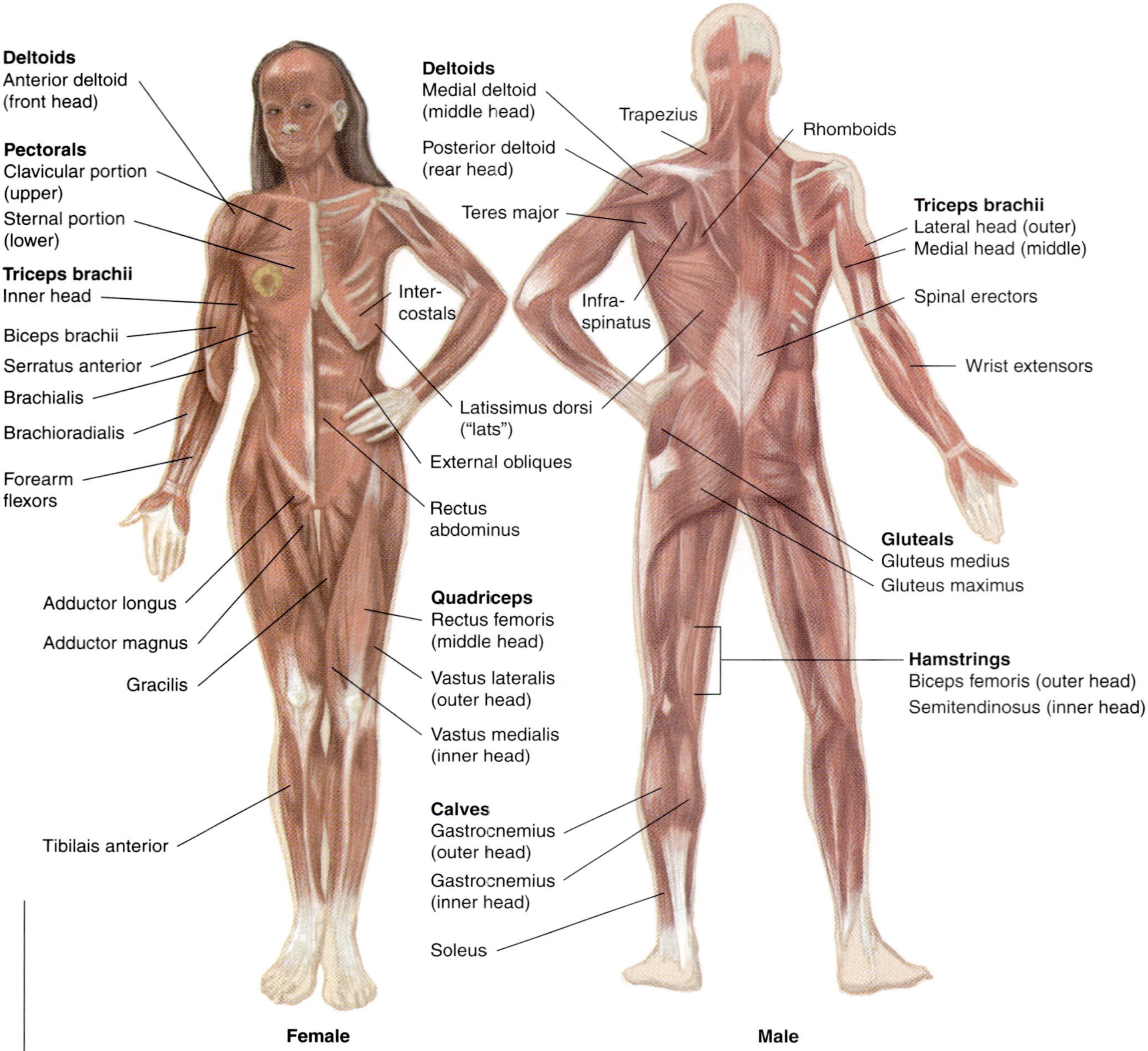

FIGURE 11.5

Muscle Groups, Front and Back.

Synergists Muscles that assist the agonist.

Neutralizer Muscle that prevents unwanted activity in muscles not directly involved in performing a movement.

If we look at the example of raising a glass from a table, the biceps muscles of the upper arm that cause the arm to bend at the elbow would be considered the agonists. The triceps muscles in the back of the upper arm resist the biceps and help keep the elbow from dislocating. In this scenario, the triceps would be acting as an antagonist.

Muscles can also act as **synergists** if they assist the agonist, but are not primarily responsible for carrying out the movement. In the above example, the brachial radialis (a muscle that crosses the elbow and connects to the forearm) would act as a synergist. A **neutralizer**, or fixator, is a muscle whose action prevents unwanted activities of muscles not directly involved in the movement you wish to carry out. For example, the abdominal muscles frequently act as neutralizers to support the spinal column when the arm is bent at the elbow.

GETTING STRONGER, BUILDING SIZE, TONING UP

In order for muscles to become stronger, they must regularly be exposed to more stress than they are exposed to under normal resting conditions. A stronger muscle is one that can produce more force. Muscles that are stressed will grow in size **(hypertrophy)** and become stronger. Hypertrophy occurs when a muscle is regularly challenged to produce near-optimal levels of force. The structure of the muscle then changes by increasing the size of its protein filaments. Once this happens, the muscle is capable of producing greater force.

3. Muscles that are stressed by resistance training get stronger and increase in size (hypertrophy), while muscles that are neglected get weaker and shrink in size (atrophy).

The degree to which hypertrophy occurs is dependent upon four factors. The first is the amount and type of resistance training you perform. The second is making sure that you are eating a nutritious diet containing adequate amounts of carbohydrate, fat, and protein. Although you must consume adequate amounts of the essential amino acids to build muscle daily, the role of protein consumption in muscle mass development is overstated. Total dietary energy, specifically carbohydrate energy, is the most important nutritional factor affecting muscle gain (Butterfield, Kleiner, Lemon, & Stone, 1995). Carbohydrate provides the main source of fuel for a muscle used to generate force. Excessive intake of protein will not speed up the development of muscle mass or cause greater muscle mass to occur.

The third factor is the genetics for large-muscle growth, and the fourth is secretion of adequate amounts of the hormones responsible for causing muscle to grow (testosterone, androgens, human growth hormone). This last factor explains one reason why some people gain more muscle mass than others. If you produce large volumes of testosterone, androgens, and human growth hormone, and combine this production with proper training, good genetics, and proper nutrition, you will have greater muscle mass development. Men produce more of these hormones, so men tend to have the capacity for more muscle mass development than women. Most women can practice regular heavy resistance training, increase their strength tremendously, and not develop large bulky muscles.

It takes approximately 8 to 12 weeks to experience signs of muscular hypertrophy. People will show improvements in strength before this time (usually 2 weeks after starting a program); however, this improvement is mainly due to improvements in lifting technique, better coordination, and **neuromuscular adaptations.** The neuromuscular adaptations include the ability selectively to recruit the muscle fibers necessary to perform a given activity, the ability to synchronize the firing of these muscle fibers, and the ability to call more muscle fibers into action. Changes in muscular endurance will begin almost immediately. In as few as 2 weeks you should see some improvement in your muscular endurance.

Some people achieve body mass increases of about 20 percent during the first year of regular heavy resistance training; however, later gains slow down substantially because we tend to approach our genetic potential relatively early in a training program. After a few years of resistance training, gains will level off at only 1 to 3 percent per year (Butterfield et al., 1995). Muscles must be regularly exposed to the stress that resistance activity supplies or the muscle fibers will become weaker and actually shrink in size. This process is called muscle **atrophy.**

Toning muscles involves training the muscle to maintain a tonic state (a state in which the muscle maintains a degree of tension). A toned muscle feels more firm than an untoned muscle. It is important to remember that *you cannot change fat to muscle* because they are different cells; however, you *can* increase the size of one while reducing the size of the other.

Hypertrophy Increase in cell size; muscle cells grow in response to resistance training.

Neuromuscular adaptations Changes in the function of the nervous and muscular systems brought on by exposure to regular resistance training. These changes include the ability to selectively recruit motor units, to synchronize the recruitment of these units, and to maintain a state of equilibrium throughout the movement.

Atrophy Decrease in cell size; muscle cells shrink in response to disuse.

4. You can develop muscular strength and endurance through a variety of resistance training programs.

Isometric Form of resistance training in which the muscle is stationary while under tension.

Isotonic Form of resistance training in which there is movement.

Isokinetic Form of resistance training in which the speed of movement is controlled.

Isotonic, Isokinetic, and Isometric Training

There are a variety of ways in which you can train a muscle to become stronger and more enduring. The three different types of training include **isometric**, **isotonic**, and **isokinetic** training. Isometric training occurs when the muscle is put under tension but the length of the muscle does not change. An example of an isometric exercise would be pushing against an immovable object such as a wall. The prefix *iso* means "the same" and *metric* refers to length, so *isometric* means the muscle maintains the same length when under tension.

Isotonic training involves muscular movement, but the resistance stays the same. An example would be lifting a barbell with 100 pounds on it. The weight stays the same throughout the lift. *Tonic* refers to tension, so *isotonic* means "the same tension." There are two types of isotonic training methods. The first involves set resistance training, in which the resistance remains the same throughout the muscular action. The best example of this type of resistance training is free weights. The second type of isotonic training involves machines that provide variable resistance as you move through the range of motion associated with a muscular activity. An example would be performing exercises on a Nautilus machine. The Nautilus camshaft causes the chain that provides resistance to move over varying lengths, thereby altering the resistance that is provided. This allows for variations in the resistance that the muscle must work against as it moves through its range of motion.

The third type of training is isokinetic training. *Kinetic* refers to the energy of movement, so *isokinetic* means "the same energy." Isokinetic training is similar to variable-resistance isotonic training with the key differences that with isokinetic training the speed of movement is controlled and the resistance is accommodating. By controlling the speed, the energy involved in the movement is regulated. *Accommodating resistance* refers to resistance that varies based on the force generated by the person performing the activity. The harder you work, the more resistance you receive. Isokinetic devices, such as the Cybex Orthotron, control the speed of motion and provide accommodating resistance through the use of hydraulics. These machines may use gas, water, or oil-based hydraulics to control speed and resistance. An example of how hydraulics can do this would be to consider a door with an automatic closer. If you allow the door to close at its preset rate, it takes little effort to move the door. However, if you try to speed the door up, the amount of resistance increases.

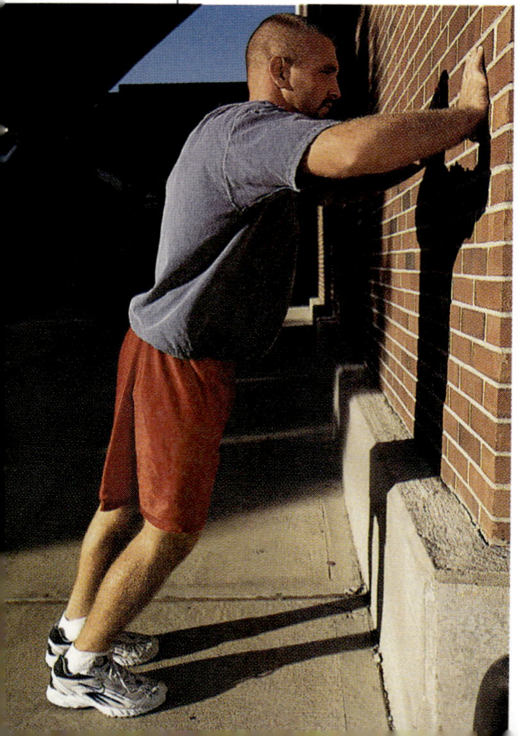

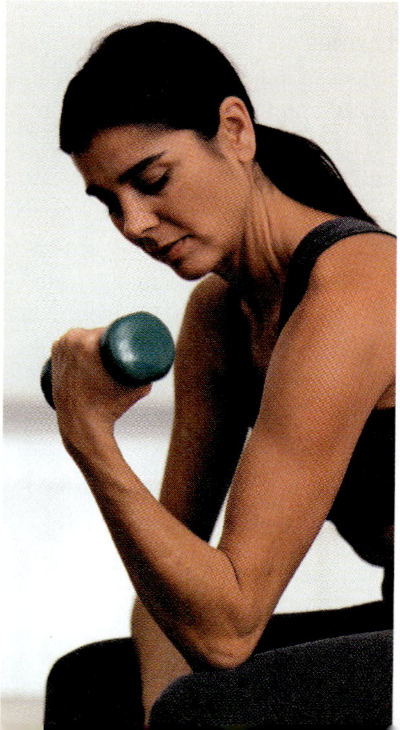

(Left) Pushing against an immovable object is a form of isometric resistance training. (Right) Lifting dumbbells is a form of isotonic resistance training.

Isometric exercises provide you with the opportunity to train anywhere. Since there is no equipment required, you are not dependent on a workout facility to perform isometric exercises. There is also no cost associated with isometric exercise. Disadvantages of isometric training include the need to perform the exercise at multiple angles to get the full range of motion involved. It's also difficult to gauge the intensity of your workout because you don't see any resistance being lifted. Isometric training may be dangerous for those with high blood pressure or cardiovascular disease. Since you are holding a position and creating tension, *isometric training raises blood pressure.*

Isotonic training is the preferred method of training for people who perform regular resist-

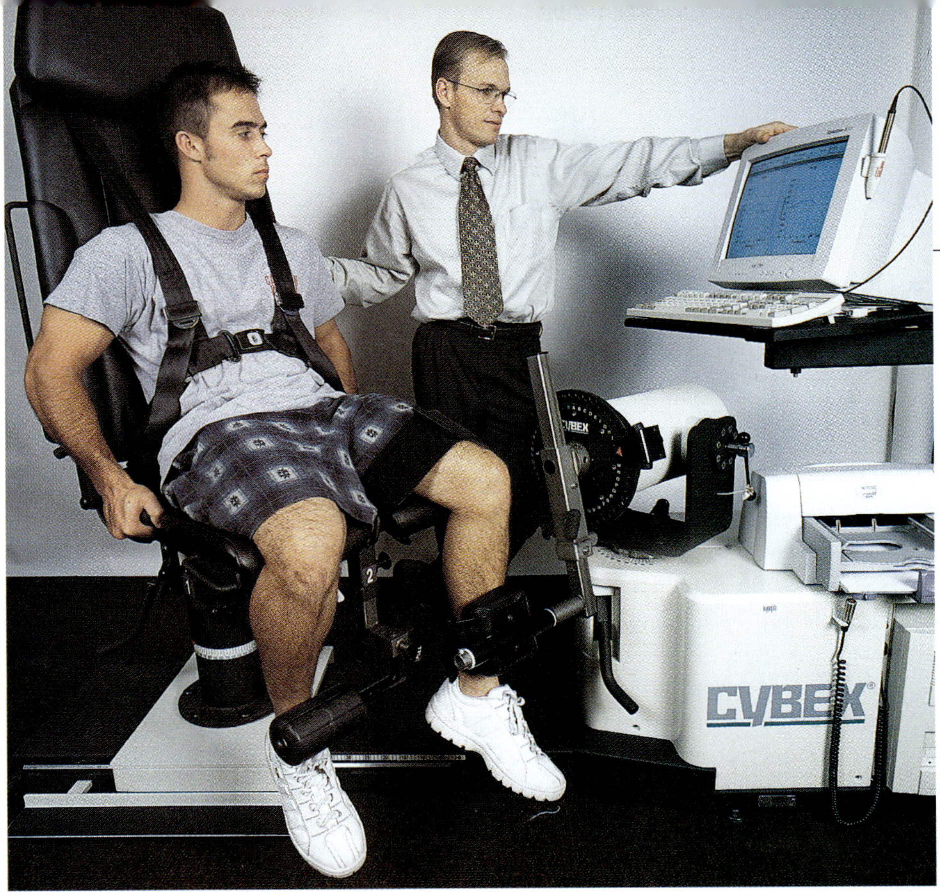

Exercise using a cybex machine is a form of isokinetic resistance training.

ance exercise and will probably be your form of choice. The advantages of isotonic training are that you can easily train through the full range of motion, you can isolate individual muscles to make sure they are properly stressed, and you can more easily gauge the intensity of your exercise by watching how much resistance you are lifting. The disadvantages of isotonic resistance training include being somewhat dependent on equipment, the cost associated with access to that equipment (either by purchasing it or by paying for membership at a health club), and the potential for injury through improper use of the equipment.

The major advantage to isokinetic training is that the resistance adjusts to the force you generate. This is important if you are rehabilitating injured or weak muscles. The disadvantages of isokinetic training include the high cost of the equipment, lack of access to this type of equipment (it is found mostly in rehabilitation clinics), and the inability to isolate individual muscle groups easily.

RESISTANCE TRAINING GUIDELINES

As with the guidelines for cardiovascular physical activity (Chapter 6), there are two sets of guidelines for resistance training. The first guideline is for those people seeking baseline health benefits. Baseline health benefits are associated with good health, but not optimal health. Some individuals only wish to perform the amount of physical activity that will bring about some protection against degenerative disease, are not overly concerned about their level of fitness, and are not willing to perform the amount of exercise required to bring about optimal health and fitness.

Others may wish to bring about optimal protection against degenerative disease and higher levels of fitness. The second set of guidelines is for those seeking optimal health and fitness benefits. The baseline health benefit guidelines require less time and effort. The optimal health and fitness guidelines build upon the baseline health benefit

Reps Repetitions; a rep occurs each time a muscle action is performed.

Sets Groups of repetitions.

Overload Principle of training under which a system (e.g., muscle) must be forced to work harder than it normally works to get stronger.

Progression Principle of training wherein overload must be applied in a logical and systematic fashion.

Specificity Principle of training under which specific activities must be performed to bring about changes in specific systems.

Recovery Principle of training wherein adequate time must be given for a stressed system to become stronger.

guidelines and require more time and effort. In either case, resistance training should be an integral part of everyone's physical activity program.

ACSM Guidelines

According to the American College of Sports Medicine (ACSM), resistance training should be progressive in nature, rhythmic, individualized, performed at a moderate-to-slow speed, involve full range of motion, provide a stimulus to all the major muscle groups, and not interfere with normal breathing (ACSM, 2000). For those seeking baseline health benefits, a single set of 8 to12 exercises that condition the major muscle groups 2 to 3 days per week are recommended (ACSM, 2000) (Table 11.1). Most people should be able to complete 8 to12 repetitions of each exercise; however, for those unaccustomed to resistance training, and for more frail people, 10 to15 repetitions with lighter loads may be more appropriate (ACSM, 2000; Pollock & Vincent, 1996). The major muscle groups include the arms, shoulders, chest, abdomen, back, hips, and legs (ACSM, 2000).

There is some debate as to how many **reps** (repetitions) and **sets** you should do. A *rep* is the number of times you perform a movement. For example, if you are performing a bicep curl (grasping a dumbbell and lifting it to your shoulder by bending your elbow), each time you take the dumbbell to your shoulder and then back to its original starting position, you have completed one rep. A *set* is a series of reps.

Eighty to 90 percent of strength gains can be achieved using single-set regimens when compared to multiple-set types of programs (Pollock & Vincent, 1996). Multiple-set types of programs may provide for optimal fitness and muscle growth, and are recommended if time allows (ACSM, 2000). However, since time is an important factor for program compliance, the single-set guidelines seem appropriate for the majority of the population (Pollock & Vincent, 1996). Multiple-set regimens may not be appropriate for older, nonathletic individuals (Pollock & Vincent, 1996).

Muscular Strength Training

Basic Principles Training for muscular strength development focuses on the physical conditioning concepts of **overload**, **progression**, **specificity**, and **recovery.** In order for a muscle to hypertrophy, or increase in size, the muscle must work against resistance

TABLE 11.1 A Sample Resistance Training Workout

Arms	Bicep curls Tricep extensions
Shoulders	Seated press Shoulder shrugs
Chest	Bench press Bent arm flys
Abdomen	Sit-ups/curl-ups/crunches
Back	Lat pull-downs Bent over rows
Groin	Lunges
Legs	Quad extensions Hamstring curls

greater than that to which it is normally exposed (overload). The best way of accomplishing this task is to have the muscle work at a level exceeding 85 percent of its maximal capacity. Exactly how much weight 85 percent of maximal capacity is will be based upon the fitness level of the individual. Someone who has previously not performed resistance exercise will be working against a much lighter load than someone who has been training for years.

The principle of progression is important in training for muscular strength development. *Progression* refers to the logical and systematic application of the overload principle. Frequently, misinformed or over-eager people will attempt to do too much too soon when they begin a physical activity program that includes resistance training. The result is pain, and potentially an injury, that will have severely negative affects on adherence. Resistance training programs must be entered into wisely and gradually. You must allow your body time to adjust to the rigors of training for muscular strength. You should undergo assessment to determine exactly how much resistance you need.

If you wish to develop strength in specific muscle groups, you must perform activities that stress those muscles. This concept (specific activities for specific outcomes) is referred to as the *principle of specificity.* Ideally, you will be able to select activities that isolate the muscles you wish to develop. By isolating muscles, you can ensure that they are being overloaded properly. For instance, if you wish to stress the chest muscle (pectorals) optimally, you should perform activities in which the chest muscles are the prime movers. Bench pressing and bent arm flies are two activities that do this (Figures 11.6, 11.7).

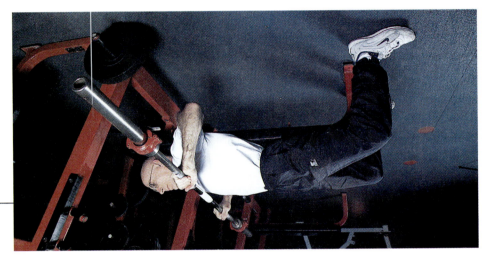

FIGURE 11.6

Principal of Specificity.
The bench press specifically stresses the chest muscles.

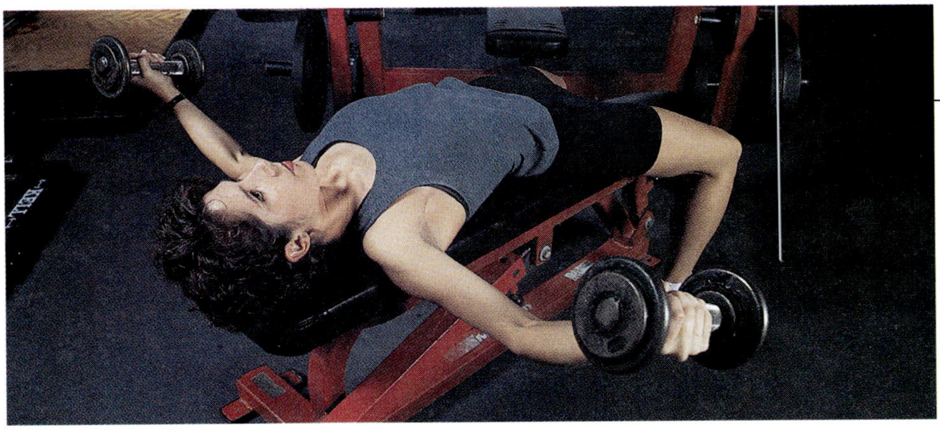

FIGURE 11.7

Principal of Specificity.
Bent-arm flies can also be used to strengthen the chest muscles.

It is also important to remember to apply the principle of recovery to your muscular strength program. Occasionally, people fall into the trap of thinking that the more frequently you perform an exercise, the more rapidly you will see improvement in fitness. This supposition does not always hold true. In fact, if you do not allow adequate recovery time, your body will not have the chance to rebuild itself and make the structural changes necessary for muscular growth to occur. It is best to allow 48 to 72 hours of recovery time between training sessions in which a muscle or group of muscles is maximally stressed. This does not mean that we must remain inactive during this time. We can perform activities that stress other parts of our bodies or other aspects of our fitness while we allow those segments that were maximally stressed time to recover.

Proper Form and Technique Any resistance training program should focus initially on proper form and technique. By doing so, you will not only improve the safety of the activities you perform but also increase the gains you receive. As stated earlier, you must stress the muscle you wish to develop in order for it to get larger and stronger. If you improperly perform a resistance training activity, you may in fact be stressing things (joints, muscles, tendons) that were not the intended target areas for improvement. At any resistance training facility you will see that many people incorrectly perform activities, putting themselves at risk for injury and reducing the possibility for achieving their desired outcomes.

Breathing It is important to remember to breathe properly when performing resistance training exercises. Improper breathing can put you at risk for injury. It is recommended that you breathe out while exerting force and breathe in when returning (not exerting force). For example, when performing the bench press exercise, you would breathe in when lowering the bar to your chest and breathe out when pressing the bar upward.

You should *never hold your breath when lifting,* particularly when you are exerting force. This may bring about a condition called the **valsalva maneuver.** The valsalva maneuver occurs when the windpipe is blocked off (as occurs when holding your breath). Pressure in your lungs begins to build up, which in turn causes an increase in blood pressure. Higher blood pressures put you at risk for a stroke, heart attack, or hemorrhage. By breathing out when exerting force, you greatly reduce this risk.

Muscular Endurance Training

Many of the same principles that govern training for muscular strength govern training for muscular endurance. The principles of overload, progression, specificity, and recovery all apply to muscular endurance training. The major differences between strength and endurance training are the amount of resistance applied and the number of repetitions performed. For optimal gains in muscular endurance, it is recommended that you train at an intensity that ranges between 50 and 65 percent of your maximal capacity. As with strength training, the amount of resistance applied will be dependent on the fitness level of the person. To gain muscular endurance benefits, you apply less stress than you would if you were seeking strength gains, but you perform more repetitions of the activity for longer periods of time.

Valsalva maneuver Condition that occurs when you hold your breath and exert force (grunting action); causes elevated blood pressure that increases the risk for stroke, heart attack, or hemorrhage.

Training for Power

Training for power is very similar to training for strength, with the major difference that power training requires greater speed. By definition, *power* means that work is accomplished at a high rate of speed. Power is best developed through explosive training. Because of the dynamic nature of power training, there is a high risk of injury. Power training is usually reserved for those individuals who have already developed a good degree of muscular fitness. When performing power training, you must try to move the resistance rapidly without forsaking proper form.

Table 11.2 contains sample regimens that may be used to train for muscular strength, endurance, or power.

Developing a Personalized Program

Explore www.pahconnection.com 11.1, 11.2

Activities & Assessments 11.1, 11.2

Engage www.pahconnection.com 11.1, 11.2

There are many variations of training routines that you can follow. The basic guidelines have been spelled out in this chapter. More information can be obtained by visiting websites that cater to those interested in strength and muscular endurance training.

Assessment As with the performance of cardiovascular physical activity (Chapter 6), you should begin any resistance training program with proper assessment. Assessment is important to establish beginning workloads, to monitor progress, and to enhance safety. Two sample assessments are included at the end of this chapter. One shows how to measure your one-repetition maximum (1-RM) for the bench press and the other shows how to measure your abdominal endurance. You can follow the same procedures to determine the 1-RM for any other muscle or to find the muscular endurance capacity of other muscle groups. Several other self-assessments are available on the Web, or you may elect to have a qualified professional help with your assessment.

Finding Qualified Professional Help When instructed by a qualified professional in the strength training field, you can learn to lift safely and effectively. A "strength coach" can teach you how to lift with proper form, demonstrate proper spotting techniques, and help you develop a sound resistance training program. You must be careful when seeking a strength coach. Don't rely on the assumption that everyone who lifts regularly knows what they are doing. We suggest that you ask at your health club to locate a person certified through one of the major professional organizations. The National Strength and Conditioning Association offers a certification for a strength and conditioning specialist (CSCS). The American College of Sports Medicine offers a certified health-fitness instructor. More information on these certifications can be found at the websites of these organizations.

TABLE 11.2 Sample Training Regimens for Strength, Endurance, or Power

TRAINING	STRENGTH	ENDURANCE	POWER
Exercises	8–12	8–12	8–12
Repetitions	8–12	10–15	8–12
Sets	1–3	3–5	3–5
Intensity	> 85% 1-RM	50–65% 1-RM	50–65% 1-RM
Days per week	2–3	2–3	2–3
Training speed	Slow to moderate	Slow to moderate	Fast, with little or no rest between sets

*These are basic guidelines. Additional sets or combinations of sets and repetitions may elicit greater gains.

Explore
www.jbpub.com/connection.com
11.3, 11.4, 11.5

Selecting Equipment and Exercises When selecting exercise equipment for resistance training, there are three overriding factors that must be considered. The first is safety. The equipment should fit your body comfortably and be sturdy enough to withstand the stress applied during a resistance training program. When using machines, the axis of rotation for any piece of equipment should be aligned with the center of the joint on your body that will be performing the activity. Safety straps should be worn to help you maintain proper body alignment. Seek out professional instruction on how to use the equipment safely and effectively.

The second factor is effectiveness. In order to develop muscular strength and endurance, your physical activity program must be designed in such a way as to optimize the time spent in training. With resistance training equipment, a great deal of time may be lost in adjusting the resistance or the equipment. The best advice we can give is to try out any piece of equipment before deciding to purchase it or incorporate it into your program.

The third factor is expense. Resistance training does not need to be expensive. Obviously, if you are interested in using gold-plated barbells or participating in the swankiest fitness facility, resistance training can be expensive. However, your muscles do not know or care what form of resistance is being applied. You can overload your muscle by pushing against an immovable object, by lifting buckets with varying amounts of sand or water, or by performing calisthenics in water. The key to developing muscular fitness is the regular application of resistance. With a little imagination, you can find a variety of ways of applying this resistance.

FIGURE 11.8

Arm Exercises.
Tricep extension.

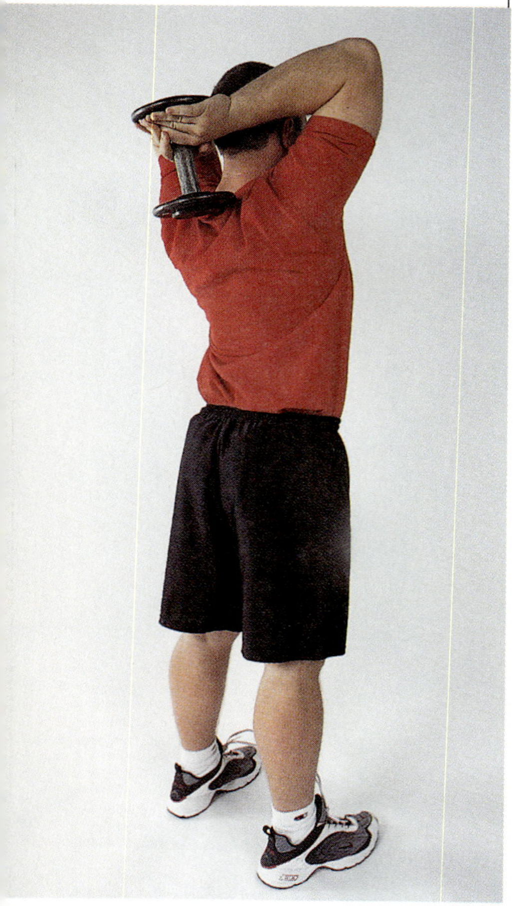

Sample Exercises As stated previously, there are a variety of activities in which you can participate to enhance your muscular strength, endurance, and power. We have subdivided some of these activities into what we refer to as *basic lifts* and *advanced lifts*. The basic lifts require little time to learn proper technique, work the major muscle groups as recommended by the ACSM (2000), and are safe if performed properly (Figures 11.8 through 11.25).

The advanced lifts are designed for those seeking optimal health and fitness goals, or those competing in sports. They require more time to learn proper technique (professional instruction is required), place a great deal of stress on specific areas of the body, and are associated with a higher risk for injury (Figures 11.26 through 11.35).

Order of Exercises For most beginners, it is better to alternate between agonists and antagonists when setting the order of exercises. It is also better to start with the large muscle groups and then move to the smaller muscle groups. For example, you might want to perform leg extensions followed by leg curls (flexion), and then move on to calf raises. Another example would be to perform bench presses followed by lat (latissimus dorsi) pulldowns, and then move on to tricep extensions.

Free Weights vs. Machines Most people who perform resistance training use either free weights or machines. Machines tend to be used more by beginners, those who may have difficulty with balance, and those who have limited space to perform resistance training. Machines allow for an application of resistance in a guided or restricted manner (Stone, 2000).

Free weights tend to be used by those who want to isolate individual muscles, are interested in developing control and balance when lifting, and want to engage in a wide variety of activities. It has been suggested that free weights allow for more mechanical specificity (more lifelike movements) than machines and therefore provide a superior method for training (Stone, 2000). Most "serious" lifters use free weights.

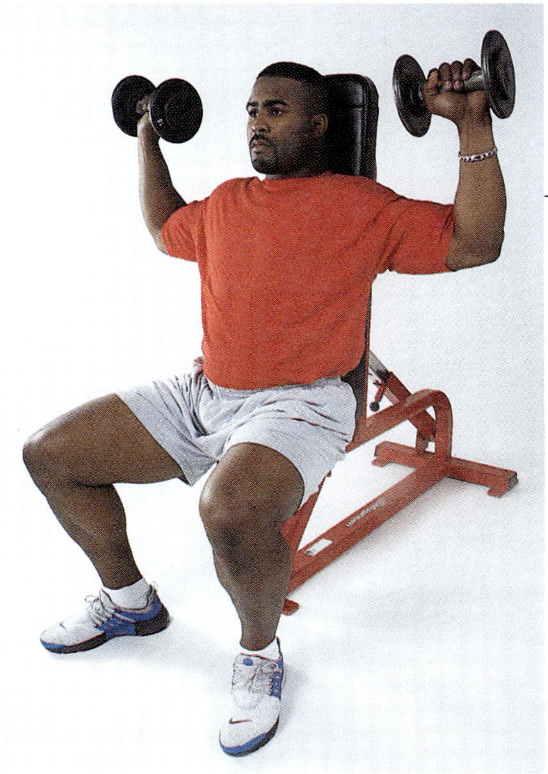

FIGURE 11.9

Shoulder Exercises.
Seated press.

FIGURE 11.11

Chest Exercises.
Bent-arm flies.

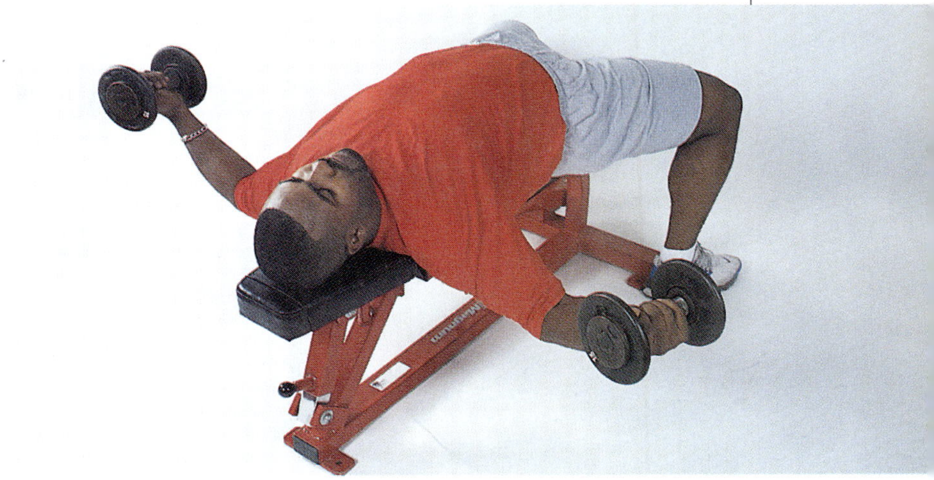

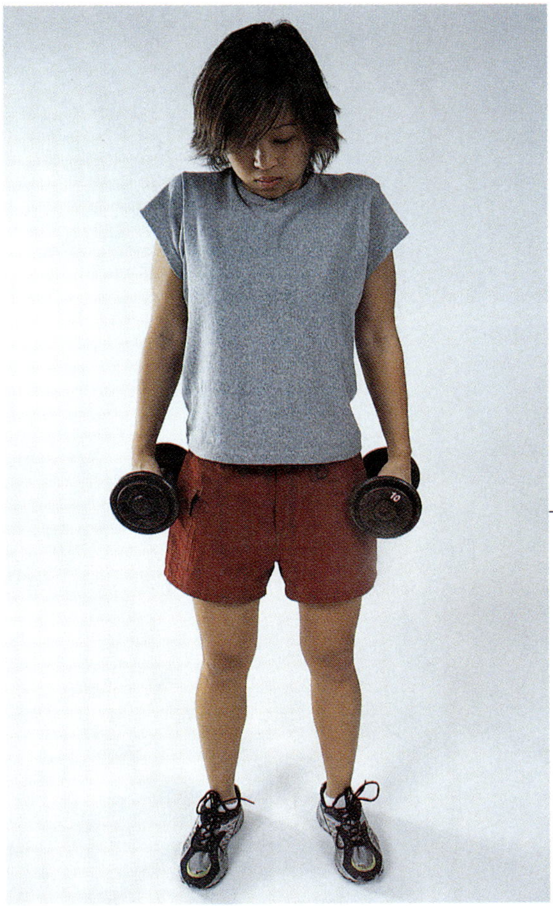

FIGURE 11.10

Neck Exercises.
Shoulder shrugs.

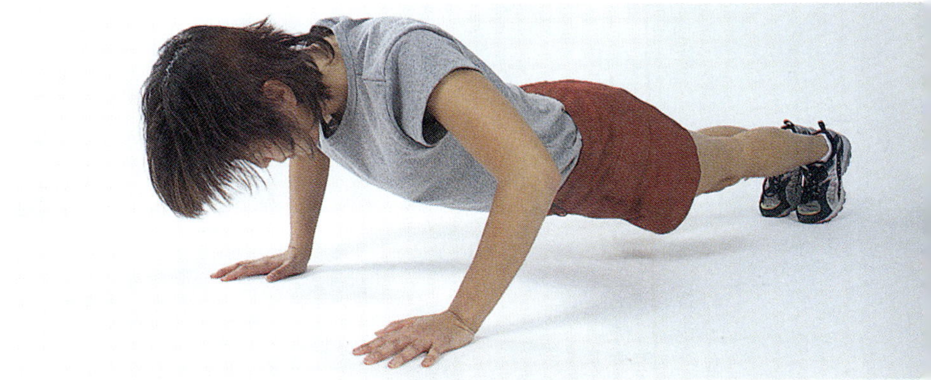

FIGURE 11.12

Chest Exercises.
Push-ups.

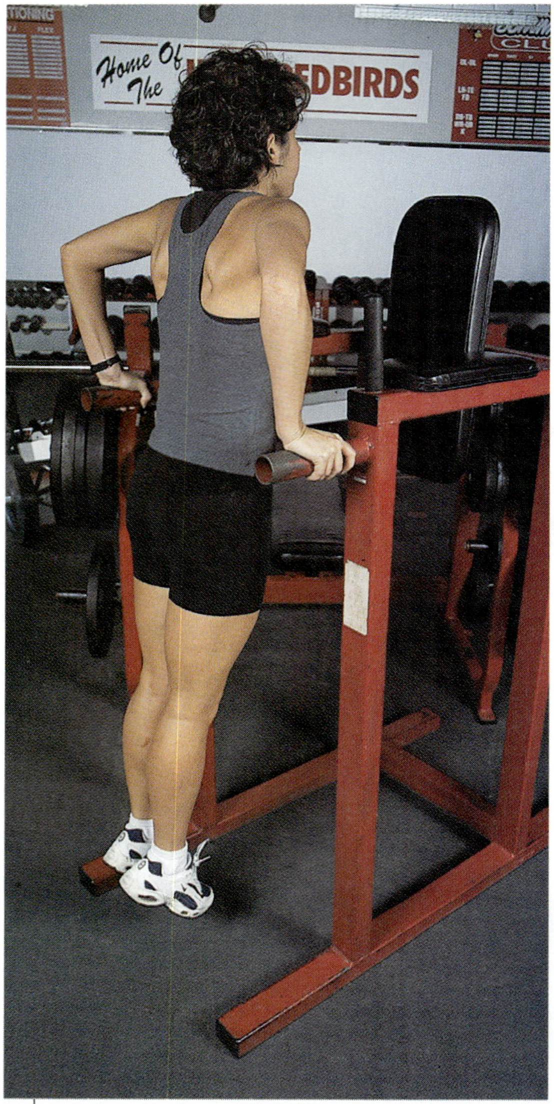

FIGURE 11.13

Chest Exercises.
Dips.

FIGURE 11.14

Abdomen Exercises.
Sit-up (upper), curl-up (lower).

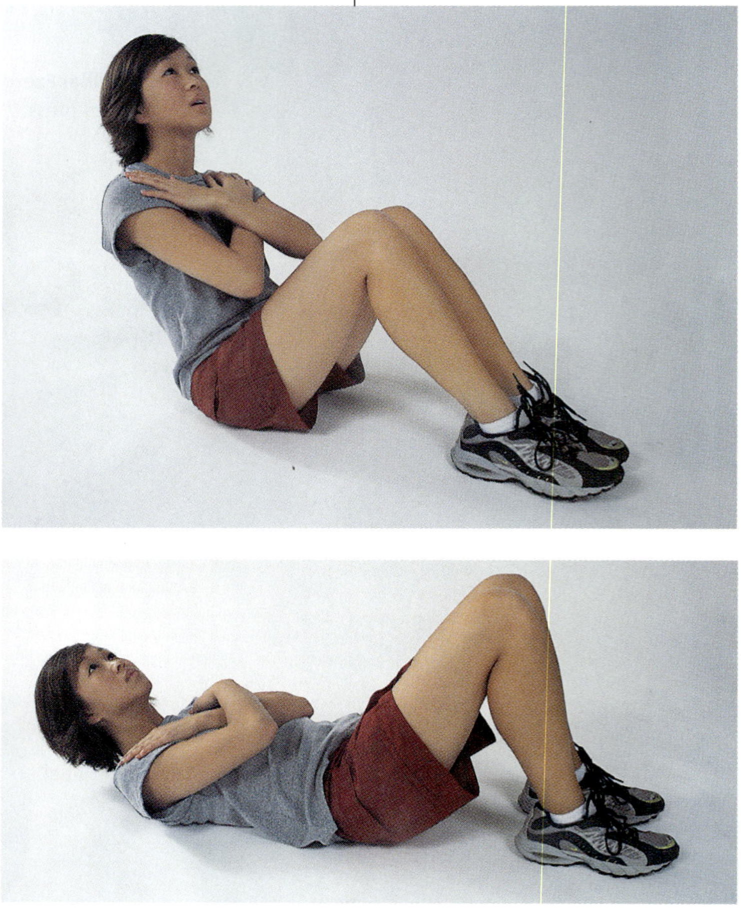

FIGURE 11.15

Back Exercises.
Lat pull down.

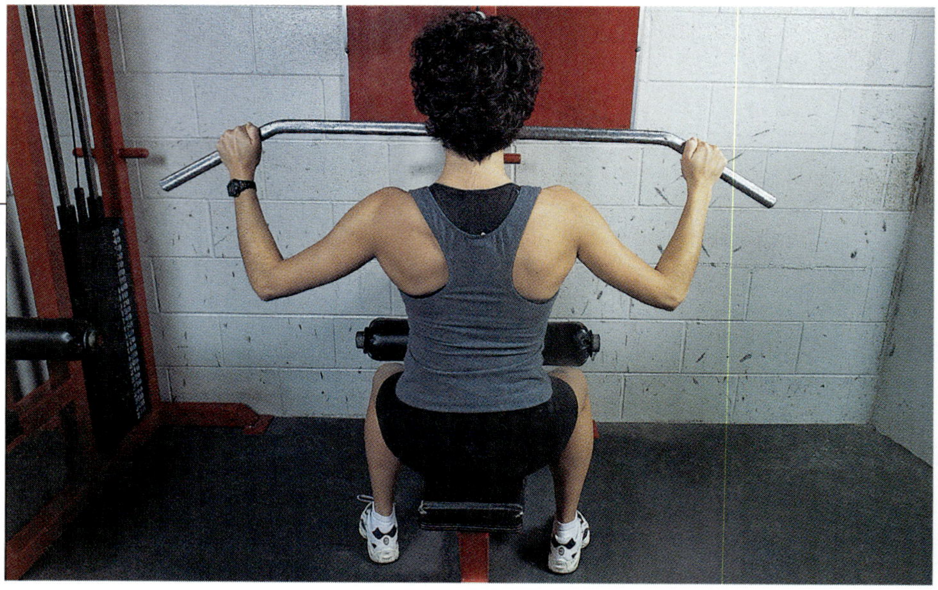

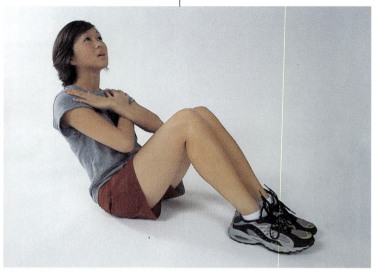

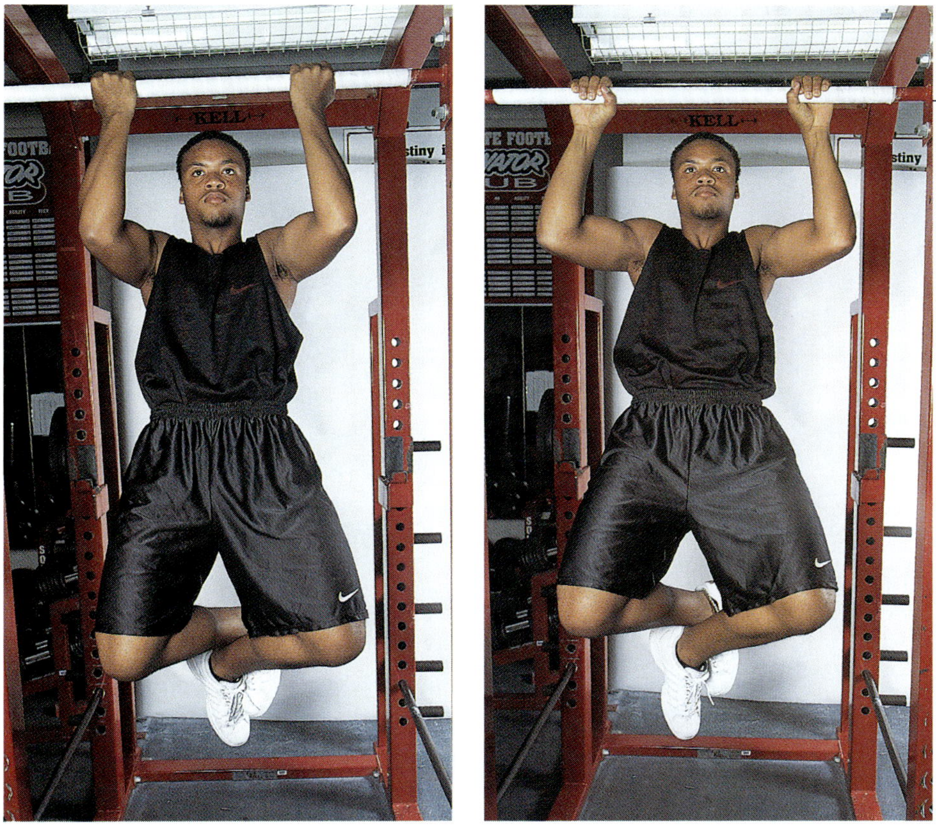

FIGURE 11.16

Back Exercises.
Curl-up (left), pull-up (right).

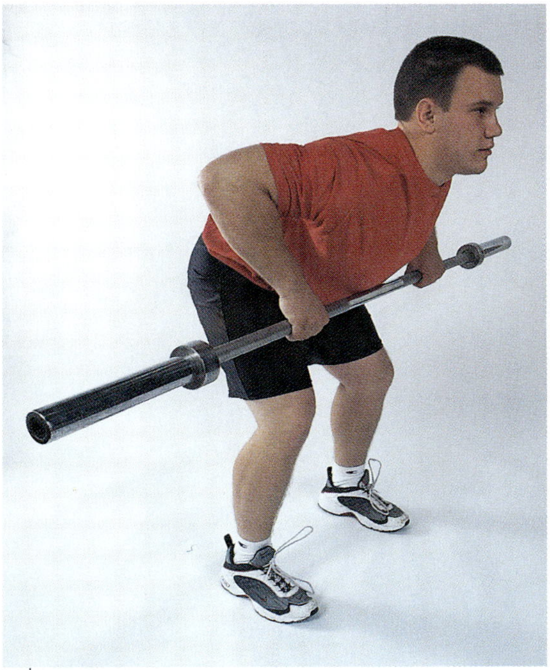

FIGURE 11.17

Back Exercises.
Bent-over rows.

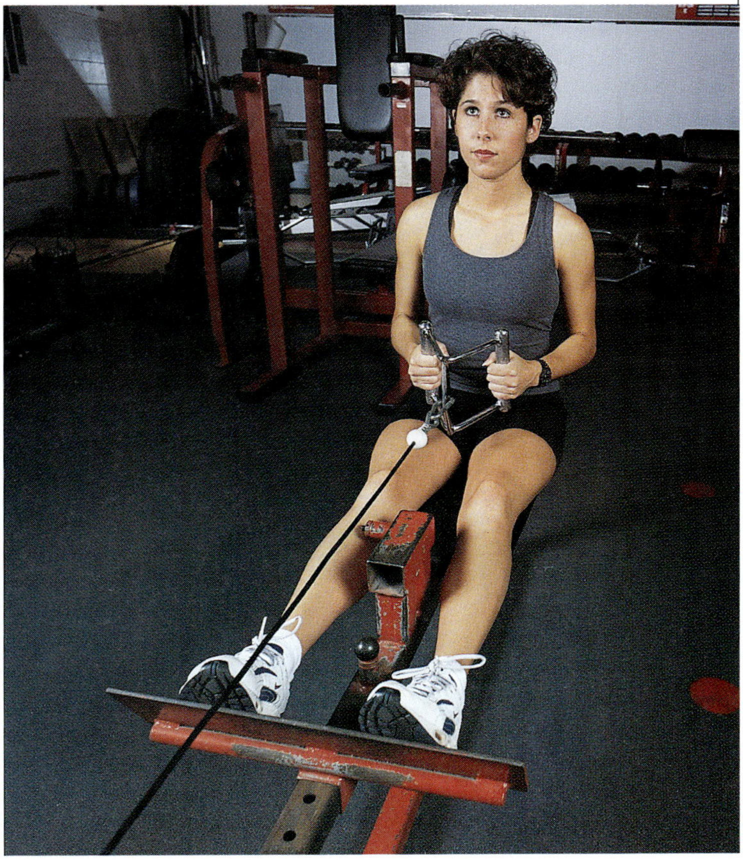

FIGURE 11.18

Back Exercises.
Seated rows.

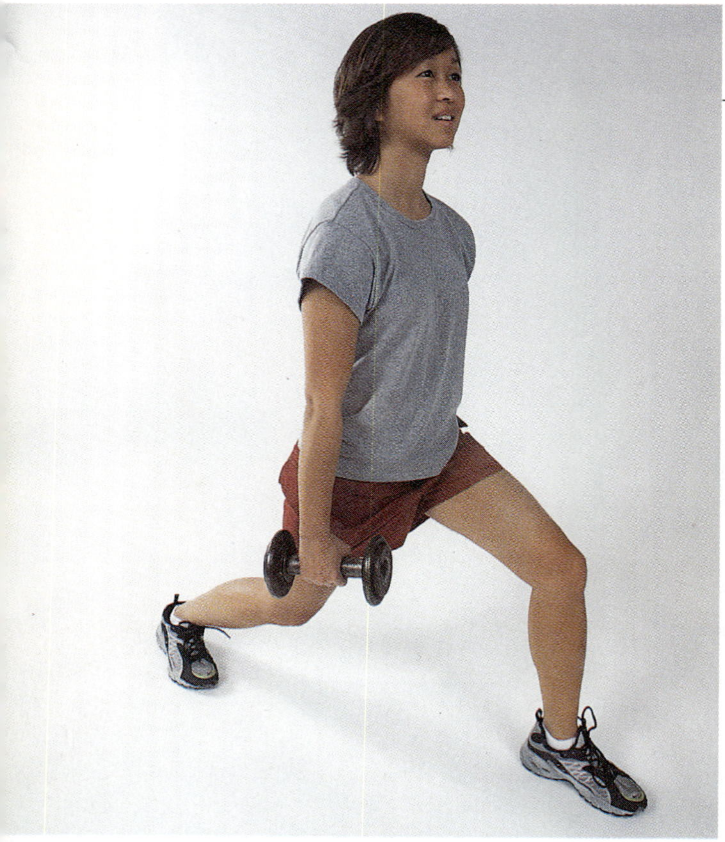

FIGURE 11.19

Groin Exercises.
Lunges.

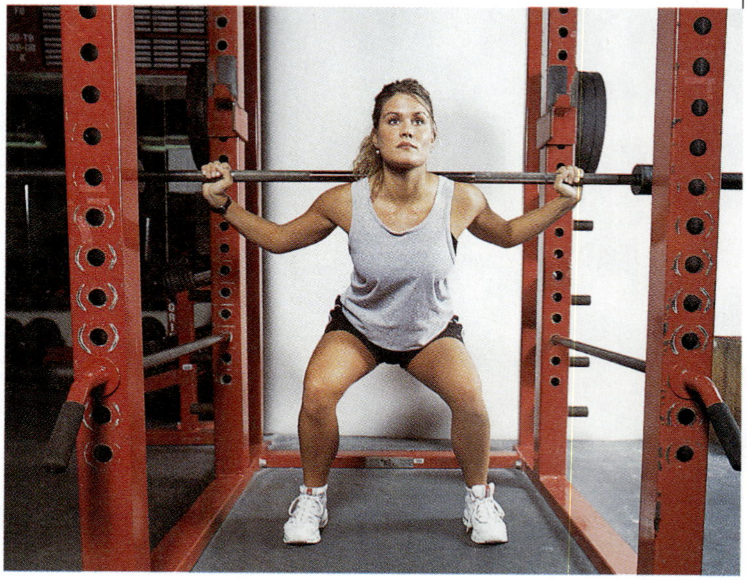

FIGURE 11.20

Leg Exercises.
Squats.

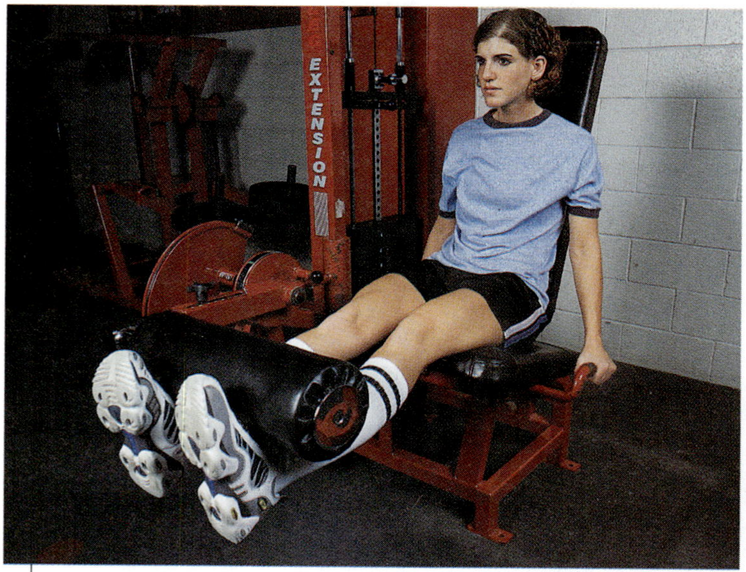

FIGURE 11.21

Leg Exercises.
Quad extension.

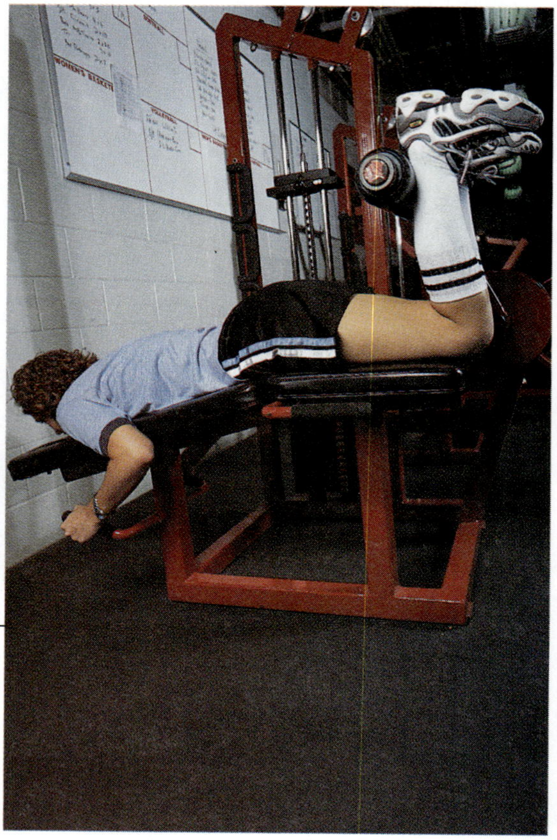

FIGURE 11.22

Leg Exercises.
Hamstring curl.

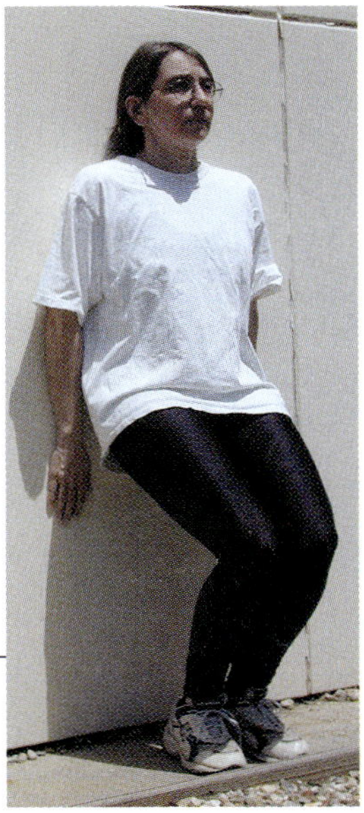

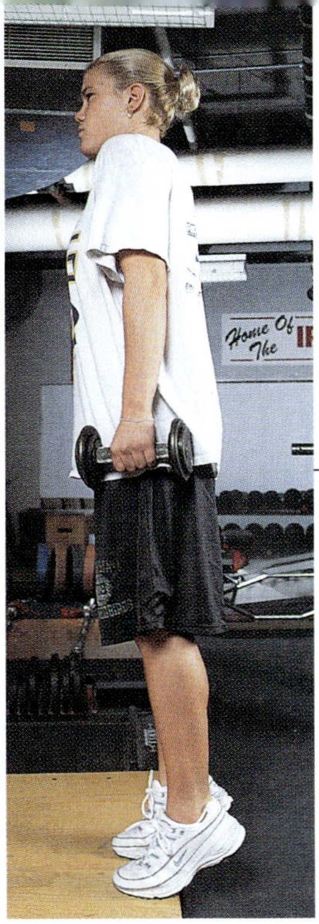

FIGURE 11.24

Leg Exercises.
Calf raise.

FIGURE 11.23

Leg Exercises.
Wall sit.

FIGURE 11.25

Leg Exercises.
Double-leg press.

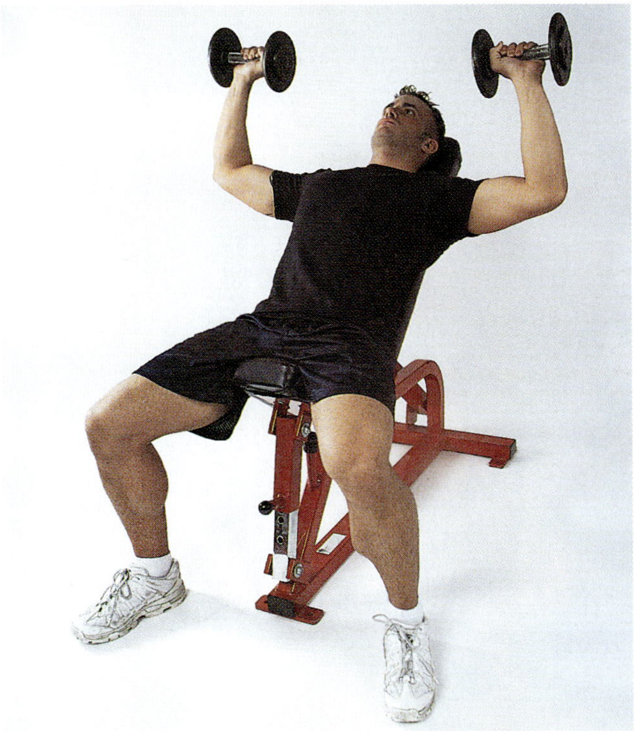

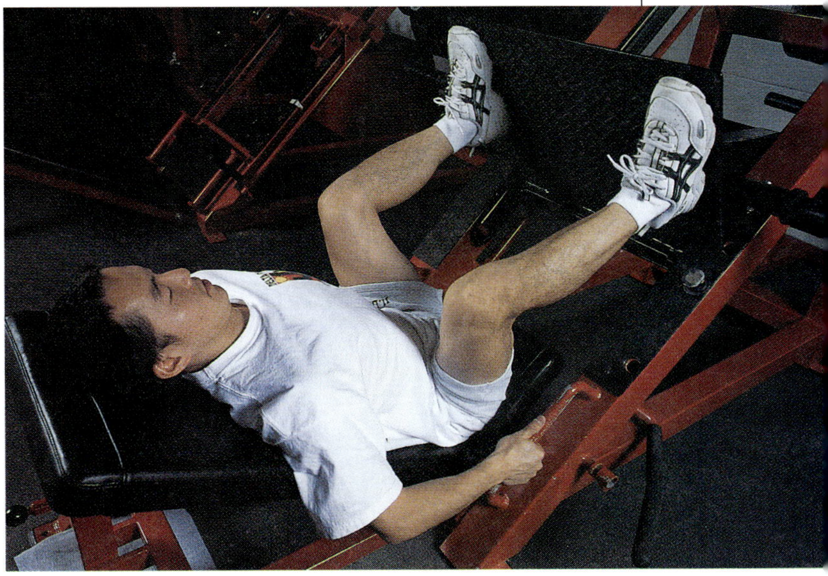

FIGURE 11.26

Advanced Lifts.
Incline bench press.

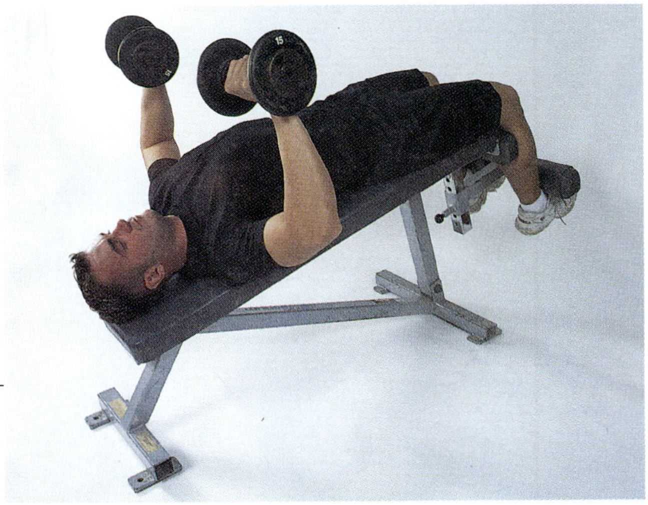

FIGURE 11.27

Advanced Lifts.
Decline bench press.

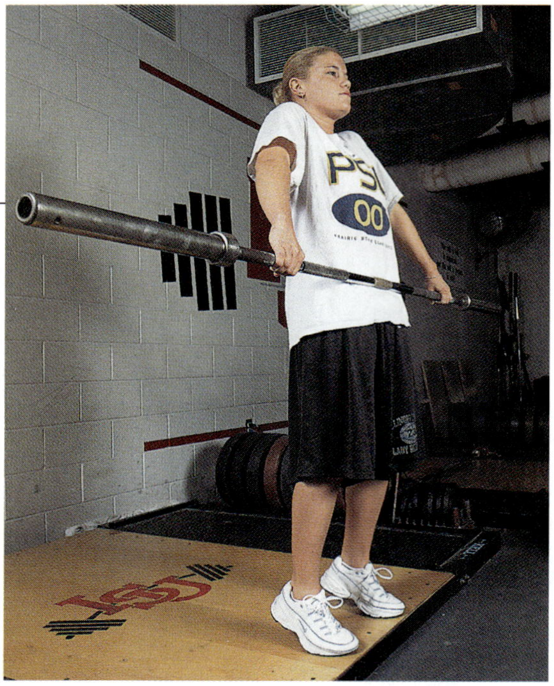

FIGURE 11.28

Advanced Lifts. Snatch pull.

FIGURE 11.30

Advanced Lifts. Dead lift.

FIGURE 11.29

Advanced Lifts. Bent-arm pullover.

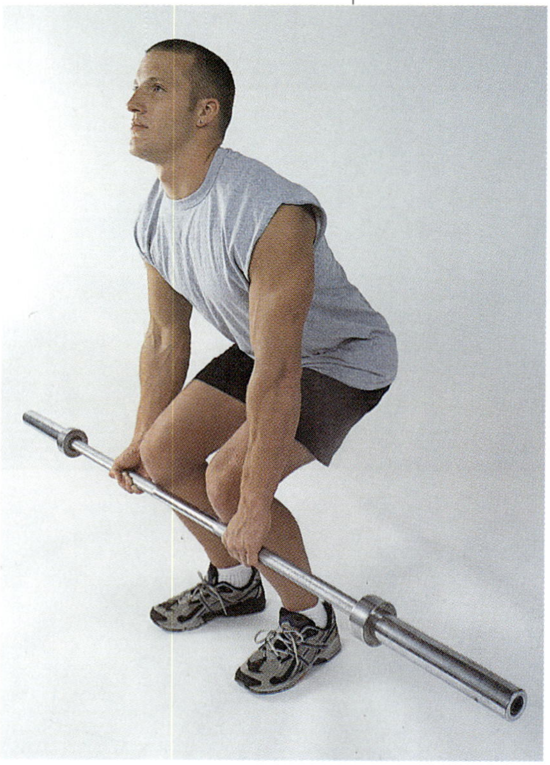

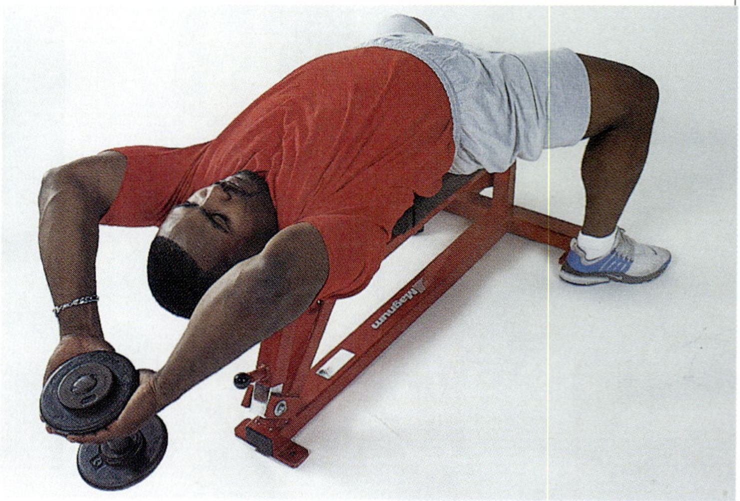

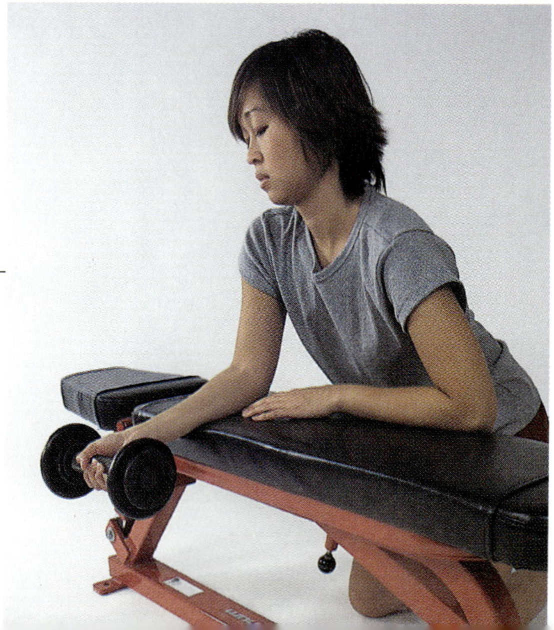

FIGURE 11.31

Advanced Lifts. Wrist curl.

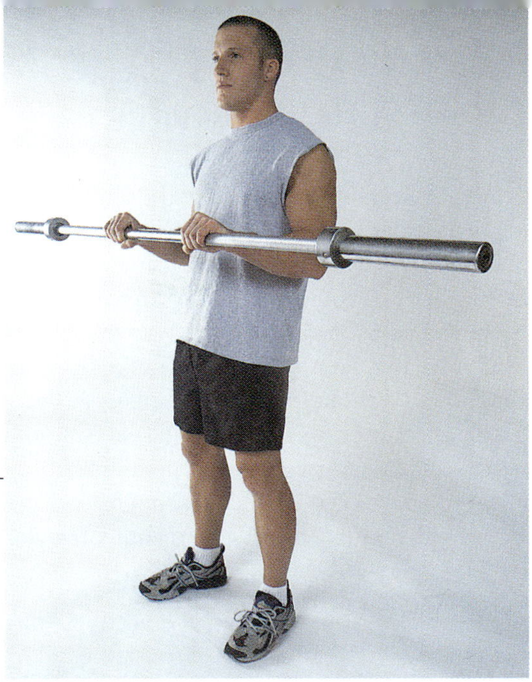

FIGURE 11.32

Advanced Lifts.
Reverse bicep curl.

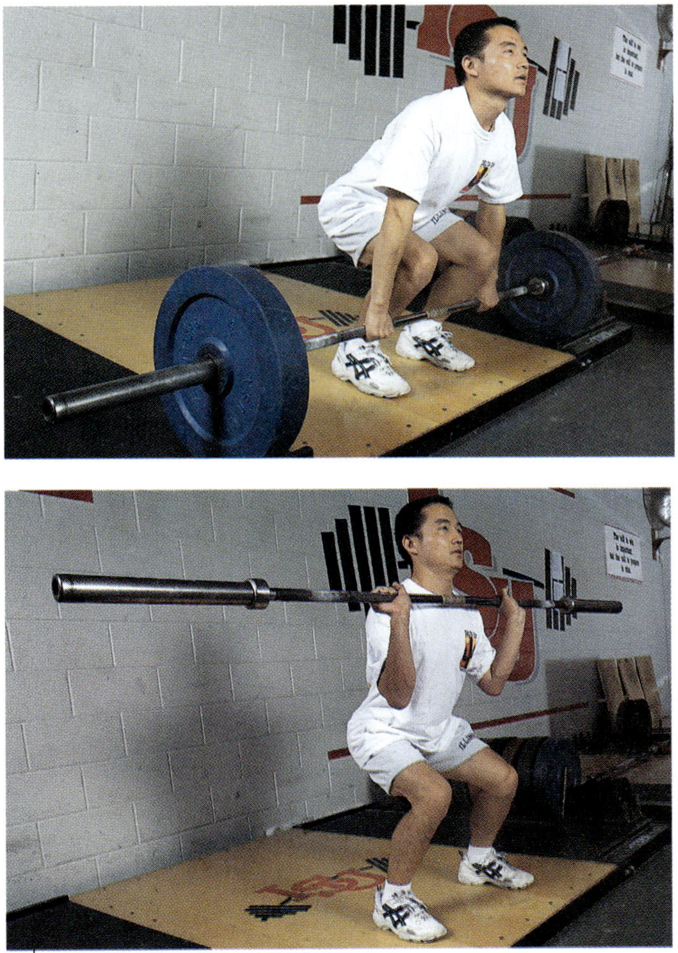

FIGURE 11.33

Advanced Lifts.
(Upper) Power clean, starting position. (Lower) Extending the bar overhead.

FIGURE 11.34

Advanced Lifts.
Preacher curl.

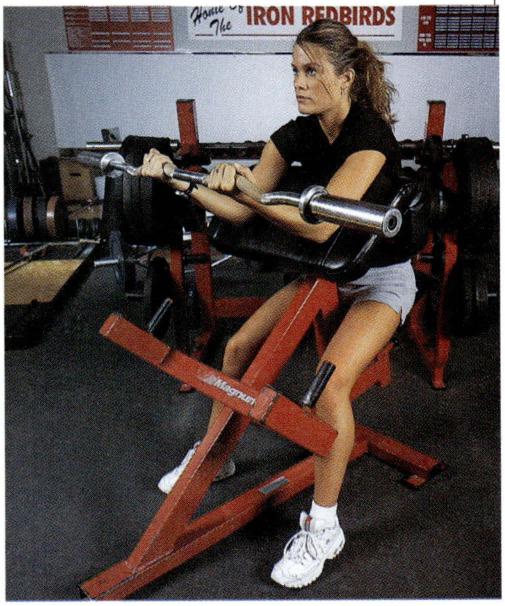

F.IGURE 11.35

Advanced Lifts.
Concentration curl.

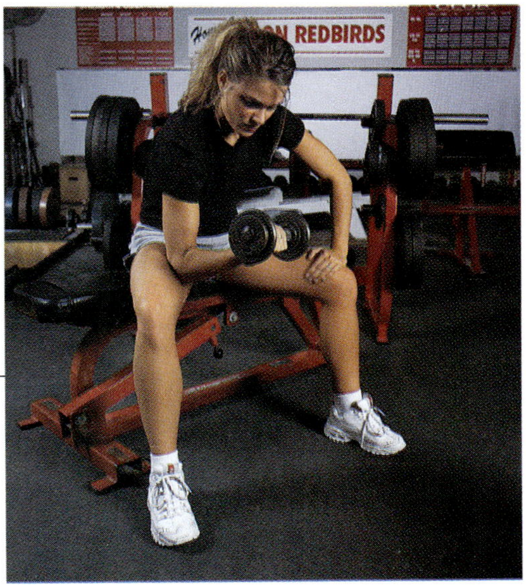

Periodization Form of resistance training in which a training program is subdivided into sections, or periods; the focus of training in each period varies, allowing for a greater overall adjustment to occur.

Pyramiding A gradual increase in the weight being lifted with a corresponding reduction in the number of repetitions until the one-repetition maximum is reached; this is followed by a gradual decrease in the resistance being lifted and an increase in the number of repetitions, until the exerciser returns to the initial load.

Plyometrics Form of resistance training that uses bounding-type exercises to overload muscles; recoil from bounding activity utilizes stored elastic energy in the connective tissue that runs through the muscle to improve performance.

Compound sets Consecutive performance of two sets of exercises that stress the same muscle group.

Tri-sets Consecutive performance of three sets of exercises that stress the same muscle group.

Supersets Consecutive performance of two sets of exercises that stress one muscle group and its antagonist without a rest period separating the sets.

Weight Room Etiquette If you elect to train in a weight room, it is important to follow the rules for safety and to maintain harmony with others who may be using the facility. Always remember to return any equipment to its proper storage place after you use it. Don't hog equipment or stations. If someone is waiting and it won't take major equipment adjustment, ask if they wish to alternate sets with you. Use a spotter to assist you with lifts. Good spotters not only make your workout safer but they also allow you to work until complete fatigue. Be aware of your environment. Pay attention to what is going on around you and keep your eyes open for equipment that may place you in danger. Always use collars on dumbbells and barbells. Don't use equipment unless you have been instructed about its use, and don't use defective equipment. In sum, have a healthy respect for the equipment and for those around you.

Specialized Training Routines

There are several variations of resistance training programs that have seen increased interest over the years. These include circuit weight training, **periodization**, **pyramiding**, **plyometrics**, and performing **compound sets**, **tri-sets**, and **supersets.**

Circuit Weight Training Circuit weight training involves setting up a series of stations at which you perform different weight training (and/or aerobic) exercises. You can use any combination of exercises included in the basic lifts outlined earlier. By limiting time between stations, you can develop muscular strength, muscular endurance, and aerobic capacity. Improvements in VO_2 max of 5 percent have been associated with circuit weight training (ACSM, 2000).

Periodization *Periodization* refers to varying the resistance training program at regular time intervals to bring about optimal gains in strength, power, motor performance, and/or muscle hypertrophy (Fleck, 1999). For example, you can subdivide the year into four cycles. During the first cycle, you may focus on the development of muscular strength. During the second cycle, you may focus on the development of muscular power. During the third cycle, you may focus on the development of muscular endurance. And, during the fourth cycle, you may focus on cross training to allow adequate recovery from the three resistance training cycles. In the case of a competitive athlete, a goal may be to bring about peak physical performance for a major competition (Fleck, 1999). The utilization of the training cycles allows the muscles to be stressed throughout the year without being stressed in the same way at all times. This will decrease the risk of injury while reducing the potential for boredom.

Advantages of programs that include periodization are greater strength gains, greater gains in lean body mass and total body weight, greater decreases in percent body fat, and greater overall fitness gains than nonperiodized multi-set and single-set programs (Fleck, 1999).

Pyramiding Pyramiding refers to a progression of sets during a resistance workout. The individual may start with a set consisting of a relatively light load and multiple repetitions (reps). For the next set, the load is increased and the number of reps decreased. This continues until the individual is lifting maximally with a minimal number of reps. The person then continues by performing mores sets during which the resistance is reduced and the number of reps increased (Figure 11.37).

Plyometrics *Plyometrics* involves the use of bounding-type exercises to overload muscle groups. For example, depth jumping involves jumping off an elevated platform, landing on a surface, and then immediately performing a maximal vertical leap. Plyo-

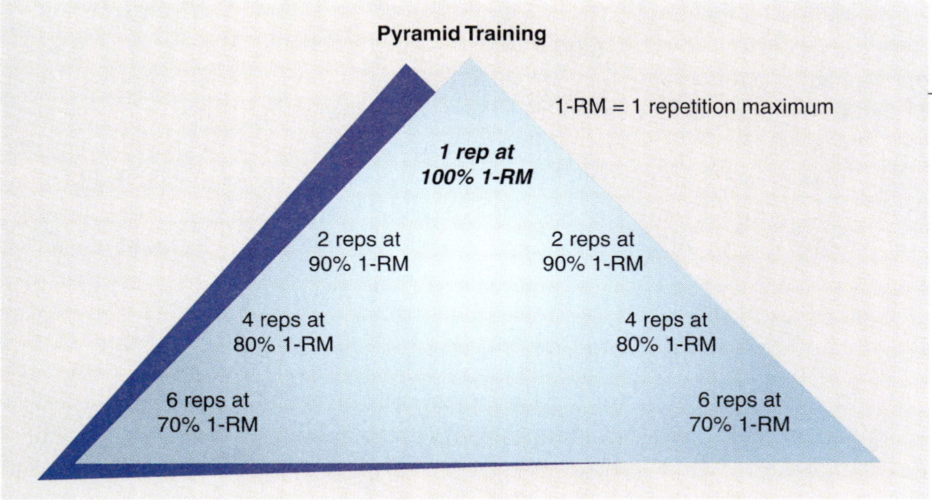

FIGURE 11.36

Pyramid Training.
The illustration is an example of using a pyramid training protocol.

metric training is favored by some athletes because it allows them to train at a normal speed of movement and overloads the muscles in a way not possible with other training techniques. The disadvantage associated with plyometric training lies in the high potential for injury, due to the ballistic nature of the activity. You must have well-conditioned muscles to perform plyometrics safely.

Compound and Tri-Sets Compound sets and tri-sets refer to performing two (compound) or three (tri) exercises in a row that stress the same muscle groups. This ensures that the muscle group is optimally fatigued and increases the likelihood that it will get stronger faster. The disadvantage to using compound and tri-sets is that you increase the likelihood of injuring a muscle or joint and increase the discomfort and pain sometimes associated with resistance training.

Supersets *Supersetting* involves performing a set of exercises for one muscle group and, with no rest period between sets, immediately performing a set of exercises for the antagonist of that group. Supersetting is designed to ensure that both muscle groups are actively fatigued. If done correctly, supersetting has the potential to speed up the development of muscular strength. The major disadvantage is the discomfort associated with this technique and its high rate of injury.

For more information on these specialized training formats, it is recommend that you check with a certified strength training professional or consult references that focus on these topics.

RESISTANCE TRAINING ACROSS THE LIFE SPAN

Resistance training can and should be performed across the life span (Brill et al., 2000). You are never too old or too young to benefit from resistance training. Infants grasping their parents fingers are performing a type of resistance training. We must remember not to fall into the trap of associating resistance training solely with weight rooms. Any type of resistance (water, body weight, free weights) can be used to bring about improvement in function.

5. Individuals of any age can benefit from resistance training.

Experience
www.pahconnection.com
11.1

Resistance training can be performed safely at any age if some commonsense guidelines are followed. In particular, pre-adolescent children should avoid maximal resistance training. In this age group, maximal resistance training (lifting at or beyond 70% of 1-RM) may bring about premature closure of the growth plate in bones. The focus of pre-adolescent programs should be on proper form and supervision. Older individuals may wish to decrease the resistance they work against and increase the number of repetitions they perform. In either case, resistance training can help to build and maintain strong and enduring muscles. It is beyond the scope of this book to provide detailed information on resistance training for the young and old.

Self Image and Training

Resistance training can have a positive impact on how we look—and how we feel about how we look. Strong, firm muscles permit better posture and a certain gracefulness of movement. Muscles that don't fatigue easily make us feel energized throughout the day. Numerous books have detailed the impact of body language upon our own moods and on how others receive us. Generally, people feel better about themselves when they are fit. Muscular fitness plays an important role in providing a healthy body image.

Resistance Training's Impact on Metabolism

Resistance training increases our lean muscle mass. Lean muscle mass is metabolically more active than any other tissue found in the body. By increasing lean body mass we can actually increase our metabolic rate. This means that we are capable of expending energy at a greater rate even when sleeping. The advantages of this state are that we can consume more food and store fewer calories.

PHYSICAL ACTIVITY AND HEALTH CONNECTION

Resistance training is an integral component in the comprehensive health program promoted by the major health organizations, including the American College of Sports Medicine, the American Heart Association, the American Association of Cardiovascular and Cardiopulmonary Rehabilitation, and the Surgeon General's Office (Feigenbaum and Pollock, 1999). Resistance training will make your muscles stronger and supply them with more endurance. Resistance training will guard against injury, prevent or rehabilitate low-back disorders, and increase metabolism, thereby having a positive impact on the body composition profile. Increased bone density and lower risk of osteoporosis are other reasons why everyone should regularly incorporate resistance training into their physical activity programs.

CONCEPT CONNECTION

1. ***Strength* refers to your muscle's ability to generate force.** Muscles generate force by contracting. Muscular strength refers to the amount of force a muscle can generate. Stronger muscles are capable of generating more force than weaker muscles.
2. **Significant health benefits are associated with resistance training.** Resistance training makes muscles stronger and more enduring. It helps guard against injury and prevents and rehabilitates low-back disorders. It will also help to increase your bone density, thereby decreasing the probability of your developing osteoporosis. It has positive effects on metabolic rate, allowing you to attain a healthy body composition profile.
3. **Muscles that are stressed by resistance training get stronger and increase in size (hypertrophy), while muscles that are neglected get weaker and shrink in size (atrophy).** A muscle will get stronger if it is physically stressed. The best way to stress a muscle physically is by incorporating resistance training into your physical activity program. A muscle that is not regularly exposed to stress atrophies and becomes weaker.
4. **You can develop muscular strength and endurance through a variety of resistance training programs.** The form of resistance you use to stress your muscles is not as important as the way in which you use the resistance. For this reason, you can perform a variety of activities using a variety of items to perform resistance training.
5. **All individuals (of any age) can benefit from resistance training.** Since muscles need to be stressed to function well, resistance training should be performed from the cradle to the grave. Infants who grasp their parent's finger are performing resistance training. To maintain functional independence as we age, resistance training should be performed throughout the life span.

TERMS

Muscular strength, 236
Muscular endurance, 236
Circuit weight training, 236
Protein filaments, 237
Actin, 237
Sarcomere, 237
Myosin, 237
Static contraction, 238
Concentric muscle action, 238
Eccentric muscle action, 238
Agonist, 239
Antagonist, 239
Synergists, 240
Neutralizer, 240
Hypertrophy, 241
Neuromuscular adaptations, 241
Atrophy, 241
Isometric, 242
Isotonic, 242
Isokinetic, 242
Reps, 244
Sets, 244
Overload, 244
Progression, 244
Specificity, 244
Recovery, 244
Valsalva maneuver, 246
Periodization, 256
Pyramiding, 256
Plyometrics, 256
Compound sets, 256
Tri-sets, 256
Supersets, 256

MAKING THE CONNECTION

Beth feels confident about her resistance training program. She has started to develop a program focused on muscular endurance. Beth understands that she must start gradually and work on proper form and safety. She has already noticed an increased feeling of self-confidence since she started resistance training.

CRITICAL THINKING

1. What are the major differences between training to improve muscular strength and training to improve muscular endurance?
2. What factors determine how large and strong a person can become?
3. What principles of training are important when developing a resistance training program?
4. In addition to using free weights, how else might one perform resistance training?
5. In what ways does resistance training improve your health?

REFERENCES

American College of Sports Medicine. (1998). The recommended quantity and quality of exercise for developing and maintaining cardiorespiratory and muscular fitness and flexibility in healthy adults. *Medicine and Science in Sports & Exercise* 30(6):975–91.

American College of Sports Medicine. (2000). *ACSM's Guidelines for Exercise Testing and Prescription,* 6th ed. Philadelphia: Lippincott, Williams & Wilkins.

Brill, P.A., Macera, C.A., Davis, D.R., Blair, S.N., & Gordon, N. (2000). Muscular strength and physical function. *Medicine & Science in Sports & Exercise* 32(2):412–16.

Butterfield, G., Kleiner, S., Lemon, P., & Stone, M. (1995). Roundtable: Methods of weight gain in athletes. *Gatorade Sports Science Exchange* 6(3).

Dolezal, B.A., Potteiger, J.A., Jacobsen, D.J., & Benedict, S.H. (2000). Muscle damage and resting metabolic rate after acute resistance exercise with an eccentric overload. *Medicine and Science in Sports & Exercise* 32(7):1202–07.

Feigenbaum, M.S., & Pollock, M.L. (1999). Prescription of resistance training for health and disease. *Medicine and Science in Sports & Exercise,* 31(1):38–45.

Fleck, S.J. (1999). Periodized strength training: A critical review. *Journal of Strength and Conditioning Research* 13(1):82–89.

Kraemer, W.J. (1992). Involvement of eccentric muscle action may optimize adaptations to resistance training. *Gatorade Sports Science Exchange* 4(41).

Mayo, J.J., & Kravitz, L. (1999). A review of the acute cardiovascular responses to resistance exercise of healthy young and older adults. *Journal of Strength and Conditioning Research* 13(1):90–96.

Pollock, M.L., & Vincent, K.R. (December 1996). Resistance Training for Health. *Research Digest,* Series 2, No. 8.

Stone, M.H., Collins, D.C., Plisk, S.P., Haff, G., & Stone, M.E. (2000). Training principles: Evaluation of modes and methods of resistance training. *Strength and Conditioning Journal* 22(3):65–76.

Activities & Assessments

NAME ______ SECTION ______ DATE ______

11.1 Finding Your One-Rep Max for the Bench Press

Max testing should take place after a few days of practicing proper technique and lifting light loads. *You should have an experienced spotter, or weight training professional, assist you.* To find your one-rep max (1-RM) for the bench press you will need a weight bench, a barbell, and weights of various denominations. After you have familiarized yourself with the proper technique to perform a bench press correctly, begin by selecting a weight that you can lift easily. Perform a light warm-up of 5 to 10 repetitions with that weight. Following a 1-minute rest with light stretching, perform 3 to 5 repetitions with a weight that you perceive is 60 to 80 percent of your maximum. You should be close to your one-RM at this point. Add a small amount of weight and try to lift the weight once. If the lift is successful, allow a rest period of 3 to 5 minutes. Then find a slightly heavier load and try again. Each attempt should be followed by a rest period. This process continues until a failed attempt occurs. The goal is to find your one-RM in your next 3 to 5 lifts. The one-RM is the last weight you successfully lift while using proper form (ACSM, 2000).

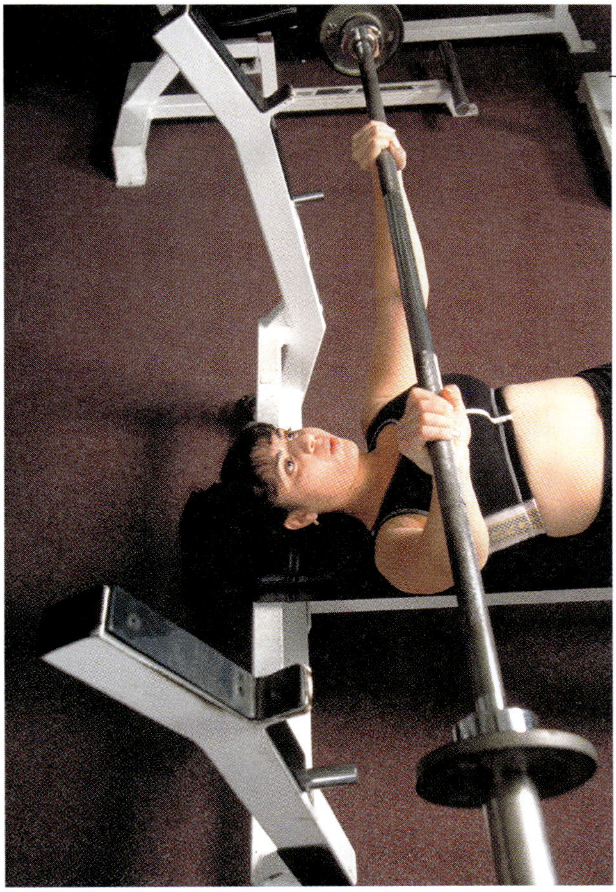

The bench-press test provides a good measure of upper-body strength.

Activities & Assessments

NAME ____________ SECTION ____________ DATE ____________

11.2 Muscular Endurance Assessment for Abdominal Fitness

The curl-up, or crunch, can be used to assess the muscular strength and endurance of the abdominal muscles. To perform this assessment, you will need some masking tape, a mat, and a metronome. First, assume a supine position (on your back) on a mat with your knees at 90 degrees. Keep your arms at your sides. Place a piece of masking tape on the mat to indicate where your fingers reach when in the starting position. A second piece of masking tape is placed 12 cm beyond the first. A metronome is set to 40 beats per minute and you perform slow, controlled curl-ups to lift the shoulder blades off the mat (your trunk should make a 30-degree angle with the mat) in time with the metronome (20 curl-ups per minute). The low back should be flattened each time before curling up again. You then perform as many curl-ups as possible without pausing, up to a maximum of 75 (ACSM, 2000). The following chart can be used to compare your results.

AGE GENDER	20–29 MEN	20–29 WOMEN	30–39 MEN	30–39 WOMEN
Well above average	75	70	75	55
Above average	41	37	46	34
Average	27	27	31	21
Below average	20	17	19	12
Well below average	4	5	0	0

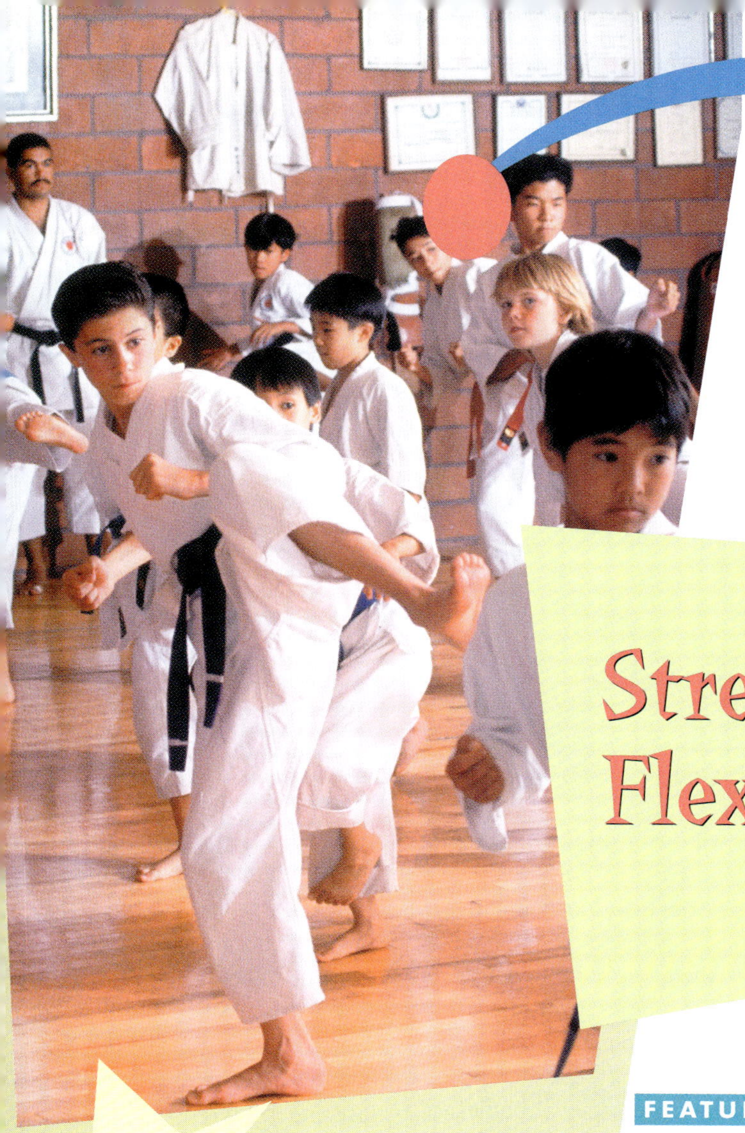

12

Stretching and Flexibility

CONCEPT CONNECTION

1. Many factors influence the amount of flexibility you have at a joint.
2. Sense receptors located in your muscles and tendons play an important role in developing good flexibility.
3. Three common categories of flexibility exercises are static, ballistic, and PNF.
4. Guidelines for improving flexibility suggest stretching a muscle and holding the position for 10–30 seconds.
5. Good flexibility protects against injury, enhances your ability to be physically active, and helps maintain an independent lifestyle.
6. Most low back pain is caused by poor muscular fitness.

FEATURES

E-Learning Tools: www.pahconnection.com

Engage www.pahconnection.com

12.1 Fitness assessment
12.2 Flexibility training: muscle map and explanation

Experience www.pahconnection.com

12.1 Alternative methods for improving flexibility
12.2 Flexibility exercises for the lower back
12.3 Recommended flexibility exercises for the elderly

Explore www.pahconnection.com

12.1 General information
12.2 Fitness online
12.3 Fitness assessment
12.4 Alternative flexibility exercises

Activities & Assessments

12.1 Sit and reach test
12.2 Trunk extension
12.3 Shoulder flexion

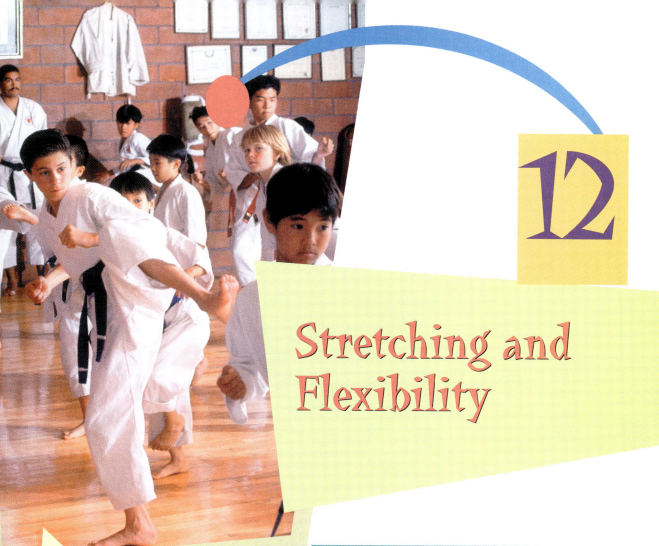

WHAT'S THE CONNECTION?

Bob works out regularly, but he has not paid much attention to incorporating flexibility exercises into his physical activity routine. Recently, Bob has noticed that his lower back gets sore in the morning following a highly active day. Bob can't remember any sudden trauma to his back and the pain subsides as he gets up and starts moving around. He remembers hearing something about low-back pain being related to poor muscular fitness and in particular, poor flexibility. Bob decides to do some investigating to see what he can find out about the relationship between low-back pain and flexibility.

1. Many factors influence the amount of flexibility you have at a joint.

Flexibility The range of motion available at a joint.

Elasticity Degree to which a material resists deformation and quickly returns to its normal shape.

Compliance Ease with which a material is elongated or stretched; the opposite of stiffness.

Tissue interference Occurs when either muscle or fat tissue physically blocks a movement, restricting a joint's full range of motion.

INTRODUCTION

This chapter will focus on the importance of maintaining good flexibility. It will provide instruction on developing a flexibility program and examples of stretching exercises. The chapter explores the relationship between good flexibility and good health.

Flexibility refers to the range of motion available at a joint. There are many factors that can influence range of motion including: anatomical structure of the joint (how the bones are aligned), muscle temperature, disease status, muscle and tendon **elasticity** and **compliance**, age, sex, activity status, and **tissue interference.** Anatomical structure varies from joint to joint in our own bodies, and there is a great deal of variation among individuals. Since range of motion is in part determined by our joint structure, this anatomical variation can have profound effects on flexibility.

Length of bone also impacts range of motion. A common test of hamstring flexibility, the sit-and-reach test, demonstrates this point. When performing the sit-and-reach, you sit down with your legs straight out in front of you (Figure 12.1). Placing your hands on top of each other, you lean as far forward as possible. Your flexibility is

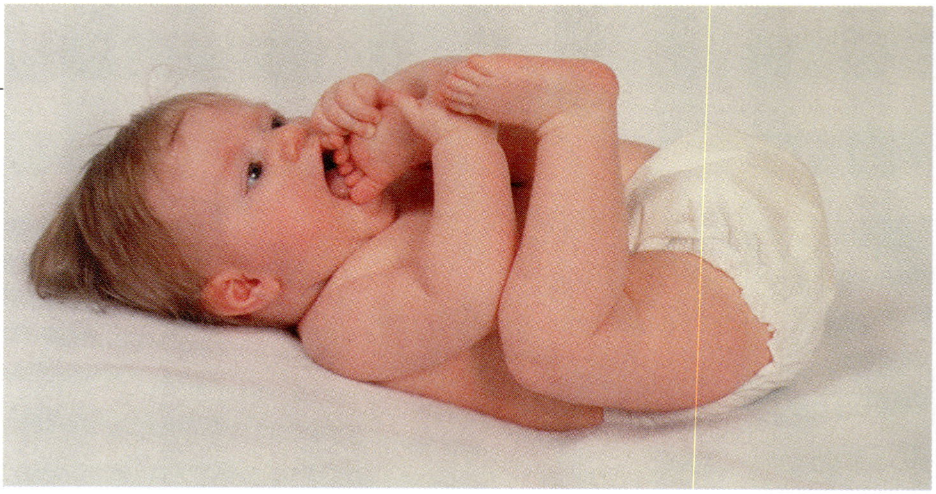

Flexibility is important throughout the life span.

assessed based on how far you can reach. If the test is not modified, limb length discrepancies may have a major impact on the results. For example, someone with short legs and long arms will score better than someone with long legs and short arms.

Muscle temperature has a direct impact on flexibility because it affects muscle elasticity and compliance. Elasticity and compliance refer to the muscle's ability to stretch beyond its normal resting length and then return to its initial length once the forces causing the stretch are removed. When a muscle is cold, its elastic and compliant properties are diminished; when it is warm, the muscle is more pliable (stretchy). If you warm a muscle, or perform stretching activities, on warm days, you will have better flexibility than if you stretch cold muscles on cold days.

Certain diseases can diminish flexibility. They can limit compliance of a muscle, of a muscle's tendon, or of the ligaments that connect the bones. We lose flexibility if we lose muscle and tendon compliance. Loss of muscle and tendon elasticity and compliance may be caused by disuse. Stretching exercises can improve muscle and tendon compliance by regularly making the muscle move through its full range of motion. Over a period of time, muscles and tendons that are stretched and then relaxed become more pliable.

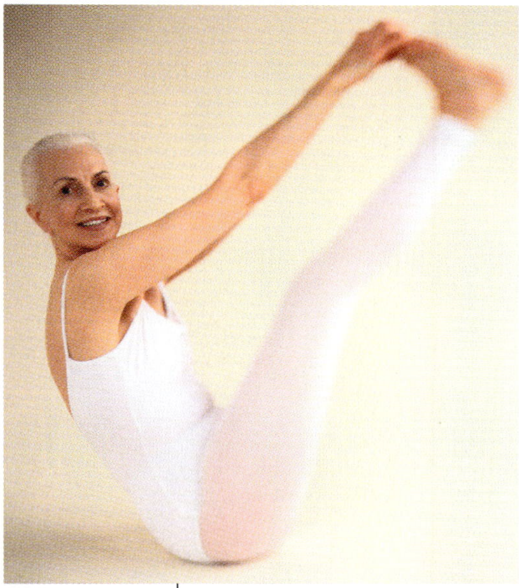

Improving your flexibility helps to maintain an independent, active lifestyle.

As we age, the elastic and compliant properties of our muscles and tendons naturally diminish. This can lead to a loss of flexibility. However, we now know that the rate and degree at which this natural aging process occurs can be limited by performing stretching activities regularly (ACSM, 2000; Knudson, Magnusson, & McHugh, 2000). We can delay the onset of age-related flexibility loss, and we can also minimize the impact of age on our functional ability.

Activities & Assessments 12.1

Engage www.pahconnection.com 12.1

In most cases, women are more flexible than men. This is due in part to anatomic differences (for example, differences in hip joint structure), but hormonal influences on muscle compliance also contributes to male/female flexibility differences.

Tissue interference refers to the possibility that either muscle or fat tissue may physically block a movement and restrict a joint's ability to provide full range of motion. For instance, an obese individual, or a person with highly developed muscle mass, may find that the fat mass or muscle mass physically blocks some movement. This can

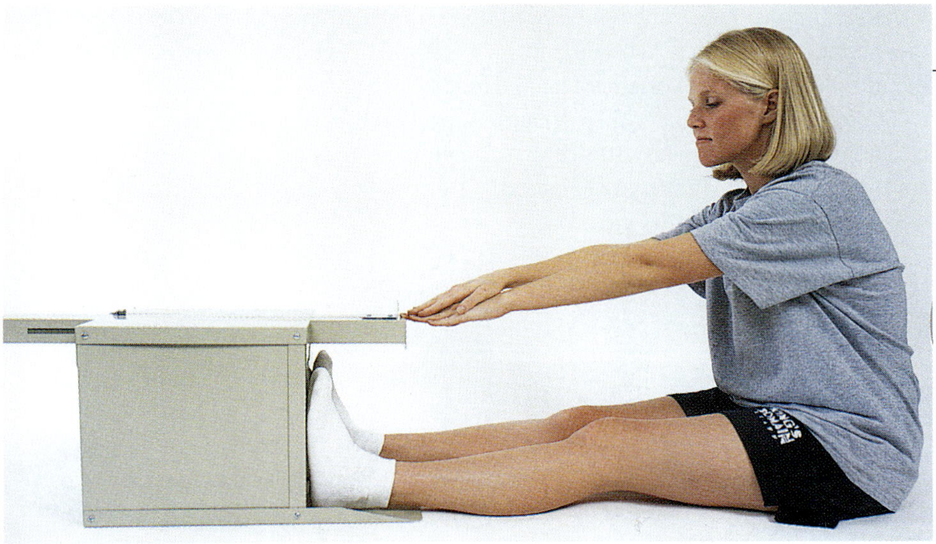

FIGURE 12.1

Sit-and-Reach Test.
A sit-and-reach test can be used to assess your hamstring flexibility.

Explore
www.pahconnection.com
12.1, 12.2

become a problem if the muscle is prevented from moving through its full range of motion. The affected muscle and tendon may shorten, thereby decreasing flexibility.

Several of these factors are beyond our control (anatomic structure, age, sex). We do, however, have the ability to manipulate other factors such as activity status, muscle temperature, disease status, muscle and tendon elasticity and compliance, and tissue interference. We can enhance our flexibility by performing stretching exercises daily and by maintaining an active lifestyle.

MUSCLE SPINDLES AND GOLGI TENDON ORGANS

2. Sense receptors located in your muscles and tendons play an important role in developing good flexibility.

Throughout the body we have **proprioceptors,** or sense receptors, that provide feedback to the central nervous system. Located within the thick center portion (belly) of our muscles are sense receptors called muscle spindles. **Muscle spindles** are sensitive to rapid forceful stretching, responding with a reflexive contraction of the muscle called the stretch reflex. A **stretch reflex** occurs when your muscle contracts in response to rapid forceful stretching. If you happen to be bouncing when performing a stretching exercise, you are more likely to elicit the stretch reflex. Bouncing has the potential to cause muscle injury.

Our tendons also have sense receptors imbedded within them that are called Golgi tendon organs. **Golgi tendon organs** are sensitive to rapid forceful contractions and cause a reflexive relaxation to occur within the muscle. As the tension increases in the muscle and tendon, these sense receptors detect the tension and regulate further muscle action. Muscle action might be inhibited to induce relaxation. This reflex inhibition can prevent injury from excessive strain and may account for short-term increases in flexibility immediately after stretching (ACSM, 1998).

MUSCLE ELASTICITY AND COMPLIANCE

Proprioceptors Sense receptors that provide feedback to our central nervous system.

Muscle spindles Sense receptors sensitive to rapid forceful stretching that cause a reflexive contraction of the muscle.

Stretch reflex Reflexive response to forceful rapid stretching that causes a muscle to contract.

Golgi tendon organs Sense receptors sensitive to rapid forceful contractions that cause a reflexive relaxation to occur within the muscle.

Our muscles are held together by a series of elastic connective tissues that both surround each muscle and are found throughout each muscle. These connective tissues come together at the ends of the muscles into tendons. It is the tendons that connect muscle to bone. When we move a muscle, we stretch these connective tissues. When the muscle relaxes, the connective-tissue recoil helps the muscle return to its original resting length.

Stretching exercises have their greatest impact on the connective tissues of the muscle and tendon. By regularly stretching these connective tissues, the elastic and compliant properties of the tissues are enhanced. Stretching results in a short-term increase in muscle and tendon length, and a lasting increase through alteration in the surrounding connective tissue matrix (ACSM, 1998).

TYPES OF STRETCHING EXERCISES

3. Three common categories of flexibility exercises are static, ballistic, and PNF.

To perform stretching exercises, there are several different methods from which you can select. All have advantages and disadvantages, so choose the one that best fits your individual needs and the type of physical activity you are about to perform.

Static Stretching

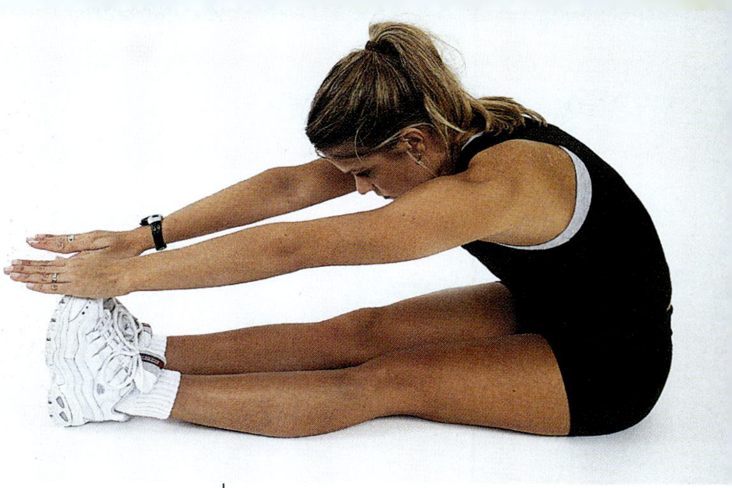

Static stretching is recommended for most people.

Static stretching moves a muscle into a position where the muscle is stretched slightly beyond its normal range of motion. A slight discomfort, but no pain, should be felt. The muscle is then held in this position for 10–30 seconds. The nonmoving state of the muscle gives static stretching its name. This type of stretching activity is recommended prior to starting physical activity. It is one of the safest methods of stretching.

A potential disadvantage of static stretching is that it may take a good deal of time to stretch out all of your muscles. For this reason, multi-joint stretching is recommended. By performing static multi-joint stretching activities, you can stretch more than one muscle group at a time.

Ballistic Stretching

Ballistic stretching, an exaggerated form of dynamic stretching, utilizes a bouncing motion to move a muscle beyond its normal range of motion. This type of stretching activity has the potential to cause injury if the muscle is not properly warmed up, or if the bouncing is too forceful and rapid. However, since most physical activity is dynamic in nature, the body can handle dynamic stretching if it is performed properly. This type of stretching is recommended only when the muscle is adequately warmed up, after static stretching has been performed, and when the dynamic stretches are performed slowly. An advantage to this type of stretching is that you can stretch rather rapidly. The major disadvantage is that you are at greater risk of injury.

Static stretching Elongating a muscle and holding that position.

Ballistic stretching Fast, momentum-assisted, pulsing movements used to stretch muscles.

PNF stretching Proprioceptive neuromuscular facilitation; utilization and integration of the nervous and muscular systems to enhance flexibility.

PNF Stretching

PNF stretching, or *proprioceptive neuromuscular facilitation,* utilizes and integrates the nervous and muscular systems to enhance flexibility. As mentioned earlier, Gogli tendon organs are located in the tendons that connect muscle to bone. They are sensitive to rapid forceful contraction and respond by causing the muscle to relax. In PNF stretching, you take advantage of the way Golgi tendon organs work and use them to enhance flexibility (Holcomb, 2000). You do this by causing a muscle to contract and then relaxing the muscle. The forced contraction aids in getting the muscle to relax.

An example of PNF stretching would be the contract-relax-contract method. In this method, you first maximally contract an agonist (prime mover, biceps). The agonist muscle then relaxes. This is followed by contraction of the antagonist (resistor, triceps) muscle. The initial forceful contraction involves Golgi tendon organ feedback. The relaxation phase and subsequent contraction of the antagonist muscle further enhances the degree of relaxation felt in the agonist muscle.

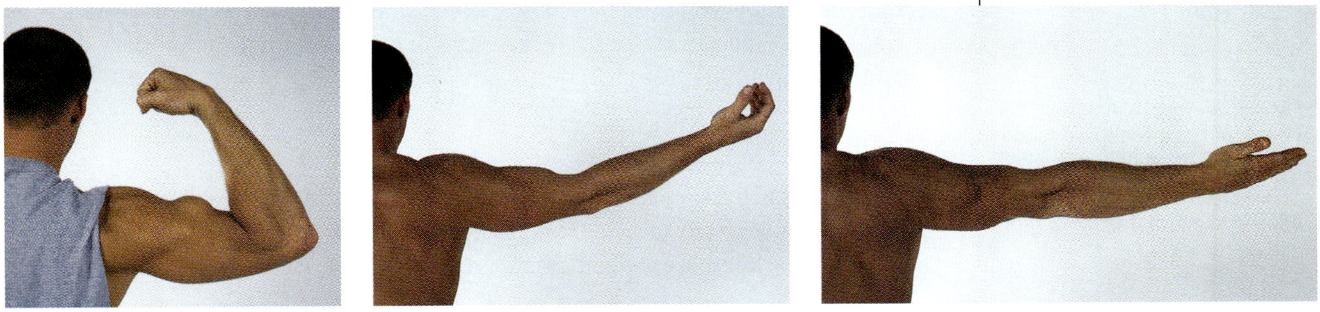

Contract, relax, antagonist-contract method of PNF stretching.

There is some evidence that PNF may bring superior results compared to the other types of exercises done to increase flexibility (ACSM, 1998, Holcomb, 2000). However, it usually takes a greater degree of training to perform PNF safely and effectively. Static stretches, therefore, are commonly used, and for many individuals represent a safer and still-effective compromise (ACSM, 1998).

PASSIVE AND ACTIVE STRETCHING

Two additional concepts that are related to stretching exercises and flexibility are the concepts of **passive** and **active stretching.** Passive stretching occurs when the individual allows the muscle and tendon to stretch naturally, without additional force being applied. This is a safer method of stretching than active stretching; however, gains in flexibility are usually not as large.

Active stretching involves taking a muscle beyond its normal range of motion with assistance. This may be facilitated by having a partner move the limb segment to the end of its normal range of motion, or by contracting antagonists to further stretch an agonist muscle. It takes a skilled partner to help you perform active stretching safely; if the muscle is moved too far, you may injure yourself.

Passive stretching A natural stretch of the muscle and tendon with no additional force applied.

Active stretching Taking a muscle beyond its normal range of motion with assistance.

FLEXIBILITY GUIDELINES

4. Guidelines for improving flexibility suggest stretching a muscle and holding the position for 10–30 seconds.

Flexibility guidelines vary based on the individuals and their needs. Generally, however, you can improve your flexibility by following some common suggestions. First of all, flexibility exercises should be just one part of an overall physical activity program. The focus of the flexibility component of your physical activity program should be to develop and maintain a healthy range of motion (ROM). Exercises that stretch the major muscle groups should be performed a minimum of 2 to 3 days per week (ACSM, 1998). Any of the previously described techniques (static, ballistic, PNF) may be used to enhance flexibility if they are performed properly.

Frequency, Intensity and Duration

It is generally suggested that slow rates of stretching allow greater stress relaxation and generate lower tensile force on the tendon. For this reason, it is recommended that you hold a position that places a muscle on stretch for 10 to 30 seconds at the point of mild discomfort (ACSM, 1998). If you perform PNF stretches, they should involve a 6-second contraction followed by a 10- to 30-second assisted stretch (ACSM, 1998). Exercises that stretch multiple muscle groups are typically suggested because they allow you to stretch more muscles, more thoroughly, and in a shorter period of time. It appears that four repetitions of a stretching activity produce the best results (ACSM, 1998).

When to Stretch

It is best to make stretching a daily part of your physical activity program. Stretching exercises can take place any time, any place. They can be performed first thing in the morning or the last thing at night. Stretching activities can be performed while watching the news or a favorite television show. In fact, you can even perform stretching exercises while you work.

As part of your workout routine, it is advisable to perform low-intensity stretching exercises before moving to more vigorous physical activity. This will help prepare your body for the activity that is to follow and decrease your chance for injury. After performing your preferred physical activity, additional stretching exercises should be done. It is during this cool-down from physical activity that the greatest improvements in flexibility are obtained. Remember that a warmer muscle stretches better and your muscle will be its warmest immediately following physical activity.

Assessment of Flexibility

Before beginning any flexibility program, it is smart to do some pre-assessment. This will help you to determine which muscle groups require the most work. Generally, it is recommended that you perform an overall stretching program that focuses on the major muscle groups and then supplement with additional activities that focus on the muscles that need more work.

When discussing the assessment of flexibility, it is important to use standardized terminology. Physical therapists often distinguish between active range of motion (unassisted) and passive range of motion (therapist assisted) in assessing static flexibility (Knudson, Magnusson, and McHugh, 2000). The type of test you perform will influence the results of the test. When results are compared, you need to know what type of flexibility was measured.

Activities & Assessments 12.2, 12.3

Single-joint flexibility tests are considered better measurements of flexibility than multiple-joint tests because they isolate specific muscles better and are less affected by limb segment length variations (Knudson et al., 2000). Goniometers are generally used to make single-joint flexibility measurements.

Explore www.pahconnection.com 12.3

Multiple-joint flexibility assessments like the sit-and-reach test are utilized by most fitness professionals (Knudson et al., 2000). In addition to the sit-and-reach, the shoulder and trunk lifts are common multiple-joint tests.

COMMON STRETCHING EXERCISES

There are numerous stretching exercises from which you can choose. These range from such exotic movements as those found in yoga and tai chi to those practiced regularly by the recreational exerciser. The websites found in this chapter contain links to many different stretching exercises that you might want to try out.

Engage www.pahconnection.com 12.2

When selecting the stretching exercises that are right for you, remember to choose those that stretch the major muscle masses of the body. Multi-joint stretches, which allow you to stretch many muscles at once, are efficient. There are a number of muscles that cross more than one joint, so they can be targeted by multi-joint stretching exercises. These would include the hamstring (back of thigh) muscles, the quadriceps (front of thigh) muscles, and the calf muscles.

Sample Stretching Program

Flexibility is specific to each joint in your body. You may have good flexibility in one region and poor flexibility in another (Knudson et al., 2000). We suggest that you focus a segment of your stretching program on each of the following: the arms, legs, shoulders, upper and lower trunk, neck, and hips. We also suggest that you perform static stretching because it is the easiest and safest method for improving flexibility (ACSM, 2000). Figures 12.2 through 12.26 illustrate suggested stretching exercises.

When performing these activities, it is recommended that you first warm your muscles with some low-intensity aerobic movement (walking). Then, take the muscle you wish to stretch to a position of mild discomfort and hold that position for 10 to 30 seconds. You should perform each stretch 3 to 4 times. Flexibility exercises should be performed a minimum of 2 to 3 days per week (ACSM, 2000).

FIGURE 12.2

Neck Stretch.
Ear to shoulder.

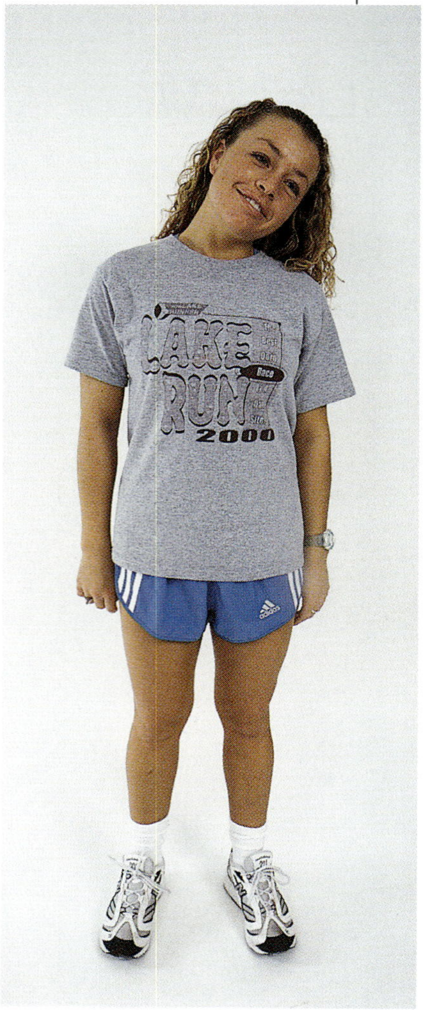

FIGURE 12.3

Neck Stretch.
Chin to chest.

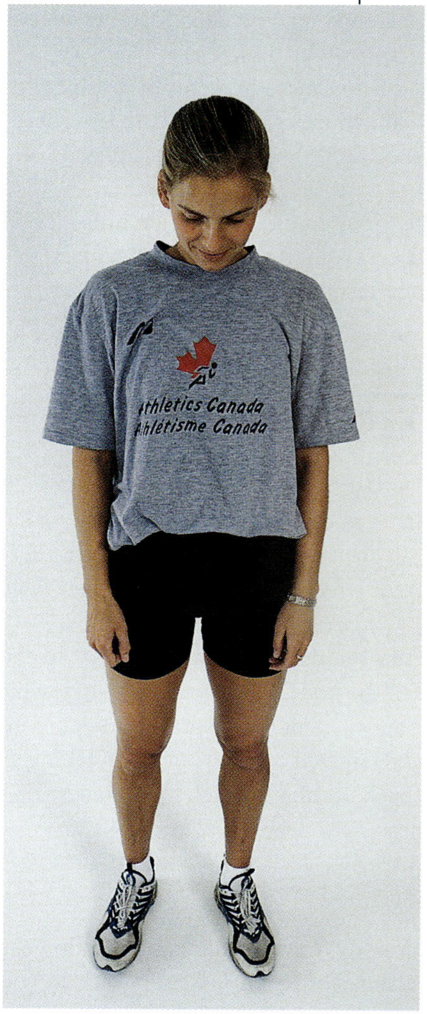

FIGURE 12.4

Neck Stretch.
Look right and left.

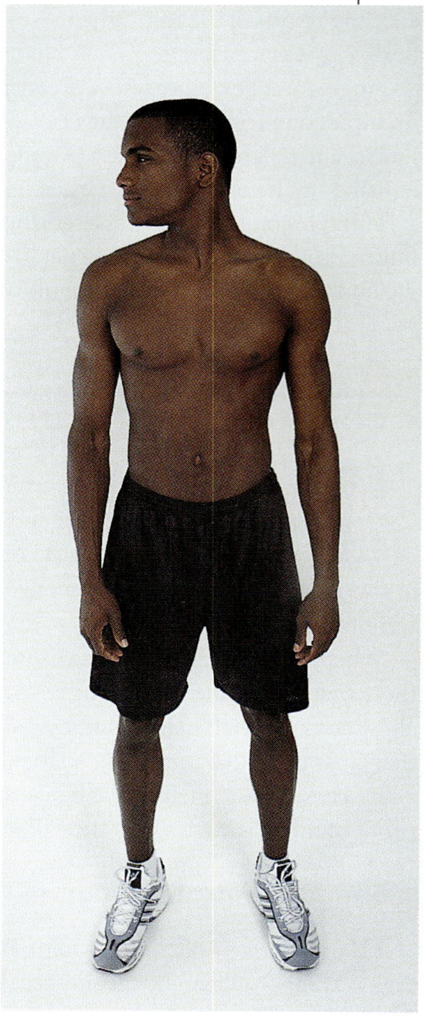

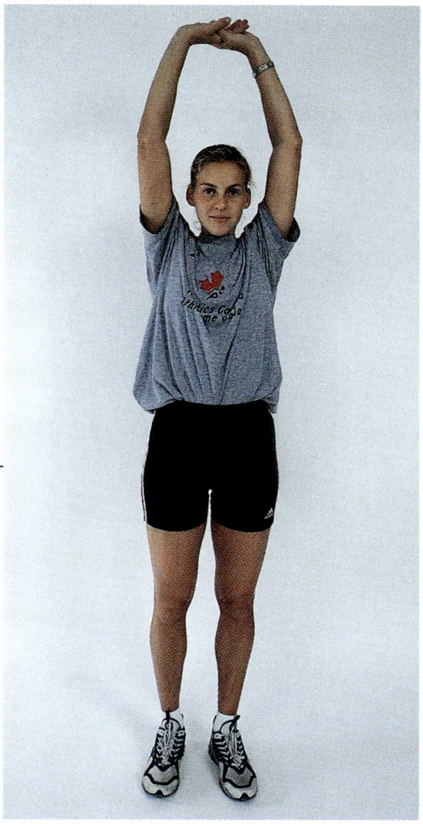

FIGURE 12.5

Shoulder, Chest, and Upper-Back Stretch. Reach up.

FIGURE 12.6

Shoulder, Chest, and Upper-Back Stretch. Slow arm circles.

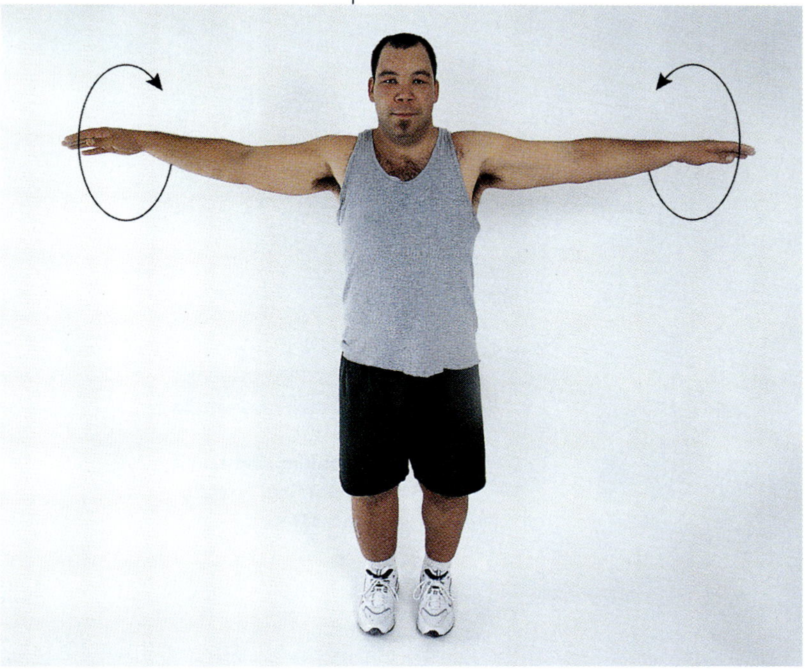

FIGURE 12.7

Shoulder and Chest Stretch. Arm across chest.

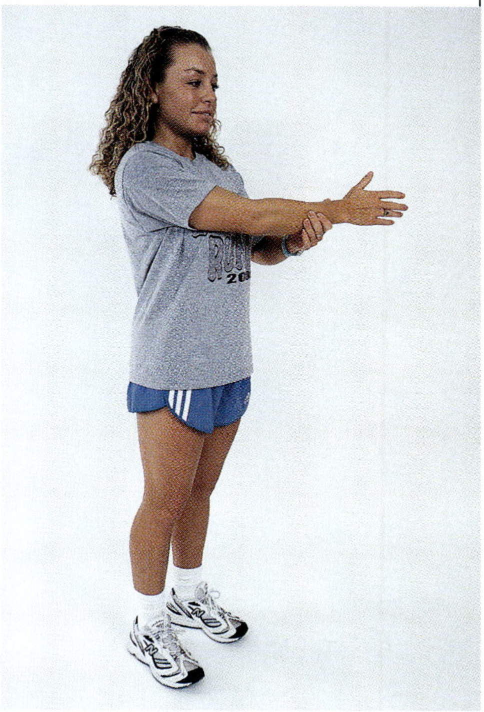

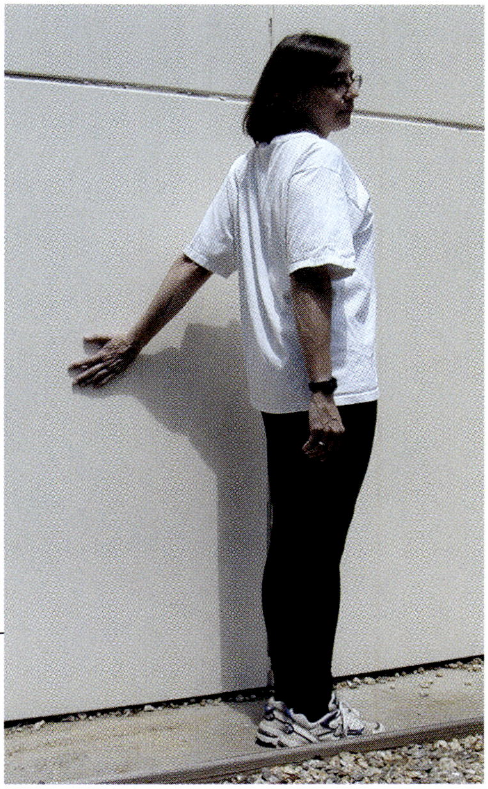

FIGURE 12.8

Shoulder and Chest Stretch. Wall chest stretch.

FIGURE 12.9

Shoulder, Chest, and Upper Back Stretch. Shoulder roll.

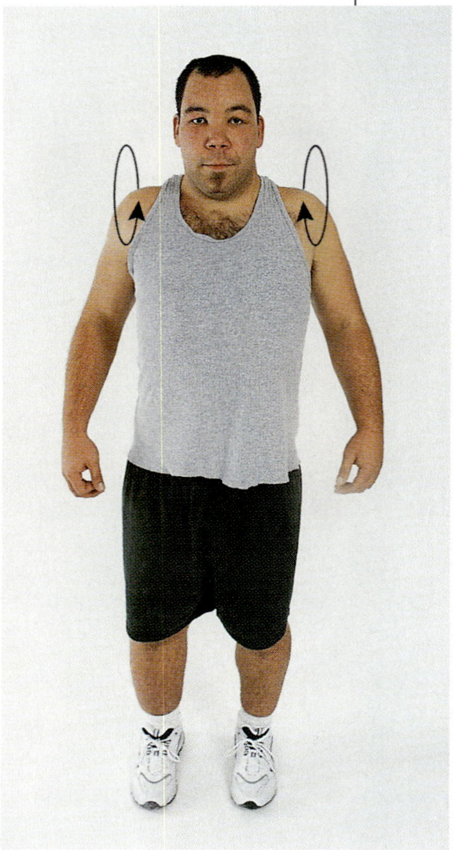

FIGURE 12.11

Shoulder, Chest, and Upper-Back Stretch. Back scratch.

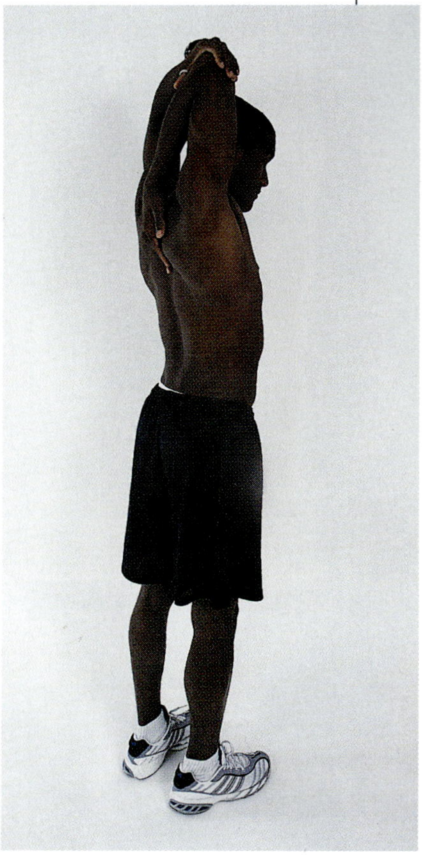

FIGURE 12.12

Shoulder, Chest, and Upper-Back Stretch. Handcuff stretch.

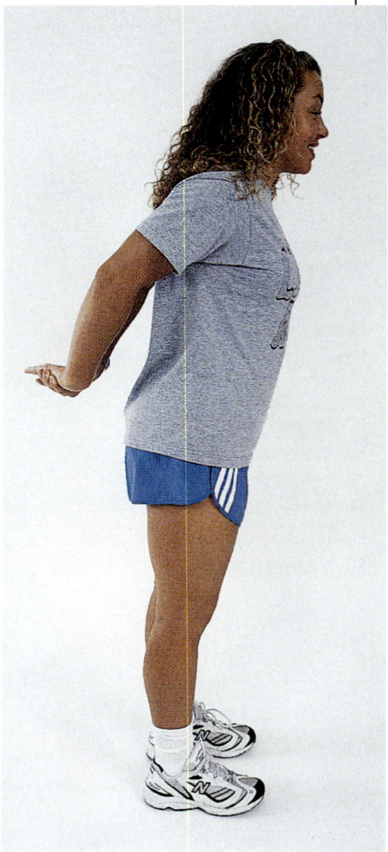

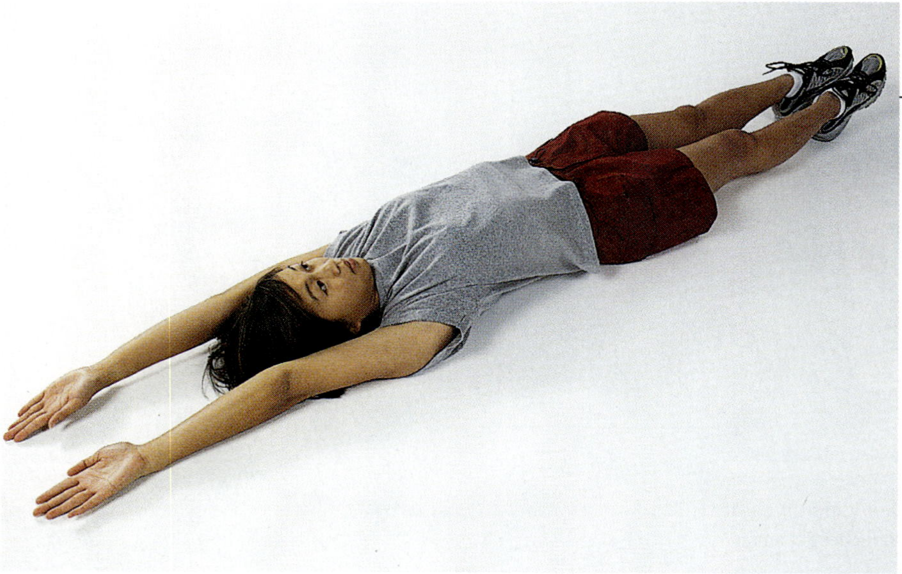

FIGURE 12.10

Shoulder, Chest, and Abdominal Stretch. Rack stretch.

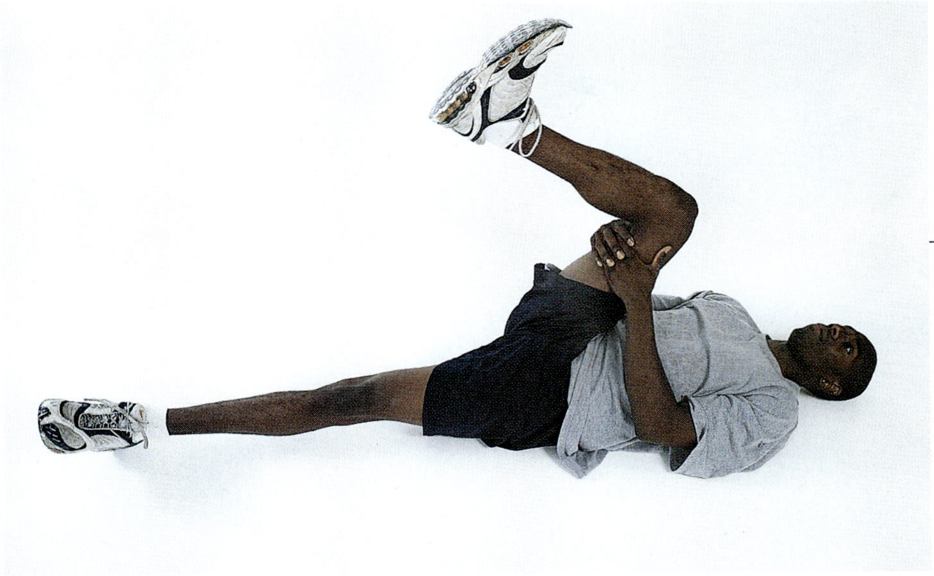

FIGURE 12.13

Hamstring Stretch.
Single bent-leg vertical.

FIGURE 12.15

Hamstring and Groin Stretch.
Modified hurdler stretch.

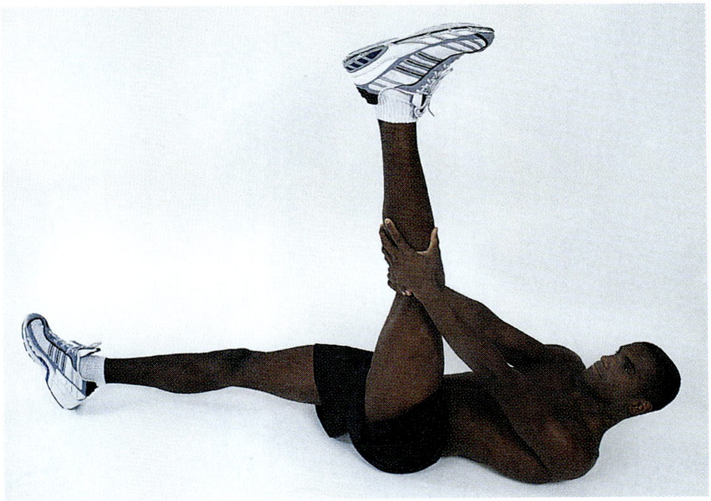

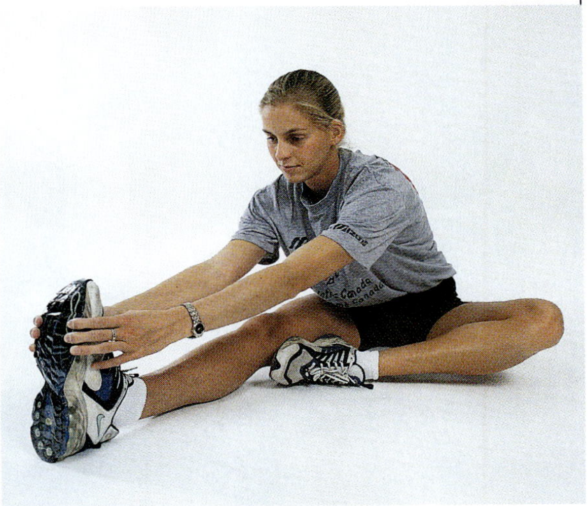

FIGURE 12.14

Hamstring Stretch.
Single straight-leg vertical.

FIGURE 12.16

Lower-Back and Hamstring Stretch.
Single knee to chest.

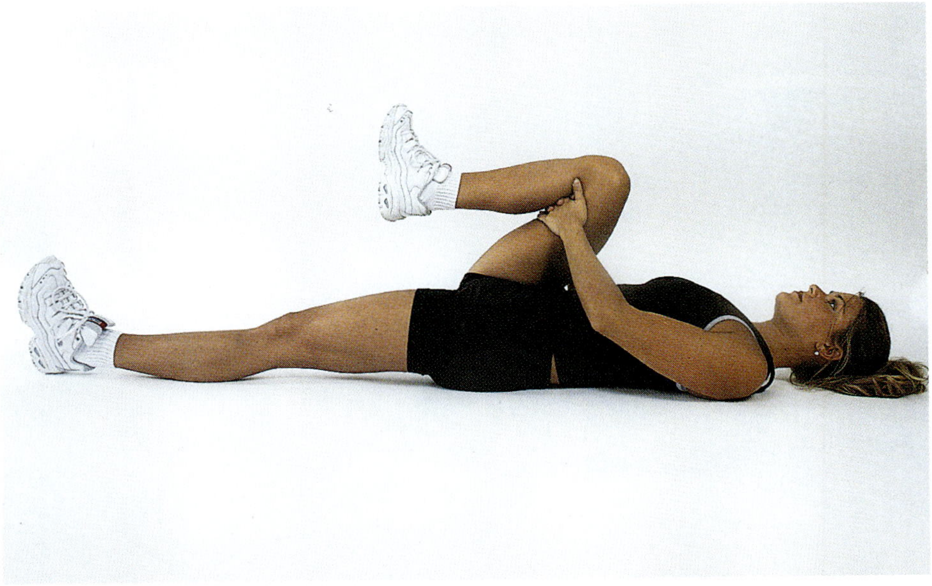

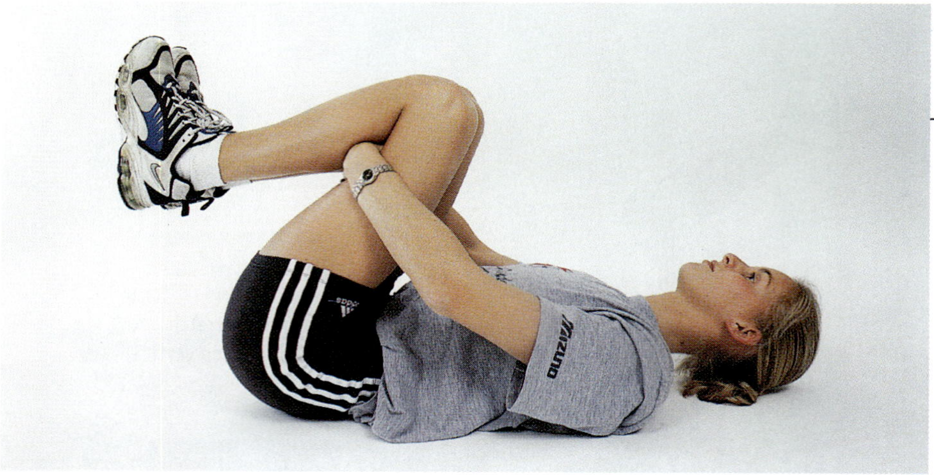

FIGURE 12.17

Lower-Back and Hamstring Stretch. Double knee to chest.

FIGURE 12.19

Lower-Back Stretch. Cat and camel.

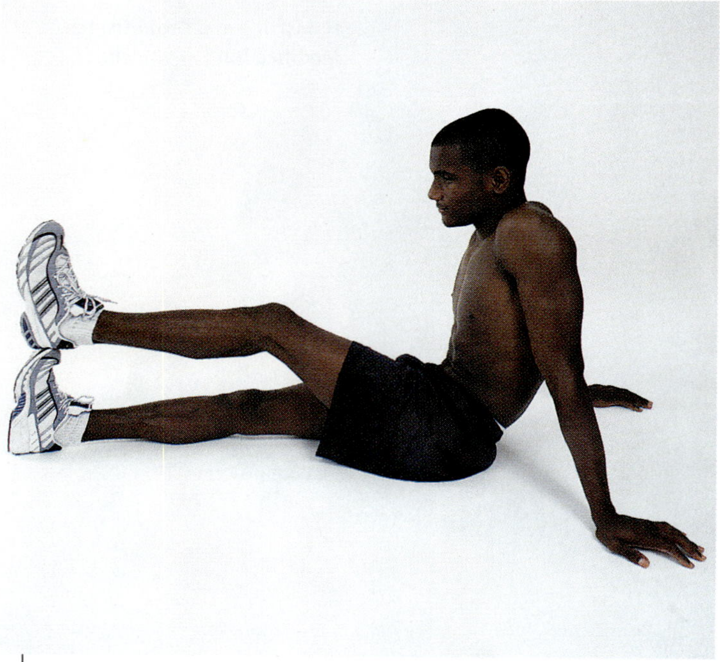

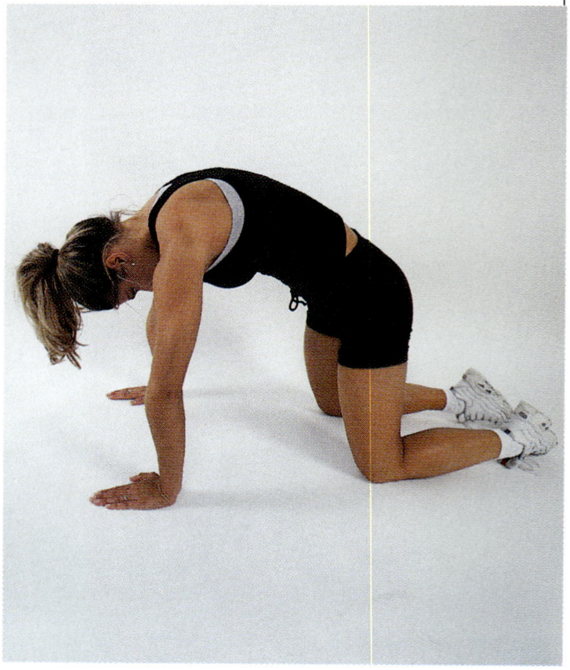

FIGURE 12.18

Calf Stretch. Seated toe stretch.

FIGURE 12.20

Lower-Back, Groin and Hamstring Stretch. V-sit stretch.

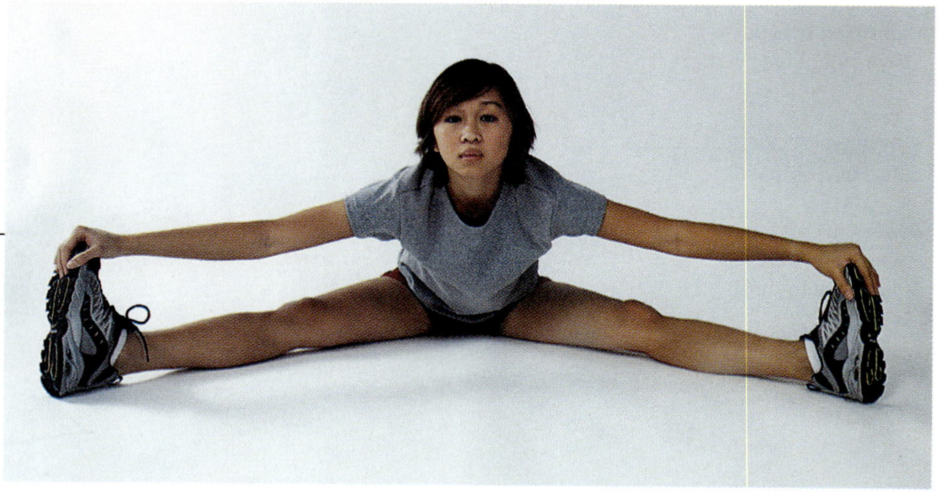

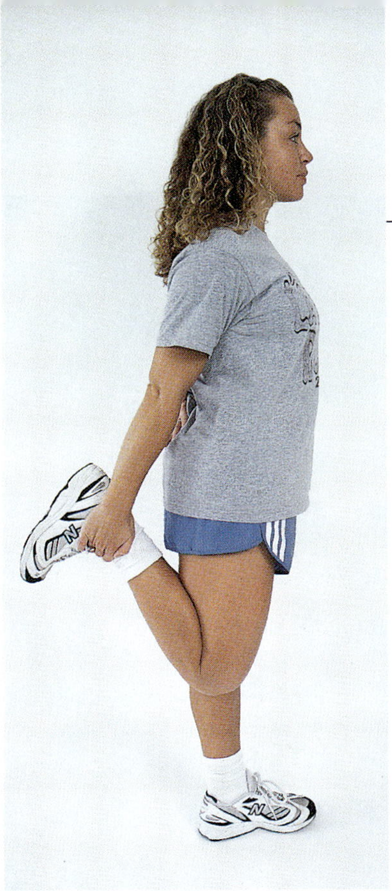

FIGURE 12.21

Quad Stretch.
Standing heel-to-buttock stretch.

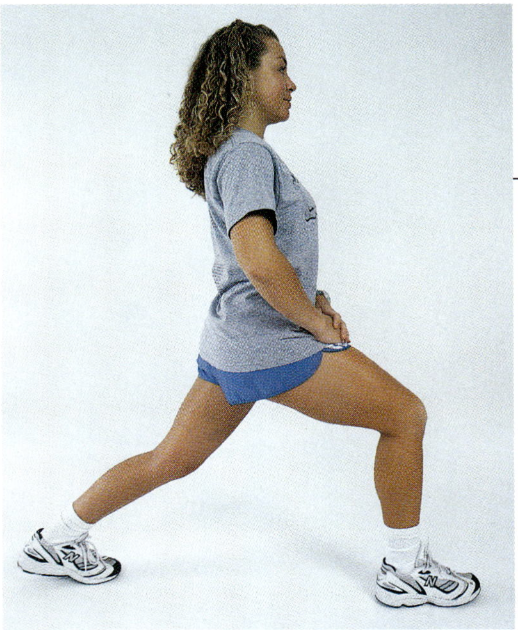

FIGURE 12.22

Inner-Thigh and Quad Stretch.
Standing lunge stretch.

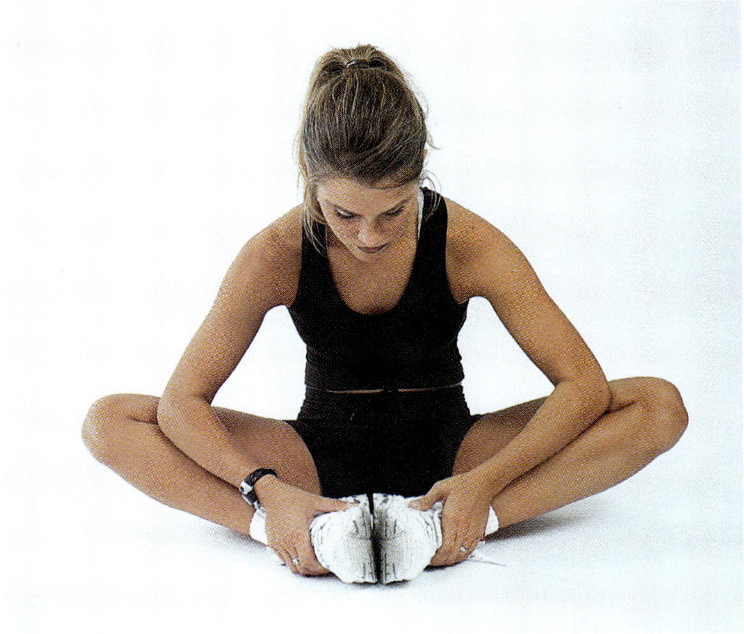

FIGURE 12.23

Inner-Thigh and Quad Stretch.
Butterfly stretch.

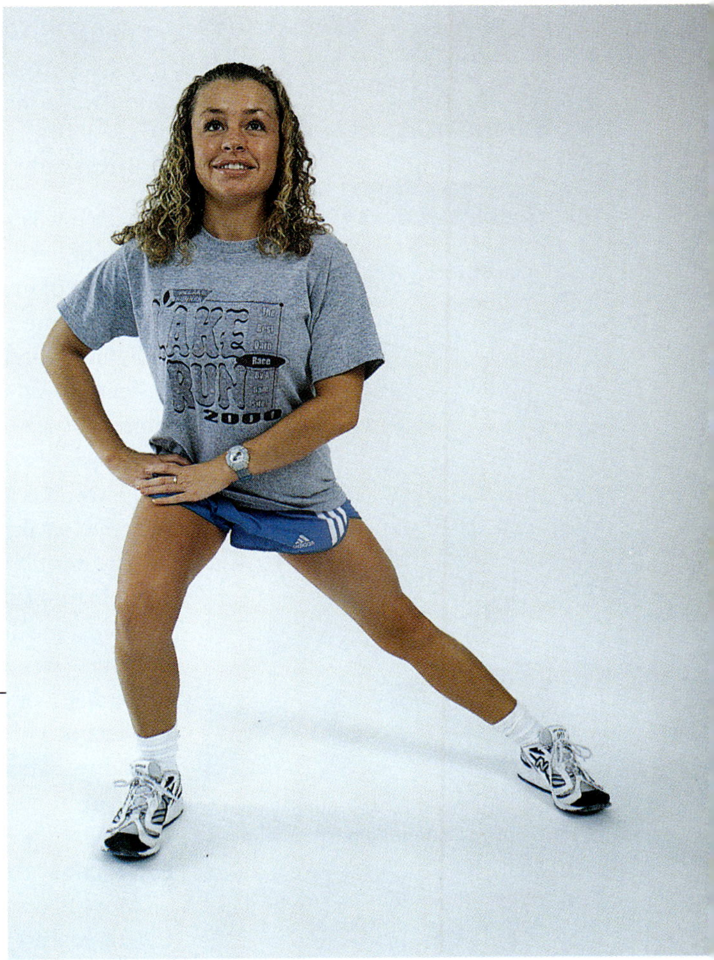

FIGURE 12.24

Inner-Thigh, Quad and Hip Stretch.
Side lunge (skater) stretch.

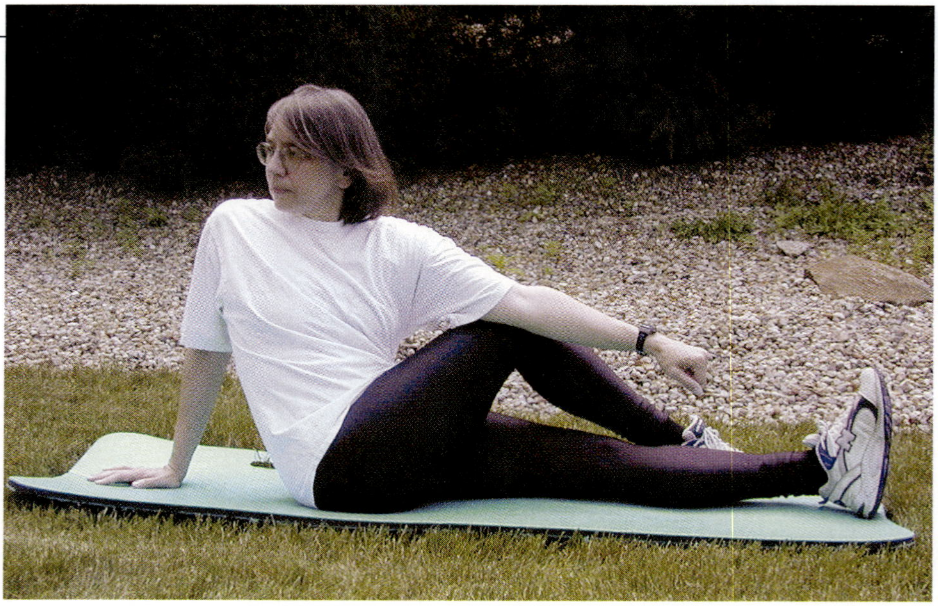

FIGURE 12.25

Gluteal and Trunk Stretch.
Elbow-to-knee stretch.

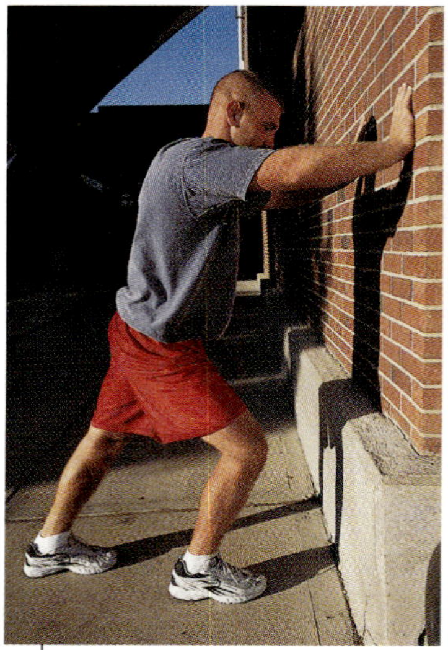

FIGURE 12.26

Calf Stretch.
Wall lean.

Alternative Flexibility Activities

Although beyond the scope of this book, there are other forms of stretching activities that you can perform to enhance flexibility. Yoga and tai chi are but two of many popular alternative flexibility activities.

Improper Stretching

When we perform activities designed to improve flexibility, it is important to remember that the primary goal is to improve muscle compliance. We can also increase the range of motion available at a joint by overstretching the ligaments that hold the joints together. Overstretching can occur when ligaments are taken beyond their normal range of motion. Ligaments connect bone to bone and do not have great elastic properties. When ligaments are stretched, they do not regain their original shape. Over time, activities that stretch the ligaments may lead to joint laxity. *Joint laxity* means that the ligaments can no longer provide the stability necessary to hold the joint together properly. This is a negative adaptation to physical activity, wherein the joint actually becomes weaker and has an increased risk for joint injury.

The positions with the greatest likelihood of causing joint laxity are those that place the joint in positions well beyond its normal range of motion. Typically these positions involve some degree of **hyperextension** or **hyperflexion.** Hyperextension occurs when a joint is extended beyond its normal range; an example would be when the leg starts in a straight or extended position and then is forced backward at the knee. Hyperflexion occurs when a joint is flexed beyond its normal range; an example would be when an individual performs a squat and bends too low, forcing the angle at the knee below 90 degrees. Ballistic (rapid, forceful) movement into or out of a hyperextended or hyperflexed position, with the addition of a load or external force being applied, further increases the risk for joint damage.

Movements that place an individual at risk for joint injury are referred to as *contraindicated* exercises, or exercises that we should avoid (Figures 12.27 through 12.31).

Explore 12.4

Hyperextension Moving beyond a normal extended position at a joint.

Hyperflexion Moving beyond a normal flexed position at a joint.

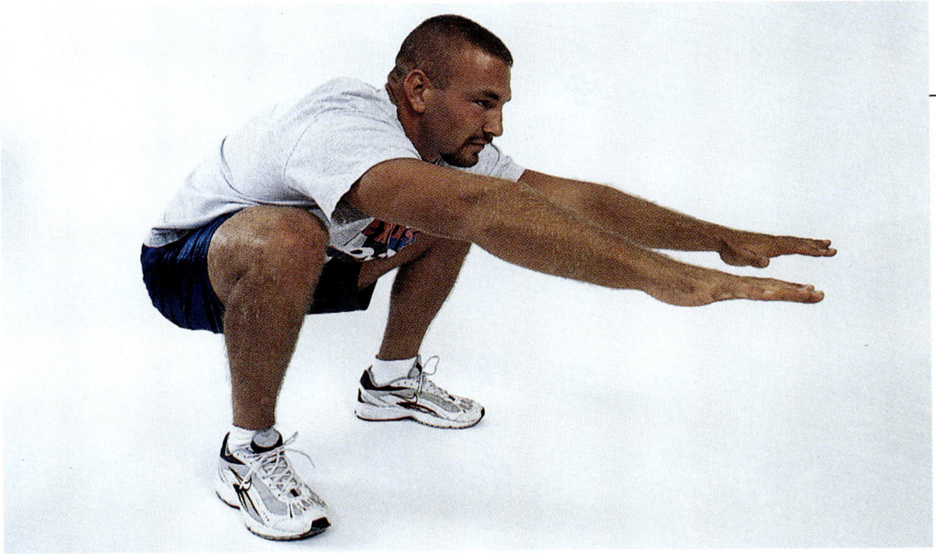

FIGURE 12.27

Contraindicated Exercise.
Full squat.

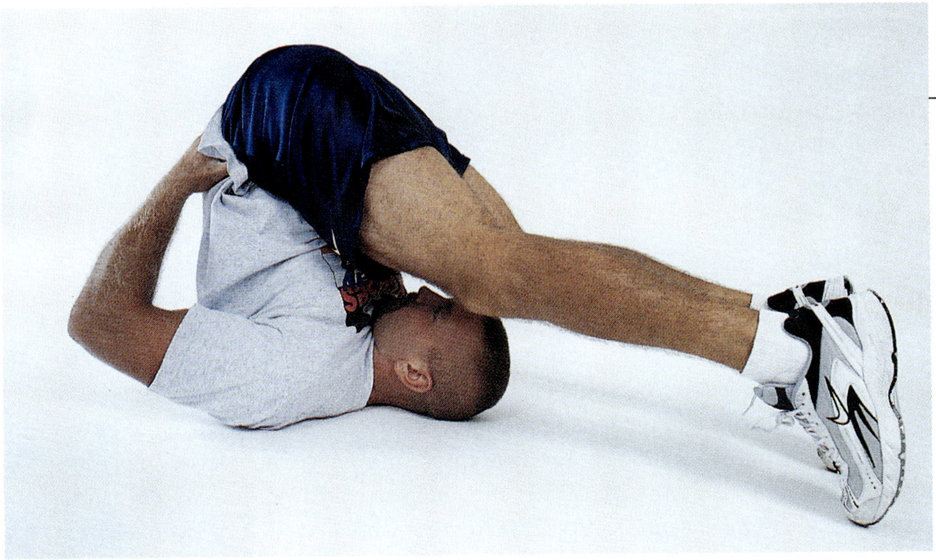

FIGURE 12.28

Contraindicated Exercise.
Plough.

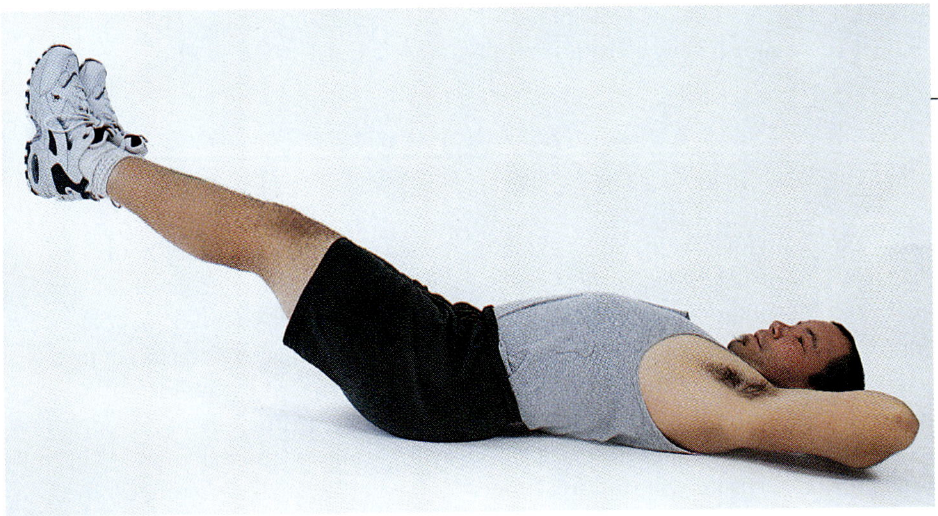

FIGURE 12.29

Contraindicated Exercise.
Double-leg raises.

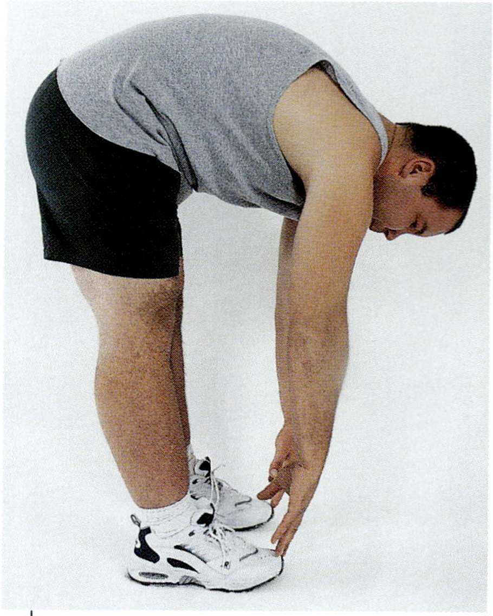

FIGURE 12.30

Contraindicated Exercise.
Standing toe touch.

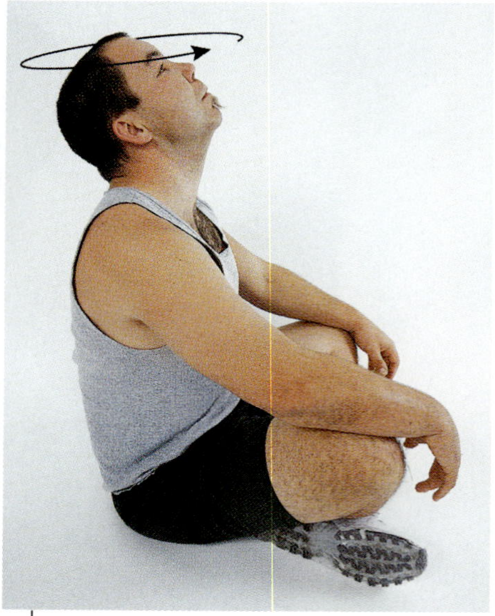

FIGURE 12.31

Contraindicated Exercise.
Full neck circles.

CHANGES IN FLEXIBILITY WITH AGE

As we age, we naturally lose some of the elasticity and compliance in our muscles and tendons. The degree and rate of loss are related to how active we are during the aging process. People who live sedentary lifestyles and those who don't perform any stretching activities lose muscle and tendon elasticity and compliance more rapidly than those who are active. A loss of elasticity and compliance will result in inflexibility and a reduction in joint range of motion (ACSM, 1998). A substantial loss of flexibility can significantly impair an individual's ability to accomplish daily activities and perform exercise (ACSM, 1998).

ROLE OF FLEXIBILITY IN INJURY PREVENTION

5. Good flexibility protects against injury, enhances your ability to be physically active, and helps maintain an independent lifestyle.

Normal levels of static flexibility are needed for a low risk of injury in most vigorous physical activities, while very high or low levels of static flexibility may represent an increased risk of injury (Knudson et al., 2000). If a muscle is constantly tightened, either through inactivity or too much activity, without proper attention to stretching, the muscle may strain or tear. A strained muscle occurs when a tight muscle is overstretched rapidly to the point where damage to the connective tissue occurs. If a strain is extreme, muscle fibers and connective tissues will rupture. If muscles are not fit, such a rupture can occur while simply performing the activities of daily living.

Flexibility and Low-Back Pain Low-back pain is a complaint common to many individuals. It is estimated that 80 percent of all Americans will experience some degree of low-back pain over the course of their lifetime. Inadequate flexibility is an important factor in the development of low-back pain. Regular stretching can both prevent and rehabilitate chronic low-back pain (ACSM, 2000).

6. The majority of low-back pain is caused by poor muscular fitness.

If you develop low-back pain, your first step should be to contact your physician. With physician approval, or as a preventive measure, you may wish to try the following activities. The muscle groups most involved in low-back pain are the abdominals, hamstrings, hip flexors, and back extensors. A combination of muscles that are inflexible and muscles that are weak may contribute to low-back pain. Usually the abdominal muscles are too weak, so exercises such as the curl-up or crunch are recommended (Figure 12.32). The hamstring muscles, through a combination of too much sitting and not enough stretching, can become too inflexible. Exercises such as the knee to the chest (Figure 12.33), or the seated toe touch (Figure 12.34), are suggested to counteract this problem. The hip flexors tend to be too tight, so exercises like the lunge stretch are recommended (Figure 12.35). The back extensors may be both weak and inflexible, so both stretching and strengthening are recommended. To stretch the back extensors, use the cat-and-camel stretch (Figure 12.36); to strengthen the back extensors, do the modified chest lift (Figure 12.37).

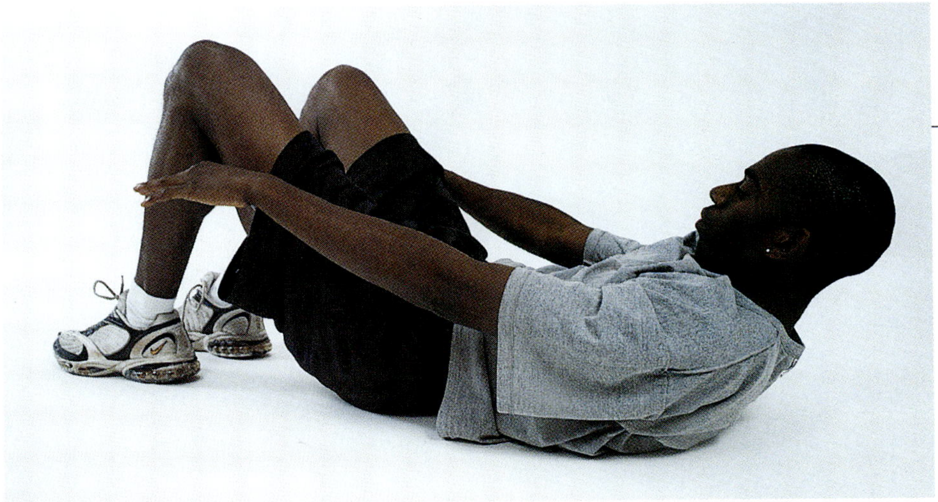

FIGURE 12.32

Low-Back Exercise. Curl-up.

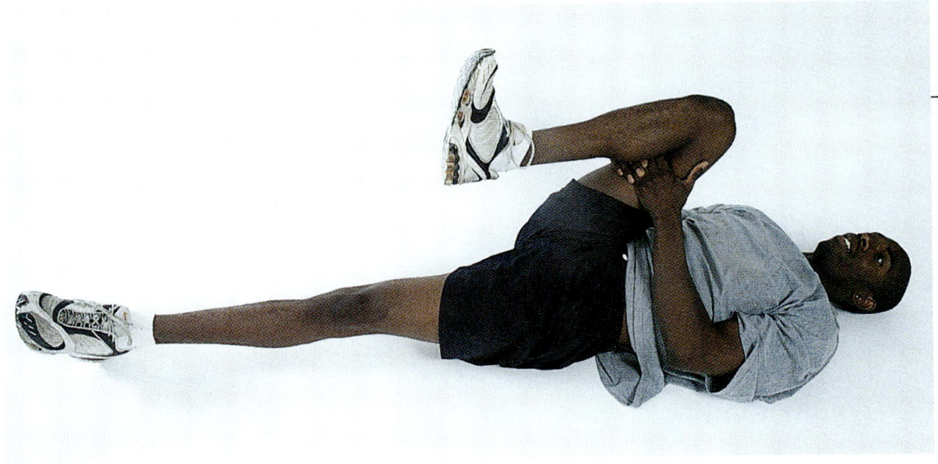

FIGURE 12.33

Low-Back Exercise. Knee to chest.

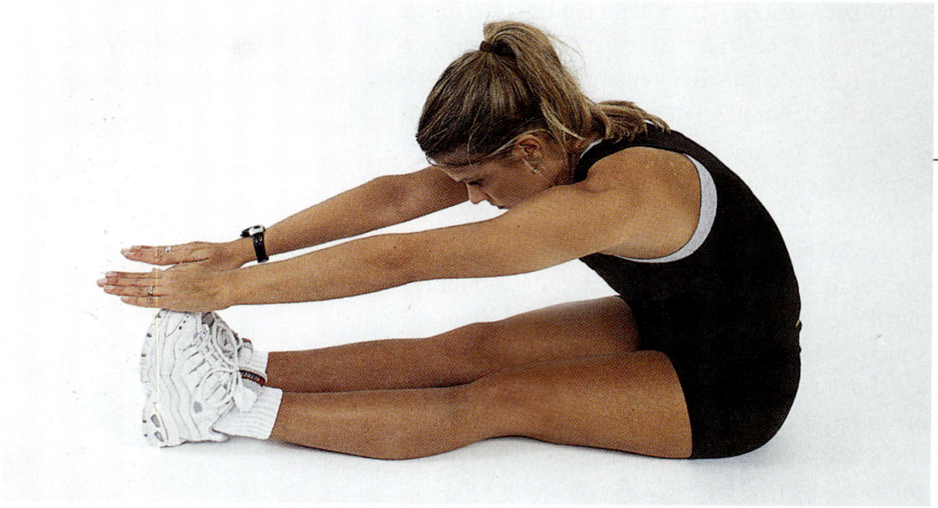

FIGURE 12.34

Low-Back Exercise. Seated toe touch.

FIGURE 12.36

Low-Back Exercise. Cat and camel.

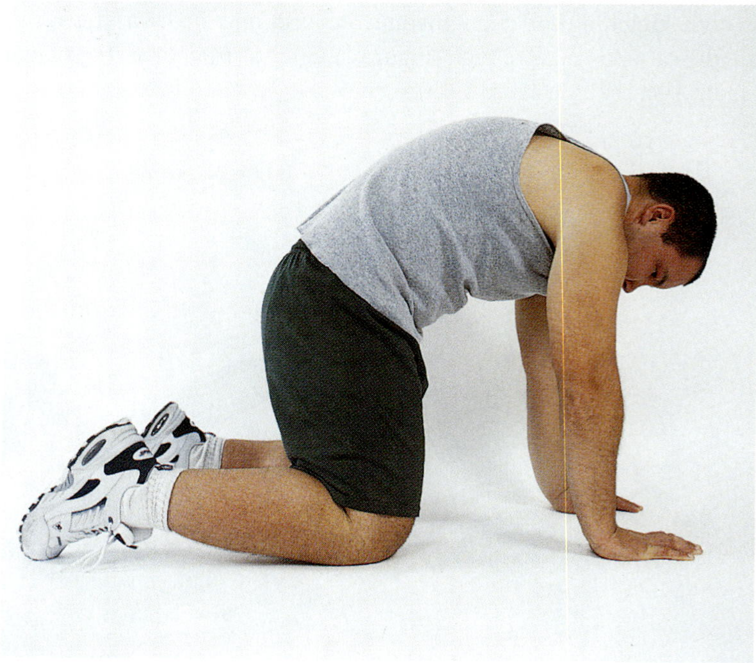

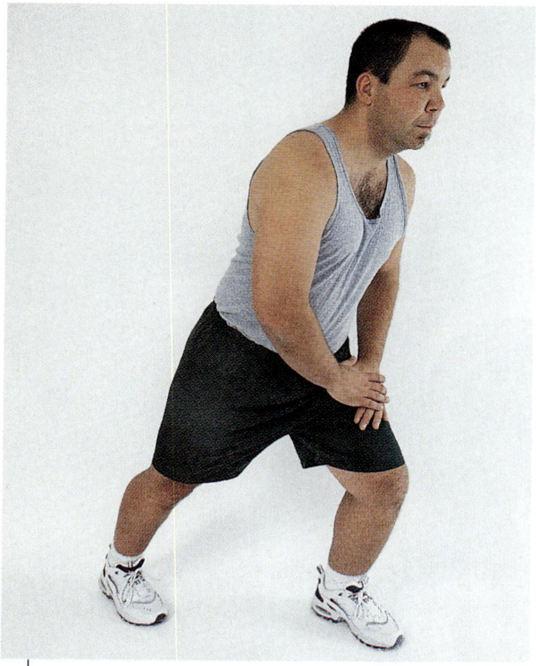

FIGURE 12.35

Low-Back Exercise. Lunge stretch.

FIGURE 12.37

Low-Back Exercise. Modified chest lift.

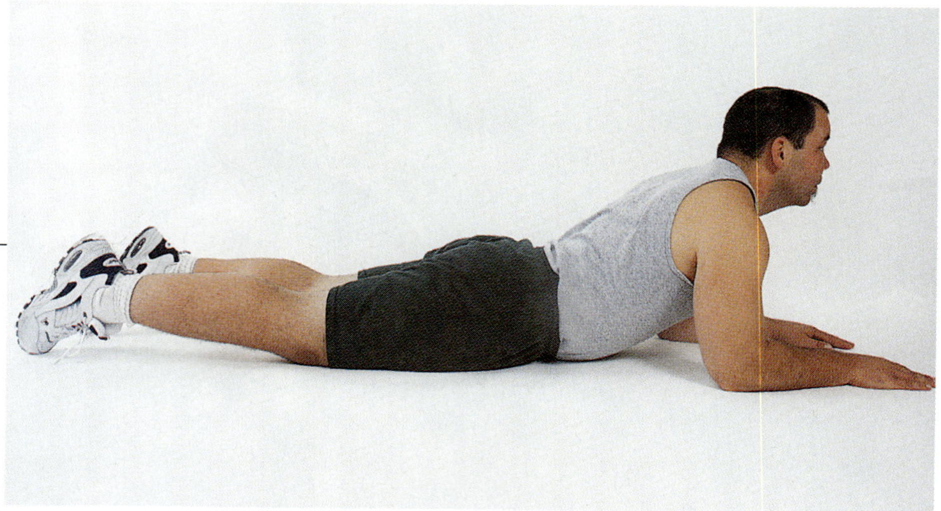

PHYSICAL ACTIVITY AND HEALTH CONNECTION

Flexibility exercises are important in enhancing your range of motion. They make muscles more pliable and resistant to injury. Good flexibility helps to guard against the development of low-back pain and enhances sport performance. Flexibility is also important in helping maintain an independently active lifestyle. By improving your flexibility, you can maintain a higher degree of functional mobility over your lifetime.

CONCEPT CONNECTION

1. **Many factors influence the amount of flexibility you have at a joint.** There are many factors that can influence range of motion, including: anatomical structure of the joint (how the bones are aligned), muscle temperature, disease status, muscle and tendon elasticity and compliance, age, sex, activity status, and tissue interference. Several of these factors are beyond our control (anatomical structure, age, sex); however, we do have the ability to manipulate other factors such as activity status, muscle temperature, disease status, muscle and tendon elasticity and compliance, and tissue interference.

2. **Sense receptors located in your muscles and tendons play an important role in developing good flexibility.** Muscle spindles and Golgi tendon organs are sense receptors that play an important role in muscle function. They control response to rapid movement. Muscle spindles cause muscles to contract in response to rapid forceful stretching. Golgi tendon organs cause muscles to relax in response to rapid forceful contractions.

3. **The three most common categories of flexibility exercises are static, ballistic, and PNF.** *Static* stretching involves putting a muscle into a stretched position and holding that position for 10–30 seconds. *Ballistic* stretching involves using pulsing or bouncing movements to stretch a muscle. *PNF* involves the use of sense receptors and forceful agonist and antagonist contractions to stretch a muscle.

4. **Guidelines for improving flexibility suggest stretching a muscle and holding the position for 10–30 seconds.** Static stretches held for 10–30 seconds provide a safe and effective way to enhance your flexibility. Perform each stretch four times for optimal benefit.

5. **Good flexibility protects against injury, enhances your ability to be physically active, and helps maintain an independent lifestyle.** Maintaining a good range of motion decreases the likelihood of injury, reduces the risk of low back pain, and enhances physical performance. Sore, inflexible muscles decrease your ability to move efficiently and increase the risk of muscle strain.

6. **Most low-back pain is caused by poor muscular fitness.** Low-back pain is most commonly the result of poor flexibility in the hamstrings, hip flexors, and back extensors. Poor muscular strength and endurance of the abdominal muscles is a contributing factor. By regularly performing stretching activities that focus on the lower back, you can reduce your risk for developing low-back pain.

TERMS

Flexibility, 264
Elasticity, 264
Compliance, 264
Tissue interference, 264
Priopriocetors, 266
Muscle spindles, 266
Stretch reflex, 266
Golgi tendon organs, 266
Static stretching, 267
Ballistic stretching, 267
PNF stretching, 267
Passive stretching, 268
Active stretching, 268
Hyperextension, 276
Hyperflexion, 276

MAKING THE CONNECTION

Bob has now learned that flexibility is important to a healthy lifestyle. He spends some time daily working to improve his flexibility. Bob has also noticed that the low-back pain he was experiencing in the morning has disappeared. What he once thought unimportant in terms of his fitness plays a much more important role than Bob had realized.

CRITICAL THINKING

1. In the vignette, Bob realized how important flexibility is to a healthy lifestyle and is spending time improving his flexibility. What types of exercises would you recommend for Bob to begin with and why? Once he has a routine in place, would you suggest that he add any flexibility exercises? If so, which ones and why?
2. Based on your current flexibility and your time commitments, identify three different types of stretching exercise you prefer and briefly explain why you selected these.
3. The last time you spoke with your parents they indicated that your grandfather was having problems getting around and that he was unable to bend over and pick things up off the floor, nor could he easily put on his shoes. Knowing what you know about flexibility diminishing when adults grow older, explain this process to your parents and make some flexibility exercise suggestions for your grandfather.

REFERENCES

American College of Sports Medicine. (1992). *ACSM Fitness Book.* Champaign, IL: Leisure Press.

American College of Sports Medicine. (1998). The recommended quantity and quality of exercise for developing and maintaining cardiorespiratory and muscular fitness and flexibility in healthy adults. *Medicine and Science in Sports and Exercise* 30(6):975–91.

American College of Sports Medicine. (2000). *ACSM's Guidelines for Exercise Testing and Prescription.* Philadelphia: Lippincott, Williams & Wilkins.

Axler, C.T., & McGill, S.M. (1997). Low back loads over a variety of abdominal exercises: Searching for the safest abdominal challenge. *Medicine and Science in Sports & Exercise* 29(6):804-810.

Holcomb, W.R. (2000). Improved stretching with proprioceptive neuromuscular facilitation. *Strength and Conditioning Journal* 22(1):59–61.

Knudson, D.V., Magnusson, P., & McHugh, M. (June 2000). Current issues in flexibility fitness. In Corbin, C., Pangrazi, B., eds., *The President's Council on Physical Fitness and Sports Research Digest,* Series 3, No. 10. Washington, DC: Department of Health and Human Services, 1–8.

Plowman, S.A. (August 1993). Physical fitness and healthy low back function. In Corbin, C., Pangrazi, B., eds., *The President's Council on Physical Fitness and Sports Research Digest,* Series 1, No. 3. Washington, DC: Department of Health and Human Services, 1–8.

Activities & Assessments

NAME ____________________ SECTION ____________ DATE ____________

12.1 Sit and Reach Test

Directions The sit-and-reach test is a commonly used assessment of hamstring flexibility. It is performed with a yardstick and length of tape, or a sit-and-reach box (see below).

1. Place a yardstick on the floor with the zero mark closest to you.
2. Tape the yardstick in place with the tape at the 15-inch mark.
3. Warm up prior to the assessment.
4. Sit on the floor with the yardstick between your legs, your feet 10–12 inches apart, and your heels even with the tape at the 15-inch mark.
5. Place one hand over the other. The tips of your two middle fingers should be on top of each other.
6. Slowly stretch forward without bouncing or jerking and slide your fingertips along the yardstick as far as possible. Reach as far as you can.
7. Keep your knees straight, but do not hyperextend them (bow the knees backward).
8. Perform these procedures three times and record your best score to the nearest inch.

(continued)

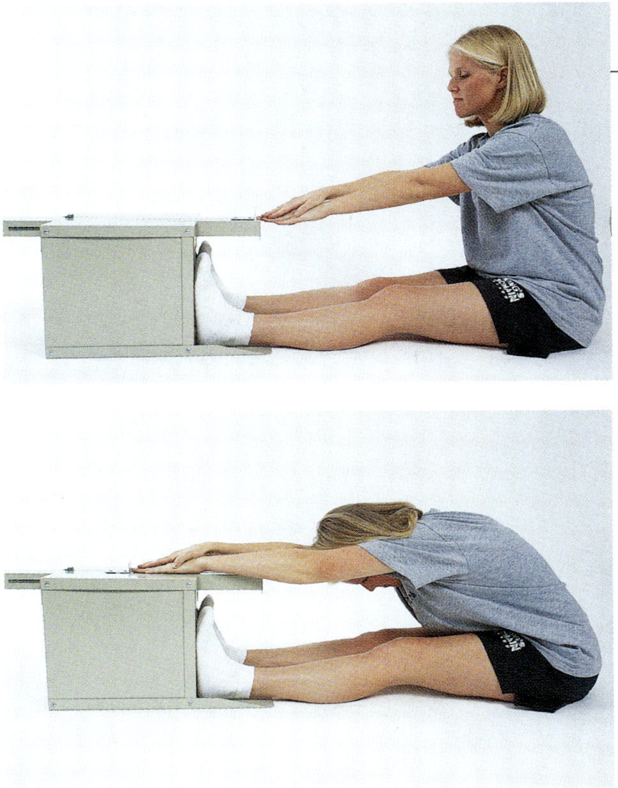

The sit-and-reach test measures hamstring flexibility.

12.1 Sit and Reach Test (cont.)

	SCORE BASED ON AGE				
AGE (YRS)	20–29	30–39	40–49	50–59	60+
Men					
High	≥ 19	≥ 18	≥ 17	≥ 16	≥ 15
Average	13–18	12–17	11–16	10–15	9–14
Below average	10–12	9–11	8–10	7–9	6–8
Low	≤ 9	≤ 8	≤ 7	≤ 6	≤ 5
Women					
High	≥ 22	≥ 21	≥ 20	≥ 19	≥ 18
Average	16–21	15–20	14–19	13–18	12–17
Below average	13–15	12–14	11–13	10–12	9–11
Low	≤ 12	≤ 11	≤ 10	≤ 9	≤ 8

SOURCE: Adapted from American College of Sports Medicine. (1992). *ACSM fitness book*. Champaign, IL: Leisure Press.

Activities & Assessments

NAME ______________ SECTION ______________ DATE ______________

12.2 Trunk Extension

Directions Use this assessment to measure the flexibility of your abdominal and hip flexor muscles.

1. Lie face down on the floor.
2. Have a partner hold down your legs (at the backs of the thighs).
3. Clasp your hands behind you at your low back.
4. Breathe in and lift your upper body as high off the floor as possible, without arching your back.
5. Hold this position for 3 sec and have someone measure the distance from the floor to your chin (rounding to the nearest inch).
6. Repeat this exercise two more times and record your scores as follows.

First attempt ________inches

Second attempt ________inches

Third attempt ________inches

Use the chart below and your best score to determine your classification.

Trunk Extension Flexibility Standards (in inches)

MEN	WOMEN	CLASSIFICATION
16	17	Poor
17–18	18–19	Average
19–21	20–23	Good
22	24	Excellent

SOURCE: Adapted from D.J. Anspaugh, M.H. Hamrick, and F.D. Rosato. (1997). *Wellness: Concepts and applications* (3rd ed.). New York: McGraw-Hill.

Activities & Assessments

NAME ____________________ SECTION ____________ DATE ____________

12.3 Shoulder Flexion

Directions Use the shoulder flexion test to measure the flexibility of your deltoids and shoulder girdle. You will need a straight edge and something to measure with (yardstick, tape measure).

1. Lie face down on the floor with your arms fully extended over your head.
2. Your chin should remain on the floor throughout the test.
3. Grasp the straight edge with both hands and raise it as high as possible off the floor.
4. Have someone measure the distance from the floor to the bottom of the straight edge (round to the nearest inch).
5. Repeat this exercise two more times and record your scores below.

First attempt ________inches

Second attempt ________inches

Third attempt ________inches

Use the chart below and your best score to determine your classification.

Shoulder Flexion Standards (in inches)

MEN	WOMEN	CLASSIFICATION
12 or lower	13 or lower	Poor
13–17	14–18	Fair
18–22	19–23	Average
23–25	24–26	Good
26 or higher	27 or higher	Excellent

SOURCE: Adapted from D.J. Anspaugh, M.H. Hamrick, and F.D. Rosato. (1997). *Wellness: Concepts and applications* (3rd ed.). New York: McGraw-Hill.

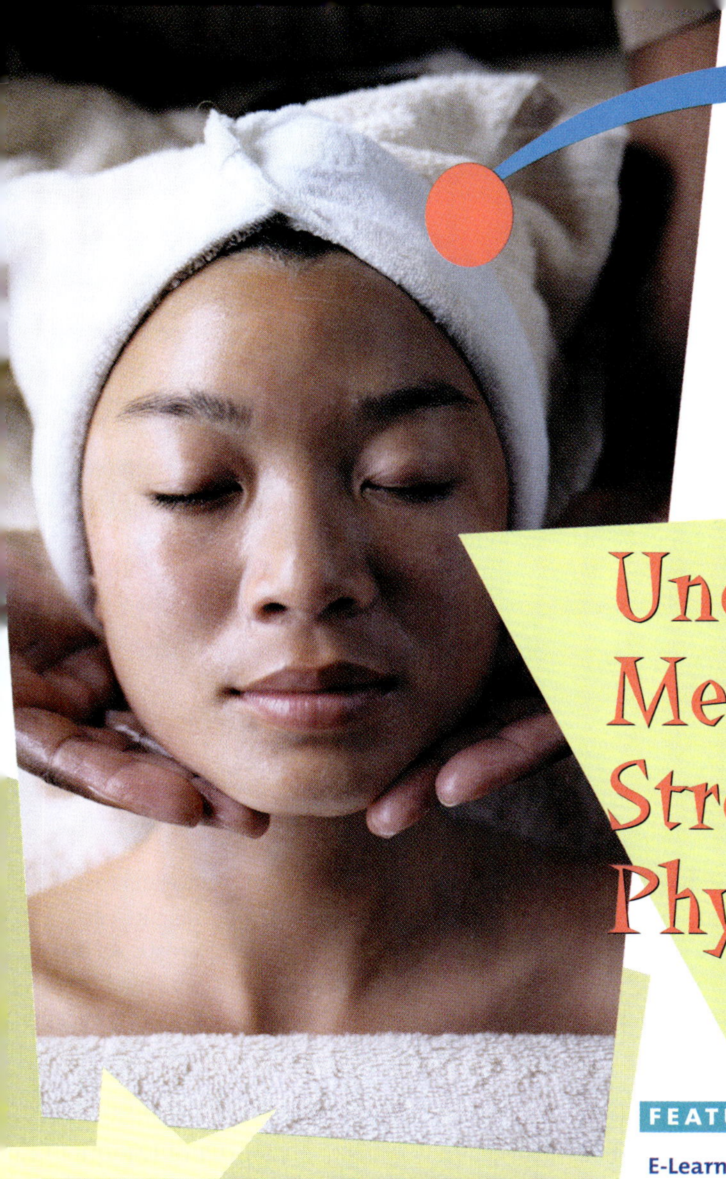

13

Understanding Mental Health, Stress, and Physical Activity

CONCEPT CONNECTION

1. People who are physically active tend to have better mental health.
2. Our mental and emotional health is central to the quality of our lives and influences our physical health.
3. Maintaining and optimizing our mental and physical health requires making countless adjustments to a variety of life's challenges.
4. The general adaptation syndrome describes the body's response to stress and the adaptability of the body to maintain homeostasis.
5. Stress is a natural process, and understanding its effects can help you use it to your own advantage.
6. The art of stress management is to keep yourself at a level of stimulation that is healthy and enjoyable.

FEATURES

E-Learning Tools: www.pahconnection.com

Engage www.pahconnection.com

13.1 Are you anxious?
13.2 Are you depressed?
13.3 Stress sources
13.4 Distress symptoms
13.5 Are you stress resistant?
13.6 Stress balancing strategies

Experience www.pahconnection.com

13.1 Mental health: a report of the Surgeon General
13.2 The anxiety disorders education program
13.3 Stress management and emotional wellness
13.4 Stress diary

Explore www.pahconnection.com

13.1 National Institute of Mental Health (NIMH)
13.2 Internet mental health
13.3 World Federation of Mental Health
13.4 The American Institute of Stress
13.5 Canadian Institute of Stress

Activities & Assessments

13.1 What are your stress reactions?
13.2 How susceptible are you to stress?
13.3 Do you have "hurry sickness"?

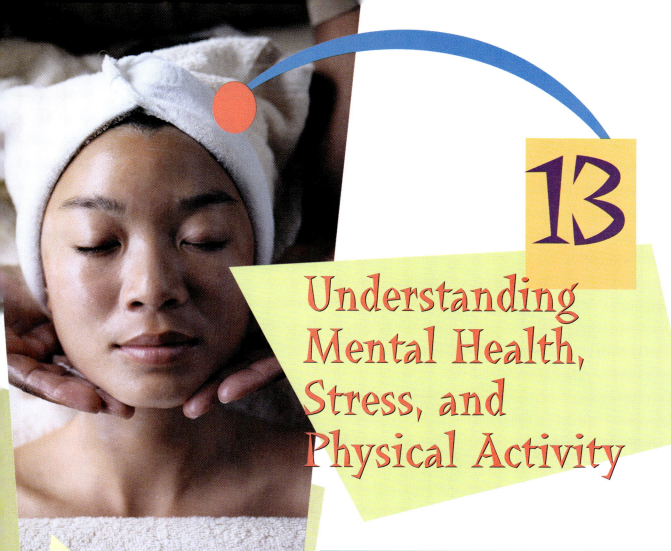

WHAT'S THE CONNECTION?

Jesse felt anxious and tense as he rehearsed a speech in his dorm room. He had spent two weeks on this English class assignment and now, the day before he was to stand up in front of the class, he was having trouble remembering and delivering his speech. Three days ago he had no trouble reciting the 30-minute presentation in front of the mirror, but now he was fretting about presenting in front of his classmates and instructor. After a number of failed attempts, Jesse decided to take a break and go out for a 45-minute jog. Halfway through the jog, the anxiety and worrying subsided and he began to recite his speech easily in his mind. When Jesse returned to the dorm, his roommate Dave was there. Jesse asked Dave to listen to the speech before they went to the cafeteria for dinner. Jesse was able to deliver his speech flawlessly in front of Dave. He then showered and got dressed for dinner. As they walked to the cafeteria, Jesse told Dave that he planned to jog before presenting his speech because he felt that the exercise had helped him deliver it with a clear head.

INTRODUCTION

1. People who are physically active tend to have better mental health.

Physical activity has been advocated throughout this book as a means to enhance health status and prevent a number of chronic illnesses like cardiovascular disease, cancer, hypertension, obesity, and osteoporosis. As discussed in Chapter 1, your health status is multidimensional and includes mental and emotional elements. Moreover, within mental and emotional health there is a physical component. Studies have shown that people who are physically active tend to have better mental health (Surgeon General's Report, 1996). The consensus is that people who are physically active score higher on important mental health factors like self-esteem, self-concept, self-worth, body image, and cognitive functioning than sedentary people. Furthermore, physical activity has been shown to be effective in treating people who report symptoms of anxiety, depression, and stress.

Improved mental health and its conservation have recently become topics of great interest in public health (Surgeon General's Report, 1999). However, given the epidemic nature of a number of mental health problems, many Americans are coming up short. For example, anxiety disorders affect as many as 19 million Americans annually and depression in some form impacts nearly 18 million people each year (Healthy People 2010). In a recent National Health Interview Survey, approximately 60 percent of U.S. adults reported experiencing at least a moderate amount of stress during the previous 2 weeks, while 20 percent experienced high stress almost every day (CDC, 1999). Each of these mental health problems erode our quality of life and contribute to the imposing $148 billion annual cost for all mental illness; this includes both direct costs (treatment) and indirect costs (lost productivity).

Explore 13.1

Mental health expenditures for treatment and rehabilitation are an important consideration when addressing mental illness. However, it has been pointed out that, similar to other public health problems in which major advances have come from in the area of prevention rather than treatment, *preventing* mental health problems is inherently better than having to treat the illness after its onset (Institute of Medicine, 1994). While there continues to be an insufficient understanding all of the biological, psychological, and sociocultural effects on mental health and illness, some successful strategies for preventive interventions have materialized. A meaningful one includes the choice of a lifestyle that incorporates regular physical activity. Increasingly, justifiable evidence advocating the role of regular physical activity as a means for preventing the onset of many mental and emotional problems, as well as serving as an effective treatment, is being encouraged among health professionals (Figure 13.1).

Many theories have been proposed to explain the positive research findings related to physical activity and mental health. To address completely these explanations related to mind and body functioning, we must first look at mental and emotional health and how it is central to the quality of our lives.

Mental and Emotional Health

2. Our mental and emotional health is central to the quality of our lives and influences our physical health.

Throughout this book, you have been exposed to the wellness continuum, which ranges from the wellness concept (quality of life) through the medical concept (absence of illness) as related to your physical health. Addressing mental function, we similarly focus on the wellness concept (fulfilling your psychological potential) and illness concept (avoiding mental disorders). As will be apparent in the following definitions, health and illness are not opposites, but points on the mental wellness continuum.

Experience www.pahconnection.com 13.1

Defining mental health is not easy because it encompasses a broad group of values across different cultures and subgroups (Cowen, 1994). The *Surgeon General's Report* defines **mental health** as a "state of successful performance of mental function, resulting in productive activities, fulfilling relationships with other people, and the ability to adapt to change and to cope with adversity" (Surgeon General's Report, 1999). Evident from the definition is that mental health doesn't just occur; we need to pay attention to our mental needs just as we do our physical needs.

Mental health A "state of successful performance of mental function, resulting in productive activities, fulfilling relationships with other people, and the ability to adapt to change and to cope with adversity" (Surgeons General's Report, 1999).

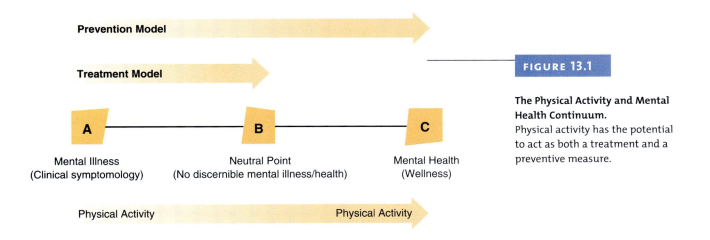

Mental health and well-being involve such factors as a sense of coherence and insight, moods, self-esteem, and coping ability. It allows us to make informed selections between alternate courses of action. We must use our cognitive abilities to make wise choices based on both previous experience and a willingness to undergo new experiences. An important part of mental health is learning to fully understand and trust the decisions we make. Mental health involves having a mind open to new ideas

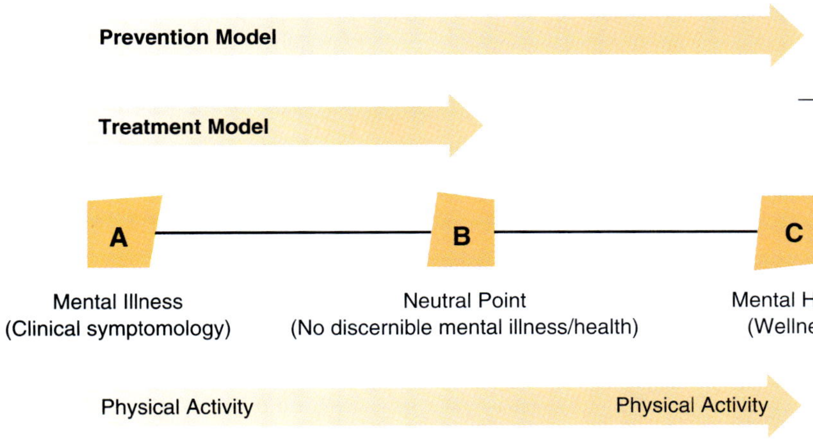

FIGURE 13.1

The Physical Activity and Mental Health Continuum.
Physical activity has the potential to act as both a treatment and a preventive measure.

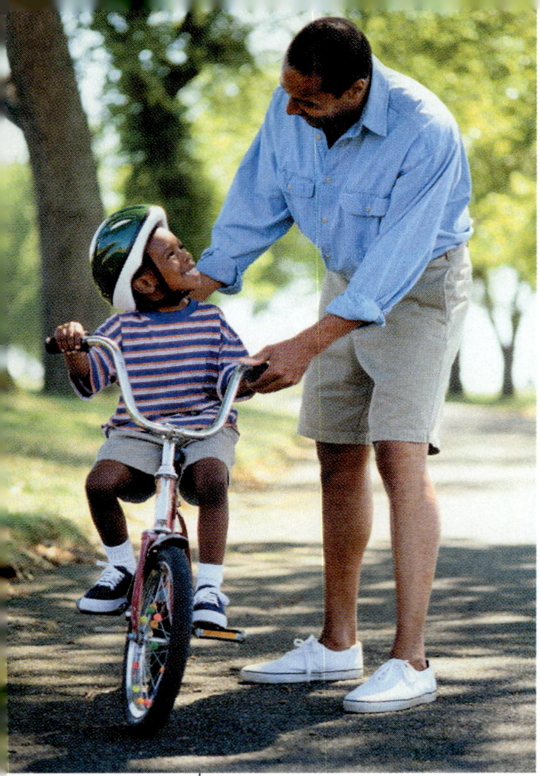

Emotional health includes feelings of joy and love.

and concepts. Mental health embodies factors not only of intellect but also of emotions, and of their relationships.

Emotional health calls for understanding our emotions and coping with changes that arise in everyday life (Chapter 1). Emotional health encompasses mental states that include feelings or subjective experiences in response to changes in our environment (Crider et al., 1993). Joy, disappointment, fear, anxiety, guilt, love, sadness, anger, jealousy, trust, empathy, and compassion describe subjective experiences that are real to us. These emotions play an important role in our overall health.

Everything you think and feel reflects who you are. An *emotion* is a thought linked to a sensation. The thought is usually about the past or the future, but the sensation is in the present. Your mind quickly links this sensation with involuntary and immediate changes in your body function. Our minds and our emotions are interrelated and interdependent. Mental functions do not exist separately from our emotions and our emotions affect our mental state. Therefore, we will speak of mental and emotional health interchangeably in this chapter.

Emotional health Encompasses mental states that include feelings or subjective experiences in response to changes in our environment.

Explore
www.jbpub.com/healthconnection.com
13.2

MIND-BODY RELATIONSHIP

Much research related to physical activity has centered on its relationship to physical health. However, holistic health perspectives emphasize mind-body unity and include the complex relationship between mental and physical function as well as the continuum between health and illness (Brown, 1990). Because of this view, there is currently a great deal of interest in the study of physical activity as it relates to mental health. The line between psychology and biology is becoming increasingly blurred. The physiological parameters of our bodies are constantly eavesdropping on our thoughts and being changed in the process. Similarly, research is now able to substantiate the proposed mental and emotional benefits of habitual physical activity, which include improved intellectual functioning, academic

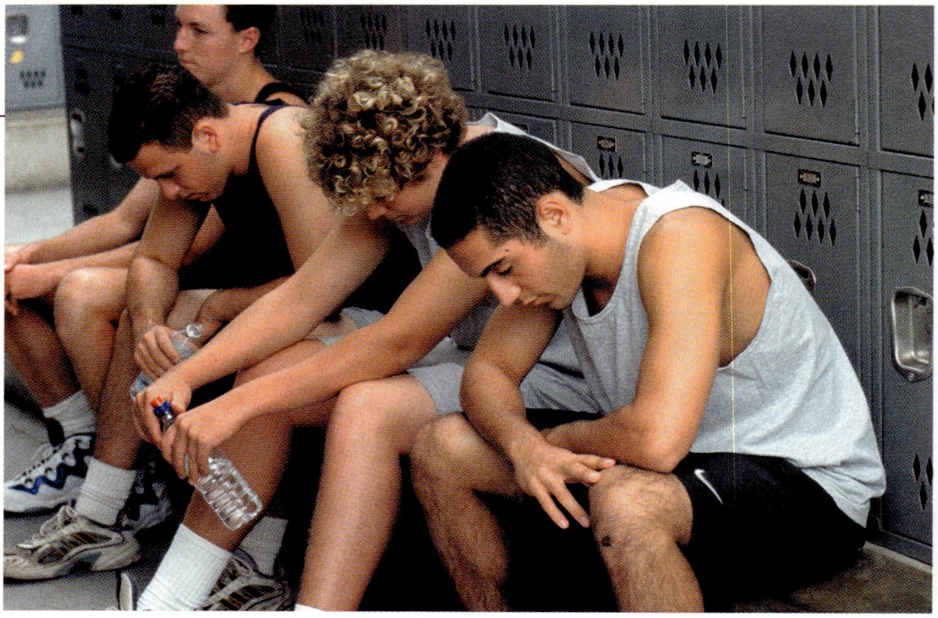

Emotional health also includes temporary feelings of sadness and disappointment.

performance, and moods (Surgeon's General Report, 1996). The old paradigm that distinguished between mental and physical health is thus somewhat unsound, in the sense that we now know mental and physical health to be highly integrated. Indeed, the *Surgeon General's Report* asserted that it is important to adopt the paradigm that mind and body are inseparable and eliminate the old idea that the mind and body are separate and independent from each other (Surgeon General's Report, 1999). The mind-body dualism we speak of today is founded in the classical connection made by the Greeks 24 centuries ago when they considered physical activity and mental health simultaneously.

Mens Sana in Corpore Sana

The Greeks long believed in the mental benefits derived from physical activity. They deemed that a healthy and fit body was positively associated with increased mental and emotional wellness. This was best exemplified by the phrase attributed to Homer: "*Mens* (mind, intellect) *sana* (sound, healthy, sane), *in corpore* (body) *sana*," which translates into "In a sound body is a sound mind." The Greeks maintained that physical activity made the mind more rational and perceptive. During the Golden Age of Greece, regular and vigorous physical activity was engaged in for its contribution to mental as well as physical health.

Former President John F. Kennedy underscored the Greek ideal of *mens sana in corpore sana* when he said:

> Physical fitness is not only one of the most important keys to a healthy body, it is the basis of dynamic and creative intellectual activity. Intelligence and skill can only function at the peak of their capacity when the body is strong. Hardy spirits and tough minds usually inhabit sound bodies.

physical activity and health connection

Many studies on the effects of physical activity on the mental health of physically active versus physically inactive people generally show positive effects (McAuley & Rudolph, 1995). The invariable findings are that, the higher the level of an individual's physical activity, the higher the level of good mental health. Mental health is defined in these studies as feelings of general well-being, positive moods, and fewer bouts of anxiety and depression. The studies conclude that physical activity may indeed play a role in maintaining or promoting positive mental health. We have seen that adequate and enhanced mental and emotional states can be associated with physical activity of the body. Is the reverse true? Can poor mental health states lead to deterioration of the body? A number of research studies seem to indicate that poor mental and emotional states can have an effect on our physical health (Raglin, 1990).

Psychosomatic Disease

Explore 13.3

Psychosomatic disease describes bodily symptoms caused by mental or emotional disturbance. The word *psychosomatic* comes from the Greek words *psyche* (the mind) and *soma* (the body). Numerous studies have confirmed that being emotionally distressed from a number of negative emotions, including chronic anxiety or depression, can lead to physical health problems such as headaches, ulcers, high blood pressure, altered insulin needs, and a suppressed immune system. These physical problems can lead to an increased risk of heart disease, stroke, cancer, and infections. The prevalence of many of these underlying emotions that begin the disease sequence are associated with life-stress circumstances (Dohrenwend & Dohrenwend, 1981). Emotionally, stress can lead to feelings of depression, anxiety, and decreased mental health (McEwen & Stellar, 1993).

Psychosomatic disease Bodily symptoms caused by mental or emotional disturbance.

Mental Illness

Mental illness encompasses all diagnosable mental disorders (Surgeon General's Report, 1999). These mental disorders are quantified by changes in our thinking, mood, or behavior that lead to impaired functioning. Our focus here will be limited to mental health concerns related to anxiety, depression, and stress. These mental problems are the most common experienced by Americans and are influenced by physical activity both as a protective factor and a therapeutic modality.

Explore www.pahconnection.com 13.2

Anxiety **Anxiety** is one of the most easily understood and responsive symptoms of mental disorders. Everyone feels anxious from time to time. Anxiety is a normal feeling that each of us experiences when a fear-eliciting situation arises in our environment. These fearful situations can be real or imagined, and the natural physiological response is "fight or flight." Anxiety is inflated worry and tension that sets off the fight-or-flight response. Most of us have felt the pounding of our heart when we think the teacher will call on us for an answer we do not know, or the muscle tension we feel when we think our parents are going to be angry with us over something we have done or not done, or that feeling of lightheadedness before calling someone for a first date (Table 13.1). A certain level of anxiety is good because it can spur us on to action. However, it is important that we be able to regulate anxiety, or it may materialize in mood disturbances (depression) and pathological physiological activity (disease).

Experiencing heightened arousal or fear over a sustained period of time can lead to **anxiety disorders,** which are debilitating and disruptive to our health. Anxiety disorders are the most common mental disorders in the United States; they include **generalized anxiety disorder (GAD),** panic disorder, obsessive-compulsive disorder, post-traumatic stress disorder (PTSD), and phobias (Healthy People 2010). Of these, GAD represents a more extended and unfounded version of anxiety.

Engage www.pahconnection.com 13.1

Generalized anxiety disorder is most often experienced as exaggerated worrying, inability to relax, and insomnia for a sustained period lasting 6 months or more. In many GAD cases, there is no immediate external situation that sets off the physiological response. Many people with GAD endure physical symptoms like fatigue and headaches. A list of anxiety symptoms is provided in Engage 13.1. This screening quiz provides information that may be indicative of the need to be evaluated by a primary care physician for the presence of mild-to-moderate anxiety symptoms. If a physician

Mental illness Diagnosable mental disorders that change our thinking, mood, or behavior and lead to impaired functioning.

Anxiety Normal response when a fear-eliciting situation arises.

Anxiety disorder Heightened arousal or fear over a sustained period of time.

Generalized anxiety disorder (GAD) Experiencing exaggerated worrying, inability to relax, and insomnia for 6 months or more.

TABLE 13.1 Common Signs of Acute Anxiety

Feelings of fear or dread
Trembling, restlessness, and muscle tension
Rapid heart rate
Lightheadedness or dizziness
Perspiration
Cold hands/feet
Shortness of breath

SOURCE: U.S. Department of Health and Human Services. (1999). *Mental health: A report of the Surgeon General* (p. 40). Rockville, MD: U.S. Department of Health and Human Services, Substance Abuse and Mental Health Services Administration, Center for Mental Health Services, National Institutes of Health, National Institute of Mental Health.

determines your symptoms are due to an anxiety disorder, the next step is referral to a mental health professional for treatment.

Depression **Depression** illustrates a mental disorder mainly noted by alterations in mood. Depression often accompanies GAD and other anxiety disorders (Barbee, 1998). Like anxiety disorders, depression can vary in severity and duration. All of us have experienced **depressive reactions** because of a disturbing event in our lives. *Depressive reactions* encompass the normal depressed feelings, such as sadness, hopelessness, dejection, and worthlessness, which arise because of a specific life situation. Fortunately, these deviations do not last long, and they lessen over time. However, when symptoms last for an extended period of time or feature one or more major depressive episodes, the condition may be serious.

Dysthymia is a chronic form of depression. *Dysthymia* is similar to *depressive reactions* in its symptoms except that the degree of suffering from its unrelenting, seething attack can lead to depressive illness, as well as increasing the susceptibility to **major depression.** *Major depression* is a serious condition that leads to an inability to function, or even to suicide. Whereas the symptoms in *dysthymia* are less intense, fewer in number, and longer-lasting, *major depression* is marked by one or more major depressive episodes over a 2-week period. Many treatments are available for depression and vary according to the cause and severity. Most people seeking help for depression visit their primary care physician. The screening test of Engage 13.2 provides indications for the need to be evaluated by a physician for presence of depressive symptoms.

Maintaining our mental health requires making countless adjustments to life's challenges. How successfully we adjust depends largely on how we view and adapt to life's challenges. Life's challenges may be viewed as **stress.** Stress includes both a mental reaction (stressor) and a physical reaction (stress response).

Stress Stress places mental and physical demands upon us. Emotionally, stress can lead to feelings of anxiety and depression (McEwen & Stellar, 1993). Just like anxiety and depressive reactions, stress is a normal part of everyone's life and should not be viewed as necessarily bad. We feel stress any time we go through some sort of change in life. All change requires adjustment by the human body. From the moment of our birth to our death, we experience a wide range of personal challenges that result in substantial emotional and physical changes. No particular level of stress is optimal for all people. As you will learn, coping and adapting to the demands of everyday life-stressors in an effective manner is of great importance for both mental and physical health.

UNDERSTANDING STRESS

Decades ago, it was pointed out that "the states of health or disease are the expressions of the success or failure experienced by the human body in its efforts to respond adaptively to environmental challenges" (Dubos 1965, p. xvii). Those who developed many of the today's concepts of stress correctly understand that different life stressors could induce helpful (**eustress;** *eu* is Greek for "good") and harmful **(distress)** outcomes. That is, good health requires the presence of eustress and also the limitation of distress to a level to which the human body can adapt (Selye, 1973). A stressor sets into motion a sequence of chemical and nervous

Engage
www.pahconnection.com
13.2

3. Maintaining and optimizing our mental and physical health requires making countless adjustments to a variety of life's challenges.

Depression A mental disorder notable for negative alteration in mood.

Depressive reactions Normal depressed feelings like sadness and hopelessness.

Dysthymia Chronic form of depression.

Major depression Serious condition that leads to inability to function and possibly suicide.

Stress Response that includes both a mental reaction (stressor) and a physical reaction (stress response).

Eustress Helpful or good stress.

Distress Harmful or bad stress.

Coping and adapting to the demands of everyday life-stressors in an effective manner is of great importance for one's health.

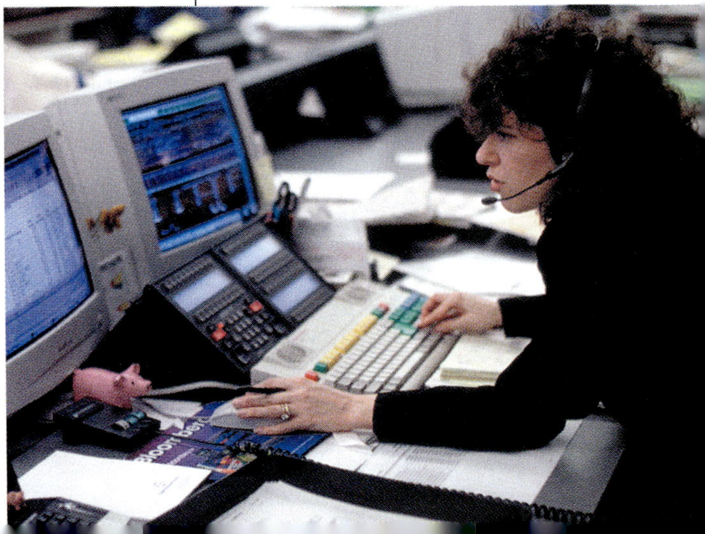

system changes that is the same regardless of the type of stressor that initiates it. This sequence has been referred to as the general adaptation syndrome.

4. The general adaptation syndrome describes the body's response to stress and the adaptability of the body to maintain homeostasis.

Explore www.pahconnection.com 13.5

General Adaptation Syndrome

Hans Selye, a pioneer in stress research, is generally recognized as the father of stress physiology and stress education. Selye coined the word *stress,* which he defined as the "nonspecific response of the body to any demand made upon it" (Selye, 1973). The key concept in Selye's definition is that there is a nonspecific response by the body to readjust itself following any demand made on it. Selye termed this nonspecific response the **general adaptation syndrome (GAS).** This syndrome is based on the principle that your body is constantly attempting to maintain homeostasis (*homeo* = similar and *statis* = position), or an internal balance. Maintaining homeostasis requires energy. Any situation or force that disturbs the body's homeostasis, or equilibrium, is a stressor. Adapting to stressors requires the body to provide the right amount of energy at the right time.

The GAS describes the body's response to stress and the adaptability of the body to maintain homeostasis. Selye's (1973) research provided evidence that the body goes through a predictable three-stage physiological response to any kind of stressor: (1) the alarm reaction, when the adrenal glands are activated in an attempt to mobilize the body's energy resources for physical action, (2) the stage of resistance, in which the readjustment occurs; and (3) if the readjustment is not complete, the stage of exhaustion may follow, leading to illness and possibly death (Figure 13.2). The demand or stimulus that elicits the GAS stress response is referred to as a stressor.

Stressors

The **stressor** itself does not actually create the body's response; it is the individual's reaction to the stressor (Figure 13.3). The stress reaction is triggered by our perception of a physical or emotional danger. It is important to underscore that it is our *perception* of each demand or stressor that makes it stressful or not stressful. What is considered a stressor for one person may not be a stressor for another. For example, the person who loves to mediate disputes and moves from job site to job site would be stressed in a job that was stable and routine, whereas the person who thrives under stable conditions would very likely be stressed on a job where duties were highly varied. Each individual will have a different response to the same stressor.

General adaptation syndrome (GAS) The body's response to stress and the adaptability of the body to maintain homeostasis.

Stressor The demand or stimulus that elicits the general adaptation syndrome.

FIGURE 13.2

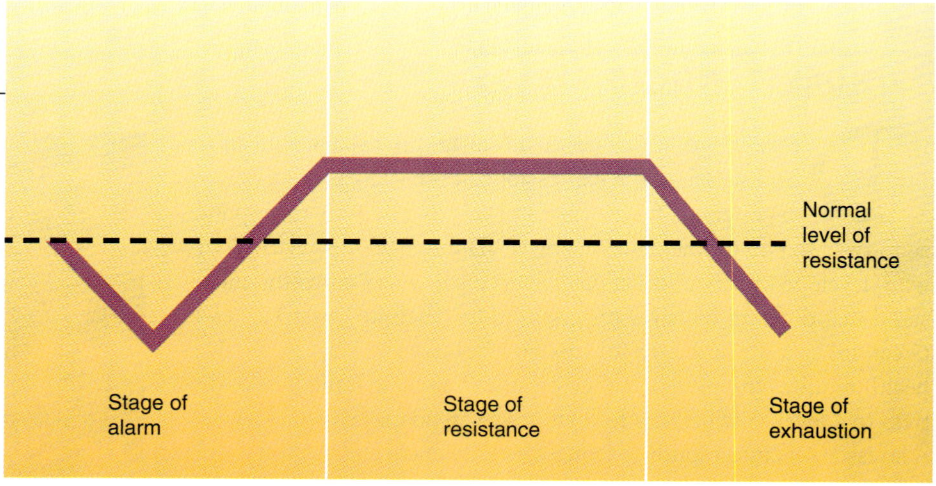

The Three Phases of the General Adaptation Syndrome. In the alarm stage, the body readies itself for action, lowering resistance. In the resistance stage the body adapts and returns to homeostatis. In the stage of exhaustion, the body's ability to resist the stressor becomes exhausted and resistance is compromised.

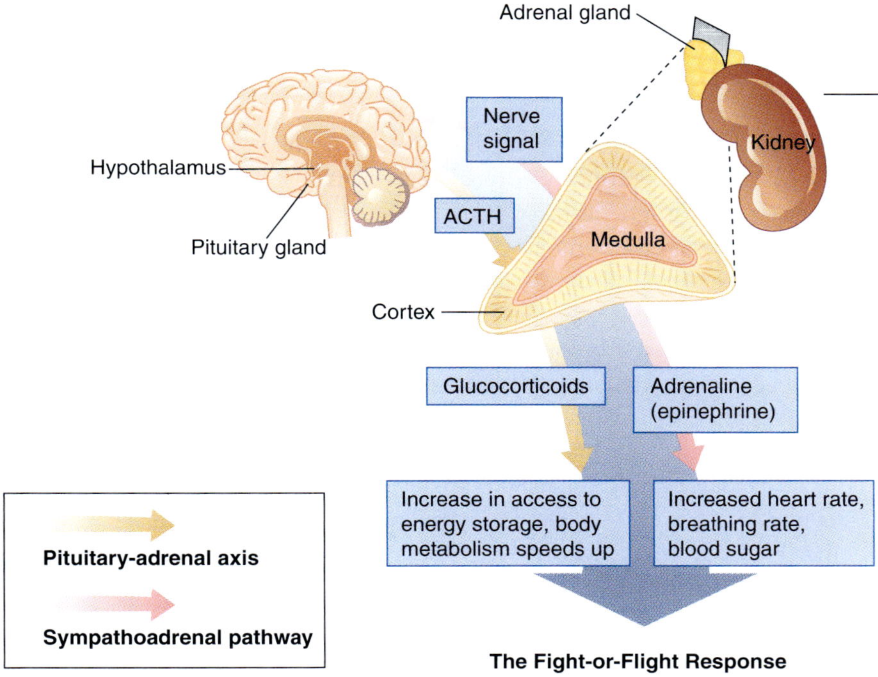

FIGURE 13.3

The Stress Response.
The physiological response to stress activates both the pituitary-adrenal axis and the sympatho-adrenal pathway.

Stressors tend to be different not only for different types of people but also for different ages. As we progress through life, each stage is accompanied by its own distinctive sources of stressors. You may want to perform Engage 13.3, "Stress Sources," at this time. This Web activity provides a comprehensive personal stress assessment designed to help you evaluate the sources of stress in your life, based on your age, sex, student status, occupation, and living arrangements. In addition to the sources of stress listed on the website, make a list of other sources of stress that you may be experiencing.

Engage www.pahconnection.com **13.3**

Our reactions to stressors can be both psychological and physiological. The psychological changes may present themselves as changes in the ways we express our emotions. One of the most frequent undesirable emotional changes is chronic worrying. Worrying too much can lead to variations in mood; you may become depressed, anxious, or irritable. These moods work against you, making finding a solution more difficult. Psychological responses to stressors can be difficult to predict. Your physiological response to stress is much more predictable.

Alarm Reaction

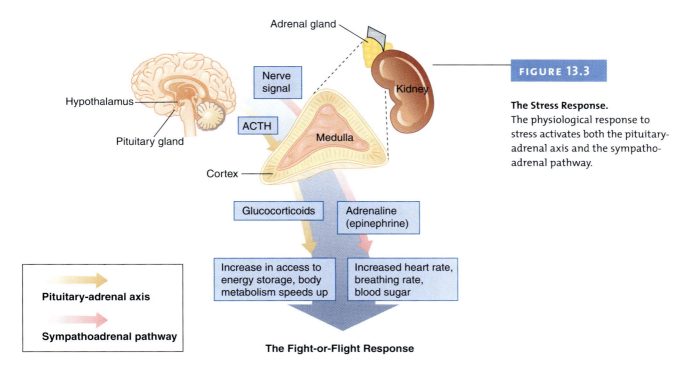

The **alarm reaction** is our immediate response to a stressor and is triggered by any threat to our physical or emotional well-being. The reason for this reaction is simple. When a danger or challenge is present, our body reacts in certain ways in order to protect ourselves. This reaction is part of our human biological makeup. The body follows a typical physiological pattern when reacting to a stressor. When a threat to our well-being is perceived, a small area of the brain known as the hypothalamus is activated (Figure 13.3). The hypothalamus stimulates a number of physiological changes, involving activity in both the **autonomic nervous system** (ANS) (nerve pathways) and the **endocrine system** (hormonal pathways). These two systems, acting in concert, alter the functioning of almost every part of the body to prepare for vigorous muscle activity. This response to stressors that challenge the body to respond physically, mentioned earlier, is referred to as the **fight-or-flight response.**

Alarm reaction Immediate response to a stressor that is triggered by any threat to our physical or emotional well-being.

Autonomic nervous system The part of the nervous system that controls smooth muscle, cardiac muscle, and glands; subdivided into sympathetic and parasympathetic.

Endocrine system The hormone-secreting cells of the body; this system is influenced in part by the nervous system.

Fight-or-flight response Response to stressors that challenge the body to respond physically.

Pituitary-adrenal axis The first pattern of the fight-or-flight response.

Glucocorticoids Chemicals responsible for speeding up the body's metabolism and increasing access to energy storage.

Sympathoadrenal system The second pattern of the fight-or-flight response.

Epinephrine The "fear hormone"; helps supply glucose for increased muscle and nervous-system activity.

Norepinephrine The "anger hormone"; helps speed the heart rate and raises blood pressure to provide more oxygen for the body.

Sympathetic nervous system The physiological system that triggers the fight-or-flight response.

Parasympathetic nervous system The counterpart to the sympathetic nervous system.

Relaxation response The opposite of the fight-or-flight response to stressful or threatening situations.

Fight-or-Flight Response The action of the sympathetic nervous system that prepares the body for intense physical activity is aptly referred to as the fight-or-flight response. The fight-or-flight response occurs when the adrenal glands are activated. The paired adrenal glands are located above each kidney and are composed of an outer adrenal cortex (layer) and an inner adrenal medulla (core). The initial pattern of the fight-or-flight response is called the **pituitary-adrenal axis** (Figure 13.3). The hypothalamus stimulates the pituitary gland, the master gland of the endocrine system, to increase the release of adrenocorticotropic hormone (ACTH) into the bloodstream. ACTH activates the outer layer of the adrenal gland, which results in the increased production of **glucocorticoids.** Glucocorticoids are chemicals responsible for speeding up the body's metabolism and increasing its access to energy storage.

Simultaneous to the activation of the pituitary-adrenal axis, the second pattern of the fight-or-flight response, called the **sympathoadrenal** system, is set in motion. The nerve impulses from the sympathetic branch of the autonomic nervous system reach the core of the adrenal glands, resulting in the increased release of **epinephrine** and **norepinephrine.** Epinephrine is referred to as the "fear hormone" and helps supply glucose to be used for increased muscle and nervous system activity. Norepinephrine is referred to as the "anger hormone" and helps speed up the heart rate and raises blood pressure in an attempt to provide more oxygen for the body. The effects of epinephrine and norepinephrine are similar to those produced by the **sympathetic nervous system,** except that the effects of the hormones last about 10 times longer.

The sum of the increased activation of the pituitary-adrenal axis and sympathoadrenal patterns (the fight-or-flight response) is to provide chemicals and hormones that permit the person to perform far more strenuous physical activity. If your response to fight-or-flight is physical activity (to fight or flee), the chemicals and hormones you have generated will be metabolized right away. If your response to the fight-or-flight response is to "sit tight" and not be physically active, the excess chemicals and hormones released in the body may cause unnecessary wear and tear. This damage, if repeated over time, may result in a number of diseases, including heart disease, stroke, and ulcerative colitis.

Stage of Resistance

Your body responds to all stress, both positive and negative, by trying to get back to normal. After the alarm reaction and the fight-or-flight responses, a stage of resistance occurs. During the resistance stage, the body attempts to adapt to the stressor and return to homeostasis. Readjustment occurs as resistance to stress rises and body functions return to normal. Physiologically, the parasympathetic nervous system is the counterpart to the sympathetic nervous system. The effects of the **parasympathetic nervous system** are the opposite of the effects of the sympathetic nervous system (Table 13.2). When no danger is perceived, the parasympathetic nervous system releases acetylcholine, a chemical that plays an inhibitory role on the effects of sympathetic stimulation of organs. This is commonly known as the **relaxation response** (Figure 13.4). The actions of both divisions of the autonomic nervous system must be balanced in order to maintain homeostasis.

Even though the body may adapt successfully to stressors in the short term, if continual major adaptation is required, or a number of adaptations are required over time, this may exact a serious toll on the body, particularly on the neuroendocrine and immune systems.

FIGURE 13.4

The Relaxation Response. The relaxation response is important because it allows the body to return to homeostatis following the fight-or-flight response.

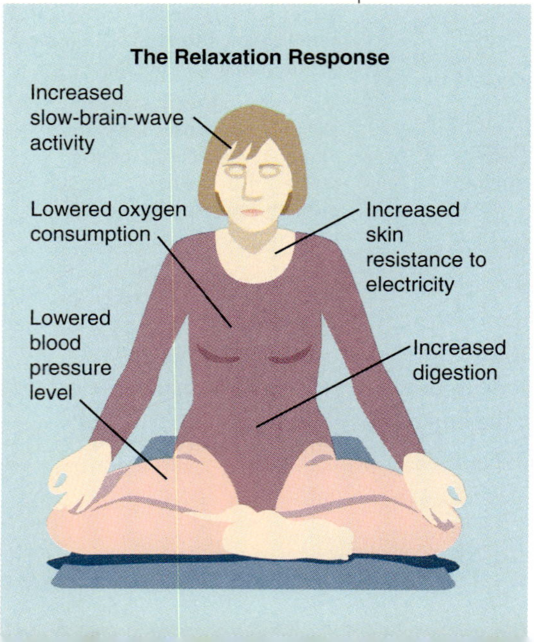

TABLE 13.2 **Effects of the autonomic nervous system on various visceral effector organs**

EFFECTOR EFFECT	SYMPATHETIC EFFECT	PARASYMPATHETIC EFFECT
Eye		
Iris (pupillary dilator muscle)	Dilation of pupil	—
Iris (pupillary sphincter muscle)	—	Contraction (for near vision)
Glands		
Lacrimal (tear)	—	Stimulation of secretion
Sweat	Stimulation of secretion	—
Salivary	Decreased secretion; saliva becomes thick	Increased secretion, saliva becomes thin
Stomach	—	Stimulation of secretion
Intestine	—	Stimulation of secretion
Adrenal medulla	Stimulation of hormone secretion	—
Heart		
Rate	Increased	Decreased
Conduction	Increased rate	Decreased rate
Strength	Increased	—
Blood vessels	Mostly constriction; affects all organs	Dilation in a few organs (e.g., penis)
Lungs		
Bronchioles (tubes)	Dilation	Constriction
Mucous glands	Inhibition of secretion	Stimulation of secretion
Gastrointestinal tract		
Motility	Inhibition of movement	Stimulation of movement
Sphincters	Closing stimulated	Closing inhibited
Liver	Stimulation of glycogen hydrolysis	—
Adipocytes (fat cells)	Stimulation of fat hydrolysis	—
Pancreas	Inhibition of exocrine secretions	Stimulation of exocrine secretions
Spleen	Stimulation of contraction	—
Urinary bladder	Muscle tone added	Stimulation of contraction
Arrector pili muscles	Stimulation of hair erection, causing goosebumps	—
Uterus	If pregnant, contraction If not pregnant, relaxation	
Penis	Ejaculation	Erection (due to vasodilation)

The ongoing level of demand for adaptation in an individual is called **allostatic load** (*allo* = all, *static* = equilibrium) on that person, and it may be an important contributor to many chronic diseases (McEwen & Stellar, 1993). The continual setting off of the alarm stage and the resultant efforts of resistance to re-establish equilibrium in the body are increasingly becoming the focal point of research on illness and disease. Repeated alarms can lead to the stage of exhaustion in which the symptoms of the alarm reaction return.

Allostatic load The ongoing level of demand for adaptation in an individual.

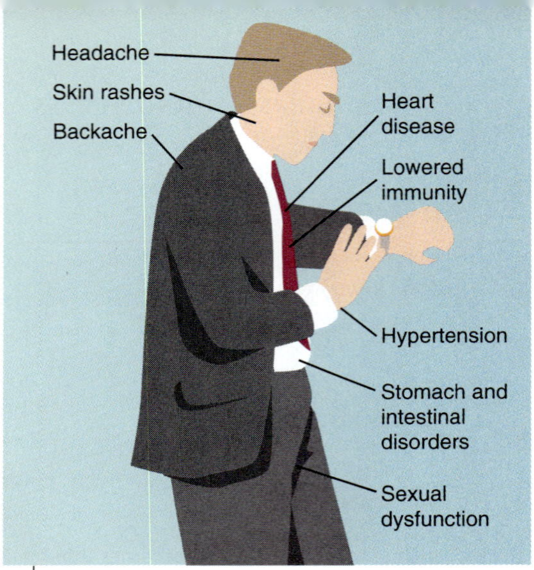

FIGURE 13.5

The Physical Toll of Stress. Unrelieved stress can cause a number of physical symptoms.

Stage of Exhaustion

The mobilization of forces during the alarm reaction, and the return to homeostasis during the resistance stage, requires a substantial amount of energy. The stage of exhaustion occurs when the body's resources become depleted and fatigued. Prolonged exposure to a stressor can cause the body organs to become weakened and increase the susceptibility to illness (Figure 13.5). If stress is unrelenting, and present long enough, it can produce permanent physical deterioration. A recent study explored the symptoms of stress and identified eight physical indicators reflecting high stress (McEwen, 1998):

- Increases in blood pressure
- Suppressed immunity
- Increased fat around the abdomen
- Bone loss
- Increases in blood sugar
- Increases in levels of cortisol
- Weaker muscles
- Increases in blood cholesterol levels

Activities & Assessments 13.1

Each person has a breaking point for dealing with stress. In addition to chronic or extended stress, stress research also indicates the cumulative adjustments required from intermittent and sequential stressors may impact the body over time. Selye (1973) observed that the number of stress responses and readjustments increases the wear and tear on the body, accelerating degenerative disease processes.

Stress and Performance

5. Stress is a natural process, and understanding its effects can help you use it to your own advantage.

Stress is a natural process, and understanding its effects can help you use it to your own advantage. Stress researchers have long recognized that some stress or stimulation is needed for optimal performance. Yerkes and Dodson described a phenomenon, known today as the **Yerkes-Dodson law**, of an inverted U–shaped function between stress and performance (Hanson, 1986). The Yerkes-Dodson law theorizes about the ways health and performance are affected as stress increases. Although the relationship between stress and performance varies from person to person, the general pattern can be expressed by viewing the curve in Figure 13.6.

The curve is divided into three sections. The far left of the curve represents **hypostress,** not enough stress, which occurs when we lack stimulation. This area is often referred to as *rustout.* Rustout is a result of decreased drive and motivation and is caused by lack of challenges in our lives. The middle of the curve represents an area of optimal productivity. This amount of increased stress or stimulation in your life can fuel creativity, create excitement, or physically energize you for important events in your life. This moderate amount of stress can be a motivator toward change and growth that brings forth good results related to our mental and physical health. Moving to the right side of the curve, we find **hyperstress,** or stress beyond that which is optimal. This condition is called *burnout,* a point where the body begins to decrease in its level of performance.

Yerkes-Dodson law Predicts an inverted U-shaped function between stress and performance.

Hypostress Too little stress or stimulation.

Hyperstress Too much stress; the body begins to decrease in its level of performance.

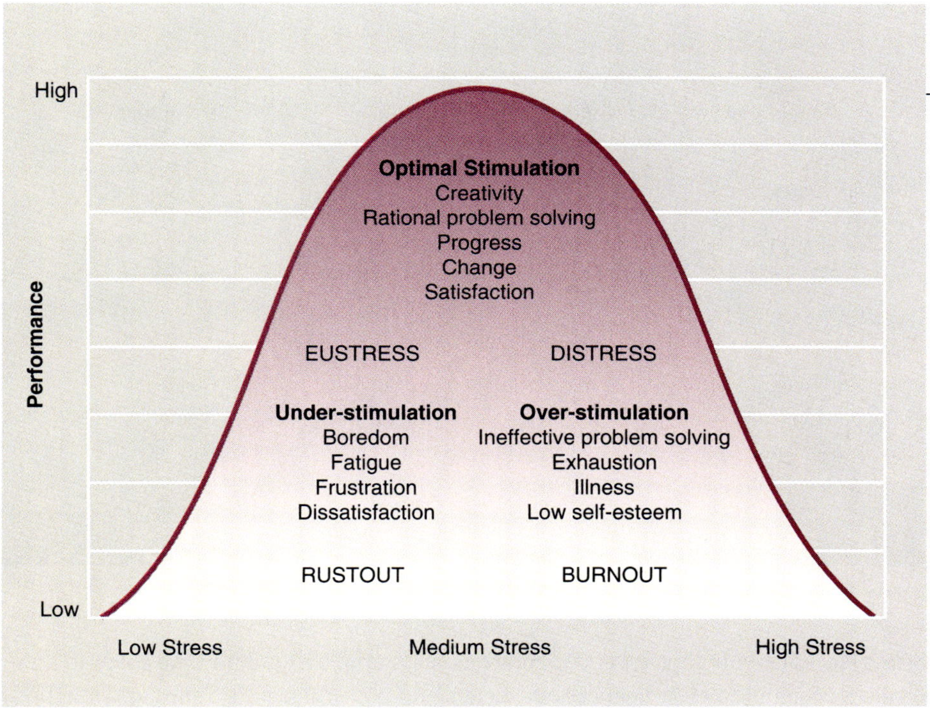

FIGURE 13.6

The Effects of Stress on Performance.

Stress becomes unmanageable and out of control at this point, and we experience impaired mental and physical capabilities.

Again, no single level of stress is optimal for all people. We are all individual beings with unique requirements. There is no way to predict conclusively how an individual will respond to different stressors. Individual differences in responding to the challenge of stress are products of our experiences, our developmental and environmental influences, and our genetics (McEwen & Stellar, 1993). Some people may cope well with stress, rising to meet the challenge, and others may be more adversely affected, responding with mental and physical fatigue. And, even when we agree that a particular event is distressing, we are likely to differ in our physiological and psychological responses to it.

It has been found that most illness is related to hyperstress and unrelieved stress. When your resistance resources are overworked, your exhausted body stops functioning smoothly. The signs of hyperstress are so pervasive in our culture that people often fail to recognize them as signs of distress. The signs may show up psychologically, physically, or behaviorally (Figure 13.7). Psychological signs may include inappropriate anger or intolerance, diminished ability to make priorities and decisions, an inability to concentrate, and a sense of hopelessness or frustration. Physical symptoms may include headaches, aching neck and back, upset stomach, and indigestion. Behavioral signs may include grinding the teeth, biting the fingernails, and overreacting to minor problems.

Complete Engage 13.4, "Distress Symptoms," at this time. This assessment will help you identify what your symptoms of stress may be. If you are experiencing stress symptoms, you have probably gone beyond your optimal stress level, and it is time to consider implementing some stress-management techniques in your life.

Engage www.pahconnection.com **13.4**

Maintaining and optimizing our mental and physical health requires making countless adjustments to a variety of life's challenges. Life's challenges are viewed as stress.

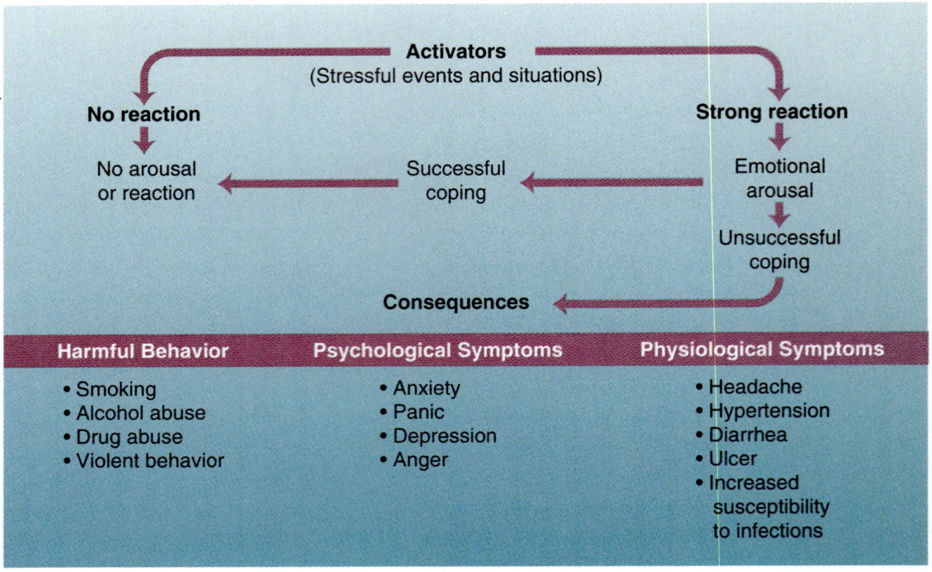

FIGURE 13.7

The Stress-Illness Relationship. It is through one's reaction that a given situation is experienced as stressful.

Stress places certain physical and mental demands upon us, and how we adapt to these challenges significantly influences our mental and physical health. Your mind and body are connected, and during stressful times it is important to understand the relationship that exists between them.

STRESS MANAGEMENT

6. The art of stress management is to keep yourself at a level of stimulation that is healthy and enjoyable.

Experience www.pahconnection.com 13.3, 13.4

The art of stress management is to keep yourself at a level of stimulation that is healthy and enjoyable. Life without stimulus would be dull and boring. Life with too many stimuli becomes unpleasant and tiring. The primary purpose for developing stress-management techniques is to reduce the potential psychological and physical illnesses that result from too much stress. There are many specific strategies available for managing hyperstress. The specific strategies found in Experience 13.3 can be categorized into three basic approaches to handing stress: (1) the environmental engineering, or "controlling your circumstances," approach; (2) the mind engineering, or "mind-over-matter," approach; and (3) the physical engineering, or the "stress-fit," approach.

These three basic stress solutions can be used singly or in any combination. Different approaches work for different stressors. Additionally, approaches vary among individuals. Before you begin reading about the three basic solutions, it may be helpful for you to have at hand the list of sources of stress in your life that you completed for Engage 13.3. You can then apply a basic approach to your source of stress and select from the wide variety of specific strategies presented at the end of the chapter.

Environmental Engineering

Environmental engineering Stress management approach that attempts to avoid it in the first place.

The **environmental engineering,** "control your circumstances," approach deals with the stressor by attempting to avoid it in the first place. This approach advocates controlling as many environmental circumstances as you can. To accomplish this, you need to analyze the situations in your environment that may lead to foreseeable stressful situations. Keeping a stress diary is a helpful way of finding out what causes you stress and when and where the event occurs. After a few weeks you should be able to analyze this information and be able to better plan a change in your environment to avoid the stressor.

For example, lately you have been feeling unprepared and tired for your Friday 8 A.M. economics class, an important class in your major field. Your journal reveals that you have routinely stayed out late with your friends on Thursday evenings and thus not studied for your economics class. You decide to take positive action by changing these circumstances; you make time to study on Thursday evening and get to bed at a reasonable hour. This new course of action leaves you feeling prepared and rested for your economics class.

Recognizing what stressors you can avoid by eliminating interaction with them is a good solution for dealing with a number of stressors. This strategy requires being able to plan ahead so that you can have the forethought to avoid the stressor. However, when a stressor is not foreseeable or avoidable, you must apply another approach to manage stress.

Mind Engineering

Mind engineering, "mind-over-matter," refers to how we deal with a stressor through the mind-body relationship. The mind and body are inseparable. Mind engineering reduces the intensity of our responses to stressors. Your mind activates your body's stress response. When your mind is healthy, your body can better resist illness. Similarly, when your mind is unhealthy, your resistance to illness decreases. The success of mind engineering depends on your attitude because the attitude you carry into a particular situation will greatly influence your perceptions of any stressor or event.

Mind engineering Stress management approach concerned with reducing the intensity of our emotional responses to stressors.

Attitude is the byproduct of our thoughts. We have explicit control over our own attitudes (see Chapter 3). It is in our attitudes that we discover strength or weakness, patience or anxiety, determination or frustration, when faced with a stressor. Our attitude about what we believe we should be, and the imagined punishment if we fail, determines how we see and react to stressors. When we view stressors positively, we are secure in our knowledge that we can make them beneficial to our growth if we choose. When we view stressors negatively, we are uncertain about our abilities to deal with them effectively and consequently feel that we are not in control.

Self-Talk. Your successes are always within your control if you understand your responsibility to your feelings and beliefs.

Are you viewing your stressors in exaggerated terms—taking a challenging situation and making it a disaster? Positive thinking is everything when it comes to managing stress. Most people carry on a silent conversation with themselves, which is referred to as *self-talk* (see Chapter 3). Positive self-talk offers many stress-reduction benefits. If you think "I know I can ace my chemistry exam," you will have a

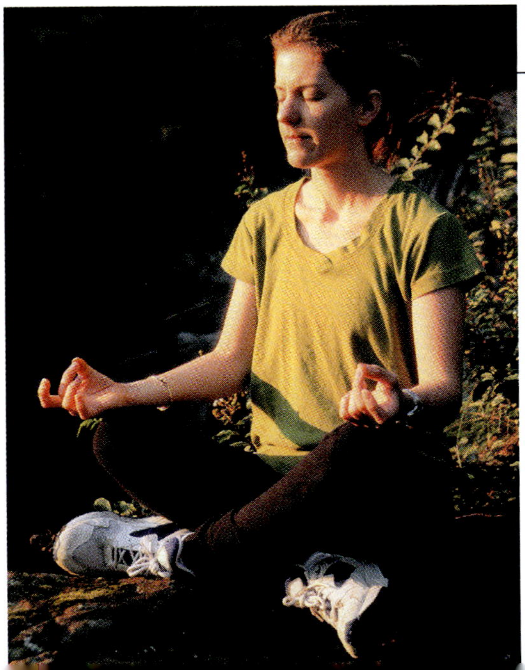

Meditation is a form of mind engineering. Mediation uses a rhythmic activity such as breath awareness to focus the mind, lifting you out of your ordinary level of consciousness into a state of "passive awareness" where the body can deal with stress problems.

better chance of success and will have made the stressor a positive one. If you engage in negative self-talk, "I can't pass that chemistry exam," you increase your chances of failure and the stressor becomes negative. As any sailor knows, "It is not the direction of the wind that determines our course so much as how we set our sails"; in sailing parlance, this is known significantly as the *attitude*.

Activities & Assessments 13.2

Engage www.pahconnection.com 13.5

Stress-Resistance While it is not possible to become totally immune to stressors, you can "inoculate" yourself against stress—make it more tolerable and reduce its intensity—by learning to resist its harmful effects. Some people are better equipped to handle and manage stress than others because they have a "risk takers" attitude. Risk takers view new situations and responsibilities as challenges for further growth rather than as opportunities for failure. Engage 13.5, "Are You Stress-Resistant?," will give you an idea of how resistant or how vulnerable you are, based on your attitudes toward various situations.

Physical Engineering

physical activity and health connection

Physical engineering Stress management approach using regular exercise to optimize your stress responses.

The **physical engineering,** "stress-fit," approach is predicated on the fact that it is easier to deal with the stress response when your body is healthy from regular physical activity. Regular physical activity is useful in removing the byproducts that occur due to the stress response and in reducing the physiological reactivity of the body to stressors.

Expending Excess Energy and Biochemicals When the body experiences the fight-or-flight reaction, it provides us with energy via stress hormones and chemicals. The result is that our bodies go into a state of high energy, but there is often nowhere for this energy to be expended, so our bodies stay in a state of arousal for hours. Additionally, the biochemicals that initiated this high state of energy are left to circulate in the body and have the capability for causing illness. During times of high stress, we can benefit from a physical outlet. Physical activity is the most logical way to expend excess energy and throw off its biochemical byproducts. When our bodies are in a high state of energy, it is healthful to expend this energy in a brisk walk or run. In addition to enjoying the available energy, the exercise is ridding the body of stress hormones and flushing the excessive biochemical buildup.

Studies show that those who experience stress-related illness, or symptoms of stress, can best reduce or eliminate those symptoms with a program of stress management that includes physical activity. Physical activity reduces many of the physical symptoms associated with stress and illness. A regular physical activity program lowers the resting heart rate and blood pressure and protects against fatigue, reduces digestive problems, and relaxes muscles.

An excellent form of physical engineering to reduce stress is to take a walk.

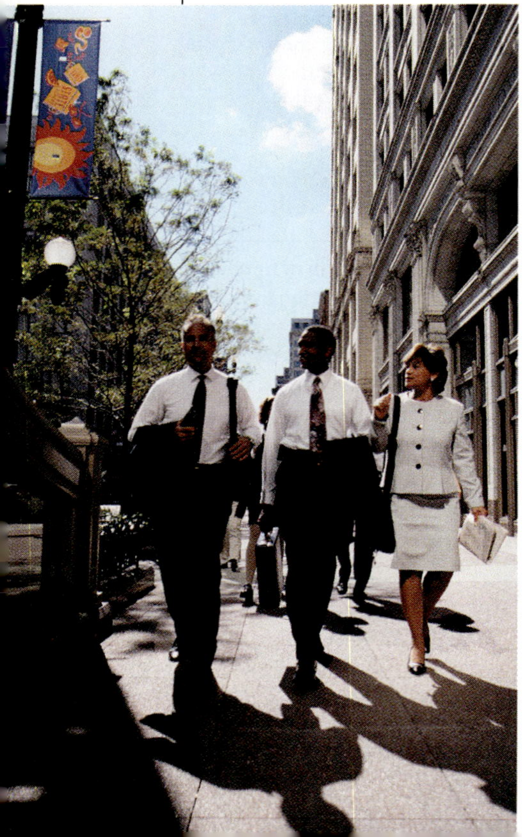

Physiological Reactivity The second part of the physical engineering approach deals with the theoretical assumption that higher levels of aerobic fitness are associated with less physiological reactivity to psychosocial stressors. This stress-buffering or inoculation effect occurs as a result of improved physiological functioning of the body. The improved cardiovascular adaptation from aerobic exercise appears to mediate and decrease an individual's physiological reactivity in response to a number of psychosocial stressors (Brown, 1990). In other words, since physical activity provides an almost identical physiological response to that which occurs with mental stress, strengthening the body to react to physical activity will strengthen the body's response to mental stress. Long-term physical activity may adjust the brain's responsiveness to chemicals associated with stress, allowing the brain to deal with stress more efficiently.

THE MENTAL HEALTH BENEFITS OF PHYSICAL ACTIVITY

You have just read about how physical activity can be therapeutic when it comes to managing stress. Interestingly, the psychological benefits from physical activity across all areas of mental well-being are advocated. There is much speculation, however, about the mechanisms by which physical activity improves mental health. What follows is a brief overview of the most frequently discussed mechanisms. Although these explanations are discussed independently, it is important to understand that they may operate interactively.

Cognitive Behavioral Theory

This explanation maintains that, as a person engages in physical activity and experiences bodily changes, self-efficacy increases. That is, participating in and mastering a specific physical task creates positive feelings because individuals perceive that they can perform activity even in tough situations. This is related to Bandura's theory of self-efficacy (see Chapter 3), in which the strength of a belief is enhanced by continued successful execution of a behavior. Feelings of mastery and control are incompatible with negative thoughts (anxiety, depression). Additionally, self-esteem is fostered when you realize that you are doing something that will ultimately benefit you. Participating in physical activity has a positive social value attached to it because it is a health-enhancing activity.

Social Interaction Theory

The buffering effects of social support are well documented when it comes to physical activity (see Chapters 2 and 3). Physical activities that are done with friends and colleagues, or in social settings, can have a net effect of improving mental health. This mental health effect is much more noticeable in groups in which people feel a collective sense of achievement and accomplishment.

Distraction Theory

The solitude experienced when performing physical activities that require a fairly consistent, repetitive motion (bicycling, jogging, hiking) can alter your state of consciousness. The regular breathing and movement associated with these activities may act as a mantra that induces feelings of calmness and tranquility similar to those obtained while practicing meditation. Physical activity provides a distraction, or time-out, from the daily worries of a stressful society. Furthermore, physical activity provides an opportunity for introspective thinking that can stimulate creativity in problem solving.

The Endorphin Hypothesis

The endorphin hypothesis represents the most popular biological explanation, despite questionable evidence. The term **endorphins** is a general classification for important body chemicals that are responsible for enhancing emotions (euphoric feelings) and providing pain relief (analgesic effect). The neurochemical reaction from endorphin release has been shown to increase following physical activity of 20 minutes or more.

The Thermogenic Hypothesis

During physical activity the body temperature rises (see Chapter 8). This body-warming effect has been shown to reduce muscle tension, thereby countering the tension that may build up in muscles from stress (neck, lower back).

endorphins Body chemicals responsible for enhancing emotions and providing pain relief.

The therapeutic benefits of regular physical activity are without rival when it comes to reducing stress and maintaining mental health. The form of physical activity you choose should be enjoyable, noncompetitive, and personally satisfying. Choose activities you like, or they will feel like a chore and you will begin to avoid them. It is also beneficial to have a variety of physical activity outlets.

QUICK RELAXATION TECHNIQUES

Others ways to reduce stress in the body are through certain disciplines that fall under the heading of relaxation techniques. The term *relaxation training* is used in the health literature to refer to various techniques that stimulate the *relaxation response* (Figure 13.4, Table 13.2). The *relaxation response* is the opposite of the fight-or-flight response to stressful or threatening situations. Just as we are all capable of heightening and sustaining a stress reaction, we have also inherited the ability to put our bodies into a state of relaxation. In this state, all the physiological events in the stress reaction are reversed: breathing and pulse slow, blood pressure declines, and muscles relax. It has been found that relaxing for just 20 minutes each day can be beneficial to both your physical and mental health. Unlike the stress reaction, which is automatic, *the relaxation response needs to be induced by intention.* Fortunately, there are many simple ways to do this. The following relaxation techniques can be practiced by anyone at any time during the day and provide instant relief from stress.

Deep Breathing

Deep breathing is a countermeasure to stress. When stressed, your breathing becomes rapid and shallow, causing an insufficient amount of oxygen to reach your lungs. The goal in deep breathing is to slow and increase the volume of air inhaled, thus providing extra oxygen to the blood. Slowly inhale through your nose, expanding your abdomen before allowing air to fill your lungs. Reverse the process by constricting your stomach and exhaling through your mouth, making a quiet, whooshing sound as you blow out calmly. Continue to take long, slow, deep breaths, focusing on the sound and feeling of breathing. After a few minutes you should become more relaxed. You may want to perform this technique a couple times a day. Deep breathing is a very effective method of relaxation and is the most basic technique used in relaxation training.

Visualization

Visualization is using your imagination to reduce stress. Find a quiet place where you feel comfortable. Sit down and close your eyes, breathing slowly. Next, try focusing on one peaceful thought, or on a goal you want to attain. If your mind strays back to the problem causing stress, make yourself return to the peaceful thought for a couple of minutes. Another variation of visualization is to create a picture in your mind of a beautiful place and imagine yourself there, using as many of your senses as you can.

Progressive Muscle Relaxation

Engage
www.pahconnection.com
13.6

Progressive muscle relaxation (PMR) is a simple technique used to induce neuromuscular relaxation by creating an awareness of the difference between muscular tension and a relaxed state. Progressive muscle relaxation is a two-step process. First, each muscle or muscle group is tensed from 5 to 10 seconds and then relaxed for 15 to 25 seconds. Repeat this procedure at least once; if the area remains tense, repeat up to 5 times.

For more long-term stress-balancing strategies, complete Engage 13.6, "Stress Balancing Strategies." These strategies provide you with long-term solutions to maintaining a healthy level of stress.

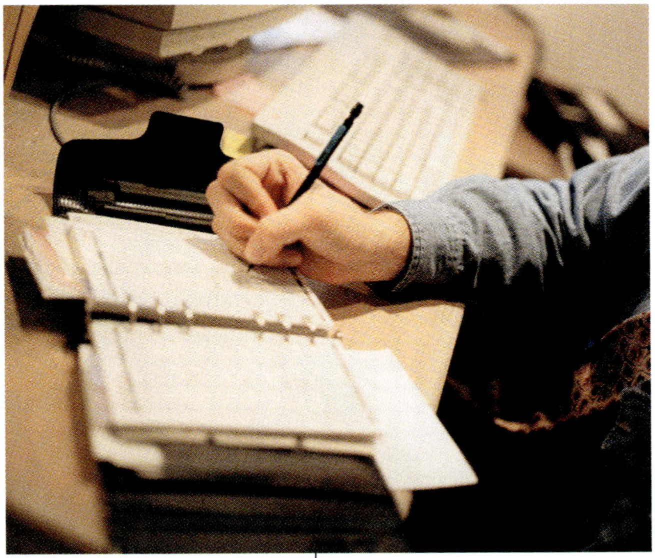

Keeping a daily log of how you spend your time is a helpful technique in time management.

Time Management

A major contributor to stress is inadequate time-management skills. Despite an image of college life being carefree and fun-filled, college life will probably require more careful and effective utilization of time than a student has ever needed to achieve before. A typical student schedules 15 or more classroom hours a week and is expected to average about 2 hours of preparation for each hour in the classroom. This means that students have at least a 45-hour work week, equivalent to a full-time job. In addition, many students find that they must balance their academic responsibilities with part-time jobs, family, and social responsibilities. Thus it is not surprising that a common concern among college students is not having enough time to get everything accomplished. The job of being a college student, like most other jobs, can be carried out more effectively with the use of time-management techniques that increase your productivity.

Activities & Assessments 13.3

Assess Current Time Use

A good place to begin is to keep track of how you currently use your time. Assess how you spend your time each day for a week by faithfully keeping a daily log of how you spend your waking hours.

Setting Priorities

Write down your goals and priorities. Divide your goals into essential, important, and trivial. Having a record of how you spend your time allows you to compare your current use of time to essential and important goals and priorities. You need to be spending virtually all of your time on essential and important priorities.

Time Scheduling

One of best techniques for developing more efficient time-use habits is to prepare a schedule. The following is a flexible way to help establish long-term, intermediate, and short-term goals. A long-term schedule consists of your fixed commitments. These include only obligations you are required to meet every week: classes, job, physical activity, church, organizational meetings. Your immediate schedule consists of a short list of major tasks to be accomplished in the next week: quiz on Monday, ballgame on Wednesday, read 60 pages in history by Friday. Finally, each evening before going to bed, write down on a small card what you must accomplish the next day. Carry this card with you during the day and cross out each item after you accomplish it.

PHYSICAL ACTIVITY AND HEALTH CONNECTION

Our mental and emotional health is essential to the quality of our lives and influences our physical health. The relationship between regular physical activity and mental wellness has been established. Much is known about the physical health benefits of physical activity as it relates to fitness, weight management, and control of a number of chronic disease conditions. Now we can also look at physical activity as an important contributor to mental health and comprehensive stress management strategies. Stress management experts increasingly regard physical activity as one the most healthful ways to reduce stress. People who are physically active tend to have better mental health. Being regularly active increases general feelings of well-being and positive moods, and decreases bouts of anxiety and depression. By engaging your body regularly in physical activity, you prepare it to deal with the physiological strains associated with emotional crises. Your body becomes better able to handle stress and the chemicals that are released during stressful situations. A sound mind and a sound body are equally important to our overall health.

CONCEPT CONNECTION

1. **People who are physically active tend to have better mental health.** The consensus is that people who are physically active have higher scores on important mental health factors like self-esteem, self-concept, self-worth, body image, and cognitive functioning than sedentary people. Furthermore, physical activity has been shown to be effective in treating people who report symptoms of anxiety, depression, and stress.
2. **Our mental and emotional health are central to the quality of our lives, and both influence our physical health.** Holistic health perspectives emphasize mind-body unity and include the complex relationship between mental and physical functioning as well as the continuum between health and illness.
3. **Maintaining and optimizing our mental and physical health requires making countless adjustments to a variety of life's challenges.** Life's challenges are perceived internally as stress. Stress places certain physical and mental demands upon us, and how we adapt to these challenges significantly influences our mental and physical health. Your mind and body are connected, and during stressful times it is important to understand the relationship that exists between them.
4. **The general adaptation syndrome describes the body's response to stress and the adaptability of the body to maintain homeostasis.** Selye's research provided evidence that the body goes through a predictable three-stage physiological response to any kind of stressor: (1) the alarm reaction, when the adrenal glands are activated in an attempt to mobilize the body's energy resources for physical action; (2) the stage of resistance, in which the readjustment occurs; and (3) if the readjustment is not complete, the stage of exhaustion may follow, leading to illness and possibly death.
5. **Stress is a natural process, and understanding its effects can help you use it to advantage.** Stress researchers have long recognized that some stress (stimulation) is needed for optimal performance.

Yerkes and Dodson described a phenomenon that is known today as the Yerkes-Dodson law, which predicts an inverted U-shaped function between stress and performance. The Yerkes-Dodson law theorizes about the way health and performance are affected as stress increases.

6. **The art of stress management is to keep yourself at a level of stimulation that is healthy and enjoyable.** Life without stimulus would be dull and boring. Life with too much stimulus becomes unpleasant and tiring. The primary purpose for developing stress management techniques is to reduce the potential psychological and physical illnesses that result from too much stress.

TERMS

Mental health, 289
Emotional health, 290
Psychosomatic disease, 291
Mental illness, 292
Anxiety, 292
Anxiety disorder, 292
Generalized anxiety disorder (GAD), 292
Depression, 293
Depressive reactions, 293
Dysthymia, 293
Major depression, 293
Stress, 293
Eustress, 293
Distress, 293
General adaptation syndrome(GAS), 294
Stressor, 294
Alarm reaction, 295
Autonomic nervous system, 295
Endocrine system, 295
Fight-or-flight response, 295
Pituitary-adrenal axis, 296
Glucocorticoids, 296
Sympathoadrenal system, 296
Epinephrine, 296
Norepinephrine, 296
Sympathetic nervous system, 296
Parasympathetic nervous system, 296
Relaxation response, 296
Allostatic load, 296
Yerkes-Dodson law, 299
Hypostress, 299
Hyperstress, 299
Environmental engineering, 300
Mind engineering, 301
Physical engineering, 302
Endorphens, 303

MAKING THE CONNECTION

Jesse now knows that research supports the idea that physical activity can enhance mental health and well-being. Therefore, his impulse to jog before he had to give the speech for English class was a good idea. The jog likely provided a distraction, or time-out, from the anxiety he was experiencing about delivering his speech.

CRITICAL THINKING

1. Jesse was able to determine that exercising helped relieve the speech anxiety he was having. Review Figures 13.4 and 13.6. Are you experiencing any of the harmful stress symptoms listed? If so, do you think stress is the cause? If yes, what are the specific stressors? What physical activities might you do to help relieve these stressors?
2. Review your list of life stress sources. Next to each source, list whether you would use environmental engineering, mind engineering, or physical engineering to manage the stressor. Would more than one strategy be useful? Do you see physical activity helping to manage the stress in your life? Why or why not?
3. Stressors can be a result of situations present on your campus or campus community. Community stressors may be problems such a crime, pollution, lack of recreation facilities, and overcrowded classrooms or residence halls. Identify what you consider to be a major stressor in your campus community. How would you go about changing this stressor?

REFERENCES

Barbee, J.G. (1998). Mixed symptoms and syndromes of anxiety and depression: Diagnostic, prognostic, and etiologic issues. *Annals of Clinical Psychiatry 10*:15–29.

Brown, D.R. (1990). Exercise, fitness, and mental health. In Bouchard, C., ed., *Exercise Fitness and Health.* Champaign, IL: Human Kinetics.

Cowan, E.L. (1994). The enhancement of psychological wellness: Challenges and opportunities. *American Journal of Community Psychology* 22:149–79.

Crider, A., Goethals, G., Kavanaugh, R., & Solloon, P. (1993). *Psychology,* 4th ed. New York: HarperCollins.

Dohrenwend, B.S., & Dohrenwend, B.T. (1981). Life, stress, and illness: Formulation of the issues. In Dohrenwend, B.S., Dohrenwend, B.T., eds., *Stressful life events and their contacts.* New York: Neal Watson Academic Publications.

Dubos, R. (1965). *Man Adapting.* New Haven: Yale University Press.

Edlin, G., Golanty, E., & McCormack Brown, K. (2000). *Essentials for Health and Wellness.* Boston: Jones & Bartlett.

Hanson, P.G. (1986). *The Joy of Stress.* Kansas City: Andrews, McMeel & Parker.

Hughes, J.R. (1984). Psychological effects of habitual exercise: A critical review. *Preventive Medicine 13*: 66–78.

Institute of Medicine. (1994). Reducing risk for mental disorders: Frontiers for preventive intervention research. Washington, DC: National Academy Press.

Lazarus, S., & Folkman, S. (1984). *Stress, Appraisal, and Coping.* New York: Springer.

McAuley, E., & Rudoph, D. (1995). Physical activity, aging, and psychological well-being. *Journal of Aging and Physical Activity* 3: 67–96.

McEwen, B.S. (1998). Protective and damaging effects of stress mediators. *New England Journal of Medicine 338*(3):171–79.

McEwen, B.S., & Stellar, E. (1993). Stress and the individual. *Archives of Internal Medicine 153*:2093–2101.

Morgan, W.P. (1985). Affective beneficence of vigorous physical activity. *Medicine and Science in Sports Exercise 17*: 94–100.

National Institutes of Mental Health. (1997). *Anxiety Disorders.* National Institutes of Health, NIH Publication No. 97-3879. Bethesda, MD.

Selye, H. (1973). The evolution of the stress concept. *American Scientist 61*:692–99.

Selye, H. (1976). *The Stress of Life.* New York: McGraw-Hill.

Stephens, T. (1988). Physical activity and mental health in the United States and Canada: Evidence from four population surveys; *Preventive Medicine 17*: 35–47.

U.S. Department of Health and Human Services. (1999). *Mental Health: A Report of the Surgeon General.* Rockville, MD.

U.S. Department of Health and Human Services. (1996). *Physical Activity and Health: A Report of the Surgeon General.* Atlanta, GA.

Activities & Assessments

NAME ______________________ SECTION ____________ DATE ____________

13.1 What Are Your Stress Reactions?

Many people experience particular physical reactions to excessive stress. Here's a list of some common stress reactions. Which ones do you frequently experience? Can you add some reactions that are not on the list?

REACTION	ONCE A DAY	ONCE EVERY 2–3 DAYS	ONCE A WEEK	ONCE A MONTH	NOT IN THE LAST 2 MONTHS
Headaches	☐	☐	☐	☐	☐
Nervous tics and twitches	☐	☐	☐	☐	☐
Blurred vision	☐	☐	☐	☐	☐
Dizziness	☐	☐	☐	☐	☐
Fatigue	☐	☐	☐	☐	☐
Coughing	☐	☐	☐	☐	☐
Wheezing	☐	☐	☐	☐	☐
Backaches	☐	☐	☐	☐	☐
Muscle spasms	☐	☐	☐	☐	☐
Itching	☐	☐	☐	☐	☐
Excessive sweating	☐	☐	☐	☐	☐
Palpitations	☐	☐	☐	☐	☐
Constipation	☐	☐	☐	☐	☐
Jaw tightening	☐	☐	☐	☐	☐
Rapid heart rate	☐	☐	☐	☐	☐
Impotence	☐	☐	☐	☐	☐
Pelvic pain	☐	☐	☐	☐	☐
Stomachache	☐	☐	☐	☐	☐
Diarrhea	☐	☐	☐	☐	☐
Frequent urination	☐	☐	☐	☐	☐
Dermatitis (rash)	☐	☐	☐	☐	☐
Hyperventilation	☐	☐	☐	☐	☐
Irregular heart rhythm	☐	☐	☐	☐	☐
High blood pressure	☐	☐	☐	☐	☐
Delayed menstruation	☐	☐	☐	☐	☐
Vaginal discharge	☐	☐	☐	☐	☐
Nail biting	☐	☐	☐	☐	☐
Heartburn	☐	☐	☐	☐	☐

SOURCE: G. Edlin, E. Golanty, and K. McCormack Brown. (1999). *Health and Wellness* (6th ed., p. 534). Boston: Jones and Bartlett.

TABLE 14.1 **Tips for Taking Medicines**

Tips for Taking Medicines

Whether prescription or over-the-counter (OTC), no medicine is without risk. Besides benefits, medicines may cause side effects, allergic reactions, and interactions with foods, drinks, or other drugs. For prescription drugs, a patient's first step to safe and effective treatment is to ask the doctor questions with each new prescription.

For example:

What is the medicine's name, and what is it supposed to do?

How and when do I take it, and for how long?

While taking this medicine, should I avoid:
- certain foods or dietary supplements?
- caffeine, alcohol, or other beverages?
- other medicines, prescription and OTC?
- certain activities, such as driving or smoking?

Will this new medicine work safely with prescription and OTC medicines I'm already taking? Are there side effects, and what do I do if they occur?

Will the medicine affect my sleep or activity level?

What should I do if I miss a dose?

Is there written information available about the medicine? (At the very least, ask the doctor or pharmacist to write out complicated directions and medicine names.)

It's wise to write down the answers to these questions immediately, to make sure you'll remember all the details.

SOURCE: U.S. Food and Drug Administration. (1997, July). Tips for taking medication.

This information is not intended to be a substitute for professional medical advice. You should not use this information to diagnose or treat a health problem or disease without consulting with a qualified healthcare provider. Please consult your healthcare provider with any questions or concerns you may have regarding your condition.

Approximately 20 percent (16 million people) of current adult drinkers drink beyond moderation. Nearly 10 percent of current drinkers (8 million people) meet alcohol-dependence criteria, and an additional 7 percent (nearly 6 million people) fulfill alcohol abuse criteria (NIAAA, 1997).

CHRONIC DRUG USE IMPLICATIONS

2. Long-term drug use can disrupt the body's normal balance, or homeostasis.

It is generally assumed that no one starts using drugs with the goal of misusing or abusing them; however, it is possible to drift from responsible use to misuse or abuse of a number of commonly used drugs. It is also clear that many chronic users eventually do experience problems with drugs and may eventually suffer negative health consequences. Addressing or rehabilitating chronic users in terms of their level of involvement with a drug is essential in forestalling a number of detrimental health effects. Therefore, it is critical to understand the processes that your body and mind undergo with chronic drug use.

Long-term drug use often unsettles the body's normal balance, or homeostasis (Pinger et al., 1998). The person who experiments with a drug once or twice and then quits experiences acute adjustments in the body and then an immediate return to homeostasis. The person who continues to use a drug moves to a level of risk one step beyond, as each exposure carries with it the possibility that the body's chemical pathways will change to adapt to repeated exposure to the drug. This can be a difficult idea to grasp, but within it lies the foundation for *tolerance, psychological dependence,* and *physical dependence with withdrawal illness.* The most extreme potential arising from chronic drug use is the threat of *drug addiction.* The next section defines each of these key terms and explains how they are related to the gradual distress of the body. This continuum of involvement with drugs is an essential issue for you to consider as you honestly examine your own drug use and evaluate its possible long-range consequences in terms of quitting or changing drug-related behaviors.

Engage
www.pahconnection.com
14.1

Tolerance

Tolerance is the adaptation of the body to a drug in such a way that repeated exposure to the same dose results in less effect on the body. To counteract the tolerance phenomenon, the individual requires increasing doses to produce the original effect. These increased doses may be dangerous to certain parts of the body, since all body parts do not become equally tolerant to the drug. For example, a higher blood alcohol concentration (higher consumption) is thought to be required to diminish a chronically heavy drinker's physical performance as compared to a moderate drinker's performance. This is because the central nervous system is less depressed in the heavy drinker, due to the nerve tissue's having become more tolerant of alcohol. Similarly, the brain and stomach do not adapt well to higher concentrations of alcohol—are not as tolerant to its toxicity—which results in blackouts (not remembering events) and acute stomach irritation and inflammation.

Another example of tolerance is with the chemical *nicotine* found in cigarettes. Nicotine produces pleasurable feelings that make the smoker want to smoke more; it also acts as a depressant by interfering with the flow of information between nerve cells. As the nervous system adapts to nicotine, smokers tend to increase the number of cigarettes they smoke and hence the amount of nicotine in their blood. After a while, the smoker develops a tolerance to the drug, which leads to an increase in smoking over time. Eventually, the smoker reaches a certain nicotine level and then smokes to maintain this level. Tolerance has been proposed as an important component in understanding drug addiction.

Explore
www.pahconnection.com
14.3

Drug Addiction

Drug addiction or dependence is a chronic, progressive, and relapsing disorder that applies to all situations in which drug users develop either a psychological or physical reliance on a drug (Figure 14.1). Drug addiction can be destructive both psychologically and physically (Cox, 1986). **Drug addiction** is a strong dependence on a drug typified by three factors: (1) tolerance to a given dose, or the need for more and more of the substance; (2) severe withdrawal symptoms; and (3) the loss of control, or the need to consume the substance at all costs. This drug abuse is characterized by a *compulsive and continued use* in spite of adverse health consequences (Leshner, 1997). Drug addiction is based on the concepts of psychological and physical dependence.

Psychological Dependence

Psychological dependence, or behavioral dependence, is a craving for a drug for primarily psychological or emotional reasons. The person begins to rely on a drug as a

Tolerance Adaptation of the body to a drug in such a way that repeated exposure to the same dose results in less effect on the body.

Drug addiction A chronic, progressive, and relapsing disorder that applies to all situations in which drug users develop either a psychological or physical reliance to a drug.

Psychological dependence Craving for a drug for primarily psychological or emotional reasons.

FIGURE 14.1

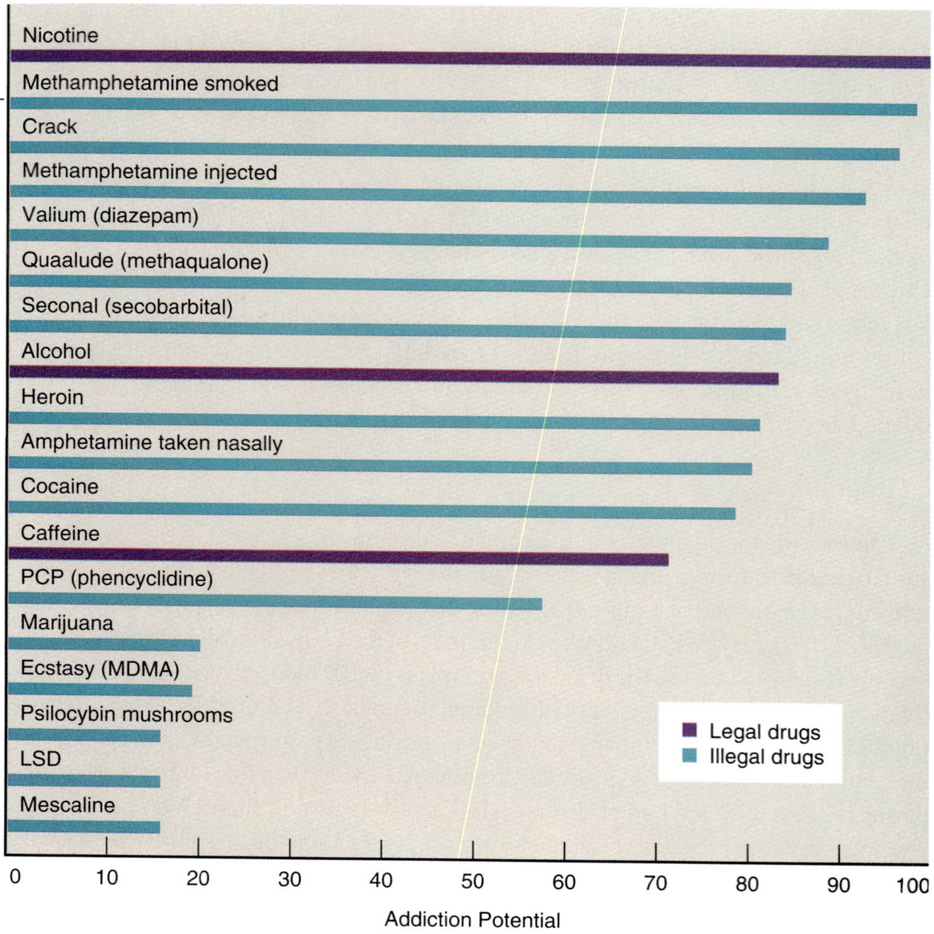

Addiction Potential of Various Drugs.
The chart shows health experts ratings of the addiction potential of various drugs, with 100 being the highest addiction potential. Note that both legal and illegal drugs can be highly addictive.

solution to a variety of emotional problems ranging from boredom to relief of anger or frustration. A good example of psychological dependence can be seen in cigarette smokers. Some smokers use the habit to enhance their moods and feelings of competency, while others use the habit to reduce their feelings of distress and anxiety. Smoking becomes a means of emotional and psychological support for many smokers and a necessary way of dealing with life. Once this happens, any attempt to quit or reduce smoking results in psychological distress. Psychological cravings for drugs may last for years after quitting.

Physical Dependence

Physical dependence is the biological adaptation to a drug by the body, in which the drug has become necessary to maintain a balance related to certain body processes. In other words, physical dependence studies investigate the motivational properties of physical withdrawal reactions. At some point the body becomes so completely adapted to the drug that it is a necessity for physiological function. The discomfort experienced during withdrawal of some drugs has long been presumed to be a factor in continued drug intake and addiction. Although physical dependence is not a necessary condition for drug addiction, it may contribute to the total reinforcing impact of some drugs. For example, in many dependent smokers, evidence suggests that the urge to smoke correlates with a low blood nicotine level, as though the smoker is trying to achieve a certain

Physical dependence The body's biological adaptation to a drug in which the drug has become necessary to maintain a balance in certain body processes.

nicotine level and avoid withdrawal symptoms. Thus smokers may be smoking to achieve the reward of nicotine effects or to avoid the pain of nicotine withdrawal. When the body has to adapt to the absence of the drug, withdrawal illness develops.

Withdrawal Illness

Withdrawal illness, or *abstinence syndrome,* displays recognizable physical signs and symptoms that result from drug abstinence. Withdrawal illness is a direct result of physical dependence. The signs and symptoms can occur within hours of drug abstinence or take several days to develop. The type and severity vary with the type of drug. For example, the nicotine found in cigarette smoke is a significant physical dependency-producing drug (Figure 14.1). Discontinuation of nicotine may result in withdrawal illness symptoms—irritability, depression, and dizziness—within hours. The physical distress of the abstinence syndrome may be of sufficient intensity to require medical intervention; it may last from 1 day up to several days (nearly 1 week in the case of alcohol). Once withdrawal sickness subsides, individuals are thought no longer to be physically dependent; however, they still may be psychologically dependent.

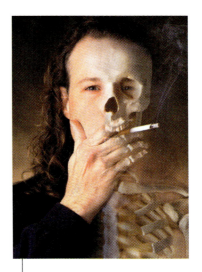

Cigarette smoking is the leading cause of preventable death in the United States.

MAKING DRUG USE DECISIONS

We have reviewed several levels of drug involvement that can occur from chronic drug use. The choice of which drug to use, the amount, and how long to use it are all important individual decisions and should not be made thoughtlessly. Therefore, it is important for an individual to practice decision-making skills related to taking drugs so that an appropriate response may be made when choosing to use drugs. Following is a six-stage decision-making strategy that you can use to evaluate your individual drug use:

1. Think about the situation and try to understand your reasons for using the drug.
2. Consider all the alternatives to using the drug by examining the reasons and thinking about alternatives for achieving your goals.
3. Attempt to identify potential difficulties associated with each of the alternatives.
4. Consider each alternative in the context of your situation, and select the one that seems best for you.
5. Take action on the alternative you have selected.
6. Assess the results, so that you may have more information available to you the next time you are faced with a similar situation. (Engs, 1979)

3. Making wise drug-use decisions is important.

Activities & Assessments 14.1

COMMONLY USED AND MISUSED SOCIAL DRUGS

The following sections examine some of the most familiar and frequently used and misused drugs—alcohol, tobacco, and caffeine—in our society. In keeping with our focus on the interconnectedness of health and physical activity, we intentionally limit our discussion to legal social drugs that have a direct application to this theme. We believe it is important for you to understand the **pharmacology** of these drugs. *Pharmacology* is the study of drugs, their sources, how

Withdrawal illness Recognizable physical signs and symptoms that result from withdrawing drug use.

Pharmacology The study of drugs, their sources, how they enter the body, how the body reacts to them, and their short-term and long-term effects on the body.

they enter the body, how the body reacts to them, and their short-term and long-term effects on the body. By understanding the positive and negative effects these common drugs have on your body, you will be able to make better-informed decisions related to their use as part of your active lifestyle.

4. Alcohol misuse and abuse is one of the most significant health problems in the United States.

Alcohol

Alcohol use in our society is widespread, and generally considered socially acceptable. Approximately 44 percent of American adults 18 and older consume alcoholic beverages on a regular basis (Alcohol and Health, 2000). People drink alcohol for many psychological reasons: to promote pleasant and carefree feelings; to reduce stress, tension, anxiety, and self-consciousness; and for social companionship (Baum-Baicker, 1985). Research also suggests that drinking small-to-moderate amounts of alcohol can decrease the risk of death from coronary heart disease (Alcohol and Health, 2000). Nevertheless, alcohol is considered to be the number one problem drug in America because of the physical, social, and emotional damage it causes (McKenzie et al., 1999) (Figure 14.2). The economic costs to the United States in health care, public safety, and social welfare total $184 billion when it comes to alcohol use and misuse, or roughly $638 for every man, woman, and child (Harwood et al., 2000).

Alcohol Properties

Alcohol is the common name for the substances with the chemical names *alcohol ethanol* or *ethyl ethanol*. Ethanol is a direct central-nervous-system depressant that causes a decreased level of consciousness and decreased motor function. At high concentrations, ethanol is toxic. Ethanol is an anesthetic and can cause autonomic dysfunction leading to death from respiratory depression and cardiovascular failure. Ethanol is produced through fermentation of sugars by yeasts and is the characteristic component of alcoholic beverages. Different sugar sources result in a variety of alcoholic beverages. The three basic types of alcoholic beverages are beer, wine, and distilled spirits.

FIGURE 14.2

Alcohol and Society.
Alcohol abuse is related to many of society's problems.

SOURCE: Prevention File. (1992). *Alcohol's grip on society.* San Diego: University of California, p. 3.

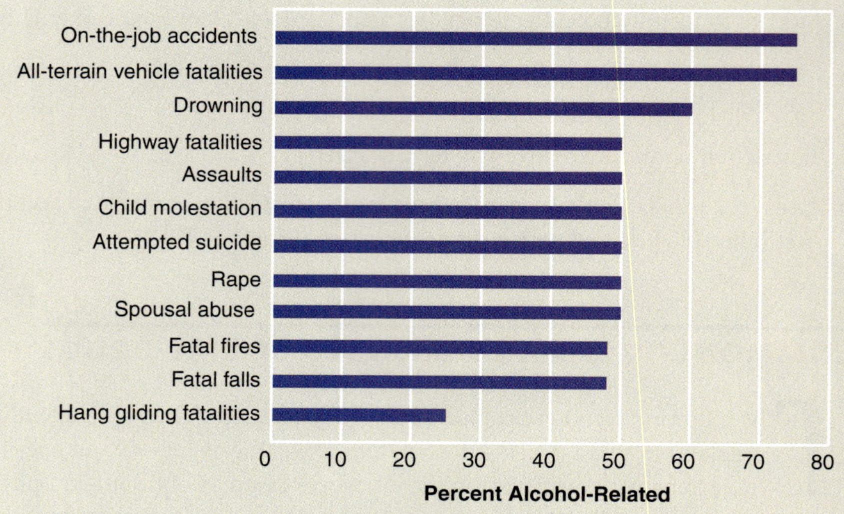

Alcohol abuse is related to many of society's problems. The statistics above underscore alcohol's influence in several problem areas.

Beer is made from fermented grains and has an alcohol content of approximately 5 percent. Light ("lite") beer, or reduced-calorie beer, has the same percent of alcohol as regular beer. Wine is made from fermented fruits and has an alcoholic content of approximately 12 percent. Some wine drinks, such as wine coolers, have lower alcohol content because of the fruit juice and sugar added to them. Fortified wines, such as port, have alcohol added to them, raising the alcohol content above 12 percent. Finally, distilled spirits, so named because liquid distillation after sugar fermentation increases their alcohol content, originate from sources of starch or sugar, including cereals, molasses from sugar beets, grapes, potatoes, cherries, plums, and other fruits. Distilled spirits (gin, rum, vodka, whiskey) produce a drink that usually contains 40 to 50 percent alcohol. The alcohol content in distilled spirits is sometimes indicated by degrees of proof, which in the United States is a figure that is twice the percentage of alcohol by volume in a beverage. Thus, 70-proof liquor is 35 percent alcohol. In general, a 12-ounce bottle of beer, a 5-ounce glass of wine, and a 1.5-ounce shot of liquor all contain the same amount of alcohol (0.5 ounce) and therefore have an identical effect on the drinker when it comes to intoxication and addiction (Figure 14.3).

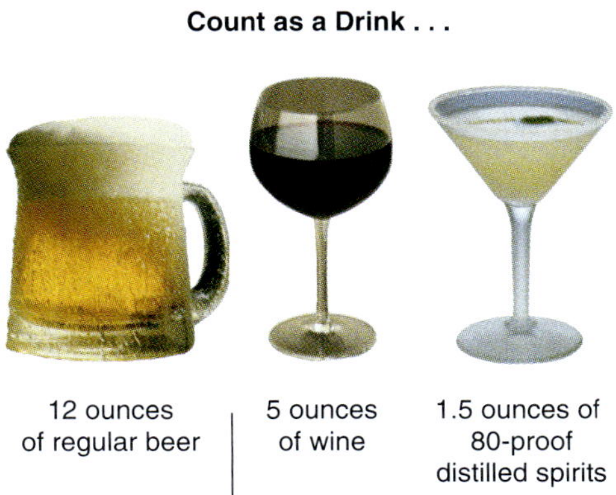

FIGURE 14.3

Alcohol Equivalents.
A can of beer, glass of wine, and a mixed drink have about the same amount of alcohol. So don't be fooled by the type of drink.

Alcohol Calories Alcohol, like fat, is a concentrated source of calories, supplying 7 kilocalories (kcal) per gram. Although alcohol is metabolized as a carbohydrate, it exhibits none of the properties of food. It is burned to the exclusion of fat and other substances. Alcohol calories supply no nutrients and therefore are considered "empty" calories. That is, alcohol calories are useless in meeting your body's nutrient needs. Alcohol does not become a protein or a carbohydrate, and does not contribute to any type of tissue except fat tissue. That's correct, alcohol consumption can make you fat! Alcoholic beverages contain a considerable number of calories. A 5-ounce glass of wine has about 100 calories, a 12-ounce beer has about 150 calories, and 1 1/2 ounces of liquor has about 105 calories (Table 14.2).

TABLE 14.2 Alcoholic Beverages and Their Alcohol and Caloric Content

BEVERAGE	ALCOHOL, BY VOLUME, APPROXIMATELY (%)	CALORIES, PER SERVING, APPROXIMATELY
Beer, regular	4.5	170
Beer, light	3	70–134
Wine, light beverage	10–14	90 calories per 4 fluid ounces
Sherry and other fortified wines	17–21	140 calories per 3.5 fluid ounces
Champagne	11–12	71 calories per 3 fluid ounces
Sake wine	14–16	39 calories per 1 fluid ounce
Tequila	40	—
Gin	40	120 calories per 1.5 fluid ounces
Brandy	35–40	60 calories per 4 fluid ounces
Vodka	40	95 calories per 1.5 fluid ounces
Rum	40	135 calories per 1.5 fluid ounces
Whiskey	40–54	130 calories per 1.5 fluid ounces

SOURCE: *Drugs and the Human Body 6/e* by Liska © 2000. Reprinted by permission of Pearson Education, Inc. Upper Saddle River, NJ 07458.

Furthermore, one prominent research study found that when alcohol, in calorically equivalent quantities, replaced other foods in the diets of healthy young men, the rate at which their bodies burned fat decreased by one-third (Suter et al., 1992). In addition to promoting fat storage, alcohol may further contribute to obesity by increasing caloric intake through depressing inhibitory nerves. Research has shown that alcohol drinkers take in more calories than nondrinkers do, and that drinkers eat more on days they drink than on days they don't drink (De Castro & Orozco, 1990). It is thought that alcohol decreases both your willpower and your desire to make healthy food choices. This could leave you susceptible to certain nutrient deficiencies. Finally, alcohol can also stimulate your appetite, so you may want to eat more.

Alcohol Consumption Patterns

Engage www.pahconnection.com 14.2

Alcohol is the most widely used *psychoactive,* or mood-changing, social drug in the United States. In this country, public health campaigns have traditionally urged people to avoid alcohol or cut back on their drinking, and appropriately so—heavy drinking is the second leading cause of preventable death in the United States, right behind cigarette smoking. Recently, the campaigns have publicized the apparent benefits of moderate drinking. These recommendations are spurred by studies that indicate small amounts of alcohol (social and moderate drinking) offer some people subtle emotional and physical benefits. People drink to relax, celebrate, have fun, and be sociable—emotional or psychological benefits that may improve health and well-being. Studies have also shown that alcohol offers some protection against heart disease, the leading cause of death in the United States. The wide range of consequences related to alcohol use is due primarily to differences in the amount, duration, and patterns of alcohol consumption, as well as to differences in genetic susceptibility (Alcohol and Health, 2000).

Social Drinking

Social use of alcohol consists of an occasional drink or two in the company of friends: a glass of champagne at a wedding or special occasion, a glass of wine with a special meal, a cold beer after a softball game. This small amount of drinking does not destroy brain cells or adversely affect any body organ.

Moderate drinking **Moderate drinking** may be defined as drinking that does not generally cause problems, either for the drinker or society (NIAAA, 1992). This definition, along with the following numerical estimates of "safe" drinking limits, must be accompanied by the understanding that a given dose of alcohol affects different people differently. Therefore, individuals making the decision to drink, or who have made the decision to drink, must be aware of the tradeoffs in alcohol use.

Current recommendations by the *Dietary Guidelines for Americans 2000,* under the basic message of Choose Sensibly, read: "If you drink alcoholic beverages, do so in moderation, with meals, and when consumption does not put you or others at risk." Moderate drinking is quantified as no more than one drink a day for most women and no more than two drinks a day for most men (Table 14.3). You may wonder why the recommendation for women is less than for men. The reason is that women have less of the enzyme (alcohol dehydrogenase) that helps break down alcohol in the body, and they have higher blood alcohol levels than men after drinking the same amount of alcohol. A standard drink contains approximately 0.5 ounces, or 12 grams, of alcohol. A standard drink is generally considered to be 12 ounces of beer, 5 ounces of wine, or 1.5 ounces of distilled spirits (Figure 14.3). This current advice about moderate drinking should be acknowl-

Moderate drinking Drinking that causes no problems, either for the drinker or for society; quantified as no more than one drink a day for most women, and no more than two drinks a day for most men.

TABLE 14.3 Criteria for Moderate and At-Risk Alcohol Use*

Moderate Drinking

Men: ≤2 drinks/day

Women: ≤1 drink/day

Over 65 (men and women): ≤1 drink/day

At-Risk Drinking

Men: >14 drinks/week, or >4 drinks/occasion

Women: >7 drinks/week, or >3 drinks/occasion

* One drink = 12 g of alcohol, which is the equivalent of 180 ml (6 oz) of wine, 360 ml (12 oz) of beer, or 45 ml (1.5 oz) of 90-proof distilled spirits.

SOURCE: G. Edlin, E. Golanty, and K. McCormack Brown. (1999). *Health and Wellness* (6th ed., p. 379). Boston: Jones and Bartlett.

edged with the understanding that there are tradeoffs involved in deciding to drink alcohol. Clearly, there are both benefits and risks associated with lower levels of drinking.

Three important points that accompany this guideline must be considered. First, *some people should not drink alcoholic beverages at all* (Table 14.4). Second, the research data used to develop the moderation guideline cannot be achieved by simply averaging the number of drinks you consume. For example, consuming seven drinks in a single day does not have the same effects as consuming one drink each day of the week. Finally, people who currently abstain from alcohol should not be advised to begin drinking.

Binge Drinking Binge drinking differs from social and moderate drinking in terms of the amount of alcohol consumed and the pattern of drinking. Binge drinkers often drink to get drunk and believe that heavy drinking is appropriate and desirable in social situations. The binge is usually planned and will not continue for more than one day. **Binge drinking** is defined for males as consuming five or more drinks in a row at one sitting, and for females as consuming four or more in a row. This amount of alcohol is approximately the amount of alcohol needed to raise the average-sized person's blood alcohol concentration to about 0.10 percent. In other words, it is the amount of alcohol consumption that would lead to the presumption of intoxication (drunkenness). Every state considers a person intoxicated and incapable of operating a vehicle safely at this level of intoxication (in many states, the highest acceptable level is 0.8 percent). Furthermore, this high level of intoxication increases the risk for hangovers, fatigue, headaches, shakiness, bloodshot eyes, nausea and vomiting, injuries from accidents, severe impairment of driving, unprotected sex, seizures, brain damage, and death from alcohol overdose.

Most binge drinkers do not feel that they are problem drinkers because they do not drink daily. After a binge, the person will be able to go for days, weeks, or months with little or no drinking before another binge occurs. It is a myth that only daily drinkers have an alcohol problem. Binge drinking is more likely in situations where people drink in groups, where they serve themselves, or where drinking games are involved. Binge drinking is most common in those aged 18 to 24 years, possibly in response to increased freedom in their lives. According to a recent study, 48 percent of college men and 39 percent of college women are binge drinkers (Wechsler et al., 2000).

Activities & Assessments 14.2

Explore www.pahconnection.com 14.4

Binge drinking Having five or more drinks at any one time.

TABLE **14.4** **Some People Should Not Drink Alcohol at All—Choose Sensibly**

Who should not drink?
Some people should not drink alcoholic beverages at all. These include:

- **Children and adolescents.**
- **Individuals of any age who cannot restrict their drinking to moderate levels.** This is a special concern for recovering alcoholics, problem drinkers, and people whose family members have alcohol problems.
- **Women who may become pregnant or who are pregnant.** A safe level of alcohol intake has not been established for women at any time during pregnancy, including the first few weeks. Major birth defects, including fetal alcohol syndrome, can be caused by heavy drinking by the pregnant mother. Other fetal alcohol effects may occur at lower levels.
- **Individuals who plan to drive, operate machinery, or take part in other activities that require attention, skill or coordination.** Most people retain some alcohol in the blood up to 2 to 3 hours after a single drink.
- **Individuals taking prescription or over-the-counter medications that can interact with alcohol.** Alcohol alters the effectiveness or toxicity of many medications, and some medications may increase blood alcohol levels. If you take medications, ask your health care provider for advice about alcohol intake, especially if you are an older adult.

Advice for Today

- If you choose to drink alcoholic beverages, do so sensibly, and in moderation.
- Limit intake to one drink per day for women or two per day for men, and take with meals to slow alcohol absorption.
- Avoid drinking before or when driving, or whenever it puts you or others at risk.

SOURCE: U.S. Department of Agriculture, Agriculture Research Service, Dietary Guidelines Advisory Committee. (2000). *Nutrition and your health: Dietary guidelines for Americans, 2000* (5th ed., p. 37). Home and Garden Bulletin No. 232. Washington, DC.

Problem Drinking

Problem drinking is the consumption of alcohol that results in significant risk of health consequences, social problems, or both (Table 14.5). Chronic abuse of alcohol can lead to a number of serious health conditions (see long-term effects of alcohol), as well as to dependence or alcoholism. *Alcohol dependence,* or *alcoholism,* refers to a disease that is characterized by abnormal alcohol-seeking behavior that leads to impaired control over drinking. Many factors contribute to alcohol dependence, including personality characteristics, stress, family environment, heredity, and the addictive nature of alcohol. Many alcoholics become able to drink ever-larger quantities of alcohol before feeling or appearing drunk. Alcohol users commonly medicate themselves with alcohol, using it, often daily, to help them relax, as a confidence booster, or in order to avoid withdrawal symptoms. Approximately 14 million American drinkers (7.4% of population) are categorized as alcohol abusers (Alcohol and Health, 2000).

Experience www.pahconnection.com 14.1

Problem drinking The consumption of alcohol that results in significant risk of health consequences, social problems, or both.

College Drinking

Alcohol has long been the drug of choice among college students of ages 18 to 25. Although it is illegal for anyone under the age of 21 to purchase, possess, and consume alcohol, many college students under age 21 drink alcoholic beverages. College

TABLE 14.5 How Do You Know if You Are Drinking Too Much?

If you are drinking too much, you can improve your life and health by cutting down.

How do you know if you drink too much?

Read these questions and answer yes or no:

- Do you drink alone when you feel angry or sad?
- Does your drinking ever make you late for work?
- Does your drinking worry your family?
- Do you ever drink after telling yourself you won't?
- Do you ever forget what you did while you were drinking?
- Do you get headaches or have a hangover after you have been drinking?

If you answered yes to any of these questions, you may have a drinking problem. Check with your doctor to be sure. Your doctor will be able to tell you whether you should cut down or abstain. If you are alcoholic or have other medical problems, you should not just cut down on your drinking—you should stop drinking completely. Your doctor will advise you about what is right for you.

SOURCE: National Institute on Alcohol Abuse and Alcoholism (NIAAA). (1996). *How to cut down on your drinking* [On-line]. Available: http://silk.gov/silk/niaaa1/publication/publication.htm; accessed 1/30/01.

students have notably high rates of heavy drinking compared to the general population and therefore are at a higher risk for alcohol-related problems (automobile accidents, crippling falls, suicide, date rape, HIV infection). Student drinking is also associated with academic problems such as missed classes and poor performance on tests and projects. Research reveals the following statistics:

- Forty-one percent of all academic problems stem from alcohol abuse.
- Twenty-eight percent of students who drop out of school may do so because of alcohol abuse.
- More than 7 percent of college freshman drop out of school for alcohol-related reasons.

Student drinking is considered to be the number one cause of health problems on college and university campuses. Therefore, personal decisions about your alcohol consumption and the associated risks and benefits should be reviewed periodically as part of your healthy lifestyle strategy. It is important that you understand the effects of alcohol before establishing potentially damaging habits of consumption.

Alcohol Absorption

When a person drinks alcohol, the alcohol is absorbed primarily by the stomach (20%) and small intestine (80%) (Figure 14.4). Since alcohol molecules are small, they are readily absorbed into the blood without being digested. Once the alcohol has been absorbed, it is rapidly carried throughout the body by the blood. A balance occurs such that blood at all points in the system contains approximately the same amount of alcohol. The amount of alcohol in your blood is expressed as **blood alcohol concentration (BAC).** Blood alcohol concentration is measured in percentages. A simple way to estimate your BAC is shown in Table 14.6.

Blood alcohol concentration (BAC) The amount of alcohol in the blood.

FIGURE 14.4

Alcohol Absorption. How alcohol is absorbed and metabolized.

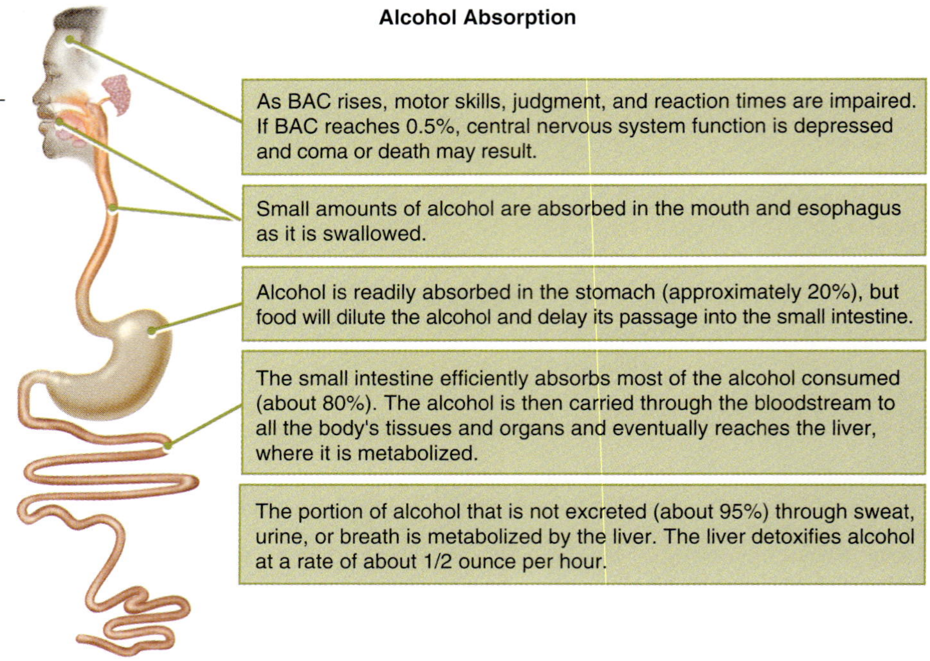
Alcohol Absorption
As BAC rises, motor skills, judgment, and reaction times are impaired. If BAC reaches 0.5%, central nervous system function is depressed and coma or death may result.
Small amounts of alcohol are absorbed in the mouth and esophagus as it is swallowed.
Alcohol is readily absorbed in the stomach (approximately 20%), but food will dilute the alcohol and delay its passage into the small intestine.
The small intestine efficiently absorbs most of the alcohol consumed (about 80%). The alcohol is then carried through the bloodstream to all the body's tissues and organs and eventually reaches the liver, where it is metabolized.
The portion of alcohol that is not excreted (about 95%) through sweat, urine, or breath is metabolized by the liver. The liver detoxifies alcohol at a rate of about 1/2 ounce per hour.

Alcohol Elimination

The body readily recognizes alcohol in the bloodstream as a toxic substance and begins to remove it from the blood as soon as it reaches the liver. The liver is responsible for eliminating 95 percent of ingested alcohol from the body though an active process of metabolism. The remainder of the alcohol is eliminated through excretion of alcohol in urine, sweat, and breath. Most of the metabolism of alcohol is performed by the enzyme alcohol dehydrogenase (ADH), which is found mostly in the liver. Alcohol dehydrogenase is also found in other tissues of the body, notably in the stomach lining, where it breaks down some of the alcohol before it ever reaches the bloodstream. The ADH enzyme is found in greater quantities and is more active in the stomachs of men than of women—meaning men break down more alcohol before it reaches their bloodstream. The liver can metabolize approximately 0.5 ounces (equivalent of one drink) per hour. Nothing can be done to speed up this process; cold showers, exercise, black coffee, fresh air, or vomiting will not help. Only time will allow the liver to break down the alcohol in the bloodstream, and unprocessed alcohol circulates through the bloodstream until the liver can process it.

If a person drinks alcohol faster than it can be eliminated from the body, the BAC rises, increasing the toxic effects of ethanol on the body. There are several important factors that a person can control related to influencing BAC. These include controlling the amount of alcohol consumed and the rate of consumption, and eating before drinking.

Amount of Alcohol As more drinks are consumed, more alcohol is readily available to be absorbed in the blood. It is important to understand the amount of alcohol in each of the three categories of alcoholic beverages. Some people attempt to distinguish among beer, wine, and liquor when explaining their drinking. But, a 12-ounce glass bottle of beer, a 5-ounce glass of wine, and a 1.5-ounce shot of liquor all contain the same amount of alcohol (0.5 ounce) and therefore have an identical effect on the drinker (Figure 14.3). The three forms of alcohol have the same potential for intoxication and addiction.

TABLE 14.6 Alcohol Impairment Chart—Never Drink and Drive!

WOMEN
APPROXIMATE BLOOD ALCOHOL PERCENTAGE
BODY WEIGHT IN POUNDS

DRINKS	90	100	120	140	160	180	200	220	240
Impairment Begins									
1	.05	.05	.04	.03	.03	.03	.02	.02	.02
Driving Skills Significantly Affected									
2	.10	.09	.08	.07	.06	.05	.05	.04	.04
3	.15	.14	.11	.10	.09	.08	.07	.06	.06
Possible Criminal Penalties									
4	.20	.18	.15	.13	.11	.10	.09	.08	.08
5	.25	.23	.19	.16	.14	.13	.11	.10	.09
Legally Intoxicated — Criminal Penalties									
6	.30	.27	.23	.18	.17	.15	.14	.12	.11
7	.35	.32	.27	.23	.20	.18	.16	.14	.13
8	.41	.38	.34	.28	.23	.20	.18	.17	.15
9	.45	.41	.34	.29	.28	.25	.23	.18	.17
10	.51	.45	.35	.32	.28	.25	.23	.21	.19

Subtract .01% for each 40 minutes of drinking.

One drink is 1.25 oz of 80-proof liquor, 12 oz of beer, or 5 oz of table wine.

MEN
APPROXIMATE BLOOD ALCOHOL PERCENTAGE
BODY WEIGHT IN POUNDS

DRINKS	100	120	140	160	180	200	220	240
Impairment Begins								
1	.04	.03	.03	.02	.02	.02	.02	.02
Driving Skills Significantly Affected — Possible Criminal Penalties								
2	.08	.06	.05	.05	.04	.04	.03	.03
3	.11	.09	.08	.07	.06	.06	.05	.05
4	.15	.12	.11	.09	.08	.08	.07	.06
5	.19	.16	.13	.12	.11	.09	.09	.08
6	.23	.19	.16	.14	.13	.11	.10	.09
Legally Intoxicated — Criminal Penalties								
7	.26	.22	.19	.16	.15	.13	.12	.11
8	.30	.25	.21	.19	.17	.15	.14	.13
9	.34	.28	.24	.21	.19	.17	.15	.14
10	.38	.31	.27	.23	.21	.19	.17	.16

Subtract .01% for each 40 minutes of drinking.

One drink is 1.25 oz of 80-proof liquor, 12 oz of beer, or 5 oz of table wine.

SOURCE: National Clearinghouse for Alcohol and Drug Information. Alcohol impairment chart [On-line]. Available: http://www.health.org:80/nongovpubs/bac-chart/index.htm; accessed 2/6/01.

Rate of Consumption The rate of drinking affects BAC due to a constant rate of alcohol metabolism or elimination by the body. Metabolism of alcohol occurs in the liver. The liver can process about 0.5 ounce (one drink) of alcohol every 1–1.5 hours. Because the body metabolizes alcohol at this constant rate, ingesting alcohol at a rate higher than the rate of elimination results in a cumulative effect of increasing BAC.

The Effect of Food The absorption of alcohol is slowed if the stomach contains food. The major reason for this is that alcohol is absorbed most efficiently in the small intestine. The presence of food in the stomach keeps the alcohol from reaching the small intestine. The pyloric valve at the bottom of the stomach remains closed to allow for the digestion of the food in the stomach. Alcohol will still be absorbed through the stomach, but at a much slower rate.

Another factor that significantly influences BAC is body weight. In general, the less you weigh, the more you will be affected by a given amount of alcohol. This is because smaller people have less blood volume than larger people and, therefore, less blood in which to distribute the alcohol. In addition to body weight, body composition also affects the distribution of alcohol. Since alcohol dissolves much more freely in water, a well-muscled individual will be less affected than someone with a higher percentage of fat because fatty tissue does not contain as much water as muscle tissue.

Immediate Effects of Alcohol

Engage www.pahconnection.com 14.3

The effects of any drug vary from person to person. The immediate effects of alcohol depend on how much you drink, whether you are used to drinking, your mood, and many other factors such as your weight, sex, and general health status.

Alcohol is considered a **depressant.** Depressants are drugs that produce a slowing of mental and physical activities. When alcohol is absorbed into the circulatory system, its effects are distributed throughout the body. The brain is remarkably sensitive to the effects of alcohol. Alcohol acts on the nerve cells deep in the brain, causing a suppressing effect on the central nervous system. The centers that control cognition, thought, judgment, and speech are depressed with the consumption of one or two drinks. As the blood alcohol concentration increases, depression occurs in the respiratory and spinal cord reflexes. An important correlation exists between the BAC and mental and physical behavior (Table 14.7). Five drinks consumed in two hours may raise the blood alcohol concentration to 0.10 percent, high enough to be considered legally intoxicated in every state. Signs and symptoms of alcohol use and intoxication include irritability, euphoria, depression, loss of consciousness, impaired short-term memory, inappropriate or violent behavior, loss of balance, unsteady gait, and decreased functioning of the cardiorespiratory system.

Alcohol Poisoning The dangerous effects of alcohol use can be seen in people who consume large amounts of alcohol relatively quickly. College students frequently engage in this type of drinking behavior, usually in the form of binge drinking. The challenge to drink to your personal limit has become a celebrated observance of college life. In one of the most extensive reports on college drinking, a recent study found that the majority (52%) of students drink "to get drunk" (Welshler, 2000). Many college students see being drunk as a primary way of socializing.

Drinking to intoxication may result in *alcohol poisoning,* which is a medical emergency that requires immediate attention. Experts estimate that excessive drinking is involved in thousands of student deaths annually. Deadly consequences from alcohol poisoning are usually the result of central nervous system and respiratory depression, or of choking to death on vomit after an alcohol overdose. Symptoms of alcohol poisoning are listed in Table 14.8. People who have overdosed on alcohol are unable to help themselves, so it is

Depressants Drugs that produce a slowing of mental and physical activities.

up to their companions to get assistance. Call for medical attention immediately. Unfortunately, there are no hard-and-fast rules on how many drinks will result in alcohol poisoning. Generally, a drinker in alcohol poisoning will have a BAC that exceeds 0.25%.

Unintentional Injuries More than 40 percent of all automobile-related deaths (the leading cause of unintentional death in the United States) are related to alcohol. Even at low blood-alcohol concentrations, alcohol impairs your judgment and dulls your reflexes. If you weigh 140 pounds, just two drinks are enough to increase your chances of having a driving accident. You should never operate any type of machinery if you have had alcohol.

TABLE 14.7 Blood Alcohol Concentration and Physical and Mental Balance

BLOOD ALCOHOL CONCENTRATION (%)	PHYSICAL AND MENTAL BEHAVIOR
0.01	Clearing of the head. Slight tingling of mucous membranes.
0.02	Mild throbbing at the back of the head. A touch of dizziness. Personal appearance of no concern. Willing to talk.
0.03	Feeling of euphoria and superiority. ("Sure am glad I came to your party." "We will always be friends.")
0.04	Talking and laughing loudly. Movements a bit clumsy. Flippant remarks. ("You don't think I'm drunk, do you?")
0.05	Normal inhibitions almost eliminated. Many liberties taken. Talkative. Some loss of motor coordination.
0.07	Feeling of remoteness. Rapid pulse. Gross clumsiness.
0.10	Legally drunk in most states. Staggering, loud singing. Drowsiness. Rapid breathing.
0.20	Blackout level. Inability to recall events later. Easily angered. Shouting, groaning, weeping.
0.30 and above	Stupor. Breathing reflex threatened. Deep anesthesia. Death is due to paralysis of the respiratory center and is generally preceded by 5–10 hours of stupor and coma.

SOURCE: *Drugs and the Human Body 6/e* by Liska © 2000. Reprinted by permission of Pearson Education, Inc. Upper Saddle River, NJ 07458.

TABLE 14.8 Symptoms of Alcohol Poisoning

Binge drinking may result in an overdose of alcohol, or alcohol poisoning—a medical emergency that requires immediate attention. It's sometimes hard to tell if someone has only "passed out" or is in serious medical danger. Here are some symptoms of alcohol poisoning:

- Does not respond to being talked to or shouted at
- Does not respond to being pinched, prodded, or poked
- Cannot stand up
- Will not wake up
- Slow, labored or abnormal breathing
- Skin has a purplish color
- Skin feels clammy
- Rapid pulse rate
- Irregular heart rhythm
- Lowered blood pressure

Long-Term Effects of Alcohol

Heavy drinking over many years has major toxic effects on the liver, heart, brain, stomach, intestines, and pancreas. These effects increase the risk for developing a number of chronic diseases, including liver disease and cirrhosis, cardiomyopathy and stroke, permanent brain damage, ulcers, pancreas inflammation, and certain forms of cancer (Healthy People 2010, 2000) (Figure 14.5).

Alcohol and Physical Activity

There are some people who believe that physical activity and exercise will offset any detrimental effects of alcohol use. While moderate drinking the night before physical activity does no real harm, it may limit in a number of ways how well you are able to perform the next day.

Alcohol has various acute and chronic metabolic and physiological effects. You need energy to work out, but the calories from alcohol are unique in that they cannot be stored in the muscles as energy; claims that alcohol provides substantial carbohydrates or energy are false. Alcohol is also a diuretic (it stimulates the production of urine). This increase in urination leads to dehydration and the loss of valuable electrolytes, such as magnesium, calcium, and potassium. These diuretic effects severely impair muscle contraction.

Some people also believe that alcohol can give them a boost during physical activity by providing instant energy. Blood glucose levels actually decrease, however, because

FIGURE 14.5

Long-Term Effects of Alcohol Use. Because excess alcohol reaches all parts of the body, it causes a wide array of physical problems.

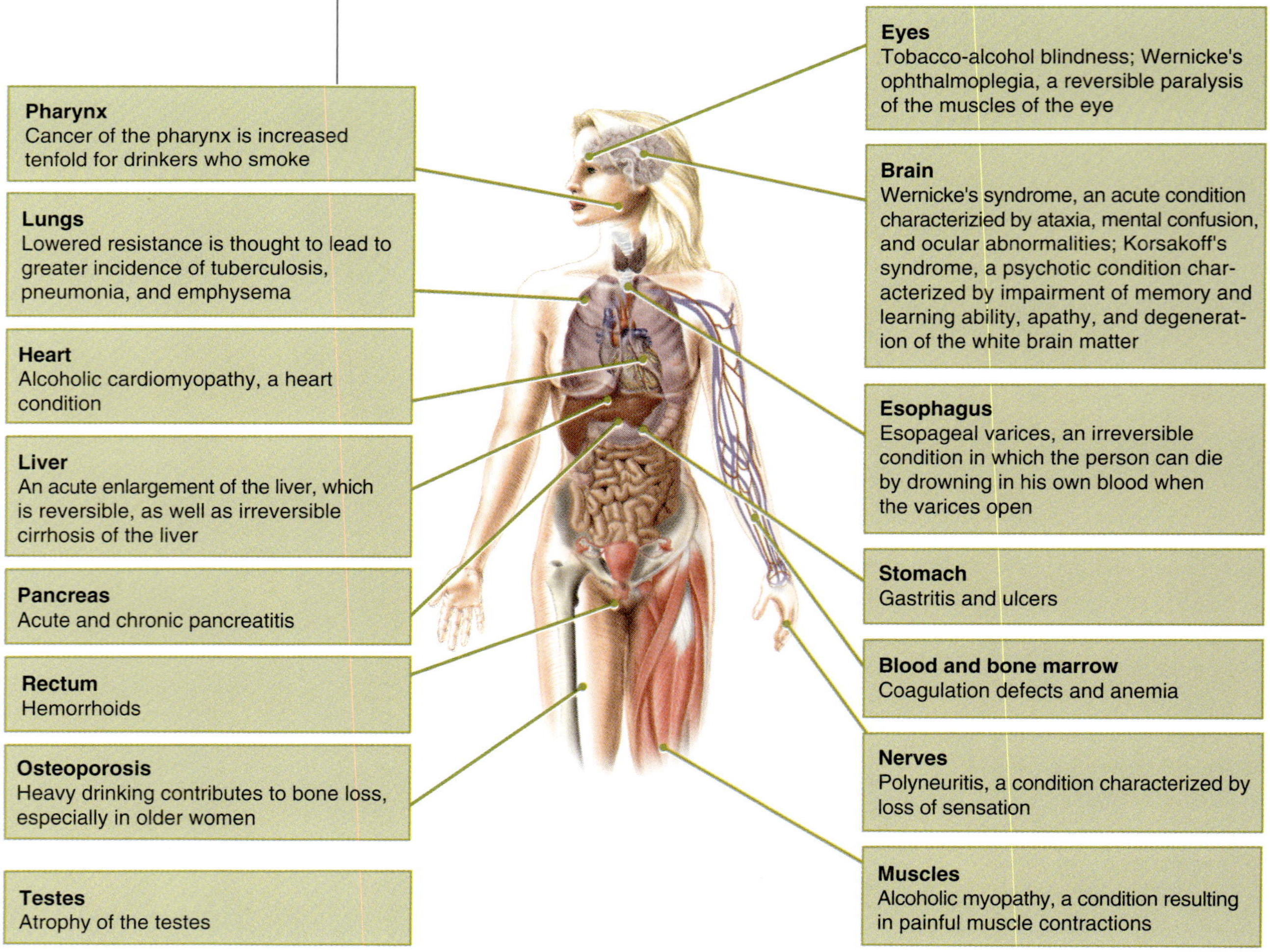
Pharynx
Cancer of the pharynx is increased tenfold for drinkers who smoke
Lungs
Lowered resistance is thought to lead to greater incidence of tuberculosis, pneumonia, and emphysema
Heart
Alcoholic cardiomyopathy, a heart condition
Liver
An acute enlargement of the liver, which is reversible, as well as irreversible cirrhosis of the liver
Pancreas
Acute and chronic pancreatitis
Rectum
Hemorrhoids
Osteoporosis
Heavy drinking contributes to bone loss, especially in older women
Testes
Atrophy of the testes
Eyes
Tobacco-alcohol blindness; Wernicke's ophthalmoplegia, a reversible paralysis of the muscles of the eye
Brain
Wernicke's syndrome, an acute condition characterizied by ataxia, mental confusion, and ocular abnormalities; Korsakoff's syndrome, a psychotic condition characterized by impairment of memory and learning ability, apathy, and degeneration of the white brain matter
Esophagus
Esopageal varices, an irreversible condition in which the person can die by drowning in his own blood when the varices open
Stomach
Gastritis and ulcers
Blood and bone marrow
Coagulation defects and anemia
Nerves
Polyneuritis, a condition characterized by loss of sensation
Muscles
Alcoholic myopathy, a condition resulting in painful muscle contractions

the liver has to metabolize the alcohol. This drop leads to hypoglycemia and early fatigue. Furthermore, when we drink more than our liver can metabolize, the remaining alcohol produces a sedating effect on the central nervous system, impairing our coordination and motor skills. This impairment of psychomotor skills makes drinking alcohol and exercising a dangerous combination.

Drinking moderate amounts of alcohol probably helps to prevent coronary heart disease in some individuals by helping boost HDL cholesterol levels (Suh et al., 1992). Moderate amounts of alcohol seem to increase the amount of HDL (good) cholesterol in the bloodstream. Scientists used to think that only red wine offered this positive effect, but recent studies have shown that beer, liquor, and white wine also increase HDL cholesterol. It is estimated that about half of alcohol's protective effect is due to its ability to raise HDL, or "good" cholesterol, levels. However, research also shows that drinking may offset the cholesterol benefits of moderate drinking related to heart disease, by increasing your risk for high blood pressure and obesity. Both high blood pressure and obesity are major contributors to heart disease (see Chapter 5). Therefore, you may be better off to increase your HDLs by using aerobic exercise and diet (see Chapters 6 and 8) and maintaining a healthy body composition (see Chapter 9) than by using alcohol (Table 14.9).

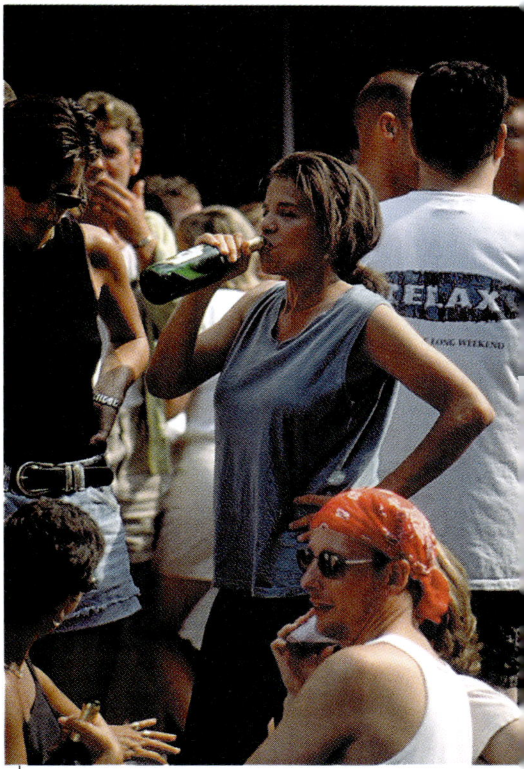

College students have notably high rates of drinking compared to the general population and therefore are at higher risk for alcohol-related problems.

TABLE 14.9 Learning to Drink Less

There are many ways you can help yourself to cut down. Try these tips:

Watch it at home. Keep a small amount or no alcohol at home. Don't keep temptations around.

Drink slowly. When you drink, sip your drink slowly. Take a break of 1 hour between drinks. Drink soda, water, or juice after a drink with alcohol. Do not drink on an empty stomach! Eat food when you are drinking.

Take a break from alcohol. Pick a day or two each week when you will not drink at all. Then, try to stop drinking for 1 week. Think about how you feel physically and emotionally on these days. When you succeed and feel better, you may find it easier to cut down for good.

Learn how to say NO. You do not have to drink when other people drink. You do not have to take a drink that is given to you. Practice ways to say no politely. For example, you can tell people you feel better when you drink less. Stay away from people who give you a hard time about not drinking.

Stay active. What would you like to do instead of drinking? Use the time and money spent on drinking to do something fun with your family or friends. Go out to eat, see a movie, or play sports or a game.

Get support. Cutting down on your drinking may be difficult at times. Ask your family and friends for support to help you reach your goal. Talk to your doctor if you are having trouble cutting down. Get the help you need to reach your goal.

Watch out for temptations. Watch out for people, places, or times that make you drink, even if you do not want to. Stay away from people who drink a lot or bars where you used to go. Plan ahead of time what you will do to avoid drinking when you are tempted. Do not drink when you are angry or upset or have a bad day. These are habits you need to break if you want to drink less.

Do not give up. Most people do not cut down or give up drinking all at once. Just like a diet, it is not easy to change. That is okay. If you do not reach your goal the first time, try again. Remember, get support from people who care about you and want to help. Do not give up!

SOURCE: National Institute on Alcohol Abuse and Alcoholism (NIAAA). (1996). *How to cut down on your drinking* [On-line]. Available: http://silk.gov/silk/niaaa1/publication/publication.htm; accessed 1/30/01.

5. Cigarette smoking is the most preventable cause of premature illness and death in the United States.

Experience
www.pahconnection.com
14.2,14.3

TOBACCO CONSUMPTION

The good news is that during the late twentieth century smoking cigarettes went from being a socially accepted behavior to being recognized as the number-one preventable cause of death and disability in the United States. Substantial public health efforts to reduce the prevalence of tobacco use began shortly after the risk was described in the 1964 landmark report *Smoking and Health: Report of the Advisory Committee to the Surgeon General,* popularly known as the *Surgeon General's Report.* These efforts have ranged from the dissemination of scientific evidence of the relationship among disease and tobacco use (health education and promotion) to changes in public policy (legislation restricting smoking in public places, taxation). These efforts have been successful. Smoking prevalence rates among adults have decreased from approximately 50 percent in the mid-1960s to 25 percent today. This was a great public health achievement with which to end the century; however, smoking remains a primary challenge as we begin the new century.

Smoking is still responsible for 1 in every 5 deaths, or more than 430,000 deaths annually, in the United States (Figures 14.6, 14.7) (McGinnis & Foege, 1993; Healthy People 2010, 2000). Forty-eight million adult Americans (25%) still smoke cigarettes, even though this single health behavior will result in disability or premature death for half of all continual users (CDC, 2000) (Figure 14.6). The current rate of smoking among young adults age 18–25 is approximately 40 percent (NHS, 2000). Moreover, even though it is illegal for anyone under 18 to purchase tobacco products, the current

FIGURE 14.6

Current Cigarette Smoking in Persons Age 18 Years or Older by Sex, 1965–1997.

SOURCE: Data compiled from Centers for Disease Control and Prevention. (1994, 1995, 1997). *Morbidity and Mortality Weekly Report (MMWR),* 45(27); *MMWR,* 46(44); *MMWR,* 48(43).

Current Cigarette Smoking
In persons age >18 years by sex, 1965–1997 (selected years)[1,2,3]

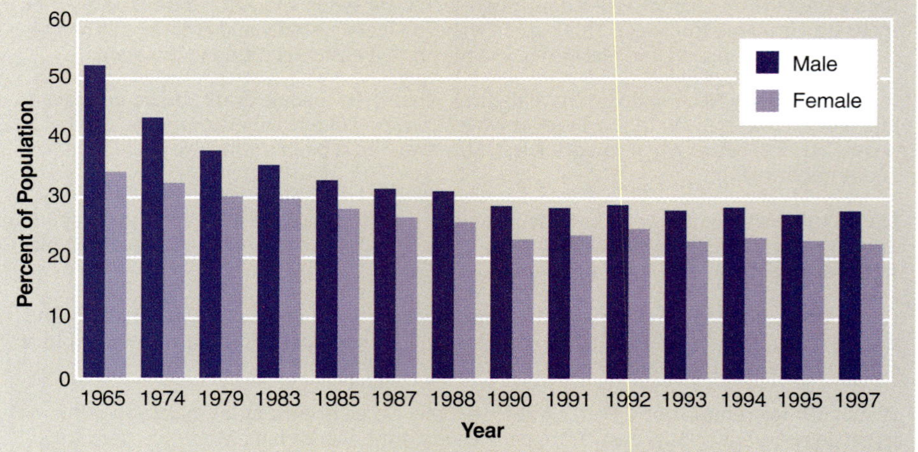

NOTES:
1. A current smoker is a person who has smoked at least 100 cigarettes and who now smokes. In 1992, the definition of current smoker was modified to include persons who smoked every day or some days.
2. Selected years are those years for which data is available.
3. Because these estimates are based on a sample, they may differ from figures that would be obtained from a census of the population. Each data point reported is an estimate of the true population value and subject to sampling variability.

smoking rate among youths age 12–17 is approximately 18 percent (4.1 million youth) (National Household Survey, 2000). This current rate is higher than rates recorded in either the 1970s or 1980s. A major concern with this increased smoking in youth is the overwhelming evidence that the nicotine found in tobacco is addictive and that addiction occurs in most smokers during the adolescent years (HHS, 1994). Using current national tobacco-use patterns, it is estimated that 5 million young persons under the age of 18 will die prematurely from a smoking-related disease (CDC, 1996).

Other forms of tobacco use are not safe alternatives to smoking cigarettes. Many people believe that cigar smoking is a safe choice. Dangerously, some cigar manufacturers claim (falsely) that cigar smokers experience little or no increased disease risk. These beliefs, along with the growing status symbolism of cigars, have contributed to a trend toward greater cigar use. Since the early 1990s, cigar sales in the United States have increased dramatically. In 1999, nearly 7 percent of the population were users of cigars (SAMHSA, 1999). According to the National Cancer Institute, "the risks of tobacco smoke exposure are similar for all sources of tobacco smoke, and the magnitude of the risks experienced by cigar smokers is proportionate to the nature and intensity of their exposure" (NCI, 1998).

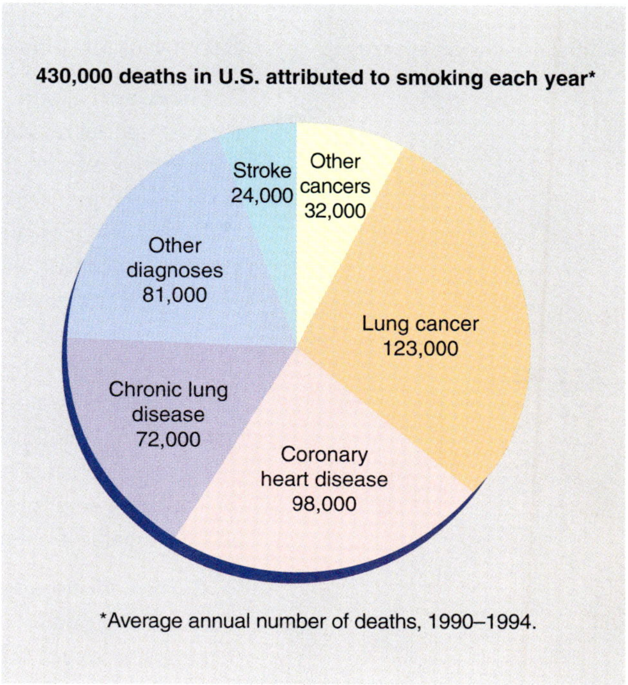

FIGURE 14.7

U.S. Deaths Attributable Each Year to Cigarette Smoking.

SOURCE: Centers for Disease Control and Prevention. (1997). *Morbidity and Mortality Weekly Report,* 46:448–51.

The smallest group of tobacco consumers uses smokeless tobacco ("spit" tobacco) in the form of snuff or chewing tobacco. In 1998, an estimated 3.1 percent of the population were users of smokeless tobacco, with the majority being male. Smokeless tobacco is more popular among *young* males, with overall use rates more than 9 percent for high school males and approximately 7 percent for males aged 18–24 (CDC, 1998). Smokeless tobacco causes a number severe health problems, including cancer of the mouth, leukoplakia, inflammation of the gums, heart disease, and tooth loss.

Few behaviors have as many—and as harmful—effects upon a person's health as tobacco use. We will now examine composition of tobacco as a drug, the damaging effects of tobacco on users, why it is habit forming, and how this habit can be defeated.

Chemicals in Tobacco Smoke

Tobacco comes from the dried leaves of the native American tobacco plant *Nicotiana tabacum*. Tobacco, in its unprocessed form, contains a number of hazardous chemicals that become increasingly dangerous as it is processed into cigarettes, cigars, or smokeless tobacco forms. The smoke from burning tobacco is the most hazardous to our health. Smoke from burning tobacco consists of a mixture of approximately 4000 chemical substances that are dangerous to living tissue. Within this immense amount of harmful matter, scientists have identified more than 40 chemicals in cigarette smoke that cause cancer. Tobacco smoke is primarily composed of droplets of **tars,** which form 40 percent of the smoke; **nicotine,** a drug that is poisonous and has addicting qualities; and a dozen gases, including **carbon monoxide.**

Tars The yellowish-brown solid, sticky materials that are inhaled as part of tobacco smoke.

Nicotine A dynamic psychoactive stimulant.

Carbon monoxide One of the most abundant and poisonous gases in cigarette smoke.

Tars Tars are the yellowish-brown solid, sticky materials that are inhaled as part of tobacco smoke. A person who smokes a pack of cigarettes a day will accumulate about 4 ounces of tar in their lungs annually. Many tars are deposited on the bronchi, contributing to chronic bronchitis and smoker's cough. Research has shown tobacco tars to be

Stimulants Drugs that increase central nervous system activity.

carcinogenic, or cancer causing (see Chapter 4). Other chemicals in tobacco tars are cocarcinogens, or stimulate the growth of cancer when combined with other carcinogens.

Nicotine Nicotine is a dynamic psychoactive **stimulant.** *Stimulants* are drugs that increase central nervous system activity. Nicotine is quickly absorbed into the blood, immediately affecting the brain and the spinal cord as well as the peripheral central nervous system. Nicotine causes a short-term increase in heart rate and blood pressure, and a narrowing or constricting of the peripheral blood vessels and bronchial airways, all of which contribute to an increased workload on the heart.

Engage www.pahconnection.com 14.4

Nicotine is a powerfully addictive drug (Figure 14.1). The *Surgeon General's Report* on the health consequences of smoking emphasized the addiction factor of nicotine (USDHHS, 1988). This means that the use of nicotine causes changes in the brain that force people to want to use more of the drug. The pharmacological and behavioral processes that reinforce tobacco addiction are similar to those for other addictive drugs. These characteristics include physical dependence and tolerance for the drug, highly controlled or compulsive use, use of the drug to restore psychoactive or physical effects, and predictable withdrawal symptoms when attempts are made to quit (APA, 1987).

Carbon Monoxide Carbon monoxide (CO) is one of the most abundant and poisonous gases in cigarette smoke. Carbon monoxide is an odorless, tasteless, and colorless gas that impairs oxygen transportation to body tissues by competing with oxygen molecules for attachment to the red blood cells. Red blood cells are responsible for carrying oxygen from the lungs to the tissues. Carbon monoxide actually has far greater attachment properties when it comes to binding with the red blood cells than does oxygen. As a result, the capacity of the blood to carry oxygen to the brain, heart, and muscles is diminished. Carbon monoxide also leads to damage of the inner walls of the arteries, a destruction that contributes to plaque buildup and arteriosclerosis (see Chapter 6).

Cigarette Smoking

Cigarette smoking is the number one preventable cause of premature mortality in the United States (Figure 14.8). Scientific research has provided decisive evidence that smoking causes coronary heart disease, stroke, and chronic lung disease, as well as cancer of the lungs, larynx, esophagus, mouth, and bladder (MMWR, 1997). The harmful effects of cigarette smoking are visited on nonsmokers as well. Each year secondhand smoke, or environmental tobacco smoke, causes 3000 lung cancer deaths in nonsmokers. More people die from tobacco-related deaths each year than from AIDS, alcoholism, cocaine, heroin, traffic accidents, fire, homicides, and suicides combined (CDC, 1999). An additional 20 million Americans suffer various debilitating and chronic diseases caused by smoking, including bronchitis, emphysema, peptic ulcer disease, and arteriosclerosis.

Deciding to Smoke Cigarettes In most cases, the decision to smoke is not made by an adult. Sixty percent of smokers start by the age of 14, and 90 percent of smokers are firmly addicted before reaching age 19. Stated another way, only 1 in 10 smokers become addicted after the age of 19, so almost no one starts smoking after age 19. Although adult smoking prevalence is at the lowest level in more than 50 years, teenage smoking has not decreased significantly since 1980, with approximately 3000 minors starting to smoke each day (Hanson, 1999). In fact, over one-third of today's young people are active smokers by the time they leave high school, and 1 in every 6 is an active smoker as early as the eighth grade (Figure 14.9).

Activities & Assessments 14.3

Smoking is particularly dangerous for teenagers because, shortly after initiating the behavior, regular use and dependency develops. This dependence on smoking can

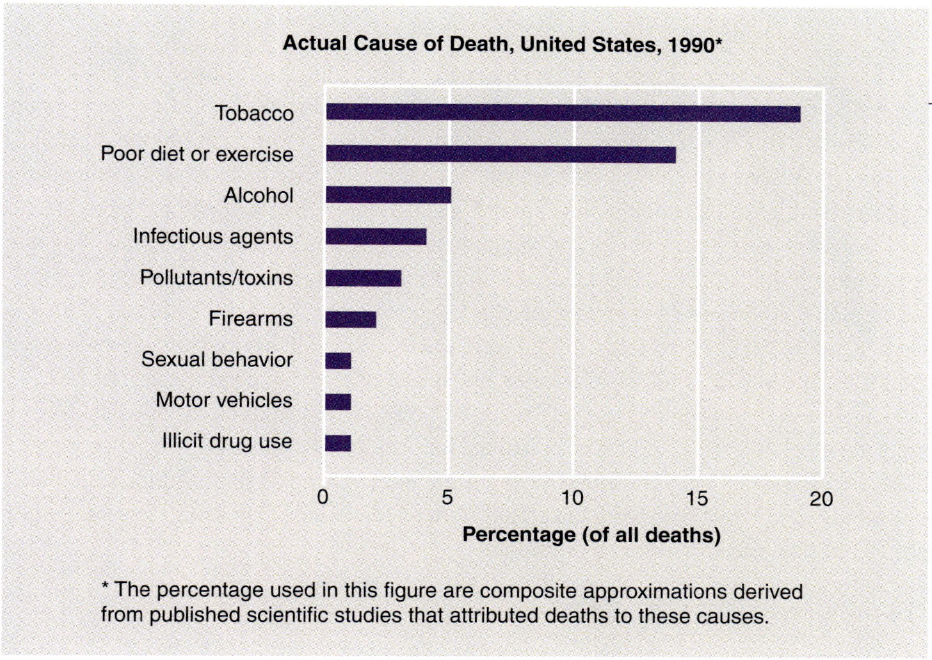

FIGURE 14.8

Actual Causes of Death, United States, 1990.

SOURCE: J.M. McGinnis and W.H. Foege. (1993). Actual causes of death in the United States. *JAMA*, 270:2207–12.

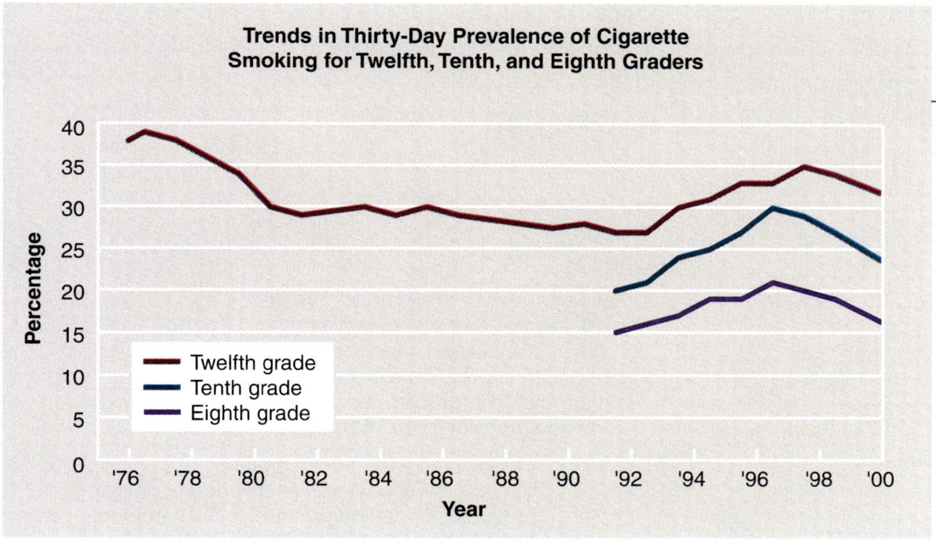

FIGURE 14.9

Cigarette Smoking Prevalence for Eighth, Tenth, and Twelfth Graders.

SOURCE: L.D. Johnston, P.M. O'Malley, J.G. Bachman. (2000, Dec.). Cigarette use and smokeless tobacco use decline substantially among teens. Monitoring the Future Institute for Social Research, University of Michigan [On-line]. Available: www.monitoringthefuture.org; accessed 01/30/01.

occur in a relatively short time and can lead to addiction. Most teens believe they will not become addicted—that they will be able to stop smoking whenever they wish. Their continuation of smoking behavior into adulthood is maintained by a variety of psychological and physiological mechanisms, including familiarity with the act and the events in which it occurs, as well as addiction to nicotine.

The younger you start smoking, the more you will smoke and the longer you will do it, all of which lead to greater impairment. Smoking doesn't do any part of the body any good, at any time, under any conditions. Think of all the positive effects of physical activity on health that you have learned; research demonstrates that cigarette smoking will wipe them out. While all organs and tissues can be damaged by the toxic chemicals present in cigarette smoke, the developing bodies of teenagers are at particular risk for chemical damage (Table 14.10). For example, cigarette smoking in teens has been shown to reduce lung growth and limit lung function.

Cigar Smoking

Americans consume over 5 billion cigars annually, compared to nearly 480 billion cigarettes annually. While cigarette sales have shown a recent decline, cigar sales are on the increase. This upward trend in cigar use has become a concern for many in public health. All available scientific evidence warrants that the magnitude of risk from cigar smoke is similar to that for cigarette smoke (NCI, 1998). The smoke from both cigars and cigarettes results largely from incomplete combustion of tobacco, and has the same toxic and carcinogenic constituents. This scientific evidence related to cigar smoking, along with the common misperception that cigar smoking may not be as dangerous as cigarette smoking, has led to the requirement that cigars sold in the United States carry health warnings (FTC, 2000). The 2000 agreement orders that cigar boxes, smaller packages, and individual cigars be labeled with one of the five different Surgeon General statements (Table 14.11). The warnings for cigars and cigar products go beyond those for cigarettes. They require a more prominent package display and include mention of the dangers of secondhand smoke. In truth, cigar smoking is bad for your health and is not a safe alternative to cigarettes.

Smoking and Physical Activity

Many studies have shown that smoking before or during exercise decreases performance, due to a number of factors. The undesirable effects of carbon monoxide become especially obvious during physical activity. Muscles require more oxygen during physical activity, but acquire less from the red blood cells because carbon monoxide has reduced the amount of oxygen the blood can carry. Consequently, muscles tire more quickly.

TABLE 14.10 Facts on Youth Smoking, Health, and Performance

Among young people, the short-term health effects of smoking include damage to the respiratory system, addiction to nicotine, and the associated risk of other drug use. Long-term health consequences of youth smoking are reinforced by the fact that most young people who smoke regularly continue to smoke throughout adulthood. (CDC. *Preventing tobacco use among young people—-A report of the Surgeon General.* 1994, p. 15)

Smoking hurts young people's physical fitness in terms of both performance and endurance—-even among young people trained in competitive running. (CDC. *Preventing tobacco use among young people,* p. 28)

Smoking among youth can hamper the rate of lung growth and the level of maximum lung function. (CDC. *Preventing tobacco use among young people,.* p. 17)

The resting heart rates of young adult smokers are two to three beats per min faster than those of nonsmokers. (CDC. *Preventing tobacco use among young people,* p. 28)

Among young people, regular smoking is responsible for cough and increased frequency and severity of respiratory illnesses. (CDC. *Preventing tobacco use among young people,* p. 9)

The younger people start smoking cigarettes, the more likely the are to become strongly addicted to nicotine. (CDC. *Preventing tobacco use among young people,* p. 9)

Teens who smoke are 3 times more likely than nonsmokers to use alcohol, 8 times more likely to use marijuana, and 22 times more likely to use cocaine. Smoking is associated with a host of other risky behaviors such as fighting and engaging in unprotected sex. (CDC. *Preventing tobacco use among young people,* pp. 36, 104)

Smoking is associated with poor overall health and a variety of short-term adverse health effects in young people and may also be a marker for underlying mental health problems, such as depression, among adolescents. High school seniors who are regular smokers and began smoking by grade nine are

- 2.4 times more likely than their nonsmoking peers to report poorer overall health
- 2.4 to 2.7 times more likely to report cough with phlegm or blood, shortness of breath when not exercising, and wheezing or gasping
- 3.0 times more likely to have seen a doctor or other health professional for an emotional or psychological complaint.

(Arday DR, Giovino GA, Schulman J, Nelson DE, Mowery P, Samet JM. Cigarette smoking and self-reported health problems among US high school seniors, 1982–1989. *Am J of Health Promotion,* 1995;10(2):111–116.)

SOURCE: Centers for Disease Control and Prevention (CDC). *CDC's tips on youth smoking, health, and performance* [On-line]. Available: http://www.cdc.gov/tobacco/ythsprt.htm; accessed 1/30/01.

Smoking also puts an extra burden on the heart and circulatory system. Combined with the effects of decreased oxygen, nicotine's constricting effects on the blood vessels requires the heart to work harder to deliver the oxygen. Breathing also becomes hindered as the lungs get irritated and accumulate more mucus from smoking, leading to increased airway resistance. Extra effort to get air in and out of the lungs occurs if a cigarette is smoked within an hour of physical activity. During heavy physical activity, the respiratory muscles are required to work twice as hard for chronic smokers compared to nonsmokers.

Quitting Smoking

Quitting smoking is the single most important step that smokers can take to enhance the length and quality of their life (Healthy People 2010, 2000). Moreover, the health benefits and physical activity benefits of quitting smoking are immediate and substantial for all smokers regardless of age, gender, disease state, or smoking history (Table 14.12).

Explore www.pahconnection.com 14.5, 14.6

Most people who have quit smoking state that they have done it on their own, without the help of a formal program. Most smokers quit a number of times before achieving long-term abstinence. If you are a present smoker who wants to quit, don't let another day go by (Table 14.13). Get help if you need it. Many groups offer programs and free materials to help smokers quit for good (Table 14.14). Your college or university health center may also be a good source for help and support.

Staying Trim after Quitting Most people who quit smoking are concerned about gaining weight. Approximately 4 out of every 5 people gain weight after quitting smoking, with the average weight gain being about 5 pounds. Changes in eating habits and in the body's processing of food leads to this weight gain.

Smoking suppresses taste-bud awareness and reduces the taste value of food. When people quit smoking they notice an improvement in the taste of food, leading to selection of higher portions and increased helpings. Increasing food consumption may also be an alternate way to deal with stress or a behavioral substitute for the oral satisfaction of smoking.

TABLE 14.11 Warning Labels on Cigar Products

June 28, 2000
Cigars and health risk warnings

Cigars sold in the United States soon will carry warnings from the Surgeon General advising users of serious health risks associated with cigar smoking.

The Federal Trade Commission (FTC) said on June 26 that it had reached settlements with the seven largest cigar manufacturers in the U.S. regarding the warnings.

In announcing the settlement, FTC Chairman Robert Pitofsky said cigar smoking "is not a harmless alternative to cigarette smoking and carries its own risk." Allowing manufacturers to sell cigars without mentioning the proven health risks from smoking "is sending the wrong message" to smokers and that misperception must be corrected, he said.

The agreement orders that cigar boxes, smaller packages, and individual cigars be labeled with one of five different Surgeon General statements: "Cigar Smoking Can Cause Cancers of the Mouth and Throat, Even If You Do Not Inhale;" "Cigar Smoking Can Cause Lung Cancer and Heart Disease;" "Tobacco Use Increases the Risk of Infertility, Stillbirth and Low Birth Weight;" "Cigars Are Not a Safe Alternative to Cigarettes;" and "Tobacco Smoke Increases the Risk of Lung Cancer and Heart Disease, Even in Nonsmokers."

The warnings will be rotated at 3-month intervals, according to the agreement.

SOURCE: MayoClinic.com. (2000, June 28). Headline watch: Cigar and health risk warnings [On-line]. Available: http://www.mayohealth.org/home?id=HQ00434; accessed 1/30/01.

Some researchers believe that the absence of nicotine influences weight gain. First, nicotine causes the liver to release glycogen, raising the blood-sugar level and making the smoker feel satiated; absence of nicotine may factor into ex-smokers' cravings for high-sugar and high-calorie foods. Second, nicotine increases the body's basic metabolic rate, making it easier for the body to expend calories and contributing to a lower body weight.

Research provides compelling evidence that people who participate in an intensive physical activity program are more likely to succeed at quitting smoking and less likely to gain weight than people who did not include physical activity as part of their cessation strategy (Marcus, 1999). This is because many people use cigarettes to help them manage their weight, moods, and stress. Clearly, physical activity is a more healthy way to deal with each of these concerns. Moreover, the health benefits derived from avoiding any tobacco use, and the subsequent risk of developing a number of debilitating chronic diseases, overwhelmingly outweigh any small weight gain.

Smokeless Tobacco

Smokeless tobacco forms include snuff and chewing tobacco. Snuff is a powdered tobacco that is generally put between the lower lip and gum. It can also be inhaled through the nose. Chewing tobacco is shredded or loose-leaf tobacco, treated with moisturizing and flavoring agents that is pressed into *plugs* and then placed inside the cheek. Both tobacco products stimulate saliva production, requiring users to spit frequently to clear the mouth of excess saliva and any tobacco that has lost its flavor. Some people refer to smokeless tobacco as "spit tobacco."

TABLE 14.12 Immediate and Long-Term Health Benefits of Stopping Smoking

Immediately
- Air around you no longer dangerous to children and other adults.

20 minutes
- Blood pressure drops to normal.
- Pulse rate drops to normal.
- Temperature in hands and feet increases to normal.

8 hours
- Carbon monoxide level in blood drops to normal.
- Oxygen level in blood increases to normal.

24 hours
- Chance of heart attack decreases.

48 hours
- Sense of smell and taste improves.

2 to 12 weeks
- Circulation improves.
- Breathing improves.
- Walking becomes easier.

1 to 9 months
- Coughing and sinus congestion decreases.
- Shortness of breath decreases.
- Overall energy increases.
- Lungs increase ability to self-clean and reduce infection.

1 year
- Risk of premature coronary heart disease is half the risk of a smoker.

5 years
- Risk of stroke comparable to that of a nonsmoker.

10 years
- Life expectancy comparable to a nonsmoker.
- Lung cancer death rate is about half the rate of a smoker.
- Risk of cancer of mouth, throat, esophagus, bladder, kidney, and pancreas decrease.

15 years
- Risk of coronary heart disease comparable to that of a nonsmoker.

Before age 50
- Risk of dying in the next 15 years decreases by 50 percent compared to continuing smokers.

SOURCE: Adapted from American Lung Association (ALA). What are the benefits of quitting smoking? [Online]. Available: http://www.lungusa.org/tobacco/quit_ben.html; accessed 3/29/01. Reprinted with permission © 2001 American Lung Association. For more information, please visit our website at www.lungusa.org or call 1-800-LUNG-USA (1-800-586-4872).

TABLE 14.13 Quit Tips

1. Don't smoke any number or any kind of cigarette. Smoking even a few cigarettes a day can hurt your health. If you try to smoke fewer cigarettes, but do not stop completely, soon you'll be smoking the same amount again.

   Smoking "low-tar, low-nicotine" cigarettes usually does little good, either. Because nicotine is so addictive, if you switch to lower-nicotine brands you'll likely just puff harder, longer, and more often on each cigarette. The only safe choice is to quit completely.

2. Write down why you want to quit. Do you want

   to feel in control of you life?
   to have better health?
   to set a good example for your children?
   to protect your family from breathing other people's smoke?

   Really wanting to quit smoking is very important to how much success you will have in quitting. Smokers who live after a heart attack are the most likely to quit for good. They're very motivated. Find a reason for quitting before you have no choice.

3. Know that it will take effort to quit smoking. Nicotine is habit forming. Half of the battle in quitting is knowing you need to quit. This knowledge will help you be more able to deal with the symptoms of withdrawal that can occur, such as bad moods and really wanting to smoke. There are many ways smokers quit, including using nicotine replacement products (gum and patches), but there is no easy way. Nearly all smokers have some feelings of nicotine withdrawal when they try to quit. Give yourself a month to get over these feelings. Take quitting one day at a time, even one minute at a time—whatever you need to succeed.

4. Half of all adult smokers have quit, so you can, too. That's the good news. There are millions of people alive today who have learned to face life without a cigarette. For staying healthy, quitting smoking is the best step you can take.

SOURCE: Centers for Disease Control and Prevention (CDC), Tobacco Information and Prevention Source (TIPS). *Quit tips* [On-line]. Available: http://www.cdc.gov/tobacco/quit/quittip.htm; accessed 1/30/01.

TABLE 14.14 National Groups Are Available to Help You Quit Smoking

Get help if you need it. Many groups offer written materials, programs, and advice to help smokers quit for good. The following national groups have toll-free telephone numbers for information and resources:

Agency for Health Care Policy and Research, Clinical Practice Guidelines on Smoking Cessation, Instant Fax 301-594-2800 [Press 1]; or call 1-800-358-9295 for physician materials and a "You Can Quit Smoking" consumer guide.

American Cancer Society, 1-800-ACS-2345

American Heart Association, 1-800-AHA-USA1

American Lung Association, 1-800-LUNG-USA

Office on Smoking and Health, 1-800-CDC-1311

National Cancer Institute, 1-800-4-CANCER

Explore 14.7

An estimated 7 million Americans (3.3 percent) use smokeless tobacco (SAMHSA, 1996). The number of smokeless users has increased over the past decade, especially among young males. Over 90 percent of smokeless tobacco users are men. Although smokeless tobacco use is not as dangerous as smoking cigarettes, it is not a safe alternative because it has many detrimental health risks.

Smokeless tobacco contains over 2000 chemicals, many of which are potent carcinogens that lead directly to cancer. The strongest association is between smokeless tobacco and oral cancer. Oral cancer risk among regular smokeless tobacco users is *up to fifty times* that of nonusers. The use of smokeless tobacco products leads to nicotine dependence and addiction; the magnitude of nicotine exposure, and its absorption, distribution, and elimination, is similar to smoking cigarettes. Other health effects include gum recession, increased tooth decay, tooth discoloration, bad breath, and a decreased sense of taste, which leads to unhealthy eating habits.

Concerns about the health risks of smokeless tobacco led to the surgeon general's sponsoring a report on the *Health Consequences of Using Smokeless Tobacco* (USDHHS, 1988). The report is a compilation of research findings that concludes that the use of smokeless tobacco products represents a significant health risk.

CAFFEINE

6. Caffeine is the most widely used drug in the United States.

Caffeine, a central nervous system stimulant, is the most widely used drug in America. Caffeine is a chemical substance that can be extracted from plants or produced synthetically. It is found naturally in the leaves, seeds, and fruits of more than 60 plants, including kola nuts, tea leaves, coffee, and cocoa beans. Many beverage and food products made with these ingredients naturally contain caffeine, including coffee, tea, chocolate, and many carbonated beverages such as colas. Caffeine has no flavor. Caffeine is also added to a number of over-the-counter medications such as appetite suppressants and cold medicines.

Americans consume nearly 80 percent of their caffeine intake from coffee, 10 percent each from tea and soft drinks, and approximately 2 percent from chocolate. On a typical day, half of the United States' population drinks an average of three cups of coffee (Ellison, 1995).

Caffeine is a celebrated American stimulant. It is a socially acceptable drug that helps people to get things done by increasing mental alertness and providing the physical capacity to do more work. Research has shown that moderate doses of caffeine enhance alertness, concentration, motivation, energy, and well-being (Consumer Reports, 1997).

Caffeine is absorbed rapidly from the gastrointestinal tract and distributed throughout the body in the bloodstream. Caffeine stimulates the central nervous system (CNS) at all levels. Effects occur in 30 minutes, with peak levels of CNS activity occurring within 2 hours of ingestion. Caffeine's effects on the brain allow for a clearer and more rapid thought pattern that increases mental attentiveness and learning. Caffeine also stimulates the CNS to increase breathing rates. Caffeine arouses the heart muscle to pump more quickly, which increases blood circulation and, along with the increased respiratory function, makes more oxygen available for the muscles. Caffeine tends to elevate fatty acids in the blood, which then can be used for energy by working muscles.

Caffeine and Health

Engage
www.pahconnection.com
14.5

The majority of research studies on caffeine indicate that there are no adverse long-term health consequences associated with moderate intake (Consumer Reports, 1997). Moderate caffeine consumption is considered to about 300 milligrams per day; that is equal to about three cups of coffee (Table 14.15). Research strongly suggests that consumption of caffeine does not contribute to cardiovascular disease (Ellison, 1995) or cancer (AICR, 1997).

Caffeine does have some acutely negative side effects in a few people. Caffeine may cause anxiety, agitation, headaches, gastrointestinal upset, increased urination, constipation or diarrhea, and insomnia, as well as irritating existing ulcers. Caffeine also causes greater excretion of calcium in the urine; therefore, it can make bones more fragile in people who don't get enough calcium from other sources. Some people become physically and psychologically dependent on their favorite caffeinated beverage. The heavy

Caffeine A natural stimulant that is present in leaves, seeds, or fruits.

Caffeinism Heavy use or preoccupation with caffeine.

use or preoccupation with caffeine is referred to as **caffeinism.** Sudden cessation of caffeine (caffeine withdrawal) in a heavy user may lead to symptoms like restlessness, irritability, and sluggishness. These symptoms can be avoided by diminishing caffeine intake gradually over a number of days. Even though short-term dependence on caffeine does develop in some users, the American Psychiatric Association's Substance Use Task Force does not classify caffeine products as addictive (APA, 1994).

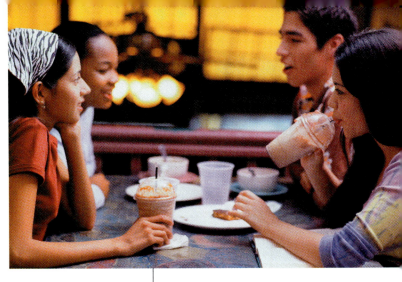

Caffeine is a celebrated American stimulant.

Caffeine and Physical Activity

A large number of studies have found that consuming moderate amounts of caffeine has positive effects on endurance activities (Graham & Spriet, 1996). The weight of evidence suggests that caffeine increases stamina in long- and mid-range events. As mentioned earlier, caffeine tends to elevate the fatty acids in the blood. The more fatty acids that are in the bloodstream at the beginning of physical activity, the more these fatty acids will be used by exercising muscles. This increased utilization of fat as an energy source slows muscle glycogen depletion, resulting in increased endurance. This energy benefit must be weighed in relationship to the possible side effects that may hinder physical activity: gastric disturbance, increased urine output contributing to dehydration, and diarrhea. According to experts, on average, healthy, physically active people who consume a moderate amount of caffeine an hour before physical activity are within safe limits.

PHYSICAL ACTIVITY AND HEALTH CONNECTION

physical activity and health connection

To develop a high level of physical activity and health in your life, you must address the issue of drug use. We live in a society that believes legal drug use is acceptable and even favorable. This notion doesn't necessarily complement a physically active or healthy lifestyle. As you increased your understanding of the physical and psychological consequences of alcohol use and cigarette smoking, you came to better understand the many negative health consequences related to their use. Your path to being physically active can be significantly impaired by the use of drugs. Before using any drug, remember that you have choices. By making responsible choices that support your goal of being physically active and healthy, you will not only enhance your present quality of life but also your future.

TABLE **14.15** Caffeine Content of Beverages and Chocolate

BEVERAGE	CAFFEINE CONTENT (MG)	AMOUNT
Brewed coffee	90–125	5 oz.
Instant coffee	14–93	5 oz.
Decaffeinated coffee	1–6	5 oz.
Tea	30–70	5 oz.
Cocoa	5	5 oz.
Coca-Cola	45	12 oz.
Pepsi-Cola	30	12 oz.
Chocolate bar	22	1 oz.

SOURCE: Hanson and Venturelli. (1998). *Drugs and Society* (p. 278). Boston: Jones and Bartlett.

CONCEPT CONNECTION

1. **Legal drug use can profoundly affect your health and your quality of life.** Legal social drugs are used by a wide percentage of the population on a regular basis and have a direct relationship to physical activity and health. The legality, as well as the annual high consumption of these drugs, does not imply that they are unrelated to major health and societal costs. The annual health care expense resulting from tobacco and alcohol use and abuse is in excess of $250 billion.

2. **Long-term drug use can disrupt the body's normal balance, or homeostasis.** It is usually assumed that no one starts using drugs to misuse or abuse them; however, it is possible to drift from responsible use to misuse or abuse. It is also clear that many chronic users eventually do experience problems with drugs and may eventually suffer negative health consequences.

3. **Making wise drug use decisions is important.** The choice of which drug to use, how much, and how long are all important individual decisions and should not be made thoughtlessly. It is important for an individual to practice decision-making skills relating to taking drugs so that an appropriate response is made.

4. **Alcohol misuse and abuse is one of the most significant health problems in the United States.** Alcohol is considered to be the number-one problem drug in America because of the physical, social, and emotional damage it causes. Dealing with alcohol-related accidents, violence, and crime consumes the majority of law-enforcement resources, while the health consequences of long-term alcohol abuse add substantially to national healthcare costs. The annual economic cost to the United States from alcohol use and abuse is estimated to be $167 billion dollars.

5. **Cigarette smoking is the most preventable cause of premature illness and death in the United States.** Smoking is the number-one preventable cause of premature mortality, responsible for 1 in every 5 deaths, or more than 430,000 deaths annually. Scientific research has provided decisive evidence that smoking causes coronary heart disease, stroke, and chronic lung disease, as well as cancer of the lungs, larynx, esophagus, mouth, and bladder.

6. **Caffeine is the most widely used drug in the United States.** Caffeine is a celebrated American stimulant. Caffeine is a socially acceptable drug that helps people to get things done by increasing mental alertness and providing the physical capacity to do more work. Research has shown that moderate doses of caffeine enhance alertness, concentration, motivation, energy, and well-being. Caffeine does have some acutely negative side effects in a few people.

TERMS

Legal drugs, 312
Illegal drugs, 313
Drug, 313
Drug use, 313
Drug misuse, 313
Drug abuse, 313
Tolerance, 315
Drug addiction, 315
Psychological dependence, 315
Physical dependence, 316
Withdrawal illness, 317
Pharmacology, 317
Moderate drinking, 320
Binge drinking, 321
Problem drinking, 322
Blood alcohol concentration, 323
Depressants, 326
Tars, 331
Nicotine, 331
Carbon monoxide, 331
Stimulants, 332
Caffeine, 338
Caffeinism, 338

MAKING THE CONNECTION

Jim has learned that alcohol has a concentrated source of calories, 7 kilocalories per gram. He also learned that, although alcohol is metabolized as a carbohydrate, it exhibits none of the properties of food. In other words, alcohol calories supply no nutrients and therefore are considered "empty." Furthermore, these empty calories contribute to the overall food calorie intake and can be stored as body fat.

CRITICAL THINKING

1. Like Jim, many people have a few drinks now and then, exercise routinely, and don't understand why they can't loose weight. Your roommate has been unsuccessfully trying to loose weigh, despite routine physical activity. You notice that he routinely has a beer or two every evening before sitting down to watch some television. Explain to your roommate why he is not losing any weight.
2. "I really don't like the taste of liquor that much, but after the first couple of shots, it doesn't taste all that bad. I know I shouldn't drink and I always have a hangover the next day but, hey, college is stressful and how else can I deal with the stress of getting the grades to keep my scholarship and making my parents happy?" What's your opinion of this person's attitude? Explain why you agree or disagree. If you disagree, how can this person deal with the stress of getting good grades?
3. College campuses often accept money from companies that sell alcoholic beverages—to support athletic events, for example. By allowing these companies to advertise at campus events, the university makes considerable money to enhance the campus environment and provide quality education. What is your campus's policy on allowing alcohol companies to advertise or sponsor events on campus? Do you agree or disagree with this policy?
4. Purchase a popular magazine and count the number of cigarette ads in the issue. In reviewing each of the ads, respond to the following questions:
   a) Who is the ad targeting (young people, older adults, women)?
   b) How is the ad appealing to the target audience (fun, sex)?
   c) What does the ad seem to promise if you smoke their brand of cigarette?

REFERENCES

American Institute for Cancer Research, (1997). Food, nutrition, and the prevention of cancer: A global perspective. *Journal of the American Medical Association 278*: 20.

American Psychiatric Association. (1994). *Diagnostic and Statistical Manual of Mental Disorders. 4th Edition, Revised.* Washington, DC.

U.S. Department of Health and Human Services. (2000). *Alcohol and Health: Tenth Special Report to the U.S. Congress.* DHHS Pub. No. (ADM). Washington, DC.

Baum-Baicker, C. (1985). The psychological benefits of moderate alcohol consumption: A review of the literature. *Drug and Alcohol Dependence 15*:303–322.

Centers for Disease Control and Prevention (CDC). (1998). Youth risk behavior survey: United States, 1997. *CDC Surveillance Summaries 47*(SS-3).

Centers for Disease Control and Prevention (CDC). (1996). Projected smoking-related deaths among youth: United States, 1993. *Morbidity and Mortality Weekly Report 45*: 971–74.

Consumer Reports. (1997). What caffeine can do for you–And to you. *Consumer Reports on Health* 9(9):97–101.

Cox, W.M. (1986). *The Encyclopedia of Psychoactive Drugs: The Addictive Personality.* New York: Chelsea House.

De Castro, J. M., & Orozco, S. (1990). Moderate alcohol intake and spontaneous eating patterns of humans: Evidence of unregulated supplementation. *American Journal of Clinical Nutrition 52*:246–53.

Douglas, K.A., et al. (1997). Results from the 1995 national college risk behavior survey. *Journal of American College Health 46*:55–64.

Ellison, R.C. (1995). Current caffeine intake of young children: Amount and source. *Journal of the American Dietetic Association 95*:802–804.

Engs, R. (1979). *Responsible Drug and Alcohol Use.* New York: Macmillan.

Graham, T.E., & Spriet, L.L. (1996). Caffeine and exercise performance. *Sports Science Exchange 9*(1). Graduate Sports Science Institute.

Hanson, M. J. (1999). Which straw will break the camel's back. *American Journal of Nursing 99*(11):63–69.

U.S. Department of Health and Human Services. (1994). *Preventing Tobacco Use among Young People: A Report of the Surgeon General.* Atlanta.

Hirsh, A.T. (1989). The effect of caffeine on exercise tolerance and left ventricle function in patients with coronary artery disease. *Annals of Internal Medicine 110*:593–98.

Johnston, L.D., O'Malley, P.M., Bachman, J.G. (December 1999). Cigarette smoking among American teens continues gradual decline. University of Michigan News and Information Services: Ann Arbor, MI. Online: www.monitoringthefuture.org [accessed 04/18/00].

Leshner, A. I. (1997). Drug abuse and addiction treatment research. *Archives of General Psychiatry 54*:691–94.

Marcus, B. (1999). Exercise helps smokers kick the habit. *Archives of Internal Medicine 159*:1169–71.

McKenzie, J. F., Pinger, R.R., & Kotecki, J.E. (1999). *An Introduction to Community Health.* Sudbury, MA: Jones and Bartlett.

Morbity and Mortality Weekly Report.(1997). Average number of deaths due to cigarette smoking. *Centers for Disease Control 46*:448–51.

Moore, R.D., & Pearson, T.A. (1986). Moderate alcohol consumption and coronary heart disease: A review. *Medicine 65*(4):242–67.

Morse, R.M., & Flavin, D.K. (1992). The definition of alcoholism. *Journal of the American Medical Association 268*(8):1012–14.

National Cancer Institute (1998). *Cigars: Health Effects and Trends.* NCI, National Institutes of Health, Monograph 9, on Smoking and Tobacco Control.

National Institute on Alcohol Abuse and Alcoholism (NIAAA). (1997). *Ninth Special Report to the U.S. Congress on Alcohol and Health from the Secretary of Health and Human Services.* NIH Pub. No. 97-4017. Rockville, MD.

National Institute on Alcohol Abuse and Alcoholism (NIAAA). (1992). Moderate drinking. *Alcohol Alert 16*:PH315.

Pinger, R.R., Payne, W., Hahn, D., & Hahn, E. (1998). *Drugs: Issues for Today.* Dubuque: WCB/McGraw-Hill.

Pomerleau, O., & Pomerleau, C. (1984). Neuroregulators and the reinforcement of smoking: Toward a biobehavioral explanation. *Neuroscience Biobehavioral Review 8*:503–513.

Powers, SK, Dodd, S. (1985). Caffeine and endurance performance. *Sports Medicine 2*:165–74.

Substance Abuse and Mental Health Services Administration. (1996). *Preliminary Estimates from the 1995 National Household Survey on Drug Abuse.* Rockville, MD.

U.S. Department of Agriculture. (1997). *Tobacco Situation and Outlook Report.* U.S. Department of Agriculture, Economic Research Service, series TBS-239.

U.S. Department of Health and Human Services. (1990). *The Health Benefits of Smoking Cessation.* DHHS Publication No. (CDC) 90-8416.

U.S. Department of Health and Human Services. (1988). *The Health Consequences of Smoking: Nicotine Addiction. A Report of the Surgeon General's Office on Smoking and Health.* DHHS Publication No. (PHS) 017-001-00468-5.

Suh, I., Shaten, B.J., Cutler, J.A., Kuller, L.H. (1992). Alcohol use and mortality from coronary heart disease: The role of high-density lipoprotein cholesterol. *Annuals of Internal Medicine 116*:881–87.

Suter, P.M. (April 1992). The effect of ethanol on fat storage in healthy subjects. *New England Journal of Medicine 326* (15: 983–87.

Wechsler, H., Lee, J.E., Kuo, M., Lee, H. (2000). College binge drinking in the 1990s, a continuing problem: Results of the Harvard School of Public Health 1999 college alcohol study. *Journal of American College Health 48*(10):199–210.

Activities & Assessments

NAME ______ SECTION ______ DATE ______

14.3 Do You Have a Drinking Problem?

This questionnaire is designed to help you determine whether you have a problem with alcohol. Answer each question yes or no and record your choice in the right-hand column.

YES	NO	
☐	☐	1. Do you believe you are a normal drinker?
☐	☐	2. Have you ever awakened after drinking the night before and found that you could not remember some part of the evening?
☐	☐	3. Does your wife, husband, a parent, or other near relative ever worry or complain about your drinking?
☐	☐	4. Can you stop drinking without a struggle after one or two drinks?
☐	☐	5. Do you ever feel bad about your drinking?
☐	☐	6. Do friends or relatives think you are a normal drinker?
☐	☐	7. Do you ever try to limit your drinking to certain times of the day or to certain places?
☐	☐	8. Are you always able to stop drinking when you want to?
☐	☐	9. Have you ever attended a meeting of Alcoholics Anonymous?
☐	☐	10. Have you gotten into fights when drinking?
☐	☐	11. Has drinking ever created problems between you and your wife, husband, boyfriend, girlfriend, a parent, or other near relative?
☐	☐	12. Has your wife, husband, boyfriend, girlfriend, a parent, or other near relative ever gone to anyone for help about your drinking?
☐	☐	13. Have you ever lost friends because of drinking?
☐	☐	14. Have you ever gotten into trouble at work because of drinking?
☐	☐	15. Have you ever lost a job because of drinking?
☐	☐	16. Have you ever neglected your obligations, your family, or your work for two or more days in a row because you were drinking?
☐	☐	17. Do you drink before noon fairly often?
☐	☐	18. Have you ever been told you have liver trouble? Cirrhosis?
☐	☐	19. After heavy drinking have you ever had delirium tremens (DTs) or severe shaking?
☐	☐	20. After heavy drinking have you ever heard voices or seen things that weren't really there?
☐	☐	21. Have you ever gone to anyone for help about your drinking?
☐	☐	22. Have you ever been in a hospital because of drinking?
☐	☐	23. Have you ever been a patient in a psychiatric hospital or in a psychiatric ward of a general hospital?
☐	☐	24. Have you ever been in a hospital to be "dried out" (detoxified) because of drinking?
☐	☐	25. Have you ever been in jail, even for a few hours, because of drunk behavior?

(continued)

14.3 Do You Have a Drinking Problem? (cont.)

SCORING

Item keying for alcoholic responses are 1. N; 2. Y; 3. Y; 4. N; 5. Y; 6. N; 7. Y; 8. N; 9–25, Y.
To score, add one point for each alcoholic response.
The total score is the number of alcoholic responses.

NUMBER OF ALCOHOLIC RESPONSES	INTERPRETATION
0–2	No problem with alcohol
3–5	Early warning signs that drinking is becoming problematic
6 or more	Problem drinker/alcoholic

If you think you have a drinking problem, seek professional help.

SOURCE: G. Edlin, E. Golanty, and K. McCormack Brown. (1999). *Health and Wellness* (6th ed., p. 401). Boston: Jones and Bartlett.

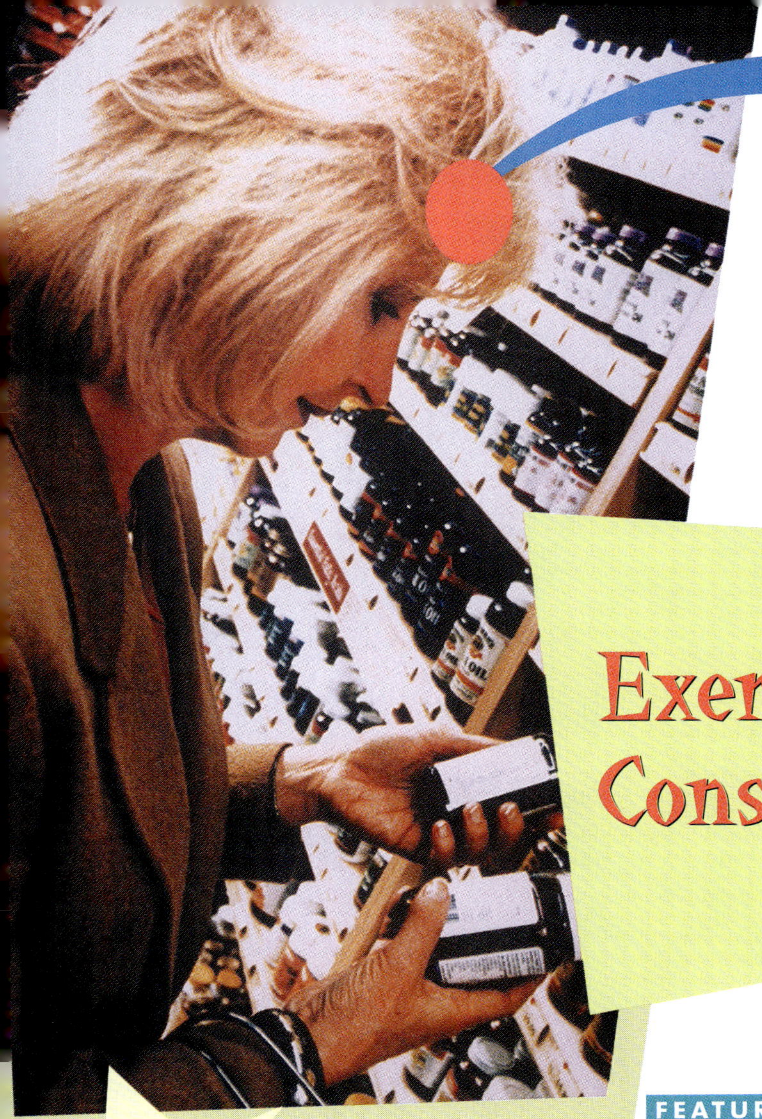

15

Exercise Consumerism

CONCEPT CONNECTION

1. To develop a quality physical activity program, you must be a wise consumer of exercise information.
2. The physical activity industry suffers from a wide range of misinformation and fraudulent claims.
3. You need to be aware of some common misconceptions, frauds, and fallacies.
4. Being a critical consumer requires knowing where to turn for valid information.
5. There are several avenues you can take in seeking redress.

FEATURES

E-Learning Tools: www.pahconnection.com

Experience www.pahconnection.com

15.1 When is a product considered questionable?
15.2 Evaluating questionable products?
15.3 Evaluating nutritional supplements

Explore www.pahconnection.com

15.1 Quackwatch
15.2 FDA
15.3 FTC
15.4 ACSM
15.5 NSCA
15.6 AAHPERD
15.7 American Council on Exercise
15.8 Fitness news
15.9 Fitness World
15.10 *Consumer Reports*
15.11 National Council Against Health Fraud

WHAT'S THE CONNECTION?

Janet's friend Kathy constantly asks her to try a new diet pill "guaranteed" to make her lose inches overnight. Kathy claims that the pill worked for her and pressures Janet into trying "just one." Janet is a bit skeptical and decides to investigate further. She asks Kathy for the ingredient list from the product and calls a registered dietitian in her town.

1. To develop a quality physical activity program, you must be a wise consumer of exercise information.

INTRODUCTION

This chapter provides information that will allow you to enhance your skills as an intelligent consumer of exercise information and products. It describes how to identify misinformation and fraud, and how to select the correct exercise equipment, products, and programs. It also provides suggestions on where to turn for factual information and how to seek redress if you think you have been a victim of fraud.

Scope of the Problem

Some people will go to any length, or take any shortcut, in the attempt to gain an edge. This statement is true in sport as well as in marketing. The exercise and fitness industry is rife with misleading advertising and fraudulent claims. Why are misleading products and statements, and even outright fraud, a problem for the consumer? First of all, misleading or fraudulent products make false promises that can lead you to develop a sense of mistrust and frustration. The result could be that you become too skeptical of all products and programs and you may miss out on the effective ones; you might decide to ignore all claims and just do nothing. Misleading claims and fraudulent products frequently turn people off from being physically active. They may also injure people. And finally, they indirectly steal money from legitimate fitness professionals. Money is spent on products that don't work rather than on programs that do work.

physical activity and health connection

Some consumers believe that certain products can make them more productive exercisers. These products are referred to as *ergogenic aids*. An **ergogenic aid** is any substance or phenomenon that enhances performance. Not all ergogenic aids are harmful. For example, endurance runners may eat a higher percentage of carbohydrates in the days leading up to a race. Carbo loading acts as an ergogenic aid by storing more fuel in your muscles. On the other hand, many body builders falsely believe that the consumption of large amounts of protein will aid in muscle development. There is no scientific evidence to support the consumption of extra protein to develop larger muscles (Wilmore & Costill, 1999). In fact, excessive intake of protein may lead to kidney and liver dysfunction (Wilmore & Costill, 1999).

Ergogenic aids Any substances or phenomena that enhance performance.

Ergolytic A substance that has a detrimental effect on performance.

Some substances generally thought to be ergogenic might actually be *ergolytic*. Instead of enhancing performance, they actually diminish performance. An **ergolytic** substance is one that has a detrimental effect on performance (Wilmore & Costill,

1999). Alcohol was once thought by many to aid sport performance by calming the nerves but we now know that alcohol adversely affects central nervous system function, coordination, and balance.

Many substances are used by people trying to gain an edge. If we add up the money spent on ergogenic aids and dietary supplements used by people in the belief that their performance will be enhanced, we would come up with a figure in the billions of dollars (Barrett, 2000). Table 15.1 includes a summary of the most commonly used substances.

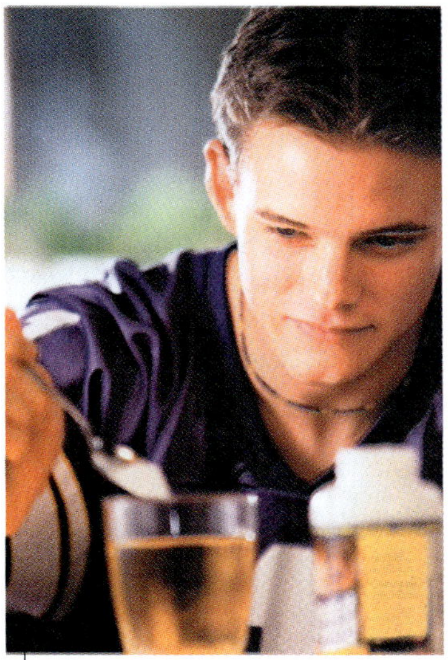

People try a wide variety of products in an attempt to enhance performance.

Fraud, Quackery, and Misinformation

To be an intelligent consumer of physical activity and fitness information, you need to know several terms. **Fraud** is a conscious promotion of unproven claims for profit. Most people hold an image of a fraudulent salesperson as one who sells watches out of a trench coat, or one who pedals snake oil on a shadowy corner. While there are certainly individuals who promote products knowing their claims cannot be true, many people promoting bad products may be unaware of the fraudulent intent of the manufacturer or distributor. Many promoters of fraudulent and misleading products are unwitting victims who themselves have been duped. They then share misinformation and personal experiences with others (Barrett & Jarvis, 2000). An example of fraudulent advertising is the "infrared body composition analyzer," which is discussed later in the chapter. **Quackery** is broadly defined as anything involving overpromotion of a product in the field of health (Barrett, 2000). This definition includes the promotion of questionable ideas as well as questionable products and services, regardless of the sincerity of their promoters (Barrett, 2000). An example of quackery would be the advertisements for "magnetic therapy," also discussed later.

2. The physical activity industry suffers from a wide range of misinformation and fraudulent claims.

Misinformation involves providing information that is not factual. In some cases, people actually believe that the products they support can produce the outcomes they are advertised to produce. They have been taken in by the marketing claims of a product and wish to share their "knowledge" with others. Friends, relatives, and neighbors who use the products and believe them to be effective typically introduce new customers to the product (Barrett & Jarvis, 2000). In these cases, there is no conscious effort to promote a useless product. Instead, misinformation is dispersed to a wider audience by people who think they know what a product can do. An example of misinformation is the common belief that shark cartilage can prevent cancer.

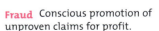

Explore www.pahconnection.com **15.1**

Common Marketing Techniques

Marketing usually involves an honest attempt to sell a product. However, we must be aware that the primary purpose of marketing is to persuade people to purchase products (Whitehead, 2000). This is true whether the person wants the product or not. There is a difference in the way products are marketed, based on the intent of the manufacturer. In some instances, marketing techniques rely on misinformation, deception, and fraud (Whitehead, 2000).

Those who seek to sell products through misleading ads, deception, or fraudulent practices use several common marketing techniques. Some examples include the misrepresentation of research, the use of testimonials ("It worked for me"), the promotion of unchallenged myths (excessive protein consumption for bigger muscles), and the quick fix (rapid weight loss, fitness is "easy"). Much of deceptive product marketing involves telling people something is bad for them (such as food additives) and selling a substitute, such as "organic" or "natural" food (Whitehead, 2000). Other common tactics can be found in Table 15.2.

Fraud Conscious promotion of unproven claims for profit.

Quackery Over-promotion of a product in the field of health.

Misinformation Information that is not factual, but is passed off as being factual.

TABLE 15.1 Proposed Ergogenic Aids and Mechanisms through Which They Might Work

	Act on heart, blood circulation, and aerobic endurance	Increase oxygen delivery	Supply fuel for muscle, and general muscle function	Act on muscle mass and strength
Pharmacological agents				
Alcohol	■	■		
Amphetamines	■			
Beta blockers	■			
Caffeine	■	■		
Cocaine and marijuana	■			
Diuretics	■			
Nicotine	■			
Hormones				
Anabolic steroids				■
Human growth hormone				■
Oral contraceptives				
Physiological agents				
Aspartic acid salts				
Bicarbonate loading				
Blood doping	■	■		
Erythropoietin	■	■		
Oxygen	■	■		
Phosphate loading	■	■		
Nutritional agents				
Amino acids	■		■	■
Chromium			■	■
Creatine			■	■
L-carnitine			■	

It is not always easy to spot misleading and fraudulent products or advertising. Marketers often use scientific jargon that can fool people not familiar with the concepts being discussed (Barrett, 2000). Even health professionals sometimes have difficulty separating fact from fiction in fields unrelated to their expertise (Barrett, 2000).

People also rely on personal experience and testimonials in deciding if a product works. If you feel better after having used a product, you usually associate those sensations with the product (Barrett, 2000). However, many ailments resolve themselves, or have symptoms that change frequently. Even serious conditions can have day-to-day variation in intensity (Barrett, 2000). An unscrupulous person can take advantage of this and mislead you into believing a fraudulent product was responsible for the temporary cessation of symptoms (Barrett, 2000).

In addition, just taking some sort of action often produces temporary relief of symptoms **(placebo effect).** You feel better because you feel that you are taking control of the situation (Barrett, 2000). Though the placebo effect is a psychological response, the body's physical response is not merely imagined—it is quite real. We know that your mental state can be effective in altering your physical state (Barrett, 2000). For example, when we get anxious, our heart begins to beat more rapidly.

TABLE 15.1 Proposed Ergogenic Aids and Mechanisms through Which They Might Work (cont.)

	Result in weight loss or weight gain	Counteract or delay onset or sensation of fatigue	Counteract CNS inhibition	Aid in relaxation and stress function
Pharmacological agents				
Alcohol				■
Amphetamines		■	■	
Beta blockers				■
Caffeine		■		
Cocaine and marijuana				■
Diuretics	■			
Nicotine				■
Hormones				
Anabolic steroids	■			
Human growth hormone	■			
Oral contraceptives				■
Physiological agents				
Aspartic acid salts		■		
Bicarbonate loading		■		
BLood doping		■		
Erythropoietin		■		
Oxygen		■		
Phosphate loading		■		
Nutritional agents				
Amino acids	■	■		
Chromium	■			
Creatine	■	■		
L-carnitine		■		

SOURCE: Adapted from E.L. Fox, R.W. Bowers, and M.L. Foss. (1988). *The physiological basis of physical education and athletics* (p. 632). Philadelphia: Saunders. Copyright © 1988 The McGraw-Hill Companies. Adapted by permission of The McGraw-Hill Companies.

Our own naiveté and gullibility often set us up for manipulation by misleading advertisers. People tend to believe what they hear often, and misleading information, particularly about nutrition, is everywhere (Barrett & Jarvis, 2000). As an example, the advertisements promoting the use of shark cartilage supplements to protect against cancer imply that sharks don't get cancer; so, if you take shark cartilage supplements, they claim you won't get cancer. In fact, sharks do get cancer and even get cancer of their cartilage.

Experience www.pahconnection.com 15.1

Individuals who have serious or chronic diseases that make them feel desperate enough to try anything that offers hope are extremely susceptible to fraudulent advertising. Alienated people, some of whom may experience paranoia, form another victim group (Barrett & Jarvis, 2000). These people may be convinced that our food supply is unsafe; that drugs do more harm than good; and that doctors, drug companies, large food companies, and government agencies are involved in conspiracies and not interested in protecting the public (Barrett, 2000). Such beliefs make them vulnerable to those who offer foods and healing approaches alleged to be "natural" (Barrett & Jarvis, 2000). For these reasons, controlled scientific studies are needed to establish whether fitness and nutrition products actually work.

TABLE 15.2 Common Deceptive Marketing Tactics Used to Promote Products

1. **Bait and switch** One product is focused on, but another is delivered.
2. **False claims (symptom free)** The claim that there are no side effects or symptoms associated with the use of a product.
3. **False expectations** The claim that the product will bring about results that sound too good to be true (they usually are!).
4. **Play upon fears (scare tactics)** Desperation marketing. Most effective for people desperately seeking change.
5. **Promise simple solutions to complex problems** "Take a pill and sleep away fat."
6. **Redundancy** Persuade you to purchase a product that might actually bring about advertised results, but is not necessary to achieve those results. An example might be an abdominal assistance contraption. A simple curl-up performed properly will provide the same result for free.
7. **Rarely provide scientific research to support claims (foreign research)** In America, the reference is to "European scientists" who have discovered some miracle product. In the rest of the world, it's "American scientists" who it is claimed have made the discovery.
8. **Rely on testimonials** It worked for me, therefore you should believe that it will work for you. Many of the people giving testimonials are being paid by the company to do so, and their objectivity must be questioned.
9. **Criticize the medical establishment (conspiracy)** Marketers tell you that the medical community doesn't want you to know about a product. They claim that there is a vast conspiracy being instigated by the medical community to withhold information from you.
10. **Money-back guarantees** Companies offer money-back guarantees with the knowledge that most people won't take the time or effort to seek their money back. In some cases, it costs more to get your money back than the total amount of money you get back.
11. **Cures or miracles** The manufacturer advertises their product in such a way as to imply that it will cure a disease or work miracles. Then, usually in small print and in a hard-to-find location, they issue a disclaimer that they don't intend to imply that the product cures any disease or causes the occurrence of a miracle.
12. **Celebrity endorsements** Companies hire famous spokespersons who tout their product. The hope is that you will connect the product with whomever the celebrity is and in some way think that the product had something to do with making this person a celebrity.
13. **Mass media marketing** The product is sold primarily through television, radio, newspaper, and magazine advertisements. You are saturated with ads pushing the product to the point that you come to associate the product with the advertising venue. Certain products are associated with certain TV shows. The intent is to get you to believe that the show (and/or actors) support the product.
14. **Buzz words (secret, rapid, etc...)** The advertising companies use buzz words to get your attention. They also try to focus your attention on the buzz words rather than on the product.
15. **Omission of facts** The marketers obscure or completely leave out certain facts that may keep you from purchasing their product. For instance, the may "forget" to tell you that there are certain side effects associated with use of the product. Another common example with weight-loss products is when the companies forget to tell you that their product only works when combined with a regular physical activity program and proper nutrition.
16. **For your eyes only** Advertising claims tell you that the product contains secret ingredients known only to a few people. This sometimes means that they don't know what is in the product, or they don't want you to know what is in the product. This method of advertising is meant to make you feel that you are being let in on the secret and are therefore special.
17. **Highly pedigreed** Individuals with multiple degrees from well-known institutions tout a product. Background checks on these individuals sometimes show that the person may never have attended, let alone graduated from, the institution from which they claim to have a degree. Another example is where someone is listed as a doctor to lend credence to a marketing claim. In many cases, the doctor is not a medical doctor, or has an area of expertise completely unrelated to the product they are pushing. One prime example is of a doctor with training in anesthesiology passing himself off as an expert in nutrition.
18. **Express mail** Many companies use express mail to deliver their product to you. One possible reason for doing this is because sending a fraudulent product through the U.S. mail constitutes mail fraud, which is a federal offense. By using express mail, the company skirts this law, since it does not apply to nongovernmental mailing agencies.
19. **Sex!** It is well known that sex is used to sell just about everything. This is also true in the physical activity and fitness industry. Remember that the product will not enhance your sex life or make members of the opposite sex desire you more just because you use it.

FACTS, FADS, AND FALLACIES

It can be very difficult to separate fact from fiction. This section provides an overview of some of the more common fallacies surrounding physical activity, exercise, and fitness.

3. You need to be aware of some common misconceptions, frauds, and fallacies.

Common Myths in Physical Activity and Fitness

Spot Reduction Myth The spot reduction myth implies that you can selectively reduce body fat in certain areas of your body by performing exercise that involves muscles in that area. The best example is performing sit-ups in an attempt to reduce abdominal fat. Spot reduction does not work. Your muscles receive energy (including energy from fat) from the bloodstream. Your body mobilizes fat from deposits throughout the body. Exercising a local muscle group does not cause your body to remove more fat from the deposits in that area. If spot reduction worked, everyone who chewed gum, or talked a lot, would have a lean face.

"Cellulite" Myth The "cellulite" myth has convinced some people that cellulite is a special type of cell that can be treated through the use of pills, lotions, and/or massage. In fact, a quick look through any anatomy book will demonstrate that there is no specific cell in the body called *cellulite*. What people refer to as cellulite is nothing more than adipose tissue (fat) that is surrounded by stretched connective tissue. Rapid onset, or rapid loss, of adipose causes the dimpling look associated with "cellulite." The connective tissue running throughout and around the fat cells take some time to adjust to the fluctuations in fat stores and appears to be stretched. The reduction of "cellulite" requires the same procedures as the reduction of body fat: expend more calories than you consume.

Muscle Stimulator/Passive Exercise Myth The muscle stimulator/passive exercise myth promotes weight loss and fitness gains without any effort by the person attempting to bring about these gains. The theory is that by applying muscle stimulators to a region of the body (for example, the abdominals) you can "get the equivalent of" a vigorous workout, or a thousand sit-ups. Other devices that promote this myth are passive motion tables that claim that all you need to do is relax on the table while the table does the work, moving your limbs to provide an effective workout. The problem with both of these types of devices is that the device does the work. The energy expended comes from the electrical outlet in the wall and not from your cells. Therefore, you are not expending any energy to bring about fat loss. In addition, there is no training effect of your neuromuscular system because using these devices does not require you to stimulate your own muscles.

Instant Gratification Myth The instant gratification myth suggests that you can take a magic pill to lose fat or improve performance. This myth is appealing to those people who do not want to put the time or effort into a physical activity program. The reality is that it takes time and effort to bring about changes in fitness. The idea that someone can take a pill to bring about these changes is just an illusion. The systems of your body (cardiovascular, muscular, skeletal) respond to regular physical activity and become stronger. A pill will not cause this response to occur.

Shake, Rattle and Roll Myth The shake, rattle and roll myth implies that you can vibrate, or massage away, unwanted fat. Adipose tissue (fat) is very resilient. Fat is designed to provide cushioning and shock absorption. In order to do this, fat must retain its structural characteristics when moved. Fat is also surrounded by connective tissue that has elastic properties allowing it to stretch and then regain its shape. In other words, fat bounces very well and is easily manipulated through massage. Shaking, rattling, or rolling fat will not make it disappear. To reduce body fat, you must expend more energy than you consume.

Torch Myth The torch myth suggests that by increasing your body temperature you can melt away fat. You will see people wearing rubberized suits, extra layers of clothing, or working out in a hot, humid environment in an attempt to lose fat. Working out like this will cause you to lose weight, but the weight lost will be almost exclusively water weight. The water lost will be replaced as soon as fluids are consumed post exercise. Additionally, losing water puts you at risk for thermal stress (heat exhaustion, heat stroke). When dehydrated, you cannot work as hard, so your rate of energy expenditure is actually lower. You need to make sure you allow your body to sweat when active and you must allow the sweat to evaporate. It takes a great deal of heat to melt fat (see how hot your grill must get to cook the fat on a piece of steak). If it were possible to raise your body temperature high enough to melt fat, other tissues and organs would also melt.

Body Beautiful Myth The body beautiful myth implies that if someone looks fit and attractive, they must be knowledgeable about physical activity and fitness. While this may be true in some instances, good genetics doesn't mean that the person has had the proper education to be an expert. Health clubs are full of people who are hired because they appear fit and because they can sell memberships. However, a brief conversation with some of these people will demonstrate that their knowledge of physical activity and fitness is extremely limited. Check to see that the person offering advice has a degree in exercise science or a related field from an accredited university. Check to see that they are certified by a reputable professional organization (American College of Sports Medicine, National Strength and Conditioning Association, American Council on Exercise).

Apples and Oranges Myth The apples and oranges myth suggests that exercise can turn fat cells to muscle cells and inactivity can turn muscle cells to fat. Fat and muscle cells are two completely different types of cells. You cannot turn one into the other. You can cause them to shrink (atrophy) or enlarge (hypertrophy) by eating too much and being inactive (fat hypertrophy), or eating in a rational way and being physically active (muscle hypertrophy).

Magical Potion Myth The magical potion myth promotes the rubbing of lotions on the skin to cause fat loss, remove lactic acid, or firm up your muscles. Fat will only be lost by expending more calories than you consume. The best way to do this is by eating wisely and maintaining a physically active lifestyle. Lactic acid is removed when oxygen becomes available in the muscle cells and bloodstream. This takes breathing and the delivery of oxygen to the cell. A good portion of the lactic acid is actually reconverted into pyruvic acid, which can then be used to supply energy to the cells (Wilmore & Costill, 1999). Lotions do not affect this process. Resistance training firms up muscles.

Vanishing Act Myth A common claim made by misleading advertisers is that their product will cause you to lose inches. This vanishing act myth suggests that the loss of inches is directly related to the loss of fat. In fact, most of what is lost in lost-inches claims is water. The water is replaced once the restrictive piece of clothing is removed, or once the person drinks fluids post exercise. Watch what happens after you remove a pair of socks with good elastic at the top. Initially you notice indentations on your skin where the elastic compressed water out of the region, but within a very short period of time the water returns and the indentations disappear. Losing inches is not important. For most people the goal is to lose fat. Losing inches does not necessarily relate to a reduction in fat.

"All Natural" Myth The "all natural" myth claims that only "natural" products are good for you. These products claim that anything that contains chemicals is bad for you. In reality, your entire body is composed of chemicals, as is everything surrounding you. Does the *All Natural* label always indicate that a product is good for you? Several substances come to mind that are all natural and are not at all good for you—things you probably don't want to ingest, including botulism, aflatoxin, salmonella, *E. coli,* rattlesnake venom, poison ivy, nicotine, and cocaine (Whitehead, 2000).

Sources of Information To be a wise consumer of physical activity, exercise, and fitness information, it pays to be skeptical about advertising claims, statements made by celebrities, "information" from info-mercials, and "breakthroughs" reported in the news media. You need to maintain a healthy degree of skepticism if you are to avoid misinformation and outright fraud.

To reduce the likelihood of becoming a victim of exercise and fitness fraud, it is important to develop the characteristics of intelligent consumer behavior. To become an intelligent consumer, you must learn to seek reliable sources of information.

Experience www.pahconnection.com 15.2

4. Being a critical consumer requires knowing where to turn for valid information.

Governmental Agencies

There are a number of places where you can get information on product safety and efficacy. The two agencies in the federal government directed to regulate product worthiness are the Food and Drug Administration (FDA) and the Federal Trade Commission (FTC). The FDA is one of our nation's oldest consumer protection agencies. It is housed within the Public Health Service, which in turn is a part of the Department of Health and Human Services. The FDA is charged with protecting American consumers by enforcing the federal Food, Drug, and Cosmetic Act and several related public health laws.

Explore www.pahconnection.com 15.2, 15.3, 15.4 15.5, 15.6, 15.7

Among other things, the FDA oversees food, medicines, and medical devices. It monitors the manufacture, import, transport, storage, and sale of approximately $1 trillion worth of products each year. The FDA is also involved in product testing, assessing risks, and weighing risks against benefits. Additionally, the FDA tests drugs and devices after they have been put on the market to monitor for any unexpected adverse reactions.

A second governmental agency involved in product safety and regulation is the Federal Trade Commission (FTC). The Federal Trade Commission enforces a variety of federal antitrust and consumer protection laws. The role of the FTC is to ensure that the nation's markets function competitively, and are vigorous, efficient, and free of undue restrictions. The FTC works to enhance the smooth operation of the marketplace by eliminating acts or practices that are unfair or deceptive.

The efforts of the FTC are directed toward stopping actions that threaten consumers' opportunities to exercise informed choice. The FTC also plays a major role in providing consumer education by making brochures available and by providing public service announcements.

Professional Health Organizations

You can also seek information from professional organizations such as the American College of Sports Medicine; the National Strength and Conditioning Association; the American Alliance for Health, Physical Education, Recreation and Dance; and the

American Council on Exercise. These organizations offer publications and videos that provide the best information available to date. They are staffed by people who research and teach about physical activity, exercise, and fitness.

Community Experts

You can also check to see if there are any experts in your local community who might be able to provide assistance. Local colleges and universities are a good place to start. Look particularly to see if they have one or more specialists in exercise science.

In addition you might be able to find someone who can help in a YM/YWCA, or in a commercial health club. Remember to check on their training, background, and credentials. Most people working in community settings are fully capable of providing accurate information, but occasionally you may run across someone who lacks the background to be an accurate source for you.

The Internet

Explore 15.8, 15.9, 15.10, 15.11

A final source of information is the Internet, which has some excellent sites providing reliable information. However, since the Internet lacks governmental regulation, you must be cautious in selecting your sources. A number of guides are available for evaluating the usefulness of websites (Kotecki & Siegel, 1998; Kotecki & Chamness, 1999).

SELECTING A PHYSICAL ACTIVITY PROGRAM

Earlier chapters in this book have outlined the components of an effective physical activity program. If you decide to follow a "canned" activity program (one developed by someone and marketed as all-inclusive), make sure the program contains all of the components covered in the preceding chapters. If you are thinking of using an exercise video, rent it first. Use caution and common sense. Don't attempt any activity that doesn't appear safe or logical.

Modify any program to fit your individual needs. If you are unsure about any claims or activities contained within the program, ask an expert to evaluate the product for you.

Not all fitness facilities are the same. Select one that meets your needs.

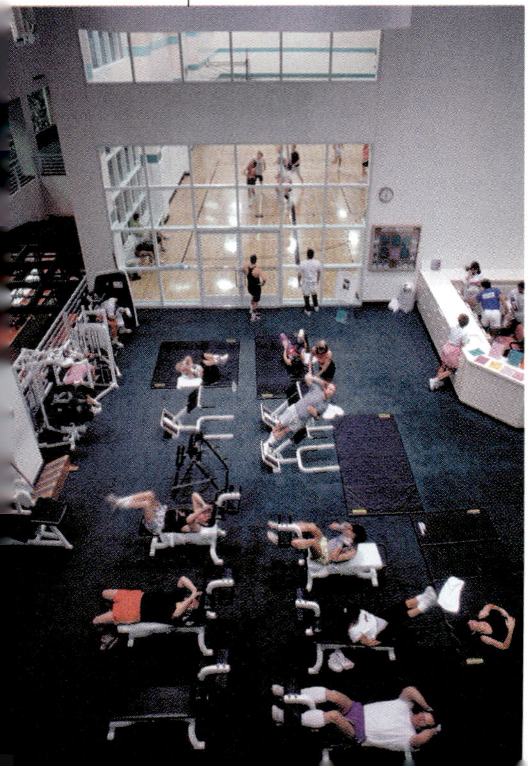

SELECTING A PHYSICAL ACTIVITY AND FITNESS FACILITY

If you choose to carry out your physical activity program in a health club or exercise facility, it is wise to do some scouting before paying membership dues. A good place to start is to make sure you understand why some of the people who join health clubs eventually leave. A common reason that someone stopped attending a health club is that they did not make sufficient use of their membership (Orejan, 2000). They might have paid dues for a certain amount of time and realized that they did not attend frequently enough to make the dues cost-effective. Rather than spending more money, they just drop out.

A second reason may be that they have lost interest or motivation (Orejan, 2000). This may be due to personal factors on the part of the member, or it may be that the facility did not provide a varied and stimulating environment. A third reason could be that they did not like the atmosphere in the facility (Orejan, 2000). It sometimes takes a while before you can determine if the facility fits your needs. You need to get to know the management and staff, of course, but realize that other customers may influence your decision as well. If you don't feel safe or feel comfortable around the other people in the facility, your adherence rate will suffer. Additionally, the physical environment of the facility may begin to wear on you and add to your dissatisfaction.

Many people quit when they realize the dreams they had when they joined have not been met by reality (Orejan, 2000). If your goals are set too high and you cannot reach them, you may become frustrated and lose interest.

You can take several steps to enhance the likelihood that you will retain your membership. Table 15.3 outlines several suggestions for selecting a health club.

TABLE 15.3 Guidelines for Selecting a Health Club

Prepare before you go.

- Identify your goals before joining a health club.
- Define your best workout environment.
- Set a budget.
- Determine the minimum amount of time you can devote to exercise and when you can do it.
- Shop around. Compare different health clubs.

Meet with the staff and get a thorough tour of the facility, its programs and amenities.

- Participate in, or at least observe, a couple of the group exercise classes.
- Check out the cardio and weight equipment. Do they have what you want?
- Visit the club at a time that you would like to work out.
- Make lists of things you like or dislike.
- Ask current members what they like and what needs improvement.
- Check the helpfulness, knowledge, and friendliness of the staff.
- See if the club is clean and well maintained.
- Is the facility crowded? Will you need to wait to work out?
- Is there sufficient variety of programs and activities?
- Is there child care, if needed?
- Is there sufficient, well-lit parking?
- Do you feel safe and comfortable?

Understand the contract agreement.

- Make sure you read and understand everything before you sign.
- Opt for shorter-term memberships.
- Find out if there is a grace period in the contract in case you change your mind.
- Do not be pressured by an aggressive sales pitch.
- Ask what the specific rules are under which you can terminate a membership, such as permanent illness, medical condition or injury, or relocation to a place not served by the club.

SOURCE: J. Orejan. (2000, March). How to select a fitness center. *Fitness Management, 16*(4), p. 48.

Once you have found a facility you like, don't hesitate to take advantage of everything it has to offer. Ask for instruction if you don't know how to use a piece of equipment. Make use of personal trainers if you need help designing a program. Exercise at your own pace; don't let someone else's pace put you at risk or act to de-motivate you (Orejan, 2000).

EXAMPLES OF MISLEADING PRODUCTS

When evaluating products for safety and efficacy, you must determine if the marketing claims made by the producer are scientifically plausible, valid, and reliable. The best way to make this determination is by investigating the scientific evidence provided through independent, rigorous research.

physical activity and health connection

One example of misleading advertising concerns the use of magnets for health and fitness. The producers of "magnet therapy" would lead you to believe that magnets can improve your health and fitness. One theory proposed by the marketers of magnet therapy is that the blood contains iron (in hemoglobin), so wearing magnets will aid in circulation and in maintaining proper blood flow because the iron in the blood draws the blood in the direction of the magnets. A second is that our body needs to be exposed to magnetic fields for good health. No scientific evidence supports these claims.

We are told that concrete and pavement and other human structures supposedly block the earth's magnetic fields. However, magnetic fields are not blocked by concrete. Simple proof can be found by taking a compass into any structure. Any place a compass works, the earth's magnetic fields are present (Gessell, 1999).

Secondly, the iron in blood is not magnetic. If it were, the human body would explode in the magnetic resonance imaging (MRI) machines commonly used in hospitals (Gessell, 1999). If the advertiser's claims were true, you would also be able to make a drop of blood on a table follow a handheld magnet as it passed over the top of the droplet.

Finally, individuals who work with magnets in industrial and research settings are exposed to magnetic field strengths 6 to 10 orders of magnitude greater than that created by the magnets promoted by supporters of magnet therapy (Gessell, 1999). We also know that DC magnetic fields have no measurable effect on the human body at levels strong enough to bend steel bars (Gessell, 1999).

Another example of misleading advertising arose from so-called infrared technology; it purported to give valid and reliable measures of body composition. The claim was that accurate measures of body fat could be made with an infrared device, and the device was found to be anything but reliable and provided no valid results. After FBI and FDA investigations, the head of the company that makes the device was sentenced in district court to 4 months home detention. He also was sentenced to 18 months' probation, a $3000 fine, and a $200 special assessment, plus settlements of $90,000 to the U.S. Customs Service and $50,000 to the U.S. Securities and Exchange Commission. The FDA's Office of Criminal Investigations received information that the clinical data used to validate the fat tester had been fabricated (Whitehead, 2000).

Dietary Supplement Health and Education Act of 1994

The nutritional supplement industry is an area frequently accused of fraud and deceptive advertising. For decades, the FDA regulated dietary supplements as foods. In most circumstances, this was done to ensure that they were safe and wholesome and that their labeling was truthful and not misleading. An important facet of ensur-

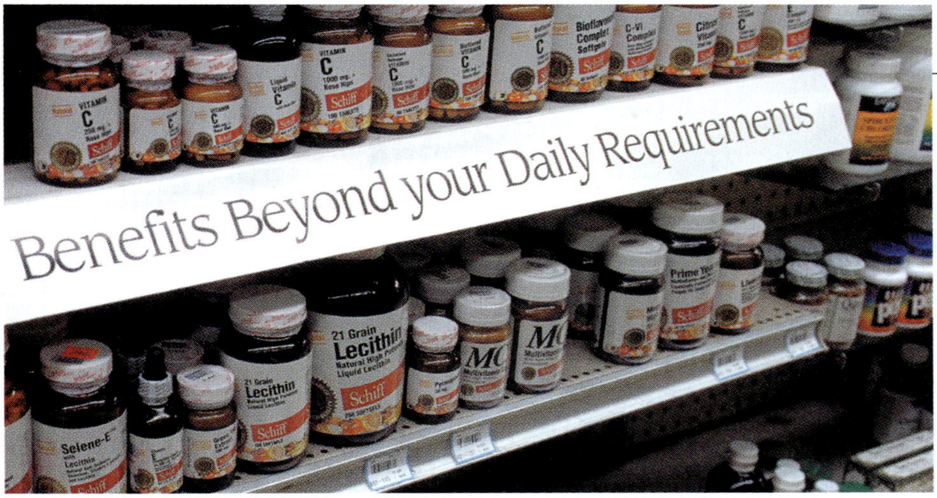

Many different products are marketed toward under-informed consumers.

ing safety was the FDA's evaluation of the safety of all new ingredients, including those used in dietary supplements, under the 1958 federal Food, Drug, and Cosmetic Act (FD&C Act).

However, with passage of the Dietary Supplement Health and Education Act of 1994 (DSHEA), Congress amended the FD&C Act to include several provisions that apply only to dietary supplements and the dietary ingredients of dietary supplements. As a result of these provisions, dietary ingredients used in dietary supplements are no longer subject to the pre-market safety evaluations required of other new food ingredients or for new uses of old food ingredients.

Several concerns have arisen with respect to DSHEA. What was supposed to provide "health freedom" for consumers has instead provided "marketing freedom" for manufacturers (Whitehead, 2000). Since there is no FDA regulation of nutritional supplements, there is no guarantee of what is actually in a product and whether the ingredients are safe or effective. Rather than controlled testing in an independent laboratory, the consumer pays to be a guinea pig (Whitehead, 2000). Regulation takes place only after a product has been shown to cause harm in humans.

Examples include the nutritional supplements containing ephedra or ma huang. Ephedrine alkaloids act as an "all natural" speed. They are banned by many sports organizations, and their side effects have been documented to kill and injure people (Whitehead, 2000). However, manufacturers of products containing ephedra still defend its use. It can be found in many dietary supplements and decongestants and puts many consumers unknowingly at risk (Whitehead, 2000).

SEEKING REDRESS

5. There are several avenues you can take in seeking redress.

When we are the victims of fraudulent or misleading advertising, we assume that we should "know better" and therefore deserve whatever we get as a consequence. This feeling is a major reason why journalists, law-enforcement officials, judges, and legislators seldom give priority to combating misleading products (Barrett, 2000).

We also operate under the false assumption that someone else is going to be looking out for us. In reality, we are on our own most of the time.

When you are seeking help, you can consult one of the agencies listed in Table 15.4. Victims of fraud often have difficulty obtaining redress through the courts. Many are afraid of lawyers. Some are embarrassed at having been fooled. Too often the victim does nothing, simply dismissing the fraud as one of life's lessons (Barrett, 2000).

One way of fighting back is to lodge a complaint with the Federal Trade Commission if you suspect that you have been victimized by fraud. The FTC may begin an investigation in a number of ways. Letters from consumers or businesses, Congressional inquiries, or articles on consumer or economic subjects may trigger FTC action. Investigations are either public or nonpublic. (Generally, FTC investigations are nonpublic in order to protect both the investigation and the company.)

If the FTC believes a violation of the law occurred, it might attempt to obtain voluntary compliance by entering into a **consent order** with the company. A company that signs a consent order need not admit that it violated the law, but it must agree to stop the disputed practices outlined in an accompanying complaint. If a consent agreement cannot be reached, the FTC may issue an **administrative complaint.** If an administrative complaint is issued, a formal proceeding that is much like a court trial begins before an administrative law judge: evidence is submitted, testimony is heard, and witnesses are examined and cross-examined.

If a law violation is found, a **cease-and-desist order** may be issued. If the company violates the order, the commission may seek civil penalties or an injunction. In some circumstances, the FTC can go directly to court to obtain an injunction, civil penalties, or consumer redress. This usually happens in cases of ongoing consumer fraud. By going directly to court, the FTC can stop the fraud before many consumers are injured. When issued, these rules have the force of law.

You can also seek to take legal action on your own. However, it is important to remember that health and nutrition fraud is not a specialty for most attorneys. Although the same general law applies, most lawyers have had no experience in dealing with such cases. Therefore dedicated, knowledgeable attorneys can be difficult to find (Barrett, 2000).

Explore 15.12

The National Council Against Health Fraud Task Force on Victim Redress helps victims of fraud obtain competent legal assistance. The services offered by this organization include: providing help in deciding whether to take the company to court; making referral to suitable attorneys; and providing information on unproven, fraudulent, and potentially dangerous treatments (Barrett, 2000). The task force can also help with locating expert witnesses, providing information on defense witnesses, and supplying reports on cases adjudicated, settled, and in progress (Barrett, 2000).

The Food and Drug Administration is another avenue for seeking redress. The FDA is responsible for performing inspections and seeking legal sanctions. If a company is found to be violating any of the laws that the FDA enforces, the FDA can encourage the firm to correct the problem voluntarily or to recall a faulty product from the market. A recall is generally the fastest and most effective way to protect the public from an unsafe product.

When a company can't or won't voluntarily correct a public health problem with one of its products, the FDA can bring legal sanctions to bear. The FDA can force a company to stop selling a product, or it can have items already produced seized and destroyed. It can also seek criminal penalties, including prison sentences.

Consent order An agreement bringing about voluntary compliance without a judicial ruling.

Administrative complaint An action that brings about a formal proceeding; much like a court trial, it takes place before an administrative law judge.

Cease-and-desist order A legal order informing a company that they must no longer advertise or market a product.

Separating Fact from Fallacy

Your best bet in separating fact from fallacy is to become an educated consumer. Staying abreast of the latest information about new products and techniques is a good way to get started. Learning to seek information from reliable sources and to question everything will make you less susceptible. Check out professional publications distrib-

TABLE 15.4 Agencies to Contact

PROBLEM	AGENCIES TO CONTACT
False advertising	FTC Bureau of Consumer Protection Council of Better Business Bureaus Editor or manager of media outlet where ad appeared
Product marketed with false or misleading claims	National or regional FDA office FDA Center for Drug Evaluation and Research State attorney general Consumer Broadcast Group State health department Local Better Business Bureau Congressional representatives
Bogus mail-order promotion	Chief Postal Inspector, U.S. Postal Service Regional postal inspector State attorney general
Adverse reaction to an herbal product or dietary supplement	FDA Special Nutritional Adverse Event Monitoring System
Dubious telemarketing	State attorney general FTC Bureau of Consumer Protection National Fraud Information Center
Improper treatment by licensed local or state professional society practitioner	Local hospital State professional licensing board National Council Against Health Fraud Task Force on Victim Redress Quackwatch.com
Improper treatment by unlicensed individual	Local district attorney State attorney general National Council Against Health Fraud Task Force on Victim Redress Consumer Broadcast Group
Advice needed about questionable product or service	National Council Against Health Fraud Consumer Health Information Research Institute Local, state, or national professional or voluntary health groups
Internet-related consumer problem	Cybercop Consumer Broadcast Group FDA Webguardian
Junk e-mail, including health-related scams and chain letters	FTC's e-mail box Consumer Broadcast Group

SOURCE: S. Barrett (2000). Quackwatch: Your guide to health fraud, quackery, and intelligent decisions. Online: http://www.quackwatch.com.

uted by professional associations. Learn how to use information available from governmental (FDA, FTC) and business organizations (Better Business Bureau). Make sure that product claims are proven to you. Be a skeptic. See if the manufacturer's claims are documented by **peer-reviewed research.** Make sure the product stands the test of time. Don't depend on others for protection.

There are certain things you can do to reduce the risk of being susceptible to misleading advertising. First, lead a healthy lifestyle. This will reduce your risk of becoming seriously ill and will lower your healthcare costs (Barrett, 2000). Living a healthy lifestyle also makes you less susceptible to desperation marketing (buying a product because you are desperate for change).

Peer-reviewed research Research articles and presentations in which experts in the field of study review material for accuracy and validity before it is disseminated to the public.

Understand the need for controlled scientific testing of products to ensure objectivity. Gather information as needed to determine which theories and practices are valid. Be wary of treatments that lack scientific support and a plausible rationale. Most treatments described as "alternative" fit the description of products whose claims have not been validated by carefully designed scientific research (Barrett, 2000).

Shop comparatively for equipment, exercise products, and nutritional aids. Report fraud, quackery, and other wrongdoing to appropriate agencies and law enforcement officials. Consumer vigilance is an essential ingredient of a healthy society (Barrett, 2000).

physical activity and health connection

Experience www.pahconnection.com 15.3

Understand the basic facts about physical activity. You must exercise to be fit. You must perform resistance training, secrete the proper hormones, and have good genetics to become strong and muscular. You must perform endurance exercise to obtain optimal cardiovascular fitness. You must combine regular exercise and sensible eating to maintain a healthy body composition. We are a product of our genetics, but we are also influenced by our environment. And finally, remember the credo of business: *Caveat emptor!* Let the buyer beware!

PHYSICAL ACTIVITY AND HEALTH CONNECTION

Regular participation in physical activity is intricately interwoven with a healthy lifestyle. To make sure your physical activity program is safe and effective, you must be a wise consumer of activity, exercise, and fitness information and products. Many products are sold to consumers that are misleading at best and fraudulent at worst. Even though there is a certain degree of governmental oversight of products available to consumers, the best defense against misleading advertising and fraudulent products is an informed consumer. Certain products can be dangerous and can lead to ill health. It is important to be vigilant when purchasing activity, exercise, and fitness products.

CONCEPT CONNECTION

1. **To develop a quality physical activity program, you must be a wise consumer of exercise information.** You must learn to protect yourself and keep yourself up-to-date on the latest information regarding what works and what doesn't work.
2. **The exercise industry suffers from a wide range of misinformation and fraudulent claims.** To avoid being misled, you need to be able to filter through advertiser claims and focus on what has been shown to work through independent research.
3. **You need to be aware of some of the more common misconceptions, fraud, and fallacies.** Many misleading and fraudulent advertisers recycle the same old exercise and nutrition myths. By learning what these myths are and why they don't make sense, you can help to protect yourself from being victimized.
4. **Being a critical consumer requires knowing where to turn for valid information.** Turn to governmental agencies such as the FDA and FTC, or professional health and fitness organizations for the straight facts on exercise and fitness products. Look for peer-reviewed research that evaluates products objectively.
5. **There are several avenues you can take in seeking redress.** Prevention is the best cure. However, if you feel that you need to seek redress, several outlets are available to you to help you take the right steps.

TERMS

Ergogenic aids, 350
Ergolytic, 350
Fraud, 351
Quackery, 351
Misinformation, 351
Consent order, 362
Administrative complaint, 362
Cease and desist order, 362
Peer-reviewed research, 363

MAKING THE CONNECTION

Janet learns that the diet pill contains mostly useless ingredients and a good deal of caffeine. The registered dietitian explains that the caffeine would temporarily increase Janet's metabolic rate and make her feel nervous, but that the effect would not last long. The impact on Janet's metabolic rate would not result in the loss of body fatness and could be dangerous for some people. She also tells Janet that she would have difficulty sleeping after taking the pill. Armed with this information, Janet feels confident about telling Kathy "Thanks, but no thanks!"

CRITICAL THINKING

1. Like Janet, we are constantly being bombarded with advertisements about a diet pill or drink that will *guarantee* losing X pounds per week. These advertisements are often seen on college and university campuses. As you walk to class, take a look around to see if you notice any of these advertisements. Record what you see. Also, review the most recent issue of your college or university newspaper. Are there any ads for fad diets or pills? If so, whom are they targeting?
2. In a popular magazine, find an advertisement that you believe might be misleading or fraudulent. Determine which of the advertising approaches are used to convince readers to purchase the product. What argument would you present to counter the advertising claims?
3. Speculate about why people often fall victim to common physical activity and health misconceptions frauds, or fallacies.
4. As a critical health consumer, where would you suggest peers go to find valid information on physical activity and health. Give three sources and explain how you determined they were valid.

REFERENCES

American College of Sports Medicine. (1998). Creatine supplementation and exercise performance. *Certified News* 8(2).

Barrett, S. (2000). Quackwatch: Your Guide to Health Fraud, Quackery, and Intelligent Decisions. Online: http://www.quackwatch.com

Barrett, S., & Jarvis, W.T. (2000). How quackery sells. *Nutrition Forum 17*(2):9–14.

Gessell, D. (1999). Magnet Therapy–Reader Response. Online: http://www.quackwatch.com/04ConsumerEducation/QA/magnet.html

Kotecki, J., & Siegel, D.E. (1998). Using a critical thinking/questioning approach to evaluate www information. *American Journal of Health Behavior* 22(1):75–76.

Kotecki, J., & Chamness B.E. (1999). A valid tool for evaluating health-related www sites. *Journal of Health Education. 30*(1):56–59.

Orejan, J. (2000). How to select a fitness center. *Fitness Management 16*(4):48.

Whitehead, J.R. (2000). *Exercise and Fitness Consumerism.* Presented at the American Alliance for Health, Physical Education, Recreation, and Dance conference. Orlando, Florida, March 21, 2000.

Wilmore, J.H., & Costill, D.L. (1999). *Physiology of Sport and Exercise,* 2nd ed. Champaign, IL: Human Kinetics.

ORGANIZATIONS TO CONTACT FOR HELP

Consumer Broadcast Group:
Online resource center for aggrieved consumers

Federal Trade Commission (FTC)
Bureau of Consumer Protection
Washington, DC 20580
Tel. (202) 326-2222

National Advertising Division
Council of Better Business Bureaus
845 Third Avenue, New York, NY 10022
Tel. (212) 753-1358

Food and Drug Administration (FDA)
5600 Fishers Lane, Rockville, MD 20857
Tel. (301) 295-8024

Chief Postal Inspector
U.S. Postal Service, Washington, DC 20260
Tel. (202) 268-4267

Consumer Health Information Resource Institute
300 E. Pinkhill Road, Independence, MO 64050
Tel. (816) 228-4595

Cybercop

Federal Bureau of Investigation (FBI)
935 Pennsylvania Avenue, N.W., Washington, D.C. 20535

National Council Against Health Fraud
P.O. Box 1276, Loma Linda, CA 92354
Tel. (909) 824-4690

Task Force on Victim Redress
Quackwatch.com
P.O. Box 1747, Allentown, PA 18105
Tel. (610) 437-1795

National Fraud Information Center
P.O. Box 65868, Washington, DC 20035
Tel. (800) 876-7060

For local or regional offices of federal agencies consult the telephone directory under U.S. Government.

Federal Government Agencies

Food and Nutrition Information Center
National Agricultural Library
10301 Baltimore Ave., Beltsville, MD 20705
(consumer inquiries)

Consumer Information Center
P.O. Box 100, Pueblo CO 81002
(free and low-cost publications)

Consumer Product Safety Commission
5401 Westbard Ave., Bethesda, MD 20207

Federal Trade Commission
6th & Pennsylvania Ave., N.W., Washington, DC 20580

President's Council on Physical Fitness and Sports
450 E. 5th St., Washington, DC 20201

Voluntary and Professional Organizations

Most of the organizations listed below are voluntary groups that draw support and members from the general public as well as professionals. Some have a single national office, while others have chapters in various cities. Most of these organizations provide educational materials on request. Some raise and distribute funds for research. Some conduct educational programs for the public and encourage and develop local support groups. Some offer individual counseling.

Business and professional groups, are composed exclusively or primarily of health professionals or other professionally trained individuals. Most of these groups publish a scientific journal and hold educational meetings for their members. Most of them also help the public by setting professional standards, disseminating information through the news media, and responding to inquiries from individual consumers.

Aerobics and Fitness Association of America
1520 Ventura Blvd., Sherman Oaks, CA 91403

American Alliance for Health, Physical Education, Recreation and Dance
1900 Association Drive, Reston, VA 22091

American College of Sports Medicine
P.O. Box 1440, Indianapolis, IN 46206

American Heart Association
7272 Greenville Ave., Dallas, TX 75231

SOURCE Barrett, 2000

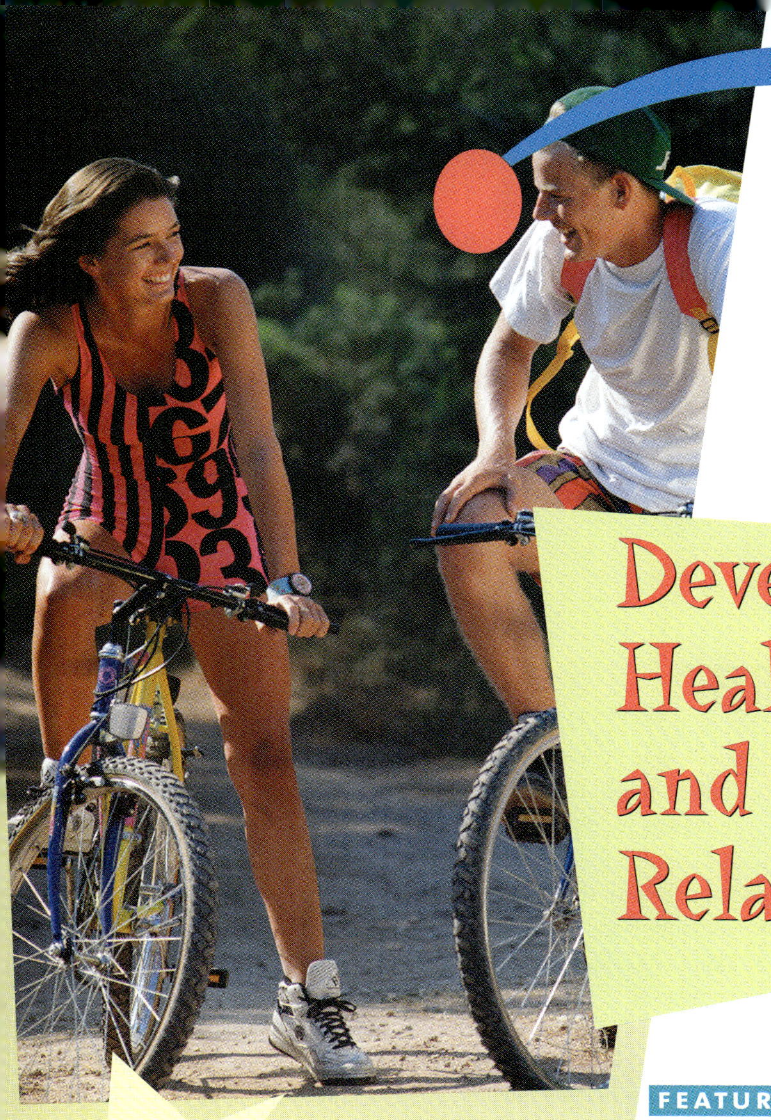

16 Developing Healthy Sexual and Intimate Relationships

CONCEPT CONNECTION

1. *Sex* refers to a person's biological classification as male or female.
2. A person's sexual biology is determined by genetic makeup, which in turn determines the nature of the sexual reproductive system.
3. A person's sexual psychology is rooted in gender identity, which guides gender role behaviors.
4. Sexual response involves four phases.
5. Effective communication is critical for developing and maintaining relationships.

FEATURES

E-Learning Tools: www.pahconnection.com

Engage www.pahconnection.com

16.1 Identification: female sexual organs
16.2 Identification: male sexual organs

Experience www.pahconnection.com

16.1 Sexuality education in the schools: issues and answers

Explore www.pahconnection.com

16.1 Sexuality Information and Education Council of the United States (SIECUS)
16.2 The Alan Guttmacher Institute
16.3 Kinsey Institute for Research in Sex, Gender, and Reproduction

Activities & Assessments

16.1 Would you say you had sex if . . .
16.2 Do you know your level of communication?

WHAT'S THE CONNECTION?

Jeff and Susan have been dating for nearly a year—long enough to take each other for granted. This is most apparent at social gatherings with others. Jeff is very outgoing. He likes to "circulate," so he leaves Susan either with her friends or by herself, and he talks to his own friends or introduces himself to strangers. This bothers Susan because she would like to be included. But even more bothersome to her is that Jeff doesn't come back to spend time with her or include her in his conversations with others. Susan resents this. She has often told Jeff how she feels, but he says she is being unreasonable. Susan feels more angry and hurt each time Jim leaves her alone at social events. When this happens now she doesn't talk to him for a day or two.

INTRODUCTION

Sexuality represents a truly holistic aspect of living, for it involves the simultaneous expression of mind, body, and spirit—the whole self. Although it is common to find sexuality represented in advertising and other media as having to do solely with physical gratification, most people are aware that sexuality involves much more than the stimulation of the body's sex organs. Sexuality involves thoughts, feelings, and identity. Sexuality is a powerful form of communication between people.

From the standpoint of physical activity and health, sexuality is an area over which you have considerable individual control. You choose when and with whom you wish to share sexual activity, and which feelings you wish to express in sexual ways. With some fundamental knowledge of sexual biology, you can conduct your sexual life responsibly, avoiding disease and freely choosing whether and when to have children. This chapter introduces the topic of sexuality and discusses the nature of the sexual self and of sexual expression.

1. *Sex* refers to a person's biological classification as male or female.

Activities & Assessments 16.1

Sex (1) An individual's classification as male or female based on anatomical characteristics, (2) a set of behaviors, (3) the experience of erotic pleasure.

Gametes Sex cells, either sperm or ova, that fuse at fertilization; gametes carry a complete set of genetic information from each parent that is passed on to the child.

Fertilization The fusion of a sperm cell and an ovum.

DEFINING SEX AND SEXUALITY

Understanding terminology is critical to good communication and relationships, including sexual relationships.

Sex

Sex can refer to (1) an individual's classification as male or female as determined by the presence of certain anatomical and physiological characteristics, (2) a set of behaviors, and (3) the experience of erotic pleasure.

At the most fundamental biological level, **sex** refers to the mating of two anatomically distinct individuals, a male and a female, each of whom manufactures specific cells, or **gametes**, which fuse to become the first cell of a new person. To facilitate the fusion process (called **fertilization**), males and females of a species possess specific organs and display certain behaviors that are intended to bring about the union of gametes.

Often the word *sex* is used to denote aspects of individuals' personal characteristics that are thought to derive from their biological classification. Thus, the biological property of femaleness is associated with the social quality of "femininity," and the biological property of maleness is associated with the social quality of "masculinity." Although most modern dictionaries still define sex as having to do with personality characteristics, this concept is more accurately referred to as *gender* to distinguish its origins in culture rather than biology.

Besides biological classification, sex is also associated with certain behaviors that are defined as **sexual.** These activities usually involve touching, in various ways, certain anatomical regions of the body, such as the genitalia and breasts, and sexual intercourse.

Sexual Characterized by, or having, sex; opposed to asexual.

Sexuality A person's sense of self, which is used to create sexual experiences.

Sexual orientation Attraction toward and interest in members of one or both genders.

Heterosexual Someone who is attracted to people of the opposite gender.

Bisexual Someone who is attracted to members of both genders.

Homosexual Someone who is attracted to people of the same gender

Gender identity Awareness and acceptance of being male or female.

Explore www.pahconnection.com 16.1, 16.2

Experience www.pahconnection.com 16.1

Sexuality

Sexuality, as distinct from sex, consists of the aspects of a person's sense of self that are used to create sexual experiences. Another term for sexuality is *the sexual self,* which has several dimensions:

1. The *physical dimension* refers to any region of the body to which an individual gives sexual meaning, including the organs and organ systems we employ to create erotic experiences (the skin, the genitals). It also includes the physical features that define us to ourselves and others as a sexual being.
2. The *psychological dimension* refers to our emotions and our conscious and unconscious beliefs that guide the interpretation of experience. This aspect of sexuality generates strategies for actions that are intended to satisfy our wants and needs.
3. The *social dimension* refers to sexual attitudes and behaviors that affect our interactions with members of the social groups to which we belong.
4. The *orientation dimension* refers to the tendency to feel "naturally" attracted to people of a particular gender, and the ability to bond emotionally with them. About 85 to 90 percent of Americans have a **sexual orientation** to members of the opposite sex **(heterosexuals)**; the rest of the population orients to individuals of either sex **(bisexuals)** or, more often, exclusively to members of the same sex **(homosexuals).** Individuals do not choose their sexual orientation; it develops as a fundamental aspect of a person's personality. Scientific studies have failed to uncover genetic, hormonal, metabolic, or psychological mechanisms underlying sexual orientation.
5. The *development dimension* is the evolution of our self throughout a lifetime. This evolution includes the body, the belief systems, and the ways sex is employed to create and maintain intimacy.
6. The *skill dimension* speaks to the physical and social skills that affect how well we meet our sexual wants and needs.

GENDER IDENTITY AND GENDER ROLE

Although anatomy and physiology explain the biological basis of human sexuality, most people's sexual experiences also involve beliefs, thoughts, feelings, and social behaviors. How individuals come to think and behave sexually is almost entirely a product of what they learn as children about the kinds of behaviors that are expected of members of one sex or the other. The development of **gender identity** and the subsequent expression of sex-specific behaviors begins with the sex typing of newborn infants. When a child is born, almost the first thing

2. A person's sexual biology is determined by genetic makeup, which in turn determines the nature of the sexual reproductive system.

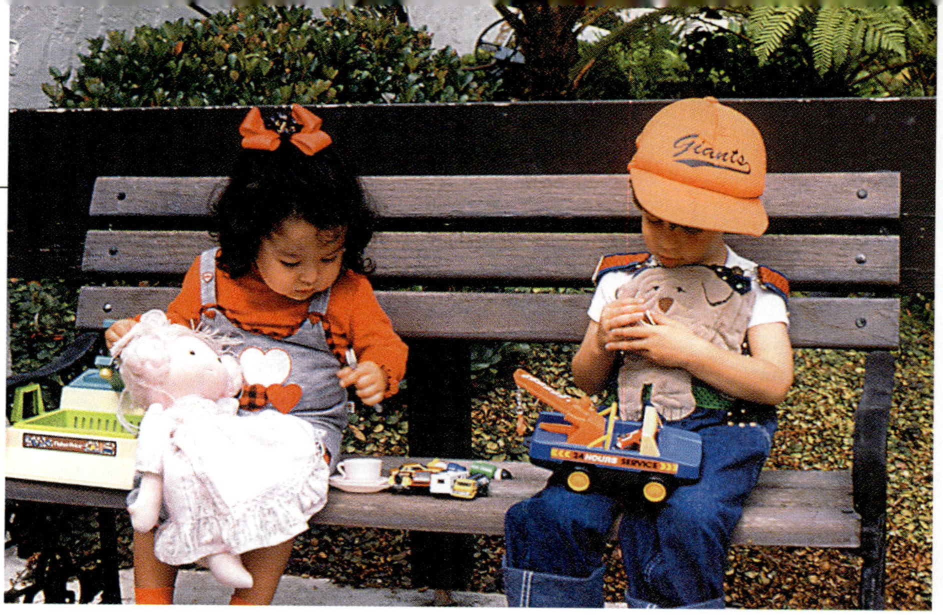

Young girls and boys learn their gender identities and roles at an early age.

noticed is its biological sex as determined by the appearance of its external genitals. If the infant is born with a penis, those attending the birth will exclaim "It's a boy!" Similarly, "It's a girl!" follows the observation of a newborn's female genitals.

Having been sex-typed at birth, the infant is thereafter treated by adults in a manner they think appropriate for a child of that sex, and eventually the infant incorporates into its self-image the awareness of being a male or a female. This awareness is called gender identity, and gender-specific behaviors are referred to as the **gender role.**

3. A person's sexual psychology is rooted in gender identity, which guides gender role behaviors.

Engage www.pahconnection.com 16.1

Gender role Complex group of behaviors expected of males and females in a given culture.

Ova, ovum Eggs, egg

Secondary sex characteristics Anatomical features appearing at puberty that distinguish males from females.

Ovaries A pair of almond-shaped organs in the female abdomen that produces egg cells (ova) and female sex hormones (estrogen and progesterone).

Fallopian tubes A pair of tube-like structures that transport ova from the ovaries to the uterus; the usual site of fertilization.

Uterus The female organ in which a fetus develops.

Vagina Female organ of copulation, and the exit pathway for the fetus at birth.

SEXUAL BIOLOGY

One of the fundamental roles of sexuality is biological reproduction. The reproductive role of the male is to produce reproductively capable sperm and to deposit them in the female reproductive tract during sexual intercourse. The reproductive role of the female is to provide reproductively capable eggs, called **ova,** and to provide a safe, nutrient-filled environment in which the fetus develops for the 9 months of pregnancy.

The genetic determination of sexual anatomy also specifies the pattern of male or female steroid hormone production, which in turn affects the **secondary sex characteristics** that distinguish adult males and females: the extent and distribution of facial and body hair, body build and stature, and the appearance of breasts (Figure 16.1).

Female Sexual Anatomy

A woman's internal sexual organs consist of two **ovaries,** which lie on either side of the abdominal cavity, the **fallopian tubes,** the **uterus,** and the **vagina;** together these structures make up a specialized receptacle and tube that goes from each ovary to the outside of the body (Figure 16.2). The function of the ovaries is to produce fertilizable ova as well as sex hormones, which control the development of the female body type, maintain normal female sexual physiology, and help regulate the course of a normal pregnancy. The fallopian tubes gather and transport the ova that are released from the ovaries (about one each month). The fallopian tubes connect to the uterus, an organ about the size of a woman's fist, which is situated just behind the pelvic bone and the bladder (Figure 16.3). The uterus is part of the passageway for sperm as they move from the vagina to the fallopian tubes to effect fertilization; after fertilization, it provides the

CONCEPT CONNECTION

1. ***Sex* refers to a person's biological classification as male or female.** Beyond the biological classification, sex is associated with sexual behaviors. Sexuality is distinct from sex and consists of aspects of a person's sense of self that are used to create sexual experiences.
2. **A person's sexual psychology is rooted in gender identity, which guides gender role behaviors.** Gender identity is the sense of *being male* or *being female*.
3. **A person's sexual biology is determined by genetic makeup, which in turns determines the nature of the sexual reproductive system.** Female and male reproductive biology is genetically determined at conception. Secondary sex characteristics externally distinguish males and females from one another. Males: testes, sperm ducts, semen-producing glands, and penis. Females: ovaries, fallopian tubes, uterus, vagina, and external genitalia.
4. **Sexual response involves four phases.** *Excitement:* person experiences sexual arousal and physiological changes begin (penile erection, vaginal lubrication). *Plateau:* physiological changes begin to level off. *Orgasm:* sexual experience climaxes. *Resolution:* physiologically, the body returns to a nonaroused state.
5. **Effective communication is critical for developing and maintaining relationships.** Communication occurs between two people: a sender and a receiver. The messages we send (verbally and by our actions) are sometimes misread; therefore, it is critical that communication between two people be clear and that both the sender and receiver establish good listening habits.

TERMS

Sex, 368
Gametes, 368
Fertilization, 368
Sexual, 369
Sexuality, 369
Sexual orientation, 369
Heterosexual, 369
Bisexual, 369
Homosexual, 369
Gender identity, 369
Gender role, 370
Ova, ovum, 370
Secondary sex characteristics, 370
Ovaries, 370
Fallopian tubes, 370
Uterus, 370
Vagina, 370
Cervix, 372
Ovulation, 372
Clitoris, 372
Labia minora, 373
Labia majora, 373
Breasts, 373
Testes, 373
Penis, 373
Copulation, 373
Scrotum, 373
Seminal vesicles, 374
Prostate gland, 374
Cowper's glands, 374
Semen, 374
Foreskin, 374
Circumcision, 374
Smegma, 374
Myotonia, 374
Vasocongestion, 374
Sexual response cycle, 374
Orgasm, 375
Self-disclosure, 376
Literal message, 379
Metamessage, 379
I-statements, 380
You-statements, 380
Feedback, 380

MAKING THE CONNECTION

Jeff and Susan realized that their relationship was very important to them and that they both needed to work on their communication skills. The communication skills they agreed to work on included sending clearer messages to one another by using I-statements and employing effective listening techniques like making eye contact, being empathic, acknowledging and praising the sender's message, and giving verbal feedback to one another.

CRITICAL THINKING

1. Read the following scenario and identify several communication problems. How could Bob and Sandy have handled this differently?

   Bob: Well, Sandy, you know that this weekend is the big reunion of all my fraternity brothers, and I'd like you to join me in celebrating our 100-year anniversary!

   Sandy: Now you ask! I've already told my theater group that we would join them for their weekend outing.

   Bob: Great, you didn't even ask me, you just went ahead and made plans for me this weekend!

   Sandy: Ask you? You have been so busy lately with work and school, I haven't even had a chance to talk to you, let alone ask you if you wanted to spend the weekend with me and the theater group.

   Bob: Oh great, now it is my fault that I've been working so hard and trying to get good grades. Go ahead, blame it on me!

   Sandy: Okay! It's your fault we never spend any time together. I'm sick of this! What will it be, *your* fraternity brothers or me?

   Bob: Well, now I'm having to choose between you and my fraternity brothers. That's easy! My fraternity brothers any day—at least they understand how hard it is to work and go to school!

2. "An intimate relationship may be sexual, but a sexual relationship is not necessarily an intimate one." Discuss the difference(s) between an intimate relationship and a sexual relationship.
3. Identify ten terms that are gender-biased. Example: fireman.
4. Identify five television shows that have characters in stereotypical male or female roles. Identify the characters and briefly explain the role they play.
5. Complete Engage 16.4, "Do You Know Your Level of Communication?" Do you feel your score accurately represents your level of communication with the person you have in mind? Why or why not?
6. Do you and/or your partner wish to increase your level of communication? If so, what steps will you take to do so?

REFERENCES

Masters, W., & Johnson, V. (1966). *Human Sexual Response.* Boston: Little, Brown.

Activities & Assessments

NAME ____________________ SECTION ____________ DATE ____________

16.1 Would You Say You Had Sex if . . .

Would you say you "had sex" with someone if the most intimate behavior you engaged in was . . .

Behavior	YES	NO
1. Deep kissing (french or tongue)	☐	☐
2. Oral contact on your breast/nipples	☐	☐
3. Person touches your breast/nipples	☐	☐
4. You touch your breast/nipples	☐	☐
5. Oral contact on other's breasts/nipples	☐	☐
6. You touch other's genitals	☐	☐
7. Person touches your genitals	☐	☐
8. Oral contact with your genitals	☐	☐
9. Penile-anal intercourse	☐	☐
10. Penile-vaginal intercourse	☐	☐

Compare your responses with your partner.

SOURCE: S.A. Sanders and J.M. Reinisch. (1999). Would you say you "had sex" if. . . ? *JAMA*, 281(3):275–277.

Activities & Assessments

NAME ____________ SECTION ____________ DATE ____________

16.2 Do You Know Your Level of Communication?

Purpose This exercise is designed to provide some indication of the level of communication in your relationship with your partner or a close friend.

Directions With one person in mind, respond to each of the following questions by checking yes or no in the column to the right.

Behavior	YES	NO
1. Do you feel that your partner does not understand you?	☐	☐
2. Do you know how to dress to please your partner?	☐	☐
3. Are you able to give constructive criticism to each other?	☐	☐
4. In appropriate places, do you openly show your affection?	☐	☐
5. When you disagree, does the same person usually give in?	☐	☐
6. Are you able to discuss money matters with each other?	☐	☐
7. Are you able to discuss religion and politics without arguing?	☐	☐
8. Do you often know what your partner is going to say before he/she says it?	☐	☐
9. Are you afraid of your partner?	☐	☐
10. Do you know where your partner wants to be in five years?	☐	☐
11. Is your sense of humor basically the same as your partner's?	☐	☐
12. Do you have the persistent feeling you do not really know each other?	☐	☐
13. Would you be able to relate an accurate biography of your partner?	☐	☐
14. Do you know your partner's secret fantasy?	☐	☐
15. Do you feel you have to avoid discussion of many topics with your partner?	☐	☐
16. Does your partner know your biggest flaw?	☐	☐
17. Does your partner know what you are most afraid of?	☐	☐
18. Do you both take a genuine interest in each other's work?	☐	☐
19. Can you judge your partner's mood accurately by watching his/her body language?	☐	☐
20. Do you know who your partner's favorite relatives are and why?	☐	☐
21. Do you know what it take to hurt your partner's feelings deeply?	☐	☐
22. Do you know the number of children your partner would like to have after getting married?	☐	☐

SCORING

Look over your responses and give yourself one point for each yes response for numbers 2, 3, 4, 6, 7, 8, 10, 11, 13, 14, and 16 to 22, and one point for each no response to 1, 5, 9, 12, and 15.

IF YOU SCORED:

1–5: This indicates there is little communication between you and your partner. However, you are together, so you must be fulfilling some need through your relationship. Perhaps the two of you simply need to develop better communication.

6–9: Your relationship is lacking in communication, but perhaps you are trying to increase the communication.

10–14: There are weak areas in your relationship, but you probably know they exist. Just keep working on the development of open and honest communication.

15–18: You have a great relationship as it is, but you do have your differences. With open communication you are learning to deal with your differences, which will strengthen the relationship.

19–22: You may be in love; at least you have a great understanding of what it takes to make a relationship continue growing and enduring.

REACTIONS

Use the space provided to respond to the following questions:

1. Do you feel your score accurately represents your level of communication with the person you have in mind? Why or why not?

____

____

____

____

____

____

____

____

(continued)

16.2 Do You Know Your Level of Communication? (cont.)

2. Do you and/or your partner wish to increase your level of communication? If so, what steps will you take to do so?

SOURCE: R.F. Valois and S. Kammerman. (1992). *Your sexuality: A self-assessment* (p. 96–97). New York: McGraw-Hill.

17

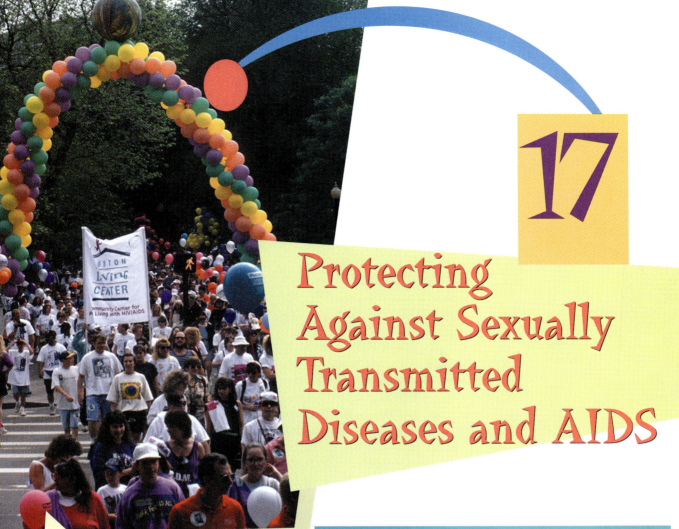

Protecting Against Sexually Transmitted Diseases and AIDS

CONCEPT CONNECTION

1. Sexually transmitted diseases (STDs) are infections passed from person to person, most frequently by sexual contact.
2. Sexually transmitted diseases (STDs) are epidemic in the United States.
3. Certain sexual behaviors increase your risk of contracting an STD.
4. Common STDs include *Trichomonas* and *Gardnerella vaginalis,* chlamydia, gonorrhea, syphilis, herpes, genital warts, pubic lice, and scabies.
5. AIDS is caused by the human immunodeficiency virus (HIV).
6. Prevention is key!

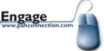

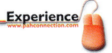

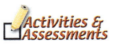

FEATURES

E-Learning Tools: www.pahconnection.com

Engage www.pahconnection.com

17.1 Unspeakable truth STD quiz
17.2 Unspeakable truth STD risk profiler

Experience www.pahconnection.com

17.1 Ask NOAH about: AIDS and HIV
17.2 CDC National Prevention Information Network (CDC NPIN)

Explore www.pahconnection.com

17.1 National Center for HIV, STD, and STD Prevention: Division of Sexually Transmitted Diseases
17.2 American Social Health Association
17.3 Expanding the response: HIV/AIDS and the World Bank
17.4 The *Journal of the American Medical Association* HIV/AIDS Information Center
17.5 Safersex

Activities & Assessments

17.1 Can you be assertive when you need to be?

WHAT'S THE CONNECTION?

Ken has a close friend, Amy, whom he loves very much. Ken has never been closer to anyone than he is to Amy. They attend the same college and get along well. Amy and Ken are best friends, and they have a close relationship, but Ken wants to take it to the level of sexual intimacy to show the depth of his love. Amy values the intimacy she has with Ken, but is not sure she is ready for sex, or that she even wants to include sexual intimacy and intercourse in their relationship. She feels uncomfortable discussing her feelings about these issues with Ken.

INTRODUCTION

Approximately twenty types of infections can be passed from person to person through sexual contact. Traditionally, these infections have been called venereal diseases, or VD—the word *venereal* is derived from Venus, the Roman goddess of love. To identify their origins more clearly, these diseases are now called **sexually transmitted diseases,** or **STDs.** You will also see them referred to as a sexually transmitted infection (STIs), which does not have such a negative connotation as STDs do. In this book we will refer to them as STDs. Diseases of sexual organs, which occur in both sexually active and sexually abstinent individuals, are referred to as **sexually related diseases (SRDs).**

1. Sexually transmitted diseases (STDs) are infections passed from person to person, most frequently by sexual contact.

The number of people infected with STDs is a major concern for our society. Throughout the world, an estimated 333 million new cases of STDs occur each year among adults—15 million in the United States (Centers for Disease Control and Prevention [CDC], 2000a; American Social Health Association [ASHA], 1998). A recent CDC study indicates that STDs account for more than 85 percent of the most common infectious diseases reported. Young people between 20 and 24 years of age make up 42 percent of the STDs (ASHA, 1998). The economic costs of STDs are enormous, especially when we include treatment for infertility (often due to STDs), treatment for pelvic inflammatory disease, and STD treatment. In addition, there are the serious human costs from lost work and study, as well as the physical suffering due to STDs.

2. Sexually transmitted diseases (STDs) are epidemic in the United States.

Explore www.pahconnection.com **17.1**

UNDERSTANDING SEXUAL BEHAVIOR

People accept different levels of risk in life. Certain sexual behaviors increase the risk of contracting an STD, so it is important to know what they are. Understanding your sexual behaviors will allow you to make the appropriate decisions and decrease your risk of contracting an STD, becoming pregnant, or impregnating someone.

3. Certain sexual behaviors increase your risk of contracting an STD.

Sexually transmitted diseases (STDs) Diseases that are primarily contracted through sexual contact.

Sexually related diseases (SRDs) Diseases of the reproductive system that occur in either sexually active or sexually inactive individuals.

Multiple Sexual Partners

There is a large pool in our society of unmarried, sexually active people because many individuals become active in late adolescence. This group consists of those who delay marriage until their mid-to-late twenties and early thirties, or later, and those who are divorced or widowed and have subsequent sexual partners. One-third of unmarried, sexually active people report having more than one sexual partner in the previous year (Kost & Forrest, 1992).

False Sense of Security

Using birth-control pills tends to decrease the use of condoms and spermicides, both of which help prevent transmission of STDs. The availability of antibiotics has made many people less fearful of sexually transmitted diseases. They believe that, as long as there is a cure for syphilis and gonorrhea, there is nothing to worry about.

Absence of Signs and Symptoms

Some STDs have very mild, or no, symptoms, which permit a worsening of the infection and the possibility of unknowingly passing it to others. Most people with chlamydia have no symptoms, for example. Approximately 80 percent of women who contract gonorrhea do not know it. People infected with the human immunodeficiency virus (HIV) can have mild or no symptoms for years, yet still be infectious.

Untreated Conditions

Some individuals lack sufficient knowledge of the signs and symptoms of STDs to know that they are infected. Those who are not accustomed to seeking health care, or who cannot afford it, are less likely to seek treatment for an infection. Furthermore, many individuals with STDs do not comply with treatment regimens. When medications are not taken for the required length of time, an infection may not be completely eradicated even though symptoms may disappear, and people who do not complete treatment may still be infectious.

Impaired Judgment

The use of drugs, including alcohol, can increase the risk of transmitting STDs because people with impaired judgment do not stop to think about using condoms. Also, people in this state may be more likely to have sex with someone they do not know; this also means they know nothing of their partner's sexual and drug history.

Lack of Immunity

Some STD-causing organisms, especially viruses, can escape the body's immune defenses, causing individuals to remain infected and to transmit the infection. This may permit re-infection and it also makes the development of vaccinations difficult to impossible.

REACTIONS TO STDS

Many people who contract a sexually transmitted disease are embarrassed or ashamed to discuss it with their healthcare provider or partner. There are usually two reactions to a sexually transmitted disease: (1) it is shameful to have one, and (2) "It won't happen to me."

Explore 17.2

Value Judgments

Unlike nearly all other kinds of infections, STDs are associated with sinfulness, dirtiness, condemnation, shame, guilt, and disgust. These negative attitudes keep people from getting check-ups, contacting partners when an STD has been diagnosed, and talking to new partners about previous exposures. In the nineteenth century, when syphilis was a scourge of Europe, rather than trying to prevent its spread (effective treatments had not yet been invented), countries blamed the disease on the weak character or immorality of their neighbors: the English referred to syphilis as the "French disease," and the French called it the "Spanish disease." This prejudice and scapegoating helped spread the disease.

Denial

With respect to contracting a STD, many people think "It can't happen to me" or "This person is too nice to have an STD" or "This isn't the type of person who would have an STD." Because there are no vaccinations against the infectious agents that cause sexually transmitted diseases, the only way to prevent them is for sexually active individuals, who are not in *monogamous* (lifelong single-partner) sexual relationships, to assume responsibility for protecting themselves and their partners. This means becoming aware of the signs and symptoms of the common STDs and seeking treatment when such signs occur. It means that sexually active people who have more than one partner within a year should obtain periodic (about every 6 months) STD check-ups. It also means knowing about and practicing "safer sex."

COMMON STDS

4. Common STDs include trichomonas and *Gardnerella vaginalis,* chlamydia, gonorrhea, syphilis, herpes, genital warts, pubic lice, and scabies.

Although many nonviral STDs can be treated with medications, the epidemic of STDs persists worldwide (Holmes, 1994; World Health Organization [WHO], 2000). There are no vaccinations for either the bacterial or viral infections that cause the most common sexually transmitted diseases. Dealing directly and responsibly with STDs is not easy. However, we owe it to the people we care about to do so. Table 17.1 outlines the major STDs, including their symptoms and treatment.

Engage www.pahconnection.com 17.1

Trichomonas and Gardnerella

Referred to as a sexually related disease (SRD), vaginal infections caused by the protozoan ***Trichomonas vaginalis*** and the bacterium ***Gardnerella vaginalis*** are transmitted during intercourse. Symptoms tend to occur only in women (vaginal itching and a cheesy, odorous discharge from the vagina), but the organisms can survive in the urethra of the penis and under the penile foreskin. A man who harbors these organisms can infect other partners or even reinfect the partner who transmitted the organisms to him. Medications can eliminate these infections, and it is essential for both partners to undergo treatment.

Trichomonas vaginalis Trichomonas is caused by a protozoan; symptoms include a foul-smelling, foamy-white or yellow-green discharge that irritates the vagina.

Gardnerella vaginalis Bacterium that causes vaginal infection; symptoms include vaginal irritation.

Chlamydia Sexually transmitted disease caused by the bacterium *Chlamydia trichomatis.*

Chlamydia

Chlamydia is caused by the bacterium *Chlamydia trichomatis,* which specifically infests certain cells lining the mucous membranes of the genitals, mouth, anus, and rectum, the conjunctiva of the eyes, and occasionally the lungs. The chlamydial bacteria bind to their surfaces and induce the host cells to engulf them. After gaining entrance to the cell, these organisms resist a host cell's defenses and eventually "steal" from the host cell the biochemical compounds required for their own survival. The

TABLE 17.1 Common Sexually Transmitted Diseases (STDs)

STD	SYMPTOMS	TREATMENT
AIDS	Flu-like symptoms followed by any of a number of diseases characteristic of immunodeficiency	New drugs may retard vital reproduction temporarily. Opportunistic infections can be treated to some degree.
Chlamydia	Usually occur within 3 weeks: infected men have a discharge from the penis and painful urination, women may have a vaginal discharge, but often are asymptomatic	Antibiotics
Gardnerella vaginalis	Yellow-green vaginal discharge with an unpleasant odor; painful urination; vaginal itching	Metronidazole
Genital warts	Usually occur within 1 to 3 months: small, dry growths on the genitals, anus, cervix, and possibly mouth	Podophyllin
Gonorrhea	Usually occur within 2 weeks: discharge from the penis, vagina, or anus; pain on urination or defecation or during sexual intercourse; pain and swelling in the pelvic region; genital and oral infections may be asymptomatic	Antibiotics
Hepatitis B	Low-grade fever, fatigue, headaches, loss of appetite, nausea, dark urine, jaundice	
Genital herpes	Usually occur within 2 weeks: painful blisters blisters on site(s) of infection (genitals, anus, cervix); occasionally itching, painful urination, and fever	None; acyclavir relieves symptoms
Pubic lice	Usually occur within 5 weeks: intense itching in the genital region; lice may be visible in pubic hair; small white eggs may be visible on pubic hair	Gamma benzene hexachloride
Syphilis	Usually occur within 3 weeks: a chancre (painless sore) on the genitals, anus, or mouth; secondary stage—skin rash—if left untreated; tertiary stage includes diseases of several body organs	Antibiotics
Trichomonas vaginalis	Yellowish-green vaginal discharge with an unpleasant odor; vaginal itching; occasionally painful intercourse	Metronidazole

SOURCE: G. Edlin, E. Golanty, and K. McCormack Brown. (1999). *Health and Wellness* (6th ed., p. 222). Boston: Jones and Bartlett.

chlamydial organisms use the stolen nutrients to reproduce and multiply, and ultimately the host cells die.

In the United States and other Western countries, chlamydia is the most prevalent sexually transmitted disease. In as many as half of all cases, chlamydia occurs simultaneously with gonorrhea.

One reason that chlamydial infections are so prevalent is that infected individuals often have extremely mild or no symptoms. Thus, infected individuals can unknowingly transmit the infection to new sex partners. When symptoms do occur, they include pain during urination in both men and women (dysuria) and a whitish discharge from the penis or vagina. Symptoms generally appear within 7 to 21 days after infection.

An infection caused by chlamydia can be readily treated with antibiotics if diagnosed early. Left untreated, the chlamydial bacteria can multiply and cause inflammation and damage of the reproductive organs in both sexes. In men, untreated chlamydia can result in inflammation of the epididymis **(epididymitis)** characterized by pain, swelling, and tenderness in the scrotum, and sometimes by mild fever. In women, untreated chlamydia can lead to **pelvic inflammatory disease (PID).**

Epididymitis Inflammation of the epididymis (structure that connects the vas deferens and the testes).

Pelvic inflammatory disease (PID) Infection of the female reproductive organs; specifically, the uterus, fallopian tubes, and pelvic cavity.

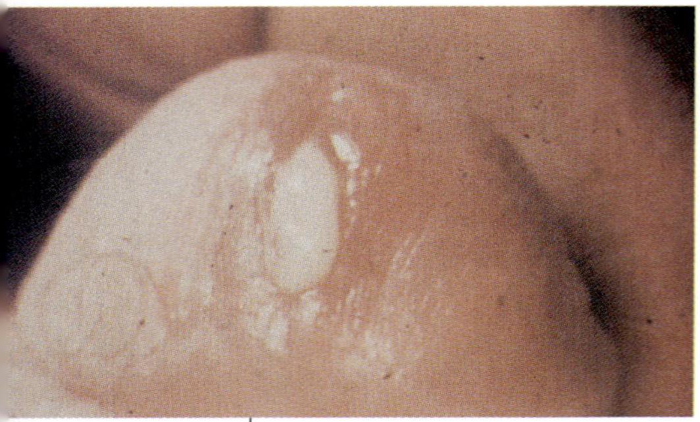

Gonorrheal discharge from the penis.

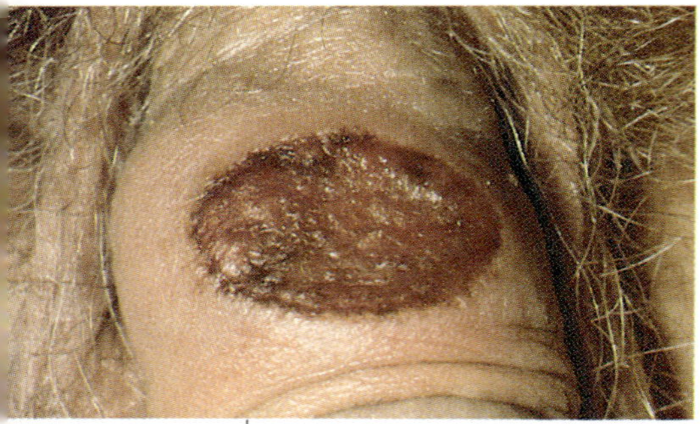

The first physical sign of a syphilis infection is an open lesion called a chancre.

Gonorrhea

Gonorrhea, also know as "the clap" or the "drip," is caused by the bacterium *Neisseria gonorrheae.* Gonorrheal organisms specifically infect the mucous membranes of the body, most often the genitals, reproductive organs, mouth and throat, anus, and eyes. *N. gonorrhea* cannot survive on toilet seats, doorknobs, bedsheets, clothes, or towels. Transmission in adults almost always occurs by genital, oral, or anal sexual contact; infection of the eyes occurs by hand (often through self-infection). Gonorrhea has seen an increase in new cases after more than a decade of declining numbers (CDC, 2000b).

Although the bacteria causing them are quite different, the symptoms of gonorrheal and chlamydial infections are very similar. Like chlamydia, many people infected with gonorrheal organisms do not develop symptoms and their infections go unnoticed. If the infection progresses, men may develop epididymitis and women may develop infections of the uterus, fallopian tubes, and pelvic region. *Such infections may cause sterility.* When symptoms appear, they include painful urination in both sexes and a yellowish discharge from the penis or vagina. Occasionally there is pain in the groin, testes, or lower abdomen. The first symptoms of gonorrhea usually appear within 7 to 10 days after exposure.

Gonorrhea can be treated with antibiotics. However, new antibiotic-resistant strains of the organism are constantly evolving. In nearly half of all cases of gonorrhea, chlamydia also is present. Individuals undergoing diagnosis for gonorrhea should also be tested for chlamydia.

Syphilis

Syphilis is caused by a spiral-shaped bacterium called *Treponema pallidum.* These organisms are transmitted from person to person through genital, oral, and anal contact, as well as being acquired from blood. Syphilis can also be transmitted from a mother to her unborn fetus, perhaps as early as the ninth week of pregnancy.

The first noticeable sign of syphilis is a painless open sore called a **chancre** (pronounced "shanker"), which can appear any time between the first week and third month after infection. If the infection is not treated within that period, the chancre will heal and the disease will enter a secondary stage, characterized by a skin rash, hair loss, and the appearance of round, flat-topped growths on most areas of the body. Left untreated, the signs of the secondary stage also disappear, and the infection enters a symptomless (latency) period during which the syphilis organisms multiply in many other regions of the body. In the final, tertiary stage, the disease damages vital organs, such as the heart or brain, causing severe symptoms and leading to death. Syphilis can be treated with antibiotics at any stage of the infection.

Herpes

Herpes is caused by the virus *Herpes simplex,* or HSV. Various strains of HSV can cause cold sores on the mouth ("fever blisters"), skin rashes, mononucleosis, and lesions on the penis, vagina, or rectum. Each year up to 500,000 adults acquire a genital herpes infection. As many as 1 out of 4 American adults have already been infected with genital herpes.

Genital herpes infections are caused most frequently by the viral strain HSV-2. Oral herpes is caused most frequently by HSV-1. However, both HSV-2 and HSV-1 can cause genital and oral infections with virtually identical symptoms. Thus people with oral herpes can transmit the infection to partners via oral sex. Once a person has been

Gonorrhea Sexually transmitted disease caused by the bacterium *Neisseria gonorrhea.*

Syphilis Sexually transmitted disease caused by spirochete bacteria *(Treponema pallidum).*

Chancre The primary lesion of syphilis, which appears as a hard, painless sore or ulcer, often on the penis or vaginal tissue; pronounced "shanker."

Herpes Sexually transmitted disease caused by *Herpes simplex* virus, or HSV.

infected, oral HSV-1 infections tend to recur much more frequently than do oral HSV-2 infections. Conversely, genital HSV-2 infections tend to recur more frequently than genital HSV-1 infections. Oral herpes can occur without sexual contact; however, genital herpes cannot occur without some form of sexual contact, either vaginal, anal, oral, or through masturbation.

A herpes lesion on the genitals usually appears within 2 to 20 days after contact with the virus. Transmission of the virus via bed linen, clothing, towels, toilet seats, and hot tubs is highly unlikely. The major symptoms of a genital herpes infection are the presence of one or more blisters, which eventually break to become wet, painful sores that last about 2 or 3 weeks; fever; and occasionally pain in the lower abdomen. Eventually these initial symptoms disappear, but the herpes virus remains dormant in certain of the body's nerve cells, permitting periodic recurrences of the symptoms, called "flare-ups," at or near the site(s) of the initial infection. Stress, anxiety, improper nutrition, sunlight, and skin irritation can bring on flare-ups.

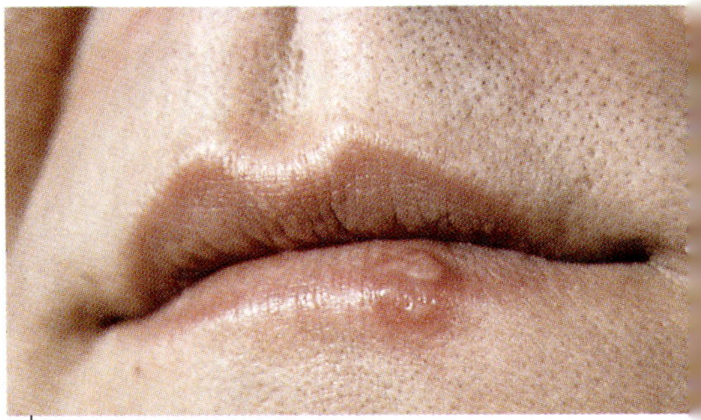

A cold sore is common among people infected by HSV.

There is no cure for herpes. Infected individuals remain so for life. The drug *acyclovir* can minimize the duration and severity of the symptoms of an initial infection or a flare-up.

Herpes is extremely contagious when a sore is present. People with open lesions should avoid sex with others until the lesions disappear. Even if no sore is present, transmission is possible, although much less likely, through the "shedding" of viral particles from the skin.

Because the herpes virus remains in the body, and because flare-ups are a persistent possibility, some people believe that infected persons can never be sexually active. This is not true. People with herpes can learn to manage the condition. In many instances, after one or two episodes, they can recognize an oncoming flare-up because they get a tingling sensation, itching, pain, or numbness at the site of the initial infection. This can be a signal to refrain from sexual contact. If used appropriately, this signal can protect against the spread of herpes.

Because genital herpes is associated with a risk of cervical cancer, women with herpes are especially urged to have annual Pap smears to ascertain the condition of the vagina and cervix.

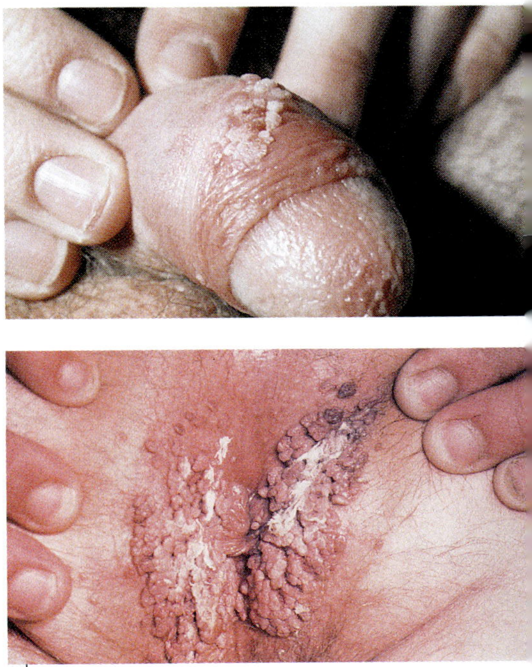

Genital warts on the penis (upper), and vaginal (lower) area.

Sexually Transmitted Warts

Sexually transmitted warts *(Condylomata acuminata)*, also known as genital or venereal warts, are hard, cauliflower-like growths that appear in men on the penis, in women on the external genitals and cervix, and in both sexes in the anal region. Warts are caused by several of the approximately sixty varieties of **human papillomavirus, HPV.** When HPV infects skin cells and cells of the genital tract, it causes them to multiply, thus forming the wart. Infection with many varieties of HPV is often more of a nuisance than it is dangerous.

Sexually transmitted warts usually appear about 3 months after contact with an infected person. They can be removed by coating the wart with a liquid containing podophyllin, which dries the wart. In severe cases, wart removal is accomplished by freezing the warts with liquid nitrogen or removing them with laser surgery.

Sexually transmitted warts Hard growths on the skin of the genitals or anus, caused by an infection with human papillomavirus, or HPV.

Human papillomavirus (HPV) Genus of viruses including those causing papillomas (small nipple-like protrusions of the skin or mucous membrane) and warts.

Hepatitis B

Hepatitis B is a disease of the liver caused by the hepatitis B virus (HBV). Hepatitis B is transmitted sexually and in blood, similar to HIV transmission, whereas other types of hepatitis are transmitted in fecally contaminated food. Hepatitis B is more easily

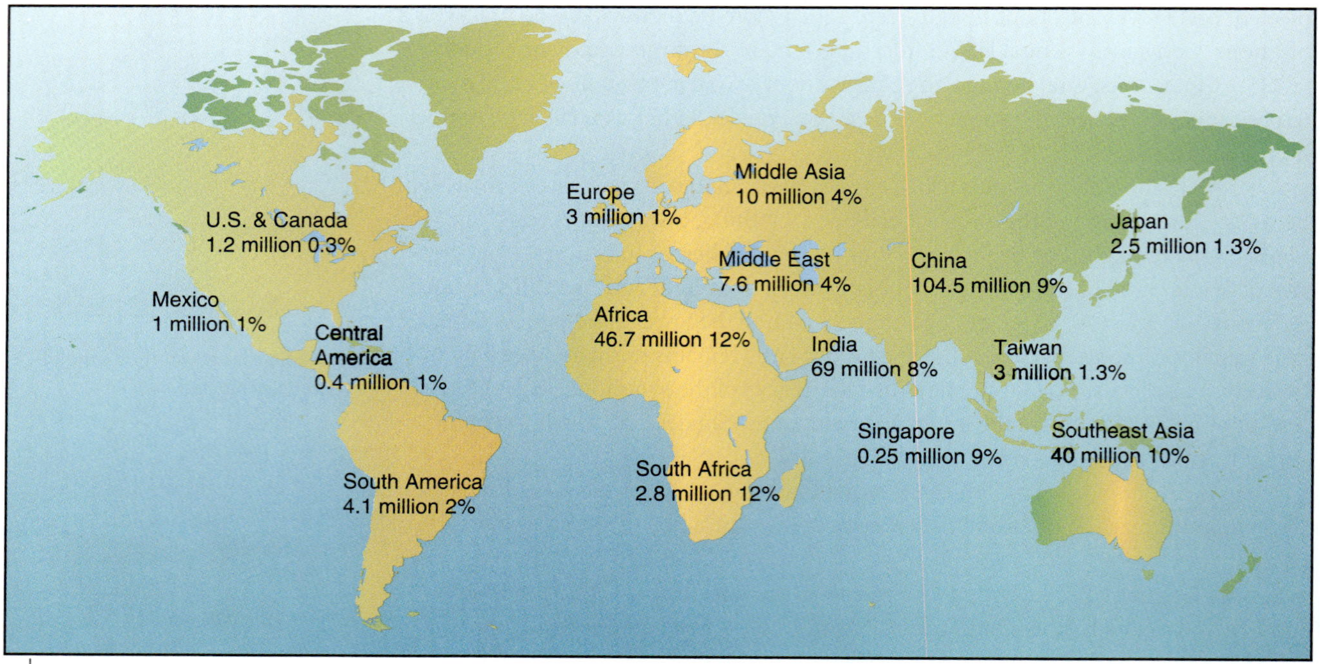

FIGURE 17.1

Hepatitis B Infection Worldwide. The number of people infected with Hepatitis B virus in 1997 in the world and the percentage infected in each region.

SOURCE: World Health Organization (1997).

transmitted than HIV and it is estimated that worldwide there are 300 million people infected with HBV (Figure 17.1). You are at increased risk of contracting HBV if you are sexually active, have unsafe sex, have sex with more than one partner, have another STD, work in healthcare, or share needles. You can also contract HBV if you are exposed to an infected person's blood via cuts or open sores. Although it is very rare in the United States, you can contract the hepatitis B virus through transfusions of infected blood or blood products.

There is no cure for HBV; however, an HBV vaccine is available and everyone is advised to be vaccinated—especially children, healthcare workers, and others who are at high risk of exposure (sexually active). The CDC recommends HBV vaccination for infants and young adults before they become sexually active.

Pubic Lice

Pubic lice *(Phthirus pubis),* also known as "crabs," are barely visible insects that live on hair shafts primarily in the genital-rectal region and occasionally on hair in the armpits, beard, and eyelashes. The organisms' claws are specifically adapted for grasping hairs with the diameter of pubic and axillary hair, which differs in diameter from the shafts of scalp hair. Thus pubic lice are not usually found on the head (scalp hair is the ecological niche of the head louse, *Pediculus humanus capitis*).

Lice feed on blood taken from tiny blood vessels in the skin, which they pierce with their mouths. Some people are sensitive to the bites and may experience itching, which is often the main symptom of infestation. The lice can also been seen; they look like small freckles. The eggs of lice are enclosed in small white pods (called "nits"), which attach to hair shafts. The presence of nits is also a sign of infestation.

Transfer of lice is via physical—usually sexually—contact. They can also be transmitted via contact with objects on which eggs might have been laid, such as towels, bed linens, and clothes. An infestation of pubic lice can be eliminated by washing the pubic hair with liquids or shampoos containing agents that specifically kill lice (pyrethrins,

Pubic lice Small insects that live in hair in the genital-rectal region.

piperonyl butoxide, and gamma benzene hydrochloride). All of an infected person's clothes, towels, and bed linens should also be washed with cleaning agents made specifically for killing lice.

Scabies

Scabies is an infestation of certain regions of the skin by extremely small (invisible to the naked eye) mites, *Sarcoptes scabiei*. The mites burrow into the skin where they live and lay eggs. The tiny lesions produced by the mites often cause intense itching, which is the major sign of a scabies infection. The mites produce tiny burrows across skin lines, which often go unnoticed. Occasionally, an infestation will produce small round nodules. The mites tend to live in the webs between the fingers, on the sides of fingers, and on the wrists, elbows, breasts, abdomen, penis, and buttocks. Rarely do mites live on the face, neck, upper back, palms, or soles.

Scabies can be transmitted both sexually and nonsexually. All that is required is close personal contact. The itching and physical symptoms often take several weeks to appear. Scabies can be treated with topical agents that kill the mites and their eggs.

Acquired Immune Deficiency Syndrome (AIDS)

Cause of AIDS AIDS is caused by **human immunodeficiency virus,** or **HIV.** HIV infection causes disease by destroying immune-system cells and weakening the body's immune system, and it also damages certain cells in the brain. Destruction of the body's immune system leaves HIV-infected individuals susceptible to a variety of bacterial, viral, and fungal infections that a person with an intact immune system could readily ward off. Individuals who are HIV-positive are also susceptible to cancer because the immune system normally protects the body against it. AIDS patients tend to develop cancer of the immune system (lymphoma) and a skin cancer called **Kaposi's sarcoma.** An HIV infection in the brain leads to loss of mental faculties (AIDS dementia).

AIDS, like cancer, is not a single disease. AIDS is defined by the CDC as having one or more of twenty-seven specific infectious diseases plus 200 or fewer CD4 T-cells in the blood. (A normal CD4 T-cell level is 800–1200 cells per milliliter of blood).

Incidence of AIDS Trends of HIV infection and AIDS in the United States indicate that as many as 1 million persons may be infected. Although the infection has occurred primarily in men, the numbers of infected women are growing. HIV infection is a public health problem not only in the United States but also around the world. About 80 percent of reported new cases now arise in developing countries where no funds are available for AIDS education and prevention programs. At the end of the century approximately three-quarter of a million people had been diagnosed with AIDS in the United States (CDC, 2000c).

A survey by the National Opinion Research Center (1995) indicated that 30 percent of adults say they changed their sexual behaviors because of AIDS. Of these, 29 percent used condoms more often, 26 percent limited their sexual activity to one partner, 25 percent are more selective in partners, 11 percent abstain from sexual intercourse, and 11 percent have reduced their number of sexual partners. Clearly, these behaviors will help reduce the risk of contracting HIV; however, everyone needs to practice "safer sex" behaviors.

Methods of Transmission The HIV virus is transmitted exclusively via blood, semen (which contains small amounts of blood), and vaginal fluids. The HIV virus is

5. AIDS is caused by the human immunodeficiency virus (HIV).

Explore www.pahconnection.com 17.3

Experience www.pahconnection.com 17.1

Scabies Infestation of the skin by microscopic mites (insects).

Human immunodeficiency virus (HIV) The virus that causes AIDS; it causes a defect in the body's immune system by invading and then multiplying within the white blood cells.

Kaposi's sarcoma Skin cancer commonly associated with HIV infection.

AIDS Acquired immune deficiency syndrome caused by HIV.

not transmitted by touching the skin or clothes of an infected person, by saliva, by shared toilets or by air, food, or water that has been touched by an infected person. Indeed, hardly any HIV transmission has been found among family members who live in intimate contact with HIV-infected hemophiliacs who received the virus from HIV-contaminated blood products used to treat their hereditary bleeding disorder.

HIV is a **retrovirus**, which means that once it gains entry to a cell it incorporates itself into the host cell's DNA. This allows HIV to manufacture many copies of itself, which eventually infect neighboring cells. Because HIV incorporates itself into host cells, it cannot be eliminated from an infected person's body. HIV infections are life-long.

Within a few weeks of individuals' becoming infected with HIV, they usually experience flu-like symptoms from which they eventually recover. Their immune systems are still intact and they produce copious antibodies to HIV. The mounting of an immune response in the early phases of an HIV infection provides the basis for HIV testing. Nearly all of the tests for HIV infection detect antibodies to HIV. A positive result ("seropositive") indicates that a person has been exposed to sufficient quantities of HIV particles to mount an immune response. The first stage of HIV infection is known as *silent infection*.

Some HIV-infected individuals will progress to the second stage of infection, *symptomatic infection*. The first signs of AIDS are usually mononucleosis-like symptoms (swollen lymph glands, fever, night sweats) and possibly headaches and impaired mental functioning caused by HIV infection of the brain. As the disease progresses, individuals often suffer weight loss, infections on the skin (shingles) or the throat ("thrush"), and one or more opportunistic infections, perhaps including cancer.

Explore www.pahconnection.com 17.4, 17.5

Because there is now no way to rid the body of HIV and hence cure AIDS, the best treatment available to infected individuals is for the opportunistic infections that result from immune suppression. In addition, there have been attempts to slow the replication of the virus. Because many viral diseases have been conquered by vaccination, much effort has gone into developing vaccines against HIV, so far without success. The only effective way to control the spread of AIDS is to prevent the transfer of HIV from person to person. This is accomplished by using condoms and spermicides (which destroy the virus), reducing exposure to infected individuals, and avoiding casual sex.

6. Prevention is key!

There are many unresolved questions about HIV and AIDS. Much more needs to be learned to reach a complete scientific understanding of HIV and its role in AIDS. In the meantime, everyone should avoid high-risk sexual behaviors and support AIDS research and prevention programs to stop the spread of this fatal disease.

Engage www.pahconnection.com 17.2

Experience www.pahconnection.com 17.2

PREVENTING SEXUALLY TRANSMITTED DISEASES

Preventing STDs requires that societies provide continuous, widespread public health programs and services for STD education and treatment. It is also crucial that infected individuals seek prompt treatment, take responsibility for not infecting other individuals, and practice "safer sex" to lower their risk of infection.

The stigma associated with STDs is a great hindrance to prevention efforts. Viewing STDs in moral terms—that is, associating them with dirtiness and immorality—makes people reluctant to think and talk about them. It also makes society want to ignore

Retrovirus A type of virus (such as the one that causes AIDS) that can invade cells and integrate its own genetic information into chromosomes.

STD epidemics. During World Wars I and II, American society supported massive gonorrhea and syphilis control programs; as a result, the incidence of these infections dropped tremendously. When the threat of a postwar STD epidemic seemed to wane, moralistic concerns thwarted the continuation of control efforts, and the incidence of STDs increased. Public health officials realize that ongoing efforts are the only way to control STDs.

Judgmental attitudes also make talking about STDs difficult. To have to tell a partner that you have an STD, or even to say that you once had an infection and are now perfectly OK, can bring feelings of guilt and shame, which can lead to avoiding the discussion altogether. Similarly, to ask about a partner's previous STDs may be interpreted as an accusation that the person is "loose" or immoral. To avoid feeling embarrassed or avoid the risk of offending a sexual partner, people are likely to dodge the topic of STDs. Prevention would be enhanced if sexually active individuals developed an open attitude about talking about STDs (and other aspects of sex) and acquired the necessary communication skills.

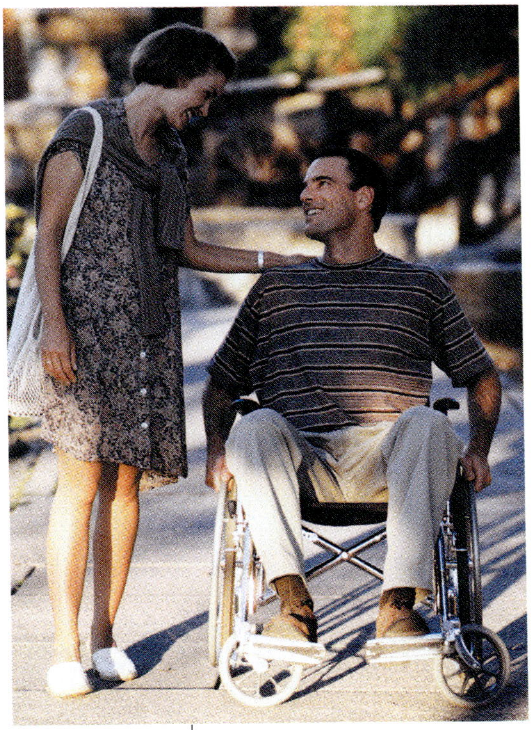

Everyone has a responsibility to practice "safer sex."

Practicing Safer Sex

The surest way to reduce the risk of acquiring a sexually transmitted disease is to abstain from sexual intercourse. This does not mean that you have to give up sexual interaction. There are many ways of giving and receiving sexual pleasure without engaging in sexual intercourse: touching, kissing, exchanging a massage, even sleeping together without intercourse.

Another way to reduce risk is to know a partner's sexual history, including all high-risk activities in which a partner may have engaged. Often this kind of information is difficult to gain early in a relationship, because exchanging information about sexual histories requires a level of trust that takes some time to develop.

Activities & Assessments 17.1

Until you have this knowledge, it is essential to protect yourself by using condoms and spermicides when having sex, even if some other form of birth control is employed. *Birth control pills offer no protection against STDs.* Women and men who are sexually active should come to accept as standard practice with new partners the use of condoms and spermicides, even if the pill is used for birth control. Sexually active women and men should carry and be prepared to use condoms and spermicides whenever the possibility of sexual activity exists. This requires overcoming the gender-role stereotypes that women who admit to being sexual are "sluts" and men who behave the same way are "studs."

You may have noticed that the commonly heard term "safe sex" has been replaced in this chapter. Health practitioners have taught for decades that, no matter the precautions, *there is no such thing as completely safe sex for individuals who are sexually active with more than one partner.* Thus, these practitioners have suggested that the more accurate phrase is *safer sex*.

Some barriers to safer sex include:

- *Denying that there is a risk.* Many people assume that STDs happen only to "dirty," "promiscuous," and "immoral" people and, since they have sex only with people who are "clean" and "nice," getting an STD is impossible. Another form of denial is to tell yourself "I eat right. I exercise. I can't get an STD."

- *Believing that the campus community is somehow insulated from STDs.* The truth is that about half of college students are sexually active before they enter college. As a result, students can arrive on campus already infected. Also, on many campuses, students in the same living groups and student organizations have sex with one another. One infected person can lead to a whole chain of infections.
- *Feeling guilty and uncomfortable about being sexual.* This prevents individuals from planning sex, so that they carry condoms and spermicides, and talking about possible risks with new partners.
- *Succumbing to social and peer pressure to be sexual.* These pressures encourage people to be sexual in situations that are potentially risky, such as one-night stands and brief relationships that are sexual virtually from the beginning. The risk of infection is lessened when individuals resist peer pressure to have sex with a relative stranger, and ask themselves instead "Is this the right relationship?" "Is this the right partner?" and "Am I going to feel OK about this afterwards?"

PHYSICAL ACTIVITY AND HEALTH CONNECTION

Although there may not appear to be a direct link between physical activity and sexually transmitted diseases, regular participation in physical activity and the avoidance of STDs are both important components of living a healthy lifestyle. If you are physically active you generally have better self-esteem, which could provide you the ability to make more positive sexual health choices.

CONCEPT CONNECTION

1. **Sexually transmitted diseases (STDs) are infections passed from person to person, most frequently by sexual contact.** Twenty different infections can be passed from person to person via sexual contact. Sexually related diseases occur among both sexually active and sexually abstinent individuals.
2. **Sexually transmitted diseases (STDs) are epidemic in the United States.** Almost 15 million people in the United States acquire an STD each year; 42 percent of STDs occur among young people between the ages of 20 and 24.
3. **Certain sexual behaviors increase your risk for contracting an STD.** Having multiple sexual partners, not practicing safer sex precautions, not recognizing STD symptoms, not treating an STD, having impaired judgement via alcohol and or other drugs, and counting on the sense of security that "I won't get an STD" or that there is a cure for an STD if I contract one, all increase your chances for contracting an STD.
4. **Common STDs include trichomonas and *Gardnerella vaginalis,* chlamydia, gonorrhea, syphilis, herpes, genital warts, pubic lice, and scabies.** Sexually transmitted diseases (STDs), although widespread, can be prevented and treated before they are transmitted to someone else. Recognizing common signs and symptoms and understanding effective treatments will be useful in decreasing the incidence and prevalence of common STDs.
5. **AIDS is caused by the human immunodeficiency virus (HIV).** AIDS and the HIV infection is pandemic. AIDS is one of the leading causes of death for both men and women of ages 25 to 44. To help reduce the incidence of AIDS, everyone should avoid high-risk sexual behaviors.
6. **Prevention is key!** Preventing STDs involves supporting public health efforts to inform people about STD prevention and treatment. It also requires individuals to practice safer sex and to comply with treatment when they are infected.

TERMS

Sexually transmitted diseases (STDs), 388
Sexually related diseases (SRDs), 388
Trichomonas vaginalis, 390
Gardnerella vaginalis, 390
Chlamydia, 390
Epididymitis, 391
Pelvic inflammatory disease (PID), 391
Gonorrhea, 392
Syphilis, 392
Chancre, 392
Herpes, 392
Sexually transmitted warts, 393
Human papillomavirus (HPV), 393
Pubic lice, 394
Scabies, 395
Human immunodeficiency virus (HIV), 395
Kaposi's sarcoma, 395
AIDS, 395
Retrovirus, 396

MAKING THE CONNECTION

Ken and Amy both realize, after a number of heart-to-heart talks, that sexual intimacy does not necessarily need to include sexual intercourse. In deciding whether to engage in intimate sexual relations, including intercourse, they understand that they must consider psychological as well physical factors. They have learned that many people choose to abstain from sexual intercourse and that they can choose among varying levels of sexual intimacy. When they decide to become sexually intimate it will be a big step in their relationship, especially since having sex involves an emotional commitment as well as a physical one. Furthermore, the decision to become sexually intimate with one another must also be considered in light of HIV and the other sexually transmitted diseases (STDs) that are prevalent among college students; many times infections may be asymptomatic, so someone may transmit the disease to another person unknowingly.

CRITICAL THINKING

1. Ken and Amy have chosen to abstain from sexual intercourse. Describe for yourself the pros and cons of sexual abstinence. Have you been able to discuss your thoughts about sexuality with your current partner?
2. As more and more people become infected with HIV, more students attending universities and colleges are infected with HIV. Many universities have residence halls with living quarters that accommodate two to four people of the same gender. Is it necessary for universities to notify students in a residence hall if a person living there is HIV-positive? If so, why? If not, why not?
3. Herpes is a sexually transmitted disease that lasts a lifetime; however, herpes can be managed with medication. Explain, in detail, how you would go about telling your new partner that you have herpes.
4. You and your best college friend are talking, and your friend confides to you that about 2 months ago he may have had sexual intercourse with someone who could be HIV-positive, but your friend is not having any symptoms. What advice would you give him?

REFERENCES

American Social Health Association. (1998). *STDs in America: How Many Cases and at What Cost?* Research Triangle Park, NC.

CDC National Prevention Information Network (NPIN). (2000a). *STD Resources: Common STDs and the Organisms that Cause them.* Online: www.cdcnpin.org/std/common.htm. [accessed June 25, 2000].

Centers for Disease Control and Prevention (2000b). Gonorrhea—United States, 1998. *Morbidity & Mortality Weekly Reports 49*(24): 538–42.

Centers for Disease Control and Prevention. (2000c). *HIV/AIDS Surveillance Report: US HIV & AIDS Cases Reported through December 1999,* Year-End Edition. Bethesda.

Holmes, K.K. (1994). Human ecology and behavior and sexually transmitted bacterial infections. *Proceedings of the National Academy of Sciences 91:* 2448–55.

Kost, K., & Forrest, J.D. (1992). American women's sexual behavior and exposure to risk of sexually transmitted diseases. *Family Planning Perspectives 24:* 244–46.

National Opinion Center Research. (1995). Behavior changed by AIDS. Snapshot. *USA Today,* 4/10/95.

World Health Organization. *Sexually transmitted diseases.* Online: www.who.org. [accessed June 28, 2000].

Activities & Assessments

NAME ______ SECTION ______ DATE ______

17.1 Can You Be Assertive When You Need to Be?

To take the necessary actions to prevent contracting a sexually transmitted disease, you will have to be assertive. That is, you will need to resist pressure to engage in sexual activity if you choose not to, and you will need to insist on the use of a condom and other safer-sex precautions if you do decide to engage in sex. Do you have assertiveness skills? To find out, write an assertive response to each of the following situations.

1. You are on a date and your partner insists on engaging in a sexual activity that you decide is not for you at that time. You say:

2. Your partner argues that condoms diminish the sensation. You respond by saying:

3. Your partner states that she or he has been tested for STDs and the test was negative. Therefore, there are no reasons for using safer-sex techniques. You respond by saying:

(continued)

17.1 Can You Be Assertive When You Need to Be? (cont.)

TO BE ASSERTIVE, YOU NEED TO:

- Specify the behavior or situation to which the statement refers.
- Relate your feelings about that situation.
- Suggest a remedy or what you would prefer to see occur.
- Identify the consequences of the change; what will happen if it occurs and what will happen if it does not occur.

Now, check your responses and revise them to be consistent with these assertiveness principles.

SOURCE: J.S. Greenberg, C.E. Bruess, and D.W. Haffner. (2000). Exploring the dimensions of human sexuality (p. 488–489). Boston: Jones and Bartlett.

NAME	SECTION	DATE

Challenge to Change

You have acquired extensive information about physical activity and health by reading this book. In addition, you have had the opportunity to make observations about your health by completing the self-assessments provided in each chapter and on the Web. The next step is to employ self-change techniques.

When planning a behavior self-change, it is important to acknowledge your level of readiness—the time before you consider making actual changes as well as the time after you have declared your willingness to change. The activities in Part I of this self-change guide can help you decide if you are ready to participate in a behavior change program; if you are ready, the activities in Part II will be more effective. The activities in Part II provide you with techniques to act on your readiness and ways to modify and enhance your health behavior.

Part I

Activity 1: Assessing readiness to change. Readiness is the state of being that precedes change. It denotes a continuum from minimal to maximal motivation across each of the assorted "stages of change" required to modify a behavior. Rate your current level of readiness by circling the stage (refer to the descriptions of each stage in the list below) that best represents your level of motivation for each of the behaviors listed in the following questionnaire.

1 = PRECONTEMPLATION: *I do not want to change this behavior at this time.*

2 = CONTEMPLATION: *I am thinking about working on this behavior in the next 6 months.*

3 = PREPARATION: *I am ready to begin work on this behavior now.*

4 = ACTION: *I have begun working on this behavior.*

5 = MAINTENANCE: *I have been practicing this behavior regularly.*

SPECIFIC HEALTH BEHAVIOR	STAGE OF CHANGE				
1. If a female, I perform a breast self-examination (BSE) every month.	1	2	3	4	5
2. If a male, I perform a testicular self-examination (TSE) every month.	1	2	3	4	5
3. I regularly protect my skin from sun exposure every time I am in the sun.	1	2	3	4	5
4. I perform a skin examination to check for cancerous spots every month.	1	2	3	4	5
5. I have my blood pressure measured by a health care professional at least twice a year.	1	2	3	4	5
6. I have my cholesterol level measured by a health care professional at 5-year intervals.	1	2	3	4	5
7. I accumulate 30 minutes daily of moderate-intensity physical activity, at least five times a week, for my cardiovascular health.	1	2	3	4	5
8. I perform moderately vigorous physical activity 3–5 days per week, at 50–85% of VO_2 maximum or heart rate reserve, for 20–60 minutes, rhythmically utilizing the large muscle masses of the body for optimizing my cardiovascular fitness.	1	2	3	4	5

SPECIFIC HEALTH BEHAVIOR	STAGE OF CHANGE				
9. I assess my cardiovascular fitness level every 2 months to determine if my physical activity program needs to be modified.	1	2	3	4	5
10. I choose a variety of grains daily (at least 6 servings), especially whole grains.	1	2	3	4	5
11. I choose a variety of fruits and vegetables daily (at least 2 servings of fruit and 3 servings of vegetables).	1	2	3	4	5
12. I choose a diet that is low in saturated fat (no more than 10% of daily calories) and cholesterol (no more than 300 mg/day) and moderate in total fat (no more than 30% of daily calories).	1	2	3	4	5
13. I perform resistive training exercises to maintain and increase my muscle mass and my metabolic rate.	1	2	3	4	5
14. I maintain a regular physical activity program (30 min daily) to avoid lowering my metabolic rate and decrease the likelihood of excessive adipose tissue storage.	1	2	3	4	5
15. I evaluate my body weight using the body mass index (BMI) periodically to assure that I am at a healthy weight.	1	2	3	4	5
16. I evaluate my waist circumference periodically to assure that fat is not accumulating around my waist.	1	2	3	4	5
17. I consume at least 1000 mg/day of calcium through calcium-rich foods such as dairy products, green leafy vegetables, and/or calcium-fortified foods.	1	2	3	4	5
18. I maintain a regular physical activity program (30 min daily) to strengthen my skeletal system.	1	2	3	4	5
19. I perform one set of 8–12 repetitions of 8–10 different exercises twice a week to maintain my muscular fitness.	1	2	3	4	5
20. I perform 8–10 exercises at least three times per week while training at an intensity that is >85% of my one-rep maximum to improve my muscular strength.	1	2	3	4	5
21. I perform 8–10 exercises at least three times per week while training at an intensity that is equal to 40–60% of my one-rep maximum to improve my muscular endurance.	1	2	3	4	5
22. I perform at least 3–4 stretching activities at least three times per week, slowly elongating the muscle and holding for 15–30 seconds, to improve my flexibility.	1	2	3	4	5
23. I regularly practice stress-management techniques when I am feeling stressed or overwhelmed.	1	2	3	4	5
24. If I choose to drink alcoholic beverages, I do so in moderation (one drink a day for women and no more than two drinks a day for men).	1	2	3	4	5
25. I choose not to smoke cigarettes.	1	2	3	4	5

SPECIFIC HEALTH BEHAVIOR	STAGE OF CHANGE				
26. I choose not to use smokeless tobacco products.	1	2	3	4	5
27. I always seek reliable sources of information related to physical activity and health.	1	2	3	4	5
28. If my partner and I have made a conscious decision to have sexual intercourse, we use a condom every time.	1	2	3	4	5
29. In communicating with my partner or close friends, I send clear messages.	1	2	3	4	5
30. In communicating with my partner or close friends, I use effective listening techniques.	1	2	3	4	5
31. Other: ____________________	1	2	3	4	5

Activity 2: Select one behavior to modify. It is best to focus on one behavior at a time. We recommend that you select a behavior from Activity 1 in which you rated yourself as being in the preparation stage.

____

Activity 3: List potential gains and losses.

GAINS	LOSSES
1. ____________________	1. ____________________
2. ____________________	2. ____________________
3. ____________________	3. ____________________
4. ____________________	4. ____________________
5. ____________________	5. ____________________
6. ____________________	6. ____________________

If the gains do not outnumber the losses at this time, you are probably in the precontemplation or contemplation stage and ambivalent about changing. Review the techniques related to these stages in Chapter 3 and rethink applying the following behavioral change techniques.

Part II: Behavioral Change Techniques

Activity 4: Monitor yourself. As a general rule, you should not begin a plan of self-change activities until after you have established a stable, reliable, detailed baseline of what you are doing now. We recommend using a structured journal. You will need to record the behavior as well as the context of the situation in which it occurred. Situations can be divided into events that come before the behavior (antecedents) and those that follow (consequences). Your journal can take on many forms depending on the type of behavior and what fits your usual habits, but should include the following information.

STEP 1: Record the behavior you want to change as soon as it occurs.

STEP 2: Record the events that preceded it (antecedents): When did it happen? Where were you? What else were you doing? Who was with you? What thoughts were you having? What feelings were you having?

STEP 3: Record the results (consequences) of the behavior or action: Was it pleasant or unpleasant?

TIME	BEHAVIOR	ANTECEDENTS	CONSEQUENCES

Keep track of your behavior until you are able to see a clear pattern (we recommend at least a week). List any patterns that you were able to identify based on the results from your baseline period.

1. ______

2. ______

3. ______

Activity 5: Make a self-contract. Complete the self-contract below. Make sure you record your goal clearly. Write exactly what you want to achieve in the most specific terms possible. Record a date to start working on the goal and another to finish it. Finally, write down an attack plan for obtaining your goal.

SELF-CONTRACT FORM

GOAL TYPE (CIRCLE ONE):

Short-Term / Mid-term / Long-term

GOAL: ______________________________

DATE GOAL SET: ______________ DATE GOAL TO BE ACCOMPLISHED: ______________

PLAN OF ATTACK:

1. ______________________________

____

____

____

2. ______________________________

____

____

____

3. ______________________________

____

____

____

SIGNED:

____

Activity 6: Practice effective time management. Effective time-management strategies go a long way toward reaching goals. In Activity 5 you made a firm written commitment about making changes. The action stage is the busiest stage of change. Planning and organizing your time will allow you to direct and focus your energy on your goal.

The first step is monitoring how you currently spend your time. An activity log is a highly effective way to do this. For a couple of days, write down the things you do as you do them, from the moment you wake up to the moment you go to bed. As well as noting activities, it is beneficial to note how energetic you feel during certain parts of the day. Your energy level depends a lot on your rest breaks, the times and amount you eat, and the quality of your nutrition.

Analyze your log after a couple of days to see how you are spending your time and how your energy levels vary throughout the day. Next to each task on which you spent time, allocate a priority rating—(1) very unimportant, (2) somewhat unimportant, (3) somewhat important, (4) very important—for each item. Based on these point allocations, complete a priority to-do list and specify when you plan to accomplish them.

PRIORITY "TO DO" LIST	TIME	ENERGY LEVEL (1 LOW TO 5 HIGH)
1.		
2.		
3.		
4.		
5.		
6.		

Activity 7: Find social support. It is important to recognize that you can't always do it alone. Create a team of people around you to encourage and reward your desirable behavior. List six people whom you trust and respect and ask them if they would be willing to assist you with your behavior change. Discuss with them specific ways that they can support you in achieving your goal.

PERSON	HOW THEY WILL SUPPORT YOU
1.	
2.	
3.	
4.	
5.	
6.	

Activity 8: Chart your progress. It is helpful to see that you are moving toward your goal. Charting your progress is a good way to accomplish this. The structured journal format you used in Activity 4 is appropriate here as well.

TIME	BEHAVIOR	ANTECEDENTS	CONSEQUENCES

Activity 9: Practice self-reinforcement. Your progress will accelerate when you reflect on your success. To reinforce your success, reward yourself. Rewards should be contingent upon the successful completion of the behavior. They should also be meaningful to you. Make a list of some meaningful rewards and when you will receive them.

	REWARD	DATE
1.		
2.		
3.		
4.		
5.		
6.		

Activity 10: Build commitment. Commitment to change is not something you have, it is something you do. Commitment is a set of behaviors. Temptations to stop your self-change project are certainly going to occur. If you have a plan for dealing with temptation, you are more likely to be successful with warding off temptations. Using reminder systems is an excellent way to avoid temptations.

Prepare a list of self-reminders when temptation arises. Include in your reminders all the advantages of practicing your new behavior.

LIST 4 WAYS YOU WILL REMIND YOURSELF.

1. ______________________________

____

____

____

2. ______________________________

____

____

____

3. ______________________________

____

____

____

4. ______________________________

____

____

____

Appendix A

Injury Prevention

INTRODUCTION

While participating in most physical activity is safe, there is always a potential risk of injury. You can prevent most injuries by following a carefully planned activity program and by following the recommended prescreening suggestions found in this book. However, accidents occasionally happen and people do get injured. This appendix addresses what to do if you become injured.

PREVENTION IS THE BEST MEDICINE

Think safety! Many injuries can be avoided by preparing carefully for physical activity. Appropriate preparation includes the following:

- Warm-up, stretch out, and cool down.
- Wear proper clothing.
- Check shoes for signs of breakdown.
- Wear appropriate protective devices including helmets, padding and eyewear.

Then, check your activity environment to ensure that the exercise area is clear of obstacles. Regularly check equipment to make sure it has been maintained and is functioning properly. If you are unsure how to use a piece of equipment, seek instruction. Learning by trial and error usually means you will suffer through some error, which could cause injury. If you are active in a remote area (rock climbing or hiking), take a cell phone.

Take a first aid class and become certified in CPR. Learn how to contact emergency medical services (EMS). In most, but not all, communities dialing 911 is the quickest way to contact EMS.

Seek professional assessment

In all cases in which there is doubt, or when an injury presents more than just minor pain, you should seek advice from your physician. In many cases, injuries that appear minor may be more damaging than initially expected. It's better to be safe than sorry.

Emergency Action

If you need to call for help, for yourself or another, be prepared to tell EMS personnel the following information:

1. Where has the emergency occurred? Give the address or names of cross streets, roads, or other landmarks if possible.

2. Provide the telephone number from which you are calling.
3. What happened? Are you (or someone else) suffering from a heart attack, a fall, or some other emergency?
4. How many people need help?
5. What is the condition of the victim?
6. What is being done for the victim?

Remember to stay on the line. In a panic, you may forget to provide important pieces of information.

SOURCE: American Heart Association, 1987

KNOWLEDGE

You can also prepare yourself by learning a bit about injuries. Here are some of the signs of serious problems:

Signals of a heart attack

Is there persistent chest pain or discomfort? Does it increase with more activity?

Is breathing difficult (abnormal)?

Is there an abnormal change in pulse rate?

Does the skin appear pale or bluish in color?

SOURCE: American Red Cross, 1993

Signs of internal bleeding

Are there tender, swollen, bruised, or hard areas of the body, such as the abdomen?

Is there a rapid, weak pulse?

Does the skin feel cool or moist or look pale or bluish?

Are you suffering from excessive thirst?

Are you becoming confused, faint, drowsy, or unconscious?

SOURCE: American Red Cross, 1993

Signs of a stroke

Is there sudden weakness or numbness of the face, arm, and leg on one side of the body?

Is there a loss of speech, or trouble speaking or understanding speech?

Are unexplained dizziness, unsteadiness, or falls occurring?

Is there dimness or loss of vision, particularly in one eye?

Was there any loss of consciousness?

SOURCE: American Heart Association, 1987

Common Injuries

You need to learn to identify and treat some common injuries. Remember, when in doubt, consult with your physician.

Tendinitis is an inflammation of a tendon. It is usually associated with overuse. Common areas affected by tendinitis include the Achilles' tendon, the elbow, and the ilio-tibial band. Tendinitis is usually treated by rest and anti-inflammatory medications.

Shin splints is a generic term that refers to any pain felt in the front portion of the lower leg. It may be caused by muscle imbalance, tendinitis, or being active on a new surface. Since this problem may be caused by a number of things, general suggestions for treatment are not possible. Occasionally stretching, cutting back on activity, and seeking better shoes may alleviate the problem. You may want to check with your physician to better define this condition.

Strains are injuries to the muscles caused by forcibly overstretching them. You can reduce the likelihood of strains by properly warming up your muscles prior to activity. Good muscular balance (symmetry) also reduces the likelihood of experiencing strains.

Sprains are injuries to the ligaments that are also caused by forceful overstretching. Sprains usually result from bending a joint into an unusual position. This can be caused by performing exercises incorrectly or by accident (sprained ankle).

Both sprains and strains are usually treated by R.I.C.E. (see below).

Fractures are broken bones. There are several degrees of fractures, from a hairline (small crack) to a compound fracture, in which the broken bone extends through the skin. If a fracture is suspected, try not to move the injured area and seek medical assistance.

Thermal stress is something those who are physically active need to learn to deal with. A few preventive steps can reduce your risk for suffering a thermal injury.

To prevent **heat injuries,** consider temperature and humidity. These two factors combine to provide a heat index. If possible, plan your activity for a climate-controlled environment. Many shopping malls will allow you to walk indoors on days with extreme temperatures. If you must be active outside on hot, humid days, wear breathable clothing, drink plenty of water, and plan your activity for the morning or evening. You might also want to lower your intensity. Wear sunscreen to reduce exposure to harmful rays.

To prevent **cold injuries,** consider temperature and wind chill. If possible, plan your activity for a climate-controlled environment. If you must be active outside on cold, windy days, wear multiple layers of clothing. You can shed layers as your body temperature rises, and you've got additional clothing to put on after your workout. Make sure you wear a hat, gloves or mittens, and protection for your nose.

SOURCE: Bristol-Myers Company, 1985

Immediate First Aid

When you suspect a muscle strain or ligament sprain, the R.I.C.E. procedure is followed for the first 72 hours: R = rest, I = ice, C = compression, E = elevation. After 72 hours, the application of heat will speed up the healing process. If a fracture is suspected, it is recommended that you immobilize the injured area and seek medical attention.

Caring for Bleeding

You can control bleeding by placing a clean covering, such as a sterile dressing, over the wound and applying pressure. Check for other injuries. If you don't find any broken bones, elevate the injured area. A bandage should be snugly applied over the dressing. If the bleeding cannot be stopped or reduced, put pressure on the nearby artery (pressure point). Always seek medical assistance for anything beyond minor bleeding.

SOURCE: American Red Cross, 1993

Follow Suggestions for Rehabilitation

To speed recovery time and to return to full health, it is critical that you follow the rehabilitation program that has been designed for you. Don't rush the program, skip steps, or fail to complete the entire rehab.

Don't Give Up the Ship

If you have an injury in one segment of your body, it doesn't mean you have to remain totally inactive. Check with your physician to see if there are any reasons you cannot be active in a modified way. For instance, if you have sprained an ankle and cannot walk comfortably, consider cycling or swimming.

REFERENCES

American Red Cross. (1993). *Community First Aid & Safety.* Boston: Stay Well.

American Heart Association. (1987). *Heart Saver Manual.* Dallas.

Bristol-Myers Company. (1985). *Sports Injuries: An Aid to Prevention and Treatment.* Coventry, CT.

Appendix B

Caloric Cost of Selected Activities

The following table shows some examples of activities and their corresponding caloric costs. You can use this information in the following ways:

- To determine level of estimated energy expenditure, multiply the figure in column three by the number of minutes you participate in the activity. (Please note that in this example the number in column three is for a person who weighs 150 pounds.)
- You can calculate your energy expenditure based on your weight in kilograms by multiplying the figure in column two by the minutes you are active and your weight in kilograms.

ACTIVITY	KCAL/MIN/KG	KCAL/MIN
Aerobics (medium intensity)	0.103	7.0
Basketball	0.138	9.4
Ballroom Dancing	0.051	3.5
Cycling		
Leisure (5.5 mph)	0.064	4.4
Golf	0.085	5.8
Jogging (9 min/mile)	0.193	13.1
Racquetball	0.178	12.1
Raking	0.054	3.7
Swimming (Breast Stroke)	0.162	11.0
Walking	0.08	5.4

A more detailed version of this chart follows in this appendix, taking into consideration variations in body weight.

APPENDIX B

Caloric Cost of Activities (cont.)

ACTIVITY	KCAL · MIN^{-1} · KG^{-1}	KG/LB 50 110	53 117	56 123	59 130	62 137	65 143	68 150	71 157	74 163	77 170	80 176	83 183	86 190	89 196	92 203	95 209	98 216
Archery	0.065	3.3	3.4	3.6	3.8	4.0	4.2	4.4	4.6	4.8	5.0	5.2	5.4	5.6	5.8	6.0	6.2	6.4
Badminton	0.097	4.9	5.1	5.4	5.7	6.0	6.3	6.6	6.9	7.2	7.5	7.8	8.1	8.3	8.6	8.9	9.2	9.5
Bakery, general (F)	0.035	1.8	1.9	2.0	2.1	2.2	2.3	2.4	2.5	2.6	2.7	2.8	2.9	3.0	3.1	3.2	3.3	3.4
Basketball	0.138	6.9	7.3	7.7	8.1	8.6	9.0	9.4	9.8	10.2	10.6	11.0	11.5	11.9	12.3	12.7	13.1	13.5
Billiards	0.042	2.1	2.2	2.4	2.5	2.6	2.7	2.9	3.0	3.1	3.2	3.4	3.5	3.6	3.7	3.9	4.0	4.1
Bookbinding	0.038	1.9	2.0	2.1	2.2	2.4	2.5	2.6	2.7	2.8	2.9	3.0	3.2	3.3	3.4	3.5	3.6	3.7
Boxing																		
in ring	0.222	6.9	7.3	7.7	8.1	8.6	9.0	9.4	9.8	10.2	10.6	11.0	11.5	11.9	12.3	12.7	13.1	13.5
sparring	0.138	11.1	11.8	12.4	13.1	13.8	14.4	15.1	15.8	16.4	17.1	17.8	18.4	19.1	19.8	20.4	21.1	21.8
Canoeing																		
leisure	0.044	2.2	2.3	2.5	2.6	2.7	2.9	3.0	3.1	3.3	3.4	3.5	3.7	3.8	3.9	4.0	4.2	4.3
racing	0.103	5.2	5.5	5.8	6.1	6.4	6.7	7.0	7.3	7.6	7.9	8.2	8.5	8.9	9.2	9.5	9.8	10.1
Card Playing	0.025	1.3	1.3	1.4	1.5	1.6	1.6	1.7	1.8	1.9	1.9	2.0	2.1	2.2	2.2	2.3	2.4	2.5
Carpentry, general	0.052	2.6	2.8	2.9	3.1	3.2	3.4	3.5	3.7	3.8	4.0	4.2	4.3	4.5	4.6	4.8	4.9	5.1
Carpet sweeping (F)	0.045	2.3	2.4	2.5	2.7	2.8	2.9	3.1	3.2	3.3	3.5	3.6	3.7	3.9	4.0	4.1	4.3	4.4
Carpet sweeping (M)	0.048	2.4	2.5	2.7	2.8	3.0	3.1	3.3	3.4	3.6	3.7	3.8	4.0	4.1	4.3	4.4	4.6	4.7
Circuit Training																		
Hydra-Fitness	0.132	6.6	7.0	7.4	7.8	8.2	8.6	9.0	9.4	9.7	10.2	10.5	10.9	11.4	11.7	12.1	12.5	12.9
Universal	0.116	5.8	6.2	6.5	6.9	7.2	7.5	7.9	8.3	8.6	8.9	9.3	9.6	10.0	10.3	10.7	11.0	11.4
Nautilus	0.092	4.6	4.9	5.2	5.5	5.8	6.0	6.3	6.6	6.8	7.1	7.4	7.7	8.0	8.2	8.5	8.8	9.1
Free Weights	0.086	4.3	4.5	4.8	5.0	5.3	5.5	5.8	6.1	6.3	6.6	6.8	7.1	7.4	7.6	7.9	8.1	8.4
Cleaning (F)	0.062	3.1	3.3	3.5	3.7	3.8	4.0	4.2	4.4	4.6	4.8	5.0	5.1	5.3	5.5	5.7	5.9	6.1
Cleaning (M)	0.058	2.9	3.1	3.2	3.4	3.6	3.8	3.9	4.1	4.3	4.5	4.6	4.8	5.0	5.2	5.3	5.5	5.7
Climbing hills																		
with no load	0.121	6.1	6.4	6.8	7.1	7.5	7.9	8.2	8.6	9.0	9.3	9.7	10.0	10.4	10.8	11.1	11.5	11.9
with 5-kg load	0.129	6.5	6.8	7.2	7.6	8.0	8.4	8.8	9.2	9.5	9.9	10.3	10.7	11.1	11.5	11.9	12.3	12.6
with 10-kg load	0.140	7.0	7.4	7.8	8.3	8.7	9.1	9.5	9.9	10.4	10.8	11.2	11.6	12.0	12.5	12.9	13.3	13.7
with 20-kg load	0.147	7.4	7.8	8.2	8.7	9.1	9.6	10.0	10.4	10.9	11.3	11.8	12.2	12.6	13.1	13.5	14.0	14.4
Coal mining																		
drilling coal, rock	0.094	4.7	5.0	5.3	5.5	5.8	6.1	6.4	6.7	7.0	7.2	7.5	7.8	8.1	8.4	8.6	8.9	9.2
erecting supports	0.088	4.4	4.7	4.9	5.2	5.5	5.7	6.0	6.2	6.5	6.8	7.0	7.3	7.6	7.8	8.1	8.4	8.6
shoveling coal	0.108	5.4	5.7	6.0	6.4	6.7	7.0	7.3	7.7	8.0	8.3	8.6	9.0	9.3	9.6	9.9	10.3	10.6
Cooking (F)	0.045	2.3	2.4	2.5	2.7	2.8	2.9	3.1	3.2	3.3	3.5	3.6	3.7	3.9	4.0	4.1	4.3	4.4
Cooking (M)	0.048	2.4	2.5	2.7	2.8	3.0	3.1	3.3	3.4	3.6	3.7	3.8	4.0	4.1	4.3	4.4	4.6	4.7
Cricket																		
batting	0.083	4.2	4.4	4.6	4.9	5.1	5.4	5.6	5.9	6.1	6.4	6.6	6.9	7.1	7.4	7.6	7.9	8.1
bowling	0.090	4.5	4.8	5.0	5.3	5.6	5.9	6.1	6.4	6.7	6.9	7.2	7.5	7.7	8.0	8.3	8.6	8.8
Croquet	0.059	3.0	3.1	3.3	3.5	3.7	3.8	4.0	4.2	4.4	4.5	4.7	4.9	5.1	5.3	5.4	5.6	5.8
Cycling																		
leisure, 5.5 mph	0.064	3.2	3.4	3.6	3.8	4.0	4.2	4.4	4.5	4.7	4.9	5.1	5.3	5.5	5.7	5.9	6.1	6.3
leisure, 9.4 mph	0.100	5.0	5.3	5.6	5.9	6.2	6.5	6.8	7.1	7.4	7.7	8.0	8.3	8.6	8.9	9.2	9.5	9.8
racing	0.169	8.5	9.0	9.5	10.0	10.5	11.0	11.5	12.0	12.5	13.0	13.5	14.0	14.5	15.0	15.5	16.1	16.6

ACTIVITY	KCAL - MIN^{-1} - KG^{-1}	KG/LB 50 110	53 117	56 123	59 130	62 137	65 143	68 150	71 157	74 163	77 170	80 176	83 183	86 190	89 196	92 203	95 209	98 216
Dancing																		
Dancing (F)																		
aerobic, medium	0.103	5.2	5.5	5.8	6.1	6.4	6.7	7.0	7.3	7.6	7.9	8.2	8.5	8.9	9.2	9.5	9.8	10.1
aerobic, intense	0.135	6.7	7.1	7.5	7.9	8.3	8.7	9.2	9.6	10.0	10.4	10.8	11.2	11.6	12.0	12.4	12.8	13.2
ballroom	0.051	2.6	2.7	2.9	3.0	3.2	3.3	3.5	3.6	3.8	3.9	4.1	4.2	4.4	4.5	4.7	4.8	5.0
choreographed		8.4	8.9	9.4	9.9	10.4	10.9	11.4	11.9	12.4	12.9	13.4	13.9	14.4	15.0	15.5	16.0	16.5
"twist," "lambada"	0.168	5.2	5.5	5.8	6.1	6.4	6.7	7.0	7.3	7.6	7.9	8.2	8.5	8.9	9.2	9.5	9.8	10.1
Digging trenches	0.145	7.3	7.7	8.1	8.6	9.0	9.4	9.9	10.3	10.7	11.2	11.6	12.0	12.5	12.9	13.3	13.8	14.2
Drawing (standing)	0.036	1.8	1.9	2.0	2.1	2.2	2.3	2.4	2.6	2.7	2.8	2.9	3.0	3.1	3.2	3.3	3.4	3.5
Eating (sitting)	0.023	1.2	1.2	1.3	1.4	1.4	1.5	1.6	1.6	1.7	1.8	1.8	1.9	2.0	2.0	2.1	2.2	2.3
Electrical work	0.058	2.9	3.1	3.2	3.4	3.6	3.8	3.9	4.1	4.3	4.5	4.6	4.8	5.0	5.2	5.3	5.5	5.7
Farming																		
barn cleaning	0.135	6.8	7.2	7.6	8.0	8.4	8.8	9.2	9.6	10.0	10.4	10.8	11.2	11.6	12.0	12.4	12.8	13.2
driving harvester	0.040	2.0	2.1	2.2	2.4	2.5	2.6	2.7	2.8	3.0	3.1	3.2	3.3	3.4	3.6	3.7	3.8	3.9
driving tractor	0.037	1.9	2.0	2.1	2.2	2.3	2.4	2.5	2.6	2.7	2.8	3.0	3.1	3.2	3.3	3.4	3.5	3.6
feeding cattle	0.085	4.3	4.5	4.8	5.0	5.3	5.5	5.8	6.0	6.3	6.5	6.8	7.1	7.3	7.6	7.8	8.1	8.3
feeding animals	0.065	3.3	3.4	3.6	3.8	4.0	4.2	4.4	4.6	4.8	5.0	5.2	5.4	5.6	5.8	6.0	6.2	6.4
forking straw bales	0.138	6.9	7.3	7.7	8.1	8.6	9.0	9.4	9.8	10.2	10.6	11.0	11.5	11.9	12.3	12.7	13.1	13.5
milking by hand	0.054	2.7	2.9	3.0	3.2	3.3	3.5	3.7	3.8	4.0	4.2	4.3	4.5	4.6	4.8	5.0	5.1	5.3
milking by machine	0.023	1.2	1.2	1.3	1.4	1.4	1.5	1.6	1.6	1.7	1.8	1.8	1.9	2.0	2.0	2.1	2.2	2.3
shoveling grain	0.085	4.3	4.5	4.8	5.0	5.3	5.5	5.8	6.0	6.3	6.5	6.8	7.1	7.3	7.6	7.8	8.1	8.3
Field hockey	0.134	6.7	7.1	7.5	7.9	8.3	8.7	9.1	9.5	9.9	10.3	10.7	11.1	11.5	11.9	12.3	12.7	13.1
Fishing	0.062	3.1	3.3	3.5	3.7	3.8	4.0	4.2	4.4	4.6	4.8	5.0	5.1	5.3	5.5	5.7	5.9	6.1
Food shopping (F)	0.062	3.1	3.3	3.5	3.7	3.8	4.0	4.2	4.4	4.6	4.8	5.0	5.1	5.3	5.5	5.7	5.9	6.1
Food shopping (M)	0.058	2.9	3.1	3.2	3.4	3.6	3.8	3.9	4.1	4.3	4.5	4.6	4.8	5.0	5.2	5.3	5.5	5.7
Football	0.132	6.6	7.0	7.4	7.8	8.2	8.6	9.0	9.4	9.8	10.2	10.6	11.0	11.4	11.7	12.1	12.5	12.9
Forestry																		
ax chopping, fast	0.297	14.9	15.7	16.6	17.5	18.4	19.3	20.2	21.1	22.0	22.9	23.8	24.7	25.5	26.4	27.3	28.2	29.1
ax chopping, slow	0.085	4.3	4.5	4.8	5.0	5.3	5.5	5.8	6.0	6.3	6.5	6.8	7.1	7.3	7.6	7.8	8.1	8.3
barking trees	0.123	6.2	6.5	6.9	7.3	7.6	8.0	8.4	8.7	9.1	9.5	9.8	10.2	10.6	10.9	11.3	11.7	12.1
carrying logs	0.186	9.3	9.9	10.4	11.0	11.5	12.1	12.6	13.2	13.8	14.3	14.9	15.4	16.0	16.6	17.1	17.7	18.2
felling trees	0.132	6.6	7.0	7.4	7.8	8.2	8.6	9.0	9.4	9.8	10.2	10.6	11.0	11.4	11.7	12.1	12.5	12.9
hoeing	0.091	4.6	4.8	5.1	5.4	5.6	5.9	6.2	6.5	6.7	7.0	7.3	7.6	7.8	8.1	8.4	8.6	8.9
planting by hand	0.109	5.5	5.8	6.1	6.4	6.8	7.1	7.4	7.7	8.1	8.4	8.7	9.0	9.4	9.7	10.0	10.4	10.7
sawing by hand	0.122	6.1	6.5	6.8	7.2	7.6	7.9	8.3	8.7	9.0	9.4	9.8	10.1	10.5	10.9	11.2	11.6	12.0
sawing, power	0.075	3.8	4.0	4.2	4.4	4.7	4.9	5.1	5.3	5.6	5.8	6.0	6.2	6.5	6.7	6.9	7.1	7.4
stacking firewood	0.088	4.4	4.7	4.9	5.2	5.5	5.7	6.0	6.2	6.5	6.8	7.0	7.3	7.6	7.8	8.1	8.4	8.6
trimming trees	0.129	6.5	6.8	7.2	7.6	8.0	8.4	8.8	9.2	9.5	9.9	10.3	10.7	11.1	11.5	11.9	12.3	12.6
weeding	0.072	3.6	3.8	4.0	4.2	4.5	4.7	4.9	5.1	5.3	5.5	5.8	6.0	6.2	6.4	6.6	6.8	7.1
Furriery	0.083	4.2	4.4	4.6	4.9	5.1	5.4	5.6	5.9	6.1	6.4	6.6	6.9	7.1	7.4	7.6	7.9	8.1
Gardening																		
digging	0.126	6.3	6.7	7.1	7.4	7.8	8.2	8.6	8.9	9.3	9.7	10.1	10.5	10.8	11.2	11.6	12.0	12.3
hedging	0.077	3.9	4.1	4.3	4.5	4.8	5.0	5.2	5.5	5.7	5.9	6.2	6.4	6.6	6.9	7.1	7.3	7.5

APPENDIX B **Caloric Cost of Activities (cont.)**

ACTIVITY	KCAL · MIN^{-1} · KG^{-1}	KG/LB 50 110	53 117	56 123	59 130	62 137	65 143	68 150	71 157	74 163	77 170	80 176	83 183	86 190	89 196	92 203	95 209	98 216
Gardening (cont.)																		
mowing	0.112	5.6	5.9	6.3	6.6	6.9	7.3	7.6	8.0	8.3	8.6	9.0	9.3	9.6	10.0	10.3	10.6	11.0
raking	0.054	2.7	2.9	3.0	3.2	3.3	3.5	3.7	3.8	4.0	4.2	4.3	4.5	4.6	4.8	5.0	5.1	5.3
Golf	0.085	4.3	4.5	4.8	5.0	5.3	5.5	5.8	6.0	6.3	6.5	6.8	7.1	7.3	7.6	7.8	8.1	8.3
Gymnastics	0.066	3.3	3.5	3.7	3.9	4.1	4.3	4.5	4.7	4.9	5.1	5.3	5.5	5.7	5.9	6.1	6.3	6.5
Horse-grooming	0.128	6.4	6.8	7.2	7.6	7.9	8.3	8.7	9.1	9.5	9.9	10.2	10.6	11.0	11.4	11.8	12.2	12.5
Horse-racing																		
galloping	0.137	6.9	7.3	7.7	8.1	8.5	8.9	9.3	9.7	10.1	10.6	11.0	11.4	11.8	12.2	12.6	13.0	13.4
trotting	0.110	5.5	5.8	6.2	6.5	6.8	7.2	7.5	7.8	8.1	8.5	8.8	9.1	9.5	9.8	10.1	10.5	10.8
walking	0.041	2.1	2.2	2.3	2.4	2.5	2.7	2.8	2.9	3.0	3.2	3.3	3.4	3.5	3.6	3.8	3.9	4.0
Ironing (F)	0.033	1.7	1.7	1.8	1.9	2.0	2.1	2.2	2.3	2.4	2.5	2.6	2.7	2.8	2.9	3.0	3.1	3.2
Ironing (M)	0.064	3.2	3.4	3.6	3.8	4.0	4.2	4.4	4.5	4.7	4.9	5.1	5.3	5.5	5.7	5.9	6.1	6.3
Judo	0.195	9.8	10.3	10.9	11.5	12.1	12.7	13.3	13.8	14.4	15.0	15.6	16.2	16.8	17.4	17.9	18.5	19.1
Jumping rope																		
70 per min	0.162	8.1	8.6	9.1	9.6	10.0	10.5	11.0	11.5	12.0	12.5	13.0	13.4	13.9	14.4	14.9	15.4	15.9
80 per min	0.164	8.2	8.7	9.2	9.7	10.2	10.7	11.2	11.6	12.1	12.6	13.1	13.6	14.1	14.6	14.6	15.6	16.1
125 per min	0.177	8.9	9.4	9.9	10.4	11.0	11.5	12.0	12.6	13.1	13.6	14.2	14.7	15.2	15.8	16.3	16.8	17.3
145 per min	0.197	9.9	10.4	11.0	11.6	12.2	12.8	13.4	14.0	14.6	15.2	15.8	16.4	16.9	17.5	18.1	18.7	19.3
Knitting, sewing (F)	0.022	1.1	1.2	1.2	1.3	1.4	1.4	1.5	1.6	1.6	1.7	1.8	1.8	1.9	2.0	2.0	2.1	2.2
Knitting, sewing (M)	0.023	1.2	1.2	1.3	1.4	1.4	1.5	1.6	1.6	1.7	1.8	1.8	1.9	2.0	2.0	2.1	2.2	2.3
Locksmith	0.057	2.9	3.0	3.2	3.4	3.5	3.7	3.9	4.0	4.2	4.4	4.6	4.7	4.9	5.1	5.2	5.4	5.6
Lying at ease	0.022	1.1	1.2	1.2	1.3	1.4	1.4	1.5	1.6	1.6	1.7	1.8	1.8	1.9	2.0	2.0	2.1	2.2
Machine-tooling																		
machining	0.048	2.4	2.5	2.7	2.8	3.0	3.1	3.3	3.4	3.6	3.7	3.8	4.0	4.1	4.3	4.4	4.6	4.7
operating lathe	0.052	2.6	2.8	2.9	3.1	3.2	3.4	3.5	3.7	3.8	4.0	4.2	4.3	4.5	4.6	4.8	4.9	5.1
operating punch press	0.088	4.4	4.7	4.9	5.2	5.5	5.7	6.0	6.2	6.5	6.8	7.0	7.3	7.6	7.8	8.1	8.4	8.6
tapping and drilling	0.065	3.3	3.4	3.6	3.8	4.0	4.2	4.4	4.6	4.8	5.0	5.2	5.4	5.6	5.8	6.0	6.2	6.4
welding	0.052	2.6	2.8	2.9	3.1	3.2	3.4	3.5	3.7	3.8	4.0	4.2	4.3	4.5	4.6	4.8	4.9	5.1
working sheet metal	0.048	2.4	2.5	2.7	2.8	3.0	3.1	3.3	3.4	3.6	3.7	3.8	4.0	4.1	4.3	4.4	4.6	4.7
Marching, rapid	0.142	7.1	7.5	8.0	8.4	8.8	9.2	9.7	10.1	10.5	10.9	11.4	11.8	12.2	12.6	13.1	13.5	13.9
Mopping floor (F)	0.062	3.1	3.3	3.5	3.7	3.8	4.0	4.2	4.4	4.6	4.8	5.0	5.1	5.3	5.5	5.7	5.9	6.1
Mopping floor (M)	0.058	2.9	3.1	3.2	3.4	3.6	3.8	3.9	4.1	4.3	4.5	4.6	4.8	5.0	5.2	5.0	5.5	5.7
Music playing																		
accordion (sitting)	0.032	1.6	1.7	1.8	1.9	2.0	2.1	2.2	2.3	2.4	2.5	2.6	2.7	2.8	2.8	2.9	3.0	3.1
cello (sitting)	0.041	2.1	2.2	2.3	2.4	2.5	2.7	2.8	2.9	3.0	3.2	3.3	3.4	3.5	3.6	3.8	3.9	4.0
conducting	0.039	2.0	2.1	2.2	2.3	2.4	2.5	2.7	2.8	2.9	3.0	3.1	3.2	3.4	3.5	3.6	3.7	3.8
drums (sitting)	0.066	3.3	3.5	3.7	3.9	4.1	4.3	4.5	4.7	4.9	5.1	5.3	5.5	5.7	5.9	6.1	6.3	6.6
flute (sitting)	0.035	1.8	1.9	2.0	2.1	2.2	2.3	2.4	2.5	2.6	2.7	2.8	2.9	3.0	3.1	3.2	3.3	3.4
horn (sitting)	0.029	1.5	1.5	1.6	1.7	1.8	1.9	2.0	2.1	2.1	2.2	2.3	2.4	2.5	2.6	2.7	2.8	2.8
organ (sitting)	0.053	2.7	2.8	3.0	3.1	3.3	3.4	3.6	3.8	3.9	4.1	4.2	4.4	4.6	4.7	4.9	5.0	5.2
piano (sitting)	0.040	2.0	2.1	2.2	2.4	2.5	2.6	2.7	2.8	3.0	3.1	3.2	3.3	3.4	3.6	3.7	3.8	3.9
trumpet (standing)	0.031	1.6	1.6	1.7	1.8	1.9	2.0	2.1	2.2	2.3	2.4	2.5	2.6	2.7	2.8	2.9	2.9	3.0

APPENDIX B

Caloric Cost of Activities (cont.)

ACTIVITY	KCAL - MIN⁻¹ - KG⁻¹	KG/LB 50 110	53 117	56 123	59 130	62 137	65 143	68 150	71 157	74 163	77 170	80 176	83 183	86 190	89 196	92 203	95 209	98 216
Music playing (cont.)																		
violin (sitting)	0.045	2.3	2.4	2.5	2.7	2.8	2.9	3.1	3.2	3.3	3.5	3.6	3.7	3.9	4.0	4.1	4.3	4.4
woodwind (sitting)	0.032	1.6	1.7	1.8	1.9	2.0	2.1	2.2	2.3	2.4	2.5	2.6	2.7	2.8	2.8	2.9	3.0	3.1
Painting, inside	0.034	1.7	1.8	1.9	2.0	2.1	2.2	2.3	2.4	2.5	2.6	2.7	2.8	2.9	3.0	3.1	3.2	3.3
Painting, outside	0.077	3.9	4.1	4.3	4.5	4.8	5.0	5.2	5.5	5.7	5.9	6.2	6.4	6.6	6.9	7.1	7.3	7.5
Planting seedlings	0.070	3.5	3.7	3.9	4.1	4.3	4.6	4.8	5.0	5.2	5.4	5.6	5.8	6.0	6.2	6.4	6.7	6.9
Plastering	0.078	3.9	4.1	4.4	4.6	4.8	5.1	5.3	5.5	5.8	6.0	6.2	6.5	6.7	6.9	7.2	7.4	7.6
Printing	0.035	1.8	1.9	2.0	2.1	2.2	2.3	2.4	2.5	2.6	2.7	2.8	2.9	3.0	3.1	3.2	3.3	3.4
Racquetball	0.178	8.9	9.4	10.0	10.5	11.0	11.6	12.1	12.6	13.2	13.7	14.2	14.8	15.3	15.8	16.4	16.9	17.4
Running, cross-country	0.163	8.2	8.6	9.1	9.6	10.1	10.6	11.1	11.6	12.1	12.6	13.0	13.5	14.0	14.5	15.0	15.5	16.0
Running, horizontal																		
11 min, 30 s per mile	0.135	6.8	7.2	7.6	8.0	8.4	8.8	9.2	9.6	10.0	10.5	10.9	11.3	11.7	12.1	12.5	12.9	13.3
9 min per mile	0.193	9.7	10.2	10.8	11.4	12.0	12.5	13.1	13.7	14.3	14.9	15.4	16.0	16.6	17.2	17.8	18.3	18.9
8 min per mile	0.208	10.8	11.3	11.9	12.5	13.1	13.6	14.2	14.8	15.4	16.0	16.5	17.1	17.7	18.3	18.9	19.4	20.0
7 min per mile	0.228	12.2	12.7	13.3	13.9	14.5	15.0	15.6	16.2	16.8	17.4	17.9	18.5	19.1	19.7	20.3	20.8	21.4
6 min per mile	0.252	13.9	14.4	15.0	15.6	16.2	16.7	17.3	17.9	18.5	19.1	19.6	20.2	20.8	21.4	22.0	22.5	23.1
5 min, 30 s per mile	0.289	14.5	15.3	16.2	17.1	17.9	18.8	19.7	20.5	21.4	22.3	23.1	24.0	24.9	25.7	26.6	27.5	28.3
Scraping paint	0.063	3.2	3.3	3.5	3.7	3.9	4.1	4.3	4.5	4.7	4.9	5.0	5.2	5.4	5.6	5.8	6.0	6.2
Scrubbing floors (F)	0.109	5.5	5.8	6.1	6.4	6.8	7.1	7.4	7.7	8.1	8.4	8.7	9.0	9.4	9.7	10.0	10.4	10.7
Scrubbing floors (M)	0.108	5.4	5.7	6.0	6.4	6.7	7.0	7.3	7.7	8.0	8.3	8.6	9.0	9.3	9.6	9.9	10.3	10.6
Shoe repair, general	0.045	2.3	2.4	2.5	2.7	2.8	2.9	3.1	3.2	3.3	3.5	3.6	3.7	3.9	4.0	4.1	4.3	4.4
Sitting quietly	0.021	1.1	1.1	1.2	1.2	1.3	1.4	1.4	1.5	1.6	1.6	1.7	1.7	1.8	1.9	1.9	2.0	2.1
Skiing, hard snow																		
level, moderate speed	0.119	6.0	6.3	6.7	7.0	7.4	7.7	8.1	8.4	8.8	9.2	9.5	9.9	10.2	10.6	10.9	11.3	11.7
level, walking speed	0.143	7.2	7.6	8.0	8.4	8.9	9.3	9.7	70.2	10.6	11.0	11.4	11.9	12.3	12.7	13.2	13.6	14.0
uphill, maximum speed	0.274	13.7	14.5	15.3	16.2	17.0	17.8	18.6	19.5	20.3	21.1	21.9	22.7	23.6	24.4	25.2	26.0	26.9
Skiing, soft snow																		
leisure (F)	0.111	4.9	5.2	5.5	5.8	6.1	6.4	6.7	7.0	7.3	7.5	7.8	8.1	8.4	8.7	9.0	9.3	9.6
leisure (M)	0.098	5.6	5.9	6.2	6.5	6.9	7.2	7.5	7.9	8.2	8.5	8.9	9.2	9.5	9.9	10.2	10.5	10.9
Skindiving, as frogman																		
considerable motion	0.276	13.8	14.6	15.5	16.3	17.1	17.9	18.8	19.6	20.4	21.3	22.1	22.9	23.7	24.6	25.4	26.2	27.0
moderate motion	0.206	10.3	10.9	11.5	12.2	12.8	13.4	14.0	14.6	15.2	15.9	16.5	17.1	17.7	18.3	19.0	19.6	20.2
Snowshoeing, soft snow	0.166	8.3	8.8	9.3	9.8	10.3	10.8	11.3	11.8	12.3	12.8	13.3	13.8	14.3	14.8	15.3	15.8	16.3
Squash	0.212	10.6	11.2	11.9	12.5	13.1	13.8	14.4	15.1	15.7	16.3	17.0	17.6	18.2	18.9	19.5	20.1	20.8
Standing quietly (F)	0.025	1.3	1.3	1.4	1.5	1.6	1.6	1.7	1.8	1.9	1.9	2.0	2.1	2.2	2.2	2.3	2.4	2.5
Standing quietly (M)	0.027	1.4	1.4	1.5	1.6	1.7	1.8	1.8	1.9	2.0	2.1	2.2	2.2	2.3	2.4	2.5	2.6	2.6
Steel mill, working in																		
fettling	0.089	4.5	4.7	5.0	5.3	5.5	5.8	6.1	6.3	6.6	6.9	7.1	7.4	7.7	7.9	8.2	8.5	8.7
forging	0.100	5.0	5.3	5.6	5.9	6.2	6.5	6.8	7.1	7.4	7.7	8.0	8.3	8.6	8.9	9.2	9.5	9.8
hand rolling	0.137	6.9	7.3	7.7	8.1	8.5	8.9	9.3	9.7	10.1	10.6	11.0	11.4	11.8	12.2	12.6	13.0	13.4
merchant mill rolling	0.145	7.3	7.7	8.1	8.6	9.0	9.4	9.9	10.3	10.7	11.2	11.6	12.0	12.5	12.9	13.3	13.8	14.2
removing slag	0.178	8.9	9.4	10.0	10.5	11.0	11.6	12.1	12.6	13.2	13.7	14.2	14.8	15.3	15.8	16.4	16.9	17.4

APPENDIX B **Caloric Cost of Activities (cont.)**

ACTIVITY	KCAL · MIN^{-1} · KG^{-1}	KG/LB 50 110	53 117	56 123	59 130	62 137	65 143	68 150	71 157	74 163	77 170	80 176	83 183	86 190	89 196	92 203	95 209	98 216
Steel mill, working in (cont.)																		
tending furnace	0.126	6.3	6.7	7.1	7.4	7.8	8.2	8.6	8.9	9.3	9.7	10.1	10.5	10.8	11.2	11.6	12.0	12.3
tipping molds	0.092	4.6	4.9	5.2	5.4	5.7	6.0	6.3	6.5	6.8	7.1	7.4	7.6	7.9	8.2	8.5	8.7	9.0
Stock clerking	0.054	2.7	2.9	3.0	3.2	3.3	3.5	3.7	3.8	4.0	4.2	4.3	4.5	4.6	4.8	5.0	5.1	5.3
Swimming																		
back stroke	0.169	8.5	9.0	9.5	10.0	10.5	11.0	11.5	12.0	12.5	13.0	13.5	14.0	14.5	15.0	15.5	16.1	16.6
breast stroke	0.162	8.1	8.6	9.1	9.6	10.0	10.5	11.0	11.5	12.0	12.5	13.0	13.4	13.9	14.4	14.9	15.4	15.9
crawl, fast	0.156	7.8	8.3	8.7	9.2	9.7	10.1	10.6	11.1	11.5	12.0	12.5	12.9	13.4	13.9	14.4	14.8	15.3
crawl, slow	0.128	6.4	6.8	7.2	7.6	7.9	8.3	8.7	9.1	9.5	9.9	10.2	10.6	11.0	11.4	11.8	12.2	12.5
side stroke	0.122	6.1	6.5	6.8	7.2	7.6	7.9	8.3	8.7	9.0	9.4	9.8	10.1	10.5	10.9	11.2	11.6	12.0
treading, fast	0.170	8.5	9.0	9.5	10.0	10.5	11.1	11.6	12.1	12.6	13.1	13.6	14.1	14.6	15.1	15.6	16.2	16.7
treading, normal	0.062	3.1	3.3	3.5	3.7	3.8	4.0	4.2	4.4	4.6	4.8	5.0	5.1	5.3	5.5	5.7	5.9	6.1
Table tennis (ping pong)	0.068	3.4	3.6	3.8	4.0	4.2	4.4	4.6	4.8	5.0	5.2	5.4	5.6	5.8	6.1	6.3	6.5	6.7
Tailoring																		
cutting	0.041	2.1	2.2	2.3	2.4	2.5	2.7	2.8	2.9	3.0	3.2	3.3	3.4	3.5	3.6	3.8	3.9	4.0
hand-sewing	0.032	1.6	1.7	1.8	1.9	2.0	2.1	2.2	2.3	2.4	2.5	2.6	2.7	2.8	2.8	2.9	3.0	3.1
machine-sewing	0.045	2.3	2.4	2.5	2.7	2.8	2.9	3.1	3.2	3.3	3.5	3.6	3.7	3.9	4.0	4.1	4.3	4.4
pressing	0.062	3.1	3.3	3.5	3.7	3.8	4.0	4.2	4.4	4.6	4.8	5.0	5.1	5.3	5.5	5.7	5.9	6.1
Tennis	0.109	5.5	5.8	6.1	6.4	6.8	7.1	7.4	7.7	8.1	8.4	8.7	9.0	9.4	9.7	10.0	10.4	10.7
Typing																		
electric	0.027	1.4	1.4	1.5	1.6	1.7	1.8	1.8	1.9	2.0	2.1	2.2	2.2	2.3	2.4	2.5	2.6	2.6
manual	0.031	1.6	1.6	1.7	1.8	1.9.	2.0	2.1	2.2	2.3	2.4	2.5	2.6	2.7	2.8	2.9	2.9	3.0
Volleyball	0.050	2.5	2.7	2.8	3.0	3.1	3.3	3.4	3.6	3.7	3.9	4.0	4.2	4.3	4.5	4.6	4.8	4.9
Walking, normal pace																		
asphalt road	0.080	4.0	4.2	4.5	4.7	5.0	5.2	5.4	5.7	5.9	6.2	6.4	6.6	6.9	7.1	7.4	7.6	7.8
fields and hillsides	0.082	4.1	4.3	4.6	4.8	5.1	5.3	5.6	5.8	6.1	6.3	6.6	6.8	7.1	7.3	7.5	7.8	8.0
grass track	0.081	4.1	4.3	4.5	4.8	5.0	5.3	5.5	5.8	6.0	6.2	6.5	6.7	7.0	7.2	7.5	7.7	7.9
plowed field	0.077	3.9	4.1	4.3	4.5	4.8	5.0	5.2	5.5	5.7	5.9	6.2	6.4	6.6	6.9	7.1	7.3	7.5
Wallpapering	0.048	2.4	2.5	2.7	2.8	3.0	3.1	3.3	3.4	3.6	3.7	3.8	4.0	4.1	4.3	4.4	4.6	4.7
Watch repairing	0.025	1.3	1.3	1.4	1.5	1.6	1.6	1.7	1.8	1.9	1.9	2.0	2.1	2.2	2.2	2.3	2.4	2.5
Window cleaning (F)	0.059	3.0	3.1	3.3	3.5	3.7	3.8	4.0	4.2	4.4	4.5	4.7	4.9	5.1	5.3	5.4	5.6	5.8
Window cleaning (M)	0.058	2.9	3.1	3.2	3.4	3.6	3.8	3.9	4.1	4.3	4.5	4.6	4.8	5.0	5.2	5.3	5.5	5.7
Writing (sitting)	0.029	1.5	1.5	1.6	1.7	1.8	1.9	2.0	2.1	2.1	2.2	2.3	2.4	2.5	2.6	2.7	2.8	2.8

Data from Bannister, E.W. and Brown, S.R.: The relative requirements of physical activity, in H.B. Falls (ed): *Exercise Physiology.* New York, Academic Press, 1968: Howley, E.T. and Glover, M.E.: The caloric costs of running and walking one mile for men and women. *Medicine and Science in Sports* 6.235, 1974; Passmore, R.. And Durnin, J.V.G.A.: Human energy expenditure. *Physiological Reviews* 35.801, 1955. Note: Symbols (M) and (F) denote experiments for males and females, respectively.

SOURCE: W.D. McArdle, F.I. Katch, and V.L. Katch. (1996). *Exercise physiology: Energy, nutrition, and human performance* (pp. 804–811). Baltimore, MD: Lippincott, Williams & Wilkins.

Index

C

Y

Credits

Unless otherwise acknowledged, all photographs are the property of Jones and Bartlett Publishers.

vi Chapter 1 spot image © Karl Weatherly/PhotoDisc, Chapter 2 spot image © Berta A. Daniels, Chapter 3 spot image © Jack Star/PhotoLink/PhotoDisc; vi Chapter 4 spot image © Ellen Shub, Chapter 5 spot image © Jonathan Nourok/PhotoEdit, Chapter 6 spot image © Jose Carillo/PhotoEdit, Chapter 7 spot image © Digital Vision, Chapter 8 spot image © Steven Peters/Stone/GettyOne; viii Chapter 9 spot image © Michael Newman/PhotoEdit, Chapter 10 spot image © Ryan McVay/PhotoDisc, Chapter 11 spot image © Chris Falkenstein/PhotoDisc, Chapter 12 spot image © Tony Freeman/PhotoEdit; ix Chapter 13 spot image © Steve Mason/PhotoDisc, Chapter 14 spot image © CMSP, Chapter 15 spot image © Alan Becker/The Image Bank/GettyOne, Chapter 16 spot image © S. Pearce/PhotoLink/PhotoDisc, Chapter 17 spot image © Ellen Shub; x (t) © Don Tremain/PhotoDisc, (ml) © Karl Weatherly/PhotoDisc, (mr) © E. Dygas/PhotoDisc, (bl) © Keith Brofsky/PhotoDisc, (br) © PhotoDisc; xi (tl) © Steve Mason/PhotoDisc, (tr) © Doug Menuez/PhotoDisc, (bl) © Bronwyn Kidd/PhotoDisc, (br) © Javier Pierini/PhotoDisc; 1 © Karl Weatherly/PhotoDisc; 4 © Steve Mason/PhotoDisc; 8 © Colin Paterson/PhotoDisc; 9 (b) © Robert Brenner/PhotoEdit, (t) © Lawrence M. Sawyer/PhotoDisc; 10 © Doug Menuez/PhotoDisc; 21 © Berta A. Daniels; 24 © Jim Cummins/FPG International/GettyOne; 25 © PhotoDisc; 26 © David Buffington/PhotoDisc; 27 © Javier Pierini/PhotoDisc; 28 © Frank Siteman/PhotoEdit; 33 © Ryan McVay/PhotoDisc; 34 © Don Tremain/PhotoDisc; 35 © Joaquin Palting/PhotoDisc; 39 © Andy Sotiriou/PhotoDisc; 40 © Ian Wyatt/PhotoDisc; 42 © Ryan McVay/PhotoDisc; 43 © Dana White/PhotoEdit; 55 © Jack Star/PhotoLink/PhotoDisc; 57 (t) © Donna Day/Stone/gettyone, (b) © Keith Brofsky/PhotoDisc; 58 © Bob Thomas/Stone; 60 © Ryan McVay/PhotoDisc; 63 © Ryan McVay/PhotoDisc; 69 © Ryan McVay/PhotoDisc; 71 © EyeWire; 79 © Ellen Shub; 86 (both) © Joel Gordon; 87 © Joel Gordon; 89 © Keith Brofsky/PhotoDisc; 90 © Frank Siteman/PhotoEdit; 91 © David Young-Wolff/PhotoEdit; 93 (all) © Logical Images Inc./CMSP; 99 © Jonathan Nourok/PhotoEdit; 100 © Karl Weatherly/PhotoDisc; 102 © Jack Star/PhotoLInk/PhotoDisc; 106 © W. Ober/ Visuals Unlimited; 111 © Gary Conner/PhotoEdit; 112 © Doug Menuez/PhotoDisc; 119 © Jose Carillo/PhotoEdit; 123 © Mary Kate Denny/PhotoEdit; 133 © Digital Vision; 141 (l) © Jess Alford/PhotoDisc, (m) © Jules Frazier/PhotoDisc, (r) © PhotoLink/PhotoDisc; 151 © Don Farrall/PhotoDisc; 175 © Steven Peters/Stone/GettyOne; 179 (l) © SW Productions/PhotoDisc, (r) © Ryan McVay/PhotoDisc; 181 © David Young-Wolff/PhotoEdit; 182 © Berta A. Daniels; 183 © SW Productions/PhotoDisc; 186 (t) © E. Dygas/PhotoDisc, (b) © Robert W. Ginn/PhotoEdit; 193 © Michael Newman/PhotoEdit; 194 © Karl Weatherly/PhotoDisc; 195 © Michael Newman/PhotoEdit; 201 © David Young-Wolff/PhotoEdit; 208 (both) © SPL/Custom Medical Stock Photo; 209 © Steve Mason/PhotoDisc; 211 © David Young-Wolff/PhotoEdit; 213 © PhotoLink/PhotoDisc; 215 © PhotoDisc; 221 © Ryan McVay/PhotoDisc; 223 © John A. Rizzo/PhotoDisc; 226 (t) © Mitch Hrdlicka/PhotoDisc, (b) © Skip Nall/PhotoDisc; 227 © Dr. Michael Klein/Peter Arnold, Inc.; 230 © Bill Aron/PhotoEdit; 231 (all) Photos reprinted with permission from Calcified Tissue Research, 1967; 235 © Chris Falkenstein/PhotoDisc; 242 (r) © Keith Brofsky/PhotoDisc; 261 © Bill Aron/PhotoEdit; 263 © Tony Freeman/PhotoEdit; 264 © Myrleen Ferguson Cate/PhotoEdit; 265 (t) © Ryan McVay/PhotoDisc; 287 © Steve Mason/PhotoDisc; 290 (t) © Ryan McVay/PhotoDisc, (b) © David Young-Wolff/PhotoEdit; 293 © Robert Brenner/PhotoEdit; 301 © David Buffington/PhotoDisc; 302 © Steve Mason/PhotoDisc; 305 © Jules Frazier/PhotoDisc; 311 © CMSP; 317 © Corbis Digital Stock; 319 © PhotoDisc; 329 © Steve Skjold/ PhotoEdit; 339 © Ryan McVay/PhotoDisc; 349 © Alan Becker/The Image Bank/GettyOne; 351 © SW Productions/PhotoDisc; 358 © Spencer Grant/PhotoEdit; 361 © Michael Newman/PhotoEdit; 367 © S. Pearce/PhotoLInk/PhotoDisc; 370 © Elizabeth Zuckerman/PhotoEdit; 376 © Steve Mason/PhotoDisc; 377 © Bronwyn Kidd/PhotoDisc; 387 © Ellen Shub; 392 (t) © Science VU/Visuals Unlimited, (b) © Biophoto Associates/Photo Researchers, Inc.; 393 (t) © CDC/Science Source/Photo Researchers, Inc.; 393 (m) © Dr. P. Marazzi/Science Photo LIbrary/Photo Researchers, Inc.; 393 (b) © Ken Greer/Visuals Unlimited; 397 © PhotoDisc.